ADVANCES IN PROSTAGLANDIN, THROMBOXANE, AND LEUKOTRIENE RESEARCH
VOLUME 10

Prostaglandins and the Cardiovascular System

Advances in Prostaglandin,
Thromboxane, and Leukotriene Research

Series Editors: Bengt Samuelsson and Rodolfo Paoletti

INTERNATIONAL ADVISORY BOARD

Advances in Prostaglandin, Thromboxane, and Leukotriene
Research Series
Volume 10

Prostaglandins
and the
Cardiovascular System

Editor

John A. Oates, M. D.
Professor of Medicine and Pharmacology
Vanderbilt University
School of Medicine
Nashville, Tennessee

Raven Press ■ New York

Raven Press, 1140 Avenue of the Americas, New York, New York 10036

International Standard Book Number 0-89004-580-1
Library of Congress Catalog Number 80-50413

Great care has been taken to maintain the accuracy of the information contained in the volume. However, Raven Press cannot be held responsible for errors or for any consequences arising from the use of the information contained herein.

(Advances in prostaglandin, thromboxane, and leukotriene research ; v. 10)
  Includes bibliographical references and index.
  1. Prostaglandins—Physiological effect.   2. Cardiovascular system.   3. Prostacyclin—Physiological effect.
4. Thromboxanes—Physiological effect.   I. Oates,
John A., 1932-   . II. Series. [DNLM: 1. Thromboxanes
—Pharmacodynamics.   2. Prostaglandins—Pharmacodynamics.
3. Cardiovascular system—Drug effects. W1 AD788.
v. 10 / QU 90 P96735]
QP801.P68P7233 1982   612'.1   82-15035

Preface

The objective of this volume is to describe the state of the science that relates thromboxane A_2, prostacyclin, and prostaglandins to cardiovascular regulation and disease. Emphasis is given to recent advances in these fields, and the authors who have participated in the book are those who have made major contributions to these scientific advances.

The biochemistry and pharmacology of thromboxane A_2, prostacyclin, and the prostaglandins are integrated with consideration of their participation in cardiovascular physiology and disease.

Particular attention has been given in this volume to elucidate concepts, to identify areas in which there is active scientific progress, and to report recent advances which provide a basis for the new approaches to the treatment and possible prevention of cardiovascular disease.

This book will be of interest to scientists and students with a variety of interests that relate to cardiovascular regulation and pathophysiology, the clinical disorders that stem from atherosclerosis, the interaction of platelets with blood vessels, and the biochemistry of the oxygenated metabolites of arachidonic acid.

John A. Oates

Contents

Contributors

Robert J. Anderson
*Department of Medicine and Division of
Renal Diseases
University of Colorado Health Sciences
Center
Denver, Colorado 80262*

Leland N. Benson
*Department of Pediatrics
University of California, Los Angeles
School of Medicine
Los Angeles, California 90024*

Robert A. Branch
*Departments of Medicine and
Pharmacology
Vanderbilt University Medical Center
Nashville, Tennessee 37232*

Alan R. Brash
*Departments of Medicine and
Pharmacology
Vanderbilt University Medical Center
Nashville, Tennessee 37232*

Kenneth L. Brigham
*Pulmonary Circulation Center and
Pulmonary Division
Department of Medicine
Vanderbilt University School of Medicine
Nashville, Tennessee 37232*

Ulf Diczfalusy
*Department of Physiological Chemistry
Karolinska Institutet
S-104 01 Stockholm, Sweden*

G. T. Dusting
*University of Melbourne
Department of Medicine
Austin Hospital
Heidelberg, Victoria 3084, Australia*

G. A. FitzGerald
*Department of Pharmacology
Vanderbilt University School of Medicine
Nashville, Tennessee 37232*

William F. Friedman
*Department of Pediatrics
University of California, Los Angeles
School of Medicine
Los Angeles, California 90024*

John G. Gerber
*Department of Medicine and Division of
Clinical Pharmacology
University of Colorado Health Sciences
Center
Denver, Colorado 80262*

Elisabeth Granström
*Department of Physiological Chemistry
Karolinska Institutet
S-104 01 Stockholm, Sweden*

Mats Hamberg
*Department of Physiological Chemistry
Karolinska Institutet
S-104 01 Stockholm, Sweden*

Göran Hansson
*Department of Physiological Chemistry
Karolinska Institutet
S-104 01 Stockholm, Sweden*

A. L. Hyman
*Departments of Pharmacology and
Surgery
Tulane University School of Medicine
New Orleans, Louisiana 70112*

Edwin K. Jackson
*Departments of Medicine and
Pharmacology
Vanderbilt University Medical Center
Nashville, Tennessee 37232*

Philip J. Kadowitz
*Departments of Pharmacology and
Surgery
Tulane University School of Medicine
New Orleans, Louisiana 70112*

H. L. Lippton
*Departments of Pharmacology and
    Surgery
Tulane University School of Medicine
New Orleans, Louisiana 70112*

Curt Malmsten
*Department of Physiological Chemistry
Karolinksa Institutet
S-104 01 Stockholm, Sweden*

D. B. McNamara
*Departments of Pharmacology and
    Surgery
Tulane University School of Medicine
New Orleans, Louisiana 70112*

Salvador Moncada
*Wellcome Research Laboratory
Langley Court
Beckenham, Kent BR3 3BS
England*

John H. Newman
*Pulmonary Circulation Center and
    Pulmonary Division
Department of Medicine
Vanderbilt University School of Medicine
Nashville, Tennessee 37232*

Alan S. Nies
*Department of Medicine and Division of
    Clinical Pharmacology
University of Colorado Health Sciences
    Center
Denver, Colorado 80262*

Bengt Nilsson
*Department of Neurology
University Hospital
S-221, 85 Lund, Sweden*

John A. Oates
*Departments of Medicine and
    Pharmacology
Vanderbilt University Medical Center
Nashville, Tennessee 37232*

Martin L. Ogletree
*Pulmonary Circulation Center and
    Pulmonary Division
Department of Medicine
Vanderbilt University School of Medicine
Nashville, Tennessee 37232*

Morton P. Printz
*Division of Pharmacology
Department of Medicine
University of California, San Diego
La Jolla, California 92037*

L. Jackson Roberts II
*Departments of Medicine and
    Pharmacology
Vanderbilt University Medical Center
Nashville, Tennessee 37232*

Bengt Samuelsson
*Department of Physiological Chemistry
Karolinska Institutet
S-104 01 Stockholm, Sweden*

Robert W. Schrier
*Department of Medicine and Division of
    Renal Diseases
University of Colorado Health Sciences
    Center
Denver, Colorado 80262*

Colin J. Schwartz
*Department of Pathology
School of Biomedical Science
University of Texas Health Science
    Center
San Antonio, Texas 78284*

Sol Sherry
*Department of Medicine
Temple University School of Medicine
Philadelphia, Pennsylvania 19140*

Bo K. Siesjö
*Laboratory of Experimental Brain
    Research
University Hospital
S-221, 85 Lund, Sweden*

Randal A. Skidgel
*Division of Pharmacology
Department of Medicine
University of California, San Diego
La Jolla, California 92037*

James R. Snapper
*Pulmonary Circulation Center and
    Pulmonary Division
Department of Medicine
Vanderbilt University School of Medicine
Nashville, Tennessee 37232*

E. W. Spannhake
Departments of Pharmacology and
  Surgery
Tulane University School of Medicine
New Orleans, Louisiana 70112

John Vane
Wellcome Research Laboratory
Langley Court
Beckenham, Kent BR3 3BS
England

Åke Wennmalm
Department of Clinical Physiology
Huddinge University Hospital
Huddinge, Sweden

Mirka Zednikova
Department of Pediatrics
University of California, Los Angeles
School of Medicine
Los Angeles, California 90024

Prostaglandins and the Cardiovascular System, edited by John A. Oates. Raven Press, New York © 1982.

Thrombosis in the Pathogenesis of Sudden Cardiac Death and Myocardial Infarction

Colin J. Schwartz

Department of Pathology, School of Biomedical Science, University of Texas Health Science Center, San Antonio, Texas 78284

In this chapter the pathologic basis of both myocardial infarction and sudden cardiac death is critically reviewed, with particular emphasis on the roles of thrombosis and platelet thromboembolic phenomena. The pathogenic significance of thrombosis in these disorders has been and remains the subject of continuing debate, in no small measure owing to an undue degree of polarization among champions of opposing viewpoints. The problem has been further magnified by nosological and semantic differences, methodological heterogeneity or inadequacies, and the biases inherent in the selection of subsets of the population for study. These various issues will emerge more clearly as the pathologic basis of transmural myocardial infarction, subendocardial infarction, and sudden cardiac death are compared and contrasted.

TRANSMURAL MYOCARDIAL INFARCTION

Occlusion Status

Patients reported here were derived from a consecutive series of necropsies performed at the Radcliffe Infirmary, Oxford, where the necropsy rate for hospital deaths was in excess of 90%. The hearts were studied by a combination of techniques including postmortem coronary stereoradiography, coupled with serial 4 mm sections of the heart and arteries, together with a Spalteholtz clearing procedure, and subsequent histologic examination of the arteries and myocardium. Infarct age was determined histologically using the criteria of Mallory et al. (44).

Table 1 summarizes the occlusion status and the nature of occlusions in 46 patients dying after their first infarct. Both the occlusion frequency and the histologic nature of occlusions are clearly related to infarct age. It is apparent that of the 25 patients dying with a single infarct of less than 4 months of age, one or more occluded arterial segments were found in excess of 90% of cases, contrasting with the 21 patients dying 4 months or more after their first infarct, where one or more occluded arterial segments were found with a frequency of only 67%. The histologic nature

1

TABLE 1.   *Occlusion status and nature of occlusion in the 46 patients with myocardial infarction dying after their first infarct[a]*

Histological age of infarct	Number of patients	Percentage with occlusions	Nature of occlusions[b](%)		
			Thrombus	Recanalizing thrombus	Plaque
Less than 2 days	10	100	94	0	6
2–13 days	11	91	88	6	6
2–4 weeks	2 ⎫	100	12	50	38
1–4 months	2 ⎭				
Over 4 months	21	67	0	80	20
All ages	46	83	44	41	15

[a]Adapted from Mitchell and Schwartz, 1965 (47).
[b]Histological nature of occluded arterial segment expressed as a percentage of the number of occluded segments within each infarct-age category. A total of 71 arterial segments was occluded.

TABLE 2.   *Occlusion status and nature of occlusions in 33 patients with more than one infarct, according to age of youngest infarct[a]*

Histological age of youngest infarct	Number of patients	Percentage with occlusions	Nature of occlusions %[b]		
			Thrombus	Recanalizing thrombus	Plaque
Less than 2 days	6	100	47	27	27
2–13 days	13	100	60	23	17
2–4 weeks	5	100	25	50	25
1–4 months	9	100	5	71	24
More than 4 months	0	—	—	—	—
All ages	33	100	39	39	22

[a]Adapted from Mitchell and Schwartz, 1965 (47).
[b]Histological nature of occluded arterial segments, expressed as a percentage of the number of occluded segments within each infarct-age category. A total of 87 arterial segments was occluded.

of occlusions also changes with survival time (Table 1), recent thrombus predominating in patients dying within 2 weeks of their first infarct, while in those patients surviving for longer periods occlusion due to recent thrombus is progressively replaced by recanalizing thrombus and atheromatous plaques. These findings serve to emphasize that the arteries of patients surviving for some months after their first infarct will exhibit the legacy of antecedent thrombotic episodes in terms of both recanalizing thrombus and plaques. This is further illustrated in Table 2, which reviews both the occlusion status and nature of occlusions found in patients who have survived one infarct, only to die with another. Even within a few days of their most recent infarct, and in contrast with the findings shown in Table 1, one finds in addition to recent thrombotic occlusion, a number of occlusions due either to recanalizing thrombus or atheromatous plaques. This complex pattern of the nature of arterial occlusions in patients not subdivided according to either the number or age of infarcts present is further illustrated in Table 3, where the findings from a

TABLE 3. *Occlusion status and nature of occlusions in 79 patients with myocardial infarction according to infarct age[a]*

Histological age of youngest infarct[b]	Number of patients	Percentage with occlusions	Nature of occlusions %[c]		
			Thrombus	Recanalizing thrombus	Plaque
Less than 2 days	16	100	69	14	17
2–13 days	24	96	69	17	14
2–4 weeks	7	100	25	56	19
1–4 months	11	100	4	64	36
Over 4 months	21	67	0	80	20
All ages	79	90	42	39	19

[a]Adapted from Mitchell and Schwartz, 1965 (47).
[b]Histological age of infarct, or youngest infarct when more than one infarct present.
[c]Histological nature of occluded arterial segments, expressed as a percentage of the number of occluded segments within each infarct-age category. A total of 158 arterial segments was occluded.

group of 79 patients are presented. Here again, as might be expected from the preceding tables, the frequency of occlusions due to recent thrombus declines with increasing histological age of the youngest infarct present, *pari passu* with an increase in the frequency of occlusions due to recanalizing thrombus or plaques alone. Such data, considered without attention to the number or age of the infarcts present, could be erroneously interpreted as reflecting a major temporal discrepancy between infarct age on the one hand, and the nature or age of occlusions on the other.

A study relating the occlusion status and nature of occlusions in 26 patients with retrosternal pain lasting more than 1 hr, in association with the development of pathological Q waves within 4 weeks of death was conducted. These patients from a clinical viewpoint had the diagnostic criteria of transmural myocardial infarction. It can be seen that 96% had an occlusion in one or more arterial segments, and of these occlusions 57% were due to recent thrombus, 25% showed the features of recanalizing thrombus, and in 18% the occlusions were of an atheromatous nature. It is also of interest that in this subset of 26 patients, 60 occluded arterial segments were observed, indicating that in myocardial infarction multiple occlusions are the rule rather than the exception (47).

Thus far, we have shown that acute transmural myocardial infarction is associated with arterial occlusion in excess of 90% of patients, and that with increasing infarct age, this frequency declines, *pari passu* with a transition in the nature of occlusions from recent thrombus, to recanalizing thrombus and atheromatous plaques. The nature of occlusions is further dependent upon the number of antecedent infarcts, a finding which reflects both the legacy of earlier thrombotic events, and the likely role which the organization and incorporation of thrombi play in plaque growth and development.

Table 4 reviews the collective experience of a number of investigators in terms of the frequency of occlusive thrombosis in acute myocardial infarction. With two

TABLE 4. *Frequency of occlusive thrombi in transmural myocardial infarction*

Reference	Number of cases studied	Frequency of occlusive coronary thrombi (%)
Chapman, 1968 (11)	282	91
Davies et al., 1976 (20)	469	95
Ehrlich and Shinohara, 1964 (22)	18	94
Sinapius, 1972 (61)	170	96.5
Spain, 1974 (62)[a]	50	90
Mitchell and Schwartz, 1965 (47)	21	94
Erhardt et al., 1973 (24)	7	100
Silver et al., 1980 (59)	62	55
Roberts and Buja, 1972 (53)	74	54
Miller et al., 1951 (46)	93	90
Caulfield et al., 1976 (8)	18	100

[a]From Chandler et al., 1974 (9).

notable exceptions, namely Roberts and Buja (53), and Silver et al. (59), most investigators report a high frequency of occlusive thrombi in acute myocardial infarction. Notwithstanding the divergent results of these latter and experienced investigators, there is an overall consensus that thrombosis plays a primary role in the pathogenesis of transmural myocardial infarction. In the report of a National Heart, Lung, and Blood Institute workshop on the role of coronary thrombosis in acute myocardial infarction (9), it was concluded that the "Multiple factors and complex relations involved in thrombus growth and extension of infarcts clearly require further study." The report continued: "Recently, a substantial body of knowledge supports the classic concept of the primary role of thrombosis in the pathogenesis of infarction. Most evidence continues to affirm the basic concept that myocardial infarction . . . can result from thrombotic occlusion of a coronary artery."

Spatial and Temporal Aspects of Occlusion

The distribution of occlusions among branches of the left and right coronary arteries is summarized in Table 5. It is apparent that occlusions are twofold more common in the left coronary artery and its branches than in the right coronary artery. Furthermore, one-half of all occlusions occurred within the left anterior descending trunk and its two main branches.

Additionally the spatial relationship of occluding coronary artery thrombi to areas of infarcted myocardium is of particular importance. In the author's experience, and in the experience of others (9), occlusive coronary artery thrombi customarily subtend the infarcted areas, this consistent anatomic dependence between the site of occlusion and the site of infarction providing good though indirect evidence for a causal relationship between thrombotic occlusion and myocardial infarction. This likely cause and effect relationship is further supported by the temporal relationships between the age of the infarct and the nature of the occlusion. As already pointed out, however, this temporal relationship may be obscured or misinterpreted partic-

TABLE 5. *Site of occlusions in each arterial segment expressed as a percentage of the total number of occluded segments[a]*

Occlusion frequency (%)			
Left coronary artery and branches	(%)	Right coronary artery and branches	(%)
Left coronary trunk	0	Right coronary trunk	11
Main left artery descending 23 ⎫		Right circumflex	14
Left artery descending branches 28 ⎭ 51		Right marginal	3
Left circumflex	12	Right posterior descending	3
Left marginal	4		
Left posterior descending	2		
All branches of left coronary arteries	69	All branches of right coronary artery	31

[a]Adapted from Mitchell and Schwartz, 1965 (47).

ularly in patients with more than one infarct. Thrombi within the coronary arteries frequently exhibit a spectrum of ages, consistent with the view that thrombosis is an episodic phenomenon, and that for some time preceding the final and acute event, earlier occlusive or nonocclusive thrombotic episodes have occurred which have left their histological footprints.

Erhardt et al. (24), in an attempt to clarify the time relationship between the onset of coronary artery thrombosis and acute myocardial infarction, studied the incorporation of ^{125}I-labeled fibrinogen into coronary artery thrombi in postinfarction patients. In all 7 patients, necropsy revealed the presence of transmural myocardial infarction, and in 6 of the 7 patients the thrombus was significantly radioactive. Their findings were interpreted as indicating that thrombosis occurs after rather than anteceding the infarction. However, they failed to recognize that a preexisting thrombus might incorporate radiofibrinogen, particularly with subsequent propagation, or alternatively, that the labeled fibrinogen may penetrate thrombi after their formation. Fulton and Sumner (28) and Erhardt et al. (25) in a more detailed morphologic study have shown that the central occlusive portion of a thrombus subtending an area of infarction is characteristically isotope-negative and, further, that the isotope is present in the propagated portion of the thrombus. These findings are consonant with the view that thrombus formation occurs at the initiation of infarction, rather than as a sequel to it.

SUBENDOCARDIAL INFARCTION

In predominantly subendocardial infarction, typically represented by circumferential necrosis and/or fibrosis in the endocardial third of the left ventricle, thrombotic occlusion of the coronary arteries is a relatively uncommon finding (Table 6). This paucity of occlusive thrombosis in subendocardial infarction was first described by Miller et al. (46) and has since been amply confirmed by a number of other investigators as summarized in Table 6 where the frequency of thrombotic coronary artery occlusion is described as ranging from 10 to 27% of patients studied. This pattern differs significantly from that in transmural myocardial infarction, where with few exceptions occlusive thrombi are found in some 90% of patients. The

TABLE 6. *Frequency of occlusive coronary thrombi in predominantly subendocardial infarction*

Reference	Number of cases studied	Frequency of occlusive thrombi
Miller et al., 1951 (46)	50	20
Ehrlich and Shinohara, 1964 (22)	20	10
Davies et al., 1976 (20)	31	13
Silver et al., 1980 (59)	11	27

principal pathologic features of so-called subendocardial infarction are generally a high degree of atherosclerotic coronary artery stenosis together with significant left ventricular hypertrophy. There is also the distinct possibility that subendocardial infarction is associated with a higher risk for sudden cardiac death than transmural myocardial infarction (42).

SUDDEN UNEXPECTED CARDIAC DEATH

The pathologic profile of sudden cardiac death (SCD) in the United States has been the subject of recent reviews (55,56). Males are more prone to SCD than females; cardiomegaly is present in approximately one-half of the cases and is associated with severe atherosclerotic disease in one or more major epicardial arteries in over 90% of patients. Between 10 and 49% of the patients exhibit recent occlusive thrombi, and recent myocardial infarction is present in from 11 to 47% of the patients.

The frequency of coronary artery thrombosis in patients dying suddenly and unexpectedly is considered in detail in Table 7. Overall, thrombotic occlusions are seen in approximately one-third of cases. Clearly then, explanations other than occlusive thrombosis of the main epicardial arteries must be considered as the precipitating cause of the lethal arrhythmias of SCD. Although the traditional risk factors such as hypertension, hypercholesterolemia, cigarette smoking, and so on do not discriminate between SCD and myocardial infarction, from a pathologic viewpoint it is clear that these should not be regarded as a single disease entity. In examining this apparent dilemma, the findings of Cobb et al. (14) are of particular interest. Of the large number of patients who have been successfully resuscitated from what would otherwise have been a lethal ventricular fibrillation, in the post-resuscitation period only 19% of the survivors went on to develop pathologic Q waves indicative of transmural infarction and, further, only some 35 to 40% of patients showed changes in their lactate dehydrogenase (LDH) isoenzymes compatible with a diagnosis of myocardial infarction. On the basis of these important findings, it was concluded that the majority of patients dying suddenly and unexpectedly (60% or more) have developed a lethal arrhythmia without traditional acute myocardial infarction as the precipitating event. These findings, in concert with a variety of pathologic studies, can be interpreted as indicating that SCD is not the

TABLE 7. *Frequency of occlusive coronary thrombi in sudden cardiac death*

Reference	Frequency of occlusive coronary artery thrombi (%)	Comments
Titus et al., 1973 (65)	19	40% with recent MI
Lie and Titus, 1972 (41)	17	33% with recent MI
Lie (unpublished)	18	31% with recent MI
Scott and Briggs, 1972 (58)	46	47% with recent MI
Liberthson et al., 1974 (40)	19	27% with recent MI
Friedman et al., 1973 (26)	49	21% with recent MI
Baba et al., 1975 (4)	38	12% with recent MI
Reichenbach et al., 1977 (52)	10	26% with recent MI
Mitchell and Schwartz, 1965 (47)	31.6	31.6% with recent MI
Kuller, 1966 (39)	31	—
Luke and Helpern, 1968 (43)	25.6	—
WHO Techn. Rep. Series, 1970 (67)	25.9	—
Crawford, 1963 (19)	41	—
Roberts and Buja, 1972 (53)	8.5	—
Spain et al., 1969 (64)	19	—
Friedman et al., 1973 (26)	4.0	Within 30 sec
Haerem, 1974 (31)	30	Within 10 min
Spain and Bradess, 1970 (63)	16	Within 1 hr
Adelson and Hoffman, 1961 (1)	33	Within 2 hr

end-result of a single disease entity, and although approximately 25% of cases may be accounted for on the basis of myocardial infarction, mechanisms other than infarction in the traditional sense must be sought to account for the remainder. These conclusions are clearly consistent with the low frequency of occlusive thrombi observed in SCD (Table 7) and the high frequency almost invariably associated with recent transmural myocardial infarction.

In a number of studies the length of the terminal episode before death has been considered in relationship to the frequency of occlusive coronary artery thrombi (Table 7). In general, the frequency of thrombosis is less in patients dying shortly after the onset of terminal symptoms or signs, but the data base remains inconclusive. Indeed a significant tautology of recent years has been and remains the facile assumption that SCD be regarded as acute myocardial infarction, before infarction has had time to become enzymically or histologically manifest. This unfortunate assumption has almost certainly contributed to heterogeneity of patients studied under the umbrella of acute myocardial infarction, and has contributed in no small way to the discrepancies observed in the frequency of occlusive thrombi reported in various studies.

Focal Myocardial Injury: Possible Role of Microvascular Lesions

Reichenbach et al. (52) in reporting the pathologic findings in 50 patients with SCD in whom cardiopulmonary resuscitation had been unsuccessful described a spectrum of myocardial changes ranging from abnormal but viable cells to frank cellular necrosis. These changes, present in 88% of patients, were focal and of histologically differing ages. They commented that the morphologic features of this focal selective myocardial injury differ from that seen in infarction and concluded that as these lesions occur in the absence of coronary artery thrombosis, factors other than permanent vascular obstruction may play a role in the pathogenesis of SCD. Lie and Titus (42), in another study, showed histologic evidence of acute focal myocardial ischemic injury in some 52 to 81% of cases of SCD. It is presumably these small foci of injured but viable cells with membrane and metabolic derangements which provide the electrical trigger for ventricular fibrillation. While some of these microscopic foci of cellular injury may be the result of regional inadequacies in perfusion, other mechanisms may also be involved including focal obliteration by microemboli or microthrombi and/or spasm of the coronary arteries.

The possible role of intravascular platelet aggregation in the pathogenesis of myocardial ischemia and SCD was addressed experimentally by Mustard and his colleagues (38). They showed that a brief intracoronary or intraventricular infusion of adenosine diphosphate, a powerful platelet aggregating agent, produces both ischemic myocardial necrosis and SCD in the pig. Infusions of adenosine monophosphate served as controls. With intracoronary adenosine diphosphate infusions, 36.1% of the animals died with lethal arrhythmias, compared to only 8% of the controls receiving adenosine monophosphate. Additionally, it was shown that thrombocytopenia prevented the development of myocardial ischemic changes produced by adenosine diphosphate, indicating the likely importance of intravascular platelet aggregation and platelet microthrombi or microemboli. Such studies lend credence to the possibility that platelet microthrombi or emboli may produce focal myocardial ischemic injury and lethal arrhythmias in man.

The role of platelet microthrombi or emboli in the pathogenesis of SCD in man has been the subject of a number of studies. Of particular importance are the reports of Haerem (29,30,31), Jørgensen et al. (37), and El Maraghi and Genton (23) in which platelet microthrombi or emboli have been observed within the myocardial microcirculation in a number of cases of SCD. In another study Frink (27) reported the findings in 5 young males dying instantaneously without any prior history of heart disease. In each of the 5 patients a nonobstructive mural coronary artery thrombus was found in a major epicardial coronary artery. Platelet-fibrin emboli were observed downstream in 2 patients, while in 4 patients the His bundle and/or bundle branches showed histologic evidence of injury. This study points to the possible importance of emboli arising from nonocclusive thrombi located proximally in the coronary arteries, but further studies are needed to clarify this issue.

Platelet aggregates within the microcirculation may exert their effects directly through mechanical obstruction to blood flow, with resulting microfoci of ischemic injury. Alternately or additionally they may release thromboxane A_2, a potent vasoconstrictor and platelet aggregating agent (32), which, in turn, may cause focal vasospasm and myocardial ischemia. Recently, Hirsh et al. (35) have shown local thromboxane A_2 release is associated with recent episodes in patients with unstable angina pectoris. Indeed, in recent years there has been increasing speculation on the role of prostaglandins and thromboxanes in so-called ischemic heart disease

(6,7). This concept has, in part, derived impetus from a number of studies showing that in some patients with angina pectoris or myocardial infarction, the reduced coronary arterial flow may be attributed to heightened coronary artery tone or spasm (12,45,51). Whether such effects of platelet-derived thromboxane A_2 are in fact modulated by prostaglandin I_2 (PGI_2), a powerful vasodilator and inhibitor of platelet aggregation (48,49), is an important question needing clarification. Additionally we should know more about factors stimulating platelet thromboxane A_2 production and release within the circulation. Exposure of platelets to atherosclerotic plaques does not appear to result in thromboxane A_2 release (35). It is feasible, however, that nonocclusive thrombi may be associated with focal thromboxane A_2 release, inducing segmental spasm which might contribute to complete obliteration of the arterial lumen. Transient coronary vasospasm would in all likelihood result in early reperfusion of areas of acute myocardial ischemic injury, a phenomenon which might itself influence the development of ventricular fibrillation. Whether thromboxane A_2 will directly influence the development of arrhythmias is unknown. Myocardial tissue is known to synthesize PGI_2, but the studies of Hirsh et al. (35) were unable to show any influence of recent anginal episodes on the coronary sinus-aortic ratios of 6 keto-$PGF_{1\alpha}$, an inactive metabolite of PGI_2.

The possible importance of intravascular platelet aggregation has been further examined by Silver et al. (60). They injected sodium arachidonate at a dosage of 1.4 mg/kg into the marginal ear vein of rabbits, a manipulation which resulted in death within 3 min. Histologic examination of these animals revealed platelet microthrombi in the microvasculature of the lungs. Of particular interest was their finding that rabbits were protected from lethal effects of arachidonic acid by pretreatment with aspirin, a known cyclooxygenase inhibitor. Further, fatty acids closely related structurally to arachidonic acid did not cause death or intravascular platelet aggregates. It is feasible that a similar phenomenon could occur within the coronary microcirculation, particularly if arachidonate is released in relatively high concentrations.

Studies examining the association of SCD and intravascular platelet aggregates are faced with a major methodologic problem, namely the evanescent nature of the platelet aggregates. This emerged as a significant factor in a study exploring the frequency and distribution of platelet microemboli arising from a pump oxygenator (57). Myocardial platelet-fibrin emboli in the microcirculation were found to be some five- to tenfold more frequent in patients surviving less than 24 hr, than in comparable patients surviving 24 to 48 hr. A similar reversibility of experimentally induced intravascular platelet aggregates was noted by Jørgensen et al. (38). Such observations indicate that the frequency of intramyocardial platelet microthrombi or emboli observed in SCD may be significantly underestimated at autopsy, and that this underestimation may be even further enhanced by postmortem lysis.

THE INITIATION OF ARTERIAL THROMBOSIS

Virchow's triad of factors predisposing to thrombogenesis continues to have important implications and, in essence, implies that thrombosis is the result of changes in (a) the vessel wall, (b) patterns or rate of blood flow, and (c) the blood itself. Each of these has assumed a new relevance as our understanding of basic mechanisms of thrombogenesis has evolved. Conceptually it is convenient and probably correct to regard thrombosis as a pathologic variant of the hemostatic plug, in which the initial stimulus is a focus of endothelial injury with exposure of circulating platelets to subendothelial components, particularly collagen and microfibrils. This collagen-platelet interaction results in a release reaction involving a number of platelet constituents, including adenosine diphosphate, serotonin, and a variety of vasoactive compounds, as described by Mustard and Packham (50). Adenosine diphosphate, a powerful aggretating agent, results in the further aggregation of platelets and growth of the thrombus. Fibrin formation, which stabilizes the structure of the thrombus, is initiated through activation of both the intrinsic and extrinsic pathways (34). The importance and relative roles of both platelet-derived thromboxane A_2, a platelet aggregating agent and vasoconstrictor, and endothelial or smooth muscle cell-derived prostaglandin I_2, an inhibitor of aggregation and a vasodilator, in the pathogenesis of thrombosis are described in detail in separate chapters. The thrombus which results from this cascade of events involving both platelet-collagen interactions, the release phenomenon, and activation of the blood coagulation mechanism, is characteristically a nonhomogenous coagulum in which there is a selective accumulation of the formed elements, particularly platelets and leukocytes, together with variable numbers of erythrocytes incorporated into a stabilizing meshwork of fibrin. In contrast, a blood clot is a homogenous coagulum in which the formed elements are present in essentially the same proportions as they occur within the circulating blood. The selective accumulation of neutrophils in a thrombus and their possible roles in both thrombogenesis and the ultimate fate of thrombi pose a number of interesting questions which have yet to be answered.

Within arteries the most frequent lesions associated with occlusions or nonocclusive thrombi are of an atherosclerotic origin. As early as 1926, Benson (5) noted that coronary thrombi typically occur in narrowed arteries in which the luminal or plaque surface is physically disrupted. The consensus now is that disruption of the surface of an atherosclerotic plaque, be it an intimal tear, surface ulceration, plaque fissure or rupture, is a significant correlate of arterial thrombosis (10,13,15), although the mechanisms responsible for plaque surface disruption are less certain. Whatever the cause, plaque rupture or ulceration exposes circulating platelets to thrombogenic elements within the arterial wall including lipids, initiating a sequence of events analogous to those which occur in the formation of an hemostatic plug.

Although the association between plaque disruption and thrombosis is impressive, it is important to recognize that this association is not universal, and thrombi may occur over plaques in the absence of plaque hemorrhage or rupture (36). This raises the possible contribution of an altered thromboresistance of morphologically intact vascular endothelium to the thrombogenic process, together with, or in addition to, changes in the thrombogenic potential of the blood itself.

FATE OF THROMBI

Although there are some differences in the fate of occlusive and nonocclusive or mural arterial thrombi, most of the changes occurring during the organization of an arterial thrombus are similar and are independent of the arterial bed involved. Changes occurring in an occlusive arterial thrombus include retraction, thrombolysis, recanalization, vascularization, endothelialization, and, ultimately, incorporation in or transformation to atherosclerotic plaques. Retraction of a thrombus occurs, presumably as a result of fibrin shortening, and also as a result of arterial relaxation occurring after transient focal vasospasm. Thrombolysis in part reflects the reversibility of aggregated platelets, and, additionally, the influence of fibrolysins on the fibrin mesh which tends to maintain thrombus stability. Some fibrin phagocytosis by neurophils and monocyte-derived macrophages is also involved in the thrombolytic process. The recanalization of an occlusive thrombus is the hallmark or *sine qua non* of the later stages of organization. Multiple small channels occur, some of which become "arterialized" with a distinct "medial" coat, which ultimately restores some degree of continuity of the circulation from proximal to distal segments. In many cases these channels are too small to be of major functional significance.

The incorporation or transformation of thrombi into atheromatous plaques was first proposed by von Rokitansky, and later brought decisively to the attention of contemporary pathologists by J. B. Duguid in the 1940s (21). For reasons which are hard to identify, the role of thrombosis as a factor contributing to plaque growth has been accepted only recently, albeit reluctantly, by many investigators. But numerous experimental studies have amply confirmed the important role which thrombosis plays in the pathogenesis of advanced atherosclerosis, a subject recently reviewed by Woolf (66). Hand and Chandler (33) demonstrated that platelet-rich artificial pulmonary thromboemboli undergo a series of transitions to lesions resembling atherosclerotic plaques, and suggested that the lipid in such lesions was derived from phagocytosed platelets. These studies were extended by Ardlie and Schwartz (2,3) who confirmed that complex fibrofatty plaques, essentially indistinguishable histologically from atherosclerotic lesions, could result from the organization of artificial platelet-rich pulmonary thromboemboli. Hyperlipidemia in these studies, induced by a dietary cholesterol-fat challenge, enhanced the amount of lipid within the lesions. Thrombi predominantly of a fibrous composition resulted in collagen-rich plaques with little or no lipid, while platelet-rich thrombi resulted in lesions containing both intra- and extracellular lipid, together with considerable fibrosis and calcification. Similar studies have been undertaken in the pig (16,17,18) where the lipid composition of the resulting lesions was described in detail. The laminated structure of many atherosclerotic plaques, and histologic transitions between organizing thrombus and plaque all support the view that platelet-rich thrombi contribute significantly to the later stages of plaque growth.

In addition to the pathogenic role of platelet-rich thrombi described above, platelets in all likelihood also contribute to atherogenesis through two other mechanisms.

Platelets have been shown to release a low molecular weight cationic protein which is mitogenic for vascular smooth muscle cells in culture. This platelet-derived growth factor, described by Ross et al. (54) may prove to be important in modulating smooth muscle cell proliferation in the atheromatous plaque. Additionally, platelets may influence endothelial structure or function, contributing to an enhanced flux of plasma constituents including low density lipoproteins into the arterial wall. Such effects may be mediated by platelet-derived serotonin or histamine, possibly other vasoactive amines, and permeability inducing proteins.

ACKNOWLEDGMENTS

This work was supported in part by NHLBI Grants HL 07446 and HL 19362.

REFERENCES

1. Adelson, L., and Hoffman, W. (1961): Sudden death from coronary disease. *JAMA*, 176:131.
2. Ardlie, N. G., and Schwartz, C. J. (1968): A comparison of the organization and fate of autologous pulmonary emboli and of artificial plasma thrombi in the anterior chamber of the eye, in normo-cholesterolaemic rabbits. *J. Pathol. Bacteriol.*, 95(1):1–18.
3. Ardlie, N. G., and Schwartz, C. J. (1968): The organization and fate of autologous pulmonary emboli in hypercholesterolaemic rabbits. *J. Pathol. Bacteriol.*, 95(1):19–29.
4. Baba, N., Bashe, W. J., Jr., Keller, M. D., Geer, J. C., and Anthony, J. R. (1975): Pathology of atherosclerotic heart disease in sudden death. I and II. *Circulation*, (Suppl. III) 52:53–63.
5. Benson, R. L. (1926): The present status of coronary arterial disease. *Arch. Pathol.*, 2:876.
6. Borer, J. S. (1980): Unstable angina: A lethal gun with an invisible trigger. *N. Engl. J. Med.*, 302:1200–1202.
7. Braunwald, E. (1978): Coronary spasm and acute myocardial infarction—new possibility for treatment and prevention. *N. Engl. J. Med.*, 299:1301–1303.
8. Caulfield, J. B., Leinbach, R., and Gold, H. (1976): The relationship of myocardial infarct size and prognosis. *AHA Monograph 48*, edited by E. Braunwald, I:141–144.
9. Chandler, A. B., Chapman, I., Erhardt, L. R., Roberts, W. C., Schwartz, C. J., Sinapius, D., Spain, D. M., Sherry, S., Ness, P. M., and Simon, T. L. (1974): Coronary thrombosis in my-ocardial infarction. *Am. J. Cardiol.*, 34(7):823–833.
10. Chapman, I. (1965): Morphogenesis of occluding coronary artery thrombosis. *Arch. Pathol.*, 80:256–261.
11. Chapman, I. (1968): Relationships of recent coronary artery occlusion and acute myocardial infarction. *J. Mt. Sinai Hosp.*, 53:149–154.
12. Chierchia, S., Brunelli, C., Simonetti, I., Lazzari, M., and Maseri, A. (1980): Sequence of events in angina at rest: Primary reduction in coronary flow. *Circulation*, 61:759–768.
13. Clark, E., Graef, I., and Chasis, H. (1936): Thrombosis of the aorta and coronary arteries, with reference to fibrinoid lesions. *Arch. Pathol.*, 22:183–212.
14. Cobb, L. A., Hallstrom, A. P., Weaver, W. D., Copass, M. K., Hedgecock, M., and Haynes, R. E. (1978): Prognostic factors in patients resuscitated from sudden cardiac death. In: *Acute and Long Term Management of Myocardial Ischemia*, edited by L. Wilhelmsen, A. Hjalmarson, A. B. Lindgren Söner, pp. 106–113. Mölndal, Sweden.
15. Constantinides, P. (1966): Plaque fissures in human coronary thrombosis. *J. Atheroscler. Res.*, 6:1–17.
16. Craig, I. H., Bell, F. P., Goldsmith, C. H., and Schwartz, C. J. (1973): Thrombosis and Ather-osclerosis: The organization of pulmonary thromboemboli in the pig. I. Microscopic observations, protein, DNA, and major lipids. *Atherosclerosis*, 18:277–300.
17. Craig, I. H., Bell, F. P., and Schwartz, C. J. (1973): Thrombosis and Atherosclerosis: The or-ganization of pulmonary thromboemboli in the pig. II. Individual phospholipids, fatty acid com-position of lecithin, sphingomyelin, esterified cholesterol and ³H-cholesterol specific activity. *Exp. Mol. Pathol.*, 18:290–304.

18. Craig, I. H., and Schwartz, C. J. (1972): Contribution of thrombus free and esterified cholesterol to atherosclerotic plaques. *Pathology*, 4(4):303–306.
19. Crawford, T. (1963): Thrombotic occlusion and the plaque. In: *Evolution of the Atherosclerotic Plaque*, edited by J. J. Jones, p. 279. University of Chicago Press, Chicago.
20. Davies, M. J., Woolf, N., and Robertson, W. B. (1976): Pathology of acute myocardial infarction with particular reference to occlusive coronary thrombi. *Br. Heart J.*, 38:659.
21. Duguid, J. B. (1946): Thrombosis as a factor in the pathogenesis of coronary atherosclerosis. *J. Pathol. Bacteriol.*, 58:207–212.
22. Erlich, J. C., and Shinohara, Y. (1964): Low incidence of coronary thrombosis in myocardial infarction. A restudy of serial block technique. *Arch. Pathol.*, 78:432.
23. El-Maraghi, N., and Genton, E. (1980): The relevance of platelet and fibrin thromboembolism of the coronary microcirculation, with special reference to sudden cardiac death. *Circulation*, 62:936–944.
24. Erhardt, L. R., Lundman, T., and Mellstedt, H. (1973): Incorporation of ^{125}I-labelled fibrinogen into coronary arterial thrombi in acute myocardial infarction in man. *Lancet*, 1:387–390.
25. Erhardt, J. R., Unge, G., and Boman, G. (1976): Formation of coronary arterial thrombi in relation to onset of necrosis in acute myocardial infarction in man. *Am. Heart J.*, 91:592–598.
26. Friedman, M., Manwaring, J. H., Rosenman, R. H., Donlow, G., Ortego, P., and Grube, S. M. (1973): Instantaneous and sudden death. Clinical and pathological differentiation in coronary artery disease. *JAMA*, 225:1319.
27. Frink, R. J. (1977): Non-obstructive mural coronary thrombosis in sudden death. In: *Atherosclerosis*, edited by G. W. Manning and M. D. Haust, pp. 124–126. Plenum, New York.
28. Fulton, W. F. M., and Sumner, D. J. (1977): Causal role of coronary thrombotic occlusion and myocardial infarction: Evidence of stereoarteriography, serial sections and ^{125}I-fibrogen autoradiography. *Am. J. Cardiol.*, 39:322.
29. Haerem, J. S. (1971): The occurrence of platelet aggregates in the epicardial arteries of man. *Atherosclerosis*, 14:417.
30. Haerem, J. W. (1972): Platelet aggregates in intramyocardial vessels of patients dying suddenly and unexpectedly of coronary artery disease. *Atherosclerosis*, 15:199.
31. Haerem, J. W. (1974): Mural platelet microthrombi and major acute lesions of main epicardial arteries in sudden coronary death. *Atherosclerosis*, 19:529.
32. Hamberg, M., Svensson, J., and Samuelsson, B. (1975): Thromboxanes: A new group of biologically active compounds derived from prostaglandin endoperoxides. *Proc. Natl. Acad. Sci. USA*, 72:2994–2998.
33. Hand, R. A., and Chandler, A. B. (1962): Atherosclerotic metamorphosis of autologous pulmonary thromboemboli in the rabbit. *Am. J. Pathol.*, 40:469–486.
34. Hirsh, J., and Cade, J. F. (1973): Haemorrhagic disorders and fibrinolysis. In: *Peripheral Vascular Surgery*, edited by M. Birnstingl, pp. 46–74. Heinemann, London.
35. Hirsh, P. D., Hillis, L. D., Campbell, W. B., Firth, B. G., and Willerson, J. T. (1981): Release of prostaglandins and thromboxane into the coronary circulation in patients with ischemic heart disease. *N. Engl. J. Med.*, 304:685–691.
36. Jørgensen, J., Chandler, A. B., and Borchgrevink, C. F. (1971): Acute lesions of coronary arteries in anticoagulant treated and untreated patients. *Atherosclerosis*, 13:21–44.
37. Jørgensen, J., Haerem, J. W., Chandler, A. B., and Borchgrevink, C. F. (1968): The pathology of acute coronary death. *Acta Anaesth. Scand.*, (Suppl.) 24:193.
38. Jørgensen, J., Rowsell, H. D., Hovig, T., Glynn, M. F., and Mustard, J. F. (1967): Adenosine diphosphate-induced platelet aggregation and myocardial infarction in swine. *Lab. Invest.*, 17:616–644.
39. Kuller, L. (1966): Sudden and unexpected non-traumatic deaths in adults. *J. Chronic Dis.*, 19:1165.
40. Liberthson, R. R., Nagel, E. L., Hirschman, J. C., Nussenfeld, S. R., Blackbourne, B. D., and Davis, J. H. (1974): Pathophysiologic observations in prehospital ventricular fibrillation and sudden cardiac death. *Circulation*, 49:790.
41. Lie, J. T., and Titus, J. L. (1972): Inapparent early myocardial ischemia in sudden death from coronary heart disease. *Proceedings of the Vth Asian-Pacific Congress of Cardiology, Singapore*, 8:13, p. 542.
42. Lie, J. T., and Titus, J. L. (1975): Pathology of the myocardium and the conduction system in sudden coronary death. *Circulation*, (Suppl. III) 52:41–52.
43. Luke, J. L., and Helpern, M. (1968): Sudden unexpected death from natural causes in young adults. *Arch. Pathol.*, 85:10.

44. Mallory, G. K., White, P. D., and Salcedo-Salgar, J. (1939): The speed of healing of myocardial infarction. A study of the pathologic anatomy in 72 cases. *Am. Heart J.*, 18:647–671.
45. Maseri, A., L'Abbate, A., and Baroldi, G. (1978): Coronary vasospasm as a possible cause of myocardial infarction: A conclusion derived from the study of "preinfarction" angina. *N. Engl. J. Med.*, 299:1271–1277.
46. Miller, R. D., Burchell, H. B., and Edwards, J. E. (1951): Myocardial infarction with and without acute coronary occlusion. *Arch. Int. Med.*, 88:597.
47. Mitchell, J. R. A., and Schwartz, C. J. (1965): *Arterial Disease*, Blackwell, Oxford.
48. Moncada, S., Gryglewski, R., Bunting, S., and Vane, J. R. (1976): An enzyme isolated from arteries transforms prostaglandin endoperoxides to an unstable substance that inhibits platelet aggregation. *Nature*, 263:663–665.
49. Moncada, S., Gryglewski, R., Bunting, S., and Vane, J. R. (1976): *Idem*. A lipid peroxide inhibits the enzyme in blood vessel microsomes that generates from prostaglandin endoperoxides the substance (prostaglandin X) which prevents platelet aggregation. *Prostaglandins*, 12:715–737.
50. Mustard, J. F., and Packham, M. A. (1970): Factors influencing platelet function—adhesion, release and aggregation. *Pharmacol. Rev.*, 22:97.
51. Oliva, P. B., and Brenkinridge, J. C. (1977): Arteriographic evidence of coronary arterial spasm in acute myocardial infarction. *Circulation*, 56:366–374.
52. Reichenbach, D. D., Moss, N. S., and Meyer, E. (1977): Pathology of the heart in sudden cardiac death. *Am. J. Cardiol.*, 39(6):865–872.
53. Roberts, W. C., and Buja, L. M. (1972): The frequency and significance of coronary arterial thrombi and other observations in fatal acute myocardial infarction. *Am. J. Med.*, 52:425.
54. Ross, R., Glomset, J., Kariya, B., and Harker, L. (1974): A platelet-dependent serum factor that stimulates the proliferation of arterial smooth muscle cells in vitro. *Proc. Natl. Acad. Sci. USA*, 71:1207–1210.
55. Schwartz, C. J. (1982): Thrombotic processes in the pathogenesis of myocardial infarction and sudden cardiac death. In: *The Thromboembolic Disorders*, edited by J. Ambrus, F. Beller, C. Prentice, and J. van de Loo. F. K. Schattauer, Stuttgart. *(in press)*.
56. Schwartz, C. J. (1982): Trigger mechanisms in the pathogenesis of sudden cardiac death. *N.H.L.B.I.*, edited by J. V. Dingell, M. B. Mock, and B. E. Sobel, Futura Publishing Co. *(in press)*.
57. Schwartz, C. J., Korns, M. E., Edwards, J. E., and Lillehei, C. W. (1970): Pathologic sequelae and complications of ventriculotomy. II. With particular reference to platelet thromboemboli in the small intramyocardial vessels. *Arch. Pathol.*, 89:56–64.
58. Scott, R. F., and Briggs, T. S. (1980): Pathologic findings in pre-hospital deaths due to coronary atherosclerosis. *Am. J. Cardiol.*, 29:782.
59. Silver, M. D., Baroldi, G., and Mariani, F. (1980): The relationship between acute occlusive coronary thrombi and myocardial infarction studied in 100 consecutive patients. *Circulation*, 61:219–227.
60. Silver, M. J., Hoch, W., Kocsis, J. J., Ingerman, C. M., and Smith, J. B. (1974): Arachidonic acid causes sudden death in rabbits. *Science*, 183:1085–1087.
61. Sinapius, D. (1972): Zur morphologie verschliessende Koronarthromben. *Dtsch. Med. Wochenschr.*, 97:544–551.
62. Spain, D. M. (1974): In: Chandler, A. B., Chapman, I., Erhardt, L. R., Roberts, W. C., Sinapius, D., Spain, D. M., Sherry, S., Ness, P. M., and Simon, T. L. Coronary thrombosis in myocardial infarction. Report of a workshop in the role of coronary thrombosis in the pathogenesis of acute myocardial infarction. *Am. J. Cardiol.*, 34:823–833.
63. Spain, D. M., and Bradess, V. A. (1970): Sudden death from coronary heart disease-survival time, frequency of thrombi, and cigarette smoking. *Chest*, 58:107.
64. Spain, D. M., Bradess, V. A., Matero, A., and Tarter, R. (1969): Sudden death due to coronary atherosclerotic heart disease. *JAMA*, 207:1347.
65. Titus, J. L., Oxman, H. A., Conolly, D. C., and Norbrega, F. T. (1973): Sudden unexpected death as the initial manifestation of coronary heart disease. Clinical and pathological observations. *Singapore Med. J.*, 14:291.
66. Woolf, N. (1978): Thrombosis and atherosclerosis. In: *The Thrombotic Process in Atherogenesis*, edited by A. B. Chandler, K. Eurenius and G. C. McMillan. p. 145. Plenum, New York.
67. World Health Organization. (1970): The pathological diagnosis of acute ischemic heart disease; Report of a WHO scientific group. *WHO Techn. Rep. Ser.*, 441.

Prostaglandins and the Cardiovascular System,
edited by John A. Oates. Raven Press,
New York © 1982.

Thromboxane A$_2$: Biosynthesis and Effects on Platelets

Elisabeth Granström, Ulf Diczfalusy, Mats Hamberg,
Göran Hansson, Curt Malmsten, and Bengt Samuelsson

*Department of Physiological Chemistry, Karolinska Institutet,
S-104 01 Stockholm, Sweden*

The discovery of thromboxane A$_2$ and its aggregating activity was made possible by previous work on prostaglandin biosynthesis. Thus, studies on the mechanism of the transformation of polyunsaturated fatty acids into prostaglandins indicated that endoperoxide structures are involved (292). When PGE$_1$ was biosynthesized from 8,11,14-eicosatrienoic acid in an atmosphere of $^{16}O_2/^{18}O_2$, it was found that the oxygens of the keto and hydroxyl groups at C-9 and C-11, respectively, originated in the same oxygen molecule and indicated the formation of a cyclic peroxide derivative that could be isomerized into a 1,3-hydroxy ketone (PGE compounds) or reduced into a 1,3-diol (PGF$_\alpha$ compounds). Further studies on the mechanism of the transformation (for review, see ref. 293) showed that the initial step consisted of a lipoxygenase-like reaction in which the pro-S hydrogen at C-13 was removed, the Δ^{11} double bond was isomerized into the Δ^{12} position, and oxygen was inserted at C-11. The subsequent steps leading to the endoperoxide were visualized to consist of attack by oxygen at C-15, shift of the Δ^{12} double bond, and formation of a new bond between C-8 and C-12.

Subsequently it was possible to isolate the methyl ester of an endoperoxide from short-time incubations of arachidonic acid with the microsomal fraction of homogenates of sheep vesicular glands (135). In an extension of these studies the endoperoxide (PGH$_2$) was obtained as the free acid; in addition, an endoperoxide carrying a hydroperoxy group at C-15 (PGG$_2$) was isolated (141,262). Two reactions are involved in the conversion of PGG$_2$ into PGE$_2$, i.e., reduction of the hydroperoxy group at C-15 into a hydroxy group (peroxidase) and isomerization of the endoperoxide structure into a β-hydroxyketone (endoperoxide isomerase) (Fig. 1).

In studies using *in vitro* preparations, it was found that the effects of the endoperoxides on gastrointestinal smooth muscle were comparable to those of PGE$_2$ and PGF$_{2\alpha}$ (Table 1). On the other hand, the effects on vascular (rabbit aorta) and airway (guinea pig trachea) smooth muscle were considerably greater than those of PGE$_2$ and PGF$_{2\alpha}$, respectively (Table 1) (134). Both endoperoxides were potent contractors of the isolated human umbilical artery. The threshold concentrations were 3 (1–4

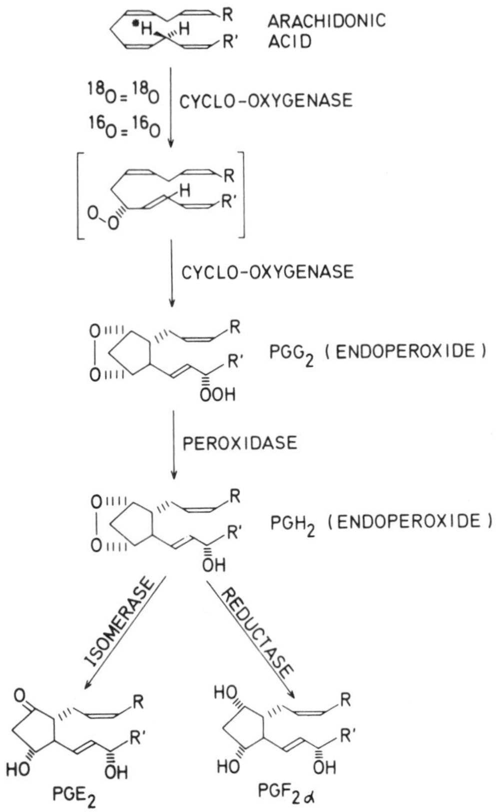

FIG. 1. Mechanism of prostaglandin biosynthesis.

TABLE 1. *Relative contractile effects of PGG₂, PGH₂, PGD₂, PGE₂, and PGF₂ₐ on some smooth muscle preparations*

Prostaglandin	Gerbil colon ($n = 5$)	Rat stomach ($n = 5$)	Rabbit aorta ($n = 5$)	Guinea pig trachea ($n = 7$)
PGG_2	1.5 ± 0.4 (n.s.)	1.9 ± 0.4 (n.s.)	80.4 ± 19.0 ($p < 0.05$)	7.5 ± 1.8 ($p < 0.05$)
PGH_2	1.2 ± 0.3 (n.s.)	3.3 ± 0.3 ($p < 0.01$)	210.4 ± 41.8 ($p < 0.01$)	9.3 ± 2.2 ($p < 0.01$)
PGD_2	0.3 ± 0.2 ($p < 0.05$)	1.4 ± 0.8 (n.s.)	—	5.2 ± 0.7 ($p < 0.01$)
PGE_2	2.9 ± 0.4 ($p < 0.05$)	5.7 ± 0.8 ($p < 0.01$)	1	relaxes[a]
$PGF_{2\alpha}$	1	1	—	1

[a]Contractions were sometimes seen with concentrations of 2 to 3 μg/ml.

ng/ml) for PGG$_2$ and one (1–12 ng/ml) for PGH$_2$ as compared to 200 (40–400 ng/ml) for PGE$_2$ (348).

Intravenous administration of PGG$_2$ and PGH$_2$ to guinea pigs (134) produced an increase in insufflation pressure which was more marked than that caused by corresponding doses of PGF$_{2\alpha}$. The cardiovascular effects of the endoperoxides showed a complex pattern. The blood pressure response was triphasic, i.e., a transient fall consistently followed by a short-lasting rise and then by a sustained reduction. These studies on vascular and airway smooth muscle demonstrated that the endoperoxides had unique effects that could not be attributed to conversion into the stable prostaglandins.

Further work from our laboratory showed that the two endoperoxides also had unique effects on platelets. Thus, PGG$_2$ and PGH$_2$ induced rapid and irreversible aggregation of human platelets (135,141,296). Since aspirin, an inhibitor of endoperoxide formation, inhibits the second wave of aggregation, it was suggested that the endoperoxides play a role in the release reaction (136). The formation of material reducible with stannous chloride to PGF$_{2\alpha}$ during aggregation by various agents also supported this view (136,313). These findings with the endoperoxides were of particular interest in relation to other studies which demonstrated that arachidonic acid caused aggregation when added to human platelets (308,355) and that aggregating material (LASS) was formed from this acid when it was incubated with preparations of sheep vesicular glands (370). LASS was considered to be due to endoperoxide but was not characterized in detail (369,372).

DISCOVERY AND STRUCTURE OF THROMBOXANE

The potency of the endoperoxides in causing contractions of the isolated rabbit aorta was of particular interest in relation to the so-called rabbit aorta contracting substance (RCS) (279). This was reported to be formed in guinea pig lung during anaphylaxis and was later suggested to be due to the endoperoxide intermediate in prostaglandin biosynthesis (126). We found that material with similar biological properties was formed after addition of arachidonic acid to human platelets. However, with the pure endoperoxides (PGG$_2$ and PGH$_2$) available we could demonstrate that the rabbit aorta contracting substance from guinea pig lung and platelets consisted of one major component with a $t_{1/2}$ of about 30 sec and a minor component of PGG$_2$ and/or PGH$_2$ with a $t_{1/2}$ of 4 to 5 min (328).

Since the short-lived major component of RCS could be generated by addition of arachidonic acid to platelets, we incubated [1-^{14}C]arachidonic acid with suspensions of washed human platelets in order to obtain structural information about RCS. Three major metabolites (I) to (III) could be demonstrated (136). Compound (I) was found to be 12L-hydroxy-5,8,10,14-eicosatetraenoic acid (HETE) (Fig. 2).

A more polar derivative, compound (II), was identified as 12L-hydroxy-5,8,10-heptadecatrienoic acid (HHT) whereas compound (III) was found to be the hemiacetal derivative of 8(1-hydroxy-3-oxopropyl)-9,12L-dihydroxy-5,10-heptadecadienoic acid (thromboxane B$_2$, PHD) (Fig. 2). The structure of the latter compound

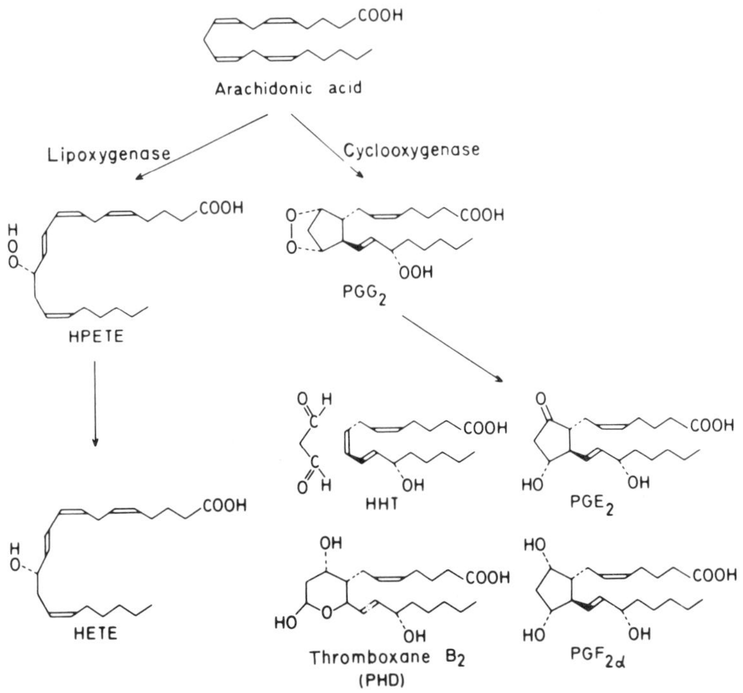

FIG. 2.　Transformation of arachidonic acid in human platelets.

was assigned mainly by mass spectrometric analysis of a number of derivatives and by oxidative ozonolysis. [1-^{14}C]PGG$_2$ added to suspensions of human platelets was rapidly converted into HHT and thromboxane B$_2$. All the identified products of arachidonic acid were stable compounds and could, therefore, not be identical with the very unstable ($t_{1/2}$ = 30 sec) RCS.

Additional biological work with the platelets involving characterization of the material formed from arachidonic acid was, therefore, carried out. When arachidonic acid was incubated with washed platelets and an aliquot of the incubate was transferred to a suspension of platelets preincubated with indomethacin, aggregation took place. This was not due to PGG$_2$ or PGH$_2$, since the amounts found in two experiments were 1.2 and 0.4 ng of PGG$_2$/PGH$_2$ per 0.1 ml and the amounts required were 110 and 68 ng of PGG$_2$/PGH$_2$ per 0.1 ml, respectively. A more detailed analysis of the appearance of the aggregating factor and the endoperoxides showed that the amount of endoperoxides was highest in the very early phase of the incubation period (maximum around 20 sec or earlier) whereas the aggregating factor had a maximum later (40–60 sec) (Fig. 3) (297). Similar results were obtained with filtrates of incubates prepared as described above. In these experiments it was noted that the aggregating factor was very unstable. When the log dose (arbitrary units) was plotted against time of incubation at 37°C, a linear relationship was obtained. The half-life of the aggregating factor calculated from this plot was 43 sec. In two

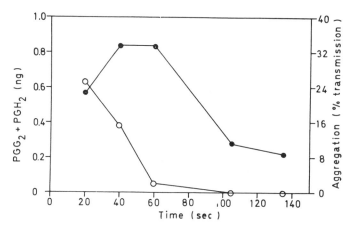

FIG. 3. Maximum aggregation induced by 0.1 ml of suspensions of washed platelets incubated for different times with 120 ng of arachidonic acid *(solid circle)*. The content of PGG₂/H₂ in these samples is also given *(open circle)*. The platelet suspension in the aggregometer tube was preincubated for 2 min with 1.4×10^{-5}M indomethacin.

other experiments, half-lives of 33 and 46 sec were obtained. A factor with similar properties was also generated from PGG₂. In addition to inducing irreversible aggregation, the unstable factor also caused release of [¹⁴C]serotonin from platelets preincubated with [¹⁴C]serotonin. These results demonstrated that the factor was distinguished from arachidonic acid, PGG₂, ADP, and serotonin, and had practically the same $t_{1/2}$ as the major component of RCS.

Additional studies involving ¹⁸O₂ experiments suggested that thromboxane B₂ (TXB₂) was formed from PGG₂ by rearrangement and subsequent incorporation of one molecule of H₂O (136). It was, therefore, conceivable that if the rearranged intermediate had an appreciable lifetime it should be trapped in the presence of nucleophilic reagents (140). As shown in Fig. 4, addition of 25 volumes of methanol to washed platelets incubated with arachidonic acid at 37°C for 30 sec gave two derivatives that were less polar than TXB₂. These derivatives were not present at longer incubation times, thus excluding the possibility that they were formed by action of methanol on one of the stable compounds in the incubation mixture, e.g., TXB₂. The mass spectral data indicated that the two compounds obtained by addition of methanol were epimers of TXB₂ methylated at the hemiacetal hydroxyl group. The two epimers also appeared when methanol was added to platelets incubated with PGG₂ for 30 sec. Similar results were obtained with ethanol and sodium azide.

These experiments showed the existence of a very unstable intermediate in the conversion of PGG₂ into TXB₂. In order to determine the half-life in aqueous medium, the platelet suspension was incubated with [1-¹⁴C]arachidonic acid for 45 sec and the reaction was stopped by filtration. The filtrate was kept at 37°C, and aliquots were removed after different times and immediately added to 25 ml of methanol containing tritium labeled mono-O-methyl thromboxane B₂. A linear relationship between the logarithms of the ¹⁴C:³H ratios of the purified methyl ester

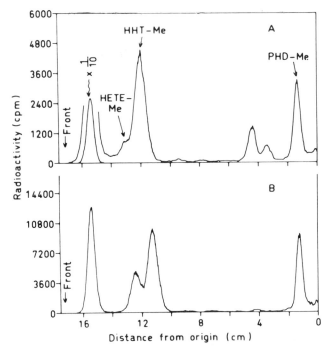

FIG. 4. Thin-layer radiochromatograms of products isolated after incubation of [1-¹⁴C] arachidonic acid (10 μg) with 1 ml of platelet suspension (10⁶ platelets/μl) for 30 sec **(upper)** and 5 minutes **(lower)**. The reactions were terminated by addition of 25 ml of methanol, and the esterified product was subjected to TLC (solvent system, organic layer of ethyl acetate-2,2,4-trimethylpentane-water 75:75:100, v/v/v).

of mono-*O*-methyl thromboxane B_2 and the times of incubation was obtained. The half-life thus obtained was 32 ± 2 (SD) sec.

The proposed structure of the unstable intermediate in the conversion of PGG_2 into TXB_2 is given in Fig. 5. The acetal carbon atom binding two oxygens should be susceptible to attack by nucleophiles, e.g., H_2O (giving TXB_2) as well as CH_3OH, C_2H_5OH, and N_3^- (giving derivatives of TXB_2 described above). This structure was also in agreement with the finding that the hydrogens at carbons 5,6,8,9,11,12,14, and 15 in arachidonic acid and PGG_2 were all retained in the conversion into TXB_2. Addition of CH_3O^2H to platelets incubated with arachidonic acid led to formation of mono-*O*-methyl thromboxane B_2 lacking carbon bound ^2H. This finding excluded an alternative structure of the unstable intermediate, i.e., an unsaturated oxane (I) in Fig. 5. Furthermore, the $t_{1/2}$ of thromboxane A_2 (TXA_2) seemed to exclude a carbonium ion structure [(II) in Fig. 5], which in aqueous medium should be considerably less stable.

The aggregating factor and the RCS were both derived from arachidonic acid or PGG_2, their formation from arachidonic acid was blocked by indomethacin, and their half-lives were similar, indicating that they were due to a single compound.

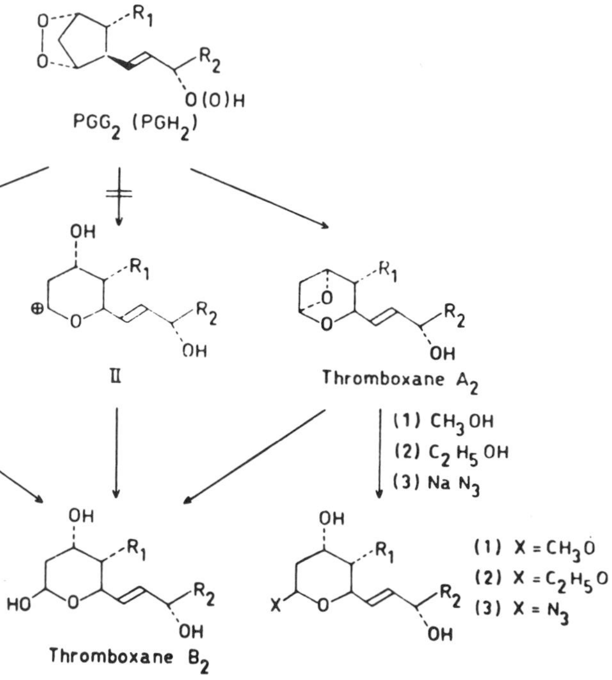

FIG. 5. Scheme of transformations of endoperoxides into thromboxane derivatives.

It was proposed that this material is identical with the unstable intermediate detected chemically in platelets (Fig. 5). This is also derived from arachidonic acid or PGG_2, its formation is blocked by indomethacin, and the half-life is close to that of the rabbit aorta contracting and platelet aggregating factors. The new oxane derivatives were named thromboxanes because of their structure and origin. TXA_2 is the highly unstable bicyclic compound and TXB_2 is the stable derivative that provisionally has been named PHD. The subscript indicates the number of double bonds, as in the prostaglandin nomenclature.

TXB_2 has been prepared synthetically by several groups (174,257,299), whereas there are no reports on the synthesis of the labile TXA_2. However, several structural analogs of TXA_2 have been synthesized. Carbocyclic TXA_2, where both oxygens in the ring systems were replaced by methylene groups, is a potent coronary vasoconstrictor but inhibits platelet aggregation (194). The basis for this separation of activities is not understood, however, it might reflect differences in receptors in platelets and vascular tissues. Replacement of the oxygen in the oxane ring of TXA_2 with sulfur afforded an analog with moderate contractile activity and no aggregating activity (183). However, substitution of sulfur for the oxygen in the oxetane ring resulted in a compound which caused contraction of isolated rabbit aorta and induced aggregation of human platelets (269).

Nomenclature

The identification of a series of metabolites of TXB$_2$ focused attention on the fact that the relatively complex systematic chemical nomenclature of the thromboxanes was not suitable for communication regarding enzymatic alterations of these molecules. A simplified nomenclature was, therefore, suggested.

The bases for the nomenclature are the parent substance *1*, thrombane, and its corresponding carboxylic acid *2*, thrombanoic acid. The oxygen of the oxane ring is designated "11a." In this way the numbering systems for thromboxanes and prostaglandins will be the same. For localization of functional groups as well as designation of dioic acid derivatives and derivatives having elongated or shortened side chain(s) the general nomenclature rules recommmended for prostaglandins should be used (256) (Fig. 6).

Biological Effects

TXA$_2$ has been shown to possess a variety of strong biological effects. The best known of these are induction of platelet aggregation and the release reaction (140,239), as well as strong constricting effects on vascular smooth muscle. The first vessel to be studied in this respect was the rabbit aorta (279,328); later similar contractile responses were observed in other vessels as well, such as coronary arteries (77,249,327,343,361), the mesenteric and celiac arteries (41,233), the umbilical artery (348), and others.

These dual effects of TXA$_2$, induction of vasoconstriction and platelet aggregation, both come into operation after a vessel has been injured. They indicate that TXA$_2$ probably plays a role in normal hemostasis *in vivo*, as well as in pathological conditions with an increased tendency to vasospasm and/or thrombosis. Several reviews have been written on the biological effects and possible roles of thromboxanes *in vivo* (e.g., refs. 123,239).

The role of TXA$_2$ in platelet function and its mode of action is discussed more in detail later.

Another well known activity of TXA$_2$ is its potent contractile effect on airways, demonstrable both *in vitro* and *in vivo* (330). When this effect was discovered, a role of TXA$_2$ as a mediator of bronchoconstriction in asthma was proposed. A large number of reports have shown an increased thromboxane production during pul-

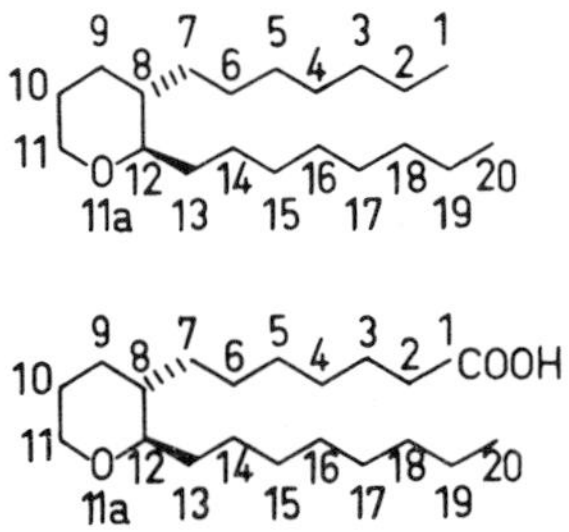

FIG. 6. Thromboxane nomenclature. **1:** Thrombane; **2:** thrombanoic acid.

monary anaphylaxis in the guinea pig (e.g., refs. 22,31,278). It is, however, beyond the scope of this chapter to cover the roles of thromboxanes in the respiratory system. Suffice it to say that after the recent development in this field, i.e., the discovery of the even more potent leukotrienes, TXA_2 is now believed to be of secondary importance in asthmatic bronchoconstriction. However, it is possible that leukotrienes, to some extent, exert their actions via release of TXA_2 (cf. ref. 88).

TXA_2 has also been shown to mediate augmented polymorphonuclear leukocyte adhesiveness (318): This is another area where thromboxanes and leukotrienes may act as agonists.

Most studies on thromboxane bioactivities have dealt with TXA_2. There are, however, reports on the effects of related compounds as well. 15-Hydroperoxy-TXA_2, the product of thromboxane synthase action on PGG_2, was found to possess biological activities similar to those of TXA_2 itself (143). PGH_3 and TXA_3, originating in 5,8,11,14,17-eicosapentaenoic acid, are somewhat less active on arterial smooth muscle than the corresponding compounds of the 2-series (250). Surprisingly, when their effects on platelets were studied, they were found to increase platelet cyclic AMP and thus act as antiaggregatory compounds (252). However, this effect was interpreted as caused by the presence of PGD_3, a break-down product of PGH_3 and a powerful antiaggregating compound.

Even TXB_2, which was originally regarded as inactive, has been shown to possess some biological activity, albeit weak. In relatively large doses it exerts some constrictor action on bronchial smooth muscle and pulmonary vasculature (90,168); even a weak chemotactic activity has been demonstrated (179).

BIOSYNTHESIS OF THROMBOXANES

Occurrence of Thromboxane Synthase

Lung

Because of the strong contractile effect of TXA_2 on airway smooth muscle (330) it was of interest to investigate lung tissue for its capability of thromboxane synthesis. In a study carried out with perfused guinea pig lung and with guinea pig lung homogenates (137), the major products formed from arachidonic acid were isolated and identified. They were found to be identical with those found in platelets, i.e., TXB_2, 12-HHT, and 12-HETE. As mentioned previously, a possible role of TXA_2 in anaphylaxis was suggested by the release of TXB_2 from sensitized guinea pig lung upon antigen challenge (138) coupled with the bronchoconstrictor effect of TXA_2 (330). On the other hand, such a mediator role of TXA_2 in causing human bronchoconstriction is not proved. Transformations of arachidonic acid in human lung (as well as rat lung) were recently found to be different from those occurring in guinea pig lung (9). Furthermore, 15-hydroperoxy-5,8,11,13-eicosatetraenoic acid (15-HPETE; isolated as the corresponding hydroxy acid) was very recently shown to be the major metabolite of arachidonic acid in human lung from an asthmatic subject (133).

Other Tissues

Thromboxane biosynthesis has been demonstrated in numerous organs and tissues apart from platelets and lung. Thromboxane formation (from endogenous and exogenous arachidonic acid) has been demonstrated in spleen (131), kidney (24,243,248, 376), brain (1,21,319,321,374), polymorphonuclear leukocytes, macrophages, and lymphocytes (60,99,242,244,362), fibroblasts (10,35,156), ocular tissues (172), vascular tissue (129,348), urinary bladder (44,45,46), the gastrointestinal tract (13,193), and in endometrial tissue (199). In the case of thromboxane formation by the kidney it is interesting to note that several conditions that lead to renal failure are accompanied by an enhanced synthesis of TXA$_2$, i.e., ureteral obstruction (243,376), renal vein constriction (248), as well as renal failure induced by glycerol (24).

Finally, TXB$_2$ has been detected in inflamed tissues [pleural fluid of carrageenin-induced pleurisy (173), human rheumatoid synovia (30), human burn blister fluid (166)] and in decidual tissue and amniotic fluid (368).

Purification of Thromboxane Synthase

The thromboxane-forming enzyme system of human platelets has been partially purified and resolved into two components, prostaglandin endoperoxide synthase (which catalyzes the conversion of arachidonic acid into PGG$_2$ and PGH$_2$) and thromboxane synthase (which catalyzes the isomerization of PGH$_2$ into TXA$_2$) (145). A microsomal fraction was prepared from washed platelets by ultrasound disruption and differential centrifugation. Treatment of the microsomes with Triton X-100 solubilized the enzymes required for thromboxane biosynthesis (145). The solubilized thromboxane synthase was reported to be fairly stable; it could be kept for weeks at 4°C (71). When the solubilized material was fractionated by DEAE-cellulose chromatography, two fractions with enzyme activity were obtained: one catalyzing the formation of PGG$_2$ and PGH$_2$ from arachidonic acid and the other catalyzing the conversion of prostaglandin endoperoxides into TXA$_2$ (145). The two enzyme activities, prostaglandin endoperoxide synthase and thromboxane synthase, had a similar subcellular distribution, suggesting that thromboxane synthase is localized in the dense tubular system of platelets. A similar scheme has been used for the partial purification of thromboxane synthase from bovine platelets (378), bovine lung (373), and sheep lung (337).

Properties of Thromboxane Synthase

PGH$_2$ is enzymatically converted into TXB$_2$ and HHT by human platelet microsomes (69,284). Kinetic studies on the formation of TXB$_2$ from arachidonic acid and PGH$_2$ indicated that the formation of the endoperoxide intermediate is the rate-limiting step in the formation of thromboxanes from arachidonic acid (340). The rate of TXB$_2$ formation was not appreciably affected by variations in the pH of the incubation medium between pH 5 to pH 8 (67,145,324), but at pH > 9 the reaction was significantly depressed (324).

When a number of compounds were screened for inhibitory action on thromboxane synthase it was found that TXB$_2$ and HHT formation was always inhibited to the same extent, irrespective of the inhibitor used. Heat inactivation of the platelet microsomes before incubation resulted in abolished TXB$_2$ and HHT forming capacity. These data suggested that TXB$_2$ and HHT are formed by the same enzyme (69). Trapping experiments with methanol, which converts TXA$_2$ into O-methyl-TXB$_2$, showed that HHT is not a breakdown product of TXA$_2$ (18,69). TXA$_2$ seemed to decompose exclusively into TXB$_2$. A reaction mechanism was proposed where the oxygen at C-9 of PGH$_2$ is first protonated, and the resulting ion then rearranges into either TXA$_2$ or HHT plus malondialdehyde (69). A similar reaction mechanism was proposed by Raz et al. (284) who, in addition, suggested an alternative pathway in which TXA$_2$ is the common intermediate for the formation of both TXB$_2$ and HHT. Kinetic studies on the conversion of PGH$_2$ by thromboxane synthase (18) suggested that TXA$_2$ formation is a bimolecular reaction; thromboxane synthase would thus not be an isomerase but rather act in a dismutase-like manner. However, when PGH$_1$ was incubated with platelet microsomes, the predominant product was 12-hydroxy-8,10-heptadecadienoic acid (HHD) and only very small amounts of TXB$_1$ were formed (69). Incubations with Δ^4-PGH$_1$, an analog of PGH$_2$ in which the double bond of the carboxyl side chain has been moved one methylene unit closer to the carboxyl group, gave a product pattern analogous to that of PGH$_1$ (67). The main product was Δ^4-HHD and only a few percent of thromboxane were formed, indicating that the position of the double bond of the carboxyl side chain is of importance for thromboxane formation. Further studies on the structural requirements for the isomerization to thromboxanes were undertaken with two C$_{21}$ analogs of PGH$_2$ (68). The two analogs, α-homo PGH$_2$ and ω-homo PGH$_2$, were both transformed into thromboxanes and hydroxy acids by platelet microsomes. The ratios of thromboxane to hydroxy acid were similar to the ratio of TXB$_2$ to HHT obtained from PGH$_2$. Thus, both the alpha and the omega chain could be elongated without interfering with thromboxane biosynthesis. However, both C$_{21}$ endoperoxides contained a double bond in the alpha-chain at the same distance from the cyclopentane ring as in PGH$_2$. As Δ^4-PGH$_1$ yielded only very small amounts of Δ^4-TXB$_1$ upon incubation with platelet microsomes, it seems likely that the double bond of the α-chain and its position relative to the cyclopentane ring are of importance for the formation of thromboxanes.

Compared to arachidonic acid, the polyunsaturated C$_{20}$ acids 8,11,14-eicosatrienoic acid and 5,8,11,14,17-eicosapentaenoic acid gave very low yields of thromboxanes when incubated with platelet suspensions (79,132). In the case of 8,11,14-eicosatrienoic acid the low yield of TXA$_1$ was explained by the poor conversion of PGH$_1$ into TXA$_1$ by thromboxane synthase (69). However, in the case of 5,8,11,14,17-eicosapentaenoic acid the low yield of TXA$_3$ was not due to a poor conversion of PGH$_3$ into TXA$_3$, but to a low conversion of the precursor acid into PGH$_3$ by the fatty acid cyclooxygenase (132,250,252). Thus, it seems that thromboxane synthase of human platelets can convert endoperoxides from the 1-, 2-, and 3-series into thromboxanes, although at different rates.

Incubation of PGG$_2$ with partially purified thromboxane synthase led to the formation of two products, 12-hydroperoxy-5,8,10-heptadecatrienoic acid and 15-hydroperoxy-TXA$_2$ (142). The thromboxane synthase was thus not associated with any peroxidase activity.

Inhibitors of Thromboxane Synthase

One aspect that has attracted great attention ever since the discovery of the thromboxane pathway is the possibility of pharmacologic inhibition of the biosynthesis of the potent TXA$_2$. A number of inhibitors effective *in vitro* on various thromboxane synthase preparations have been found. (For a discussion on *in vivo* inhibition of thromboxane biosynthesis, see below.) Among the first to be described were benzydamine (237) and sodium *p*-benzyl-4-[1-oxo-2-(4-chlorobenzyl)-3-phenyl propyl] phenyl phosphonate (N-0164) (74,185). However, benzydamine was not very selective, since it also inhibited prostaglandin biosynthesis in ram seminal vesicle microsomes with an IC$_{50}$ of 250 μg/ml, whereas thromboxane synthase (from horse platelet microsomes) was inhibited to 50% at a concentration of 100 μg/ml (237). When incubated with human platelet microsomes, benzydamine showed no inhibitory action on thromboxane synthesis at concentrations $<1 \cdot 10^{-3}$M (66). N-0164 selectively inhibited thromboxane synthesis in human platelet microsomes (IC$_{50}$ = $2,2 \cdot 10^{-5}$M) but has also been shown to be a prostaglandin receptor antagonist (75,203).

The nonacidic antiinflammatory compound 2-isopropyl-3-nicotinylindole (L-8027) was reported to be a selective inhibitor of thromboxane biosynthesis (116,127,128). Later, a report appeared which claimed that L-8027 is not a specific thromboxane synthase inhibitor, since a simultaneous inhibition of TXB$_2$ and PGE formation was found (281).

Imidazole was reported to selectively inhibit thromboxane synthesis in human platelet (232,251,260) and 1-methyl imidazole was found to be an even more potent inhibitor than imidazole itself (232). This finding led to extensive research on substituted imidazoles. 1-*n*-Butyl-imidazole was found to be a potent and selective inhibitor of thromboxane synthase (28), as was 1-(3-phenyl-2-propenyl)-1H-imidazole [(SQ 80,338); ref. 147]. Clotrimazole [1-(1-0-chlorophenyl-1,1-diphenyl methyl)-imidazole] inhibited thromboxane formation selectively and at lower concentrations than imidazole (186). A systemic study of 1-substituted imidazoles as well as of some imidazoles substituted in other positions was carried out by Tai and Yuan (339). They found that substitution at the 1-position retained the inhibitory action of imidazole, while introduction of substituents at other positions resulted in loss of the inhibitory effect. Screening of a series of 1-substituted imidazoles showed that the inhibitory potency increased with increasing chain length of the substituent. Maximum inhibition was obtained with 1-nonylimidazole. However, other authors found that 1-nonylimidazole blocked platelet aggregation in guinea pig platelet-rich plasma without interfering with TXA$_2$ formation, and they concluded that this compound should not be considered a selective inhibitor of thromboxane synthase

(281). Yoshimoto et al. (377) found that 1-carboxyalkylimidazoles were potent and selective inhibitors of thromboxane formation. Analogous to the case of 1-alkyl-imidazoles they found that the degree of inhibition varied with the chain length of the substituent; maximum inhibition was obtained with 1-carboxy-heptylimidazole. They also noted that 1-alkylimidazoles inhibited thromboxane formation, but the compounds with longer alkyl chains also inhibited prostaglandin endoperoxide synthase. Another imidazole compound, burimamide, an antagonist of histamine H$_2$ receptors, was reported to be as potent as imidazole as an inhibitor of thromboxane synthase (8,14).

When other heterocyclic compounds were screened for inhibitory action on thromboxane synthase, pyridine and some of its derivatives were shown to be active (230,335). Hydrophobic substituents in the 3- and 4-positions resulted in increased inhibitory effect, while 2-substituted pyridines were ineffective (335,336). Nicotinic acid (pyridine-3-carboxylic acid) inhibited thromboxane formation (335,359) but was less potent than pyridine (335). The pyridine derivative β-[4-(2-carboxy-1-propenyl) benzyl]-pyridine hydrochloride (OKY 1555) was shown to be a very potent (IC$_{50}$ = 3 nM) and selective inhibitor of thromboxane synthase (230). Hydralazine, dipyridamole, and diazoxide, three vasodilating agents, also inhibited thromboxane formation in human platelets (8,16,114,115). They were, however, not very potent, since hydralazine, the most active of the three, caused only 65% inhibition at the very high concentration of $1 \cdot 10^{-3}$M. Dipyridamole was shown to be an inhibitor of 3′:5′-cyclic AMP phosphodiesterase of platelets (228).

It has been reported that extracellular calcium ions inhibit TXB$_2$ formation in human platelets (26). Ionophore A23187-induced thromboxane production in human platelet-rich plasma was enhanced in the presence of ethyldiaminetetraacetate (EDTA). This suggests that extracellular calcium may be involved in the control of thromboxane biosynthesis.

Neither soluble nor microsomal fractions of rabbit myocardium were able to synthesize thromboxanes (49). When these fractions were added to other thromboxane-synthesizing systems they inhibited thromboxane formation. The chemical structure of the active principle responsible for inhibition has not yet been elucidated.

Manku et al. (214) observed similarities in action of UV-light and 8-methoxypsoralen with three thromboxane synthase inhibitors on the rat mesenteric vascular bed and, therefore, suggested that these factors may inhibit thromboxane biosynthesis as well.

A number of synthetic PGH$_2$ analogs were screened as potential thromboxane inhibitors. Two PGH$_2$ analogs were synthesized in which a methylene group had been substituted for each of the endoperoxide oxygens, 9,11-epoxymethano-15-hydroxyprosta-5,13-dienoic acid and 9,11-methano-epoxy-15-hydroxyprosta-5,13-dienoic acid (40). The 9,11-epoxymethano analog was a potent inhibitor, while the 9,11-methanoepoxy analog was much less effective (66,324). 9,11-Epoxymethano prostanoic acid was still more potent, with an IC$_{50}$ of 7 μM (324). The azo-analog 9,11-azo-15-hydroxy-prosta-5,13-dienoic acid was shown to be a powerful mimic of the prostaglandin endoperoxides PPG$_2$ and PGH$_2$ with regard to platelet aggregation and release of serotonin when added to platelet rich plasma (57). This compound also inhibited thromboxane formation by platelet microsomes with an IC$_{50}$ of 2 μM (66). Unlike the azo-analog above, the corresponding 15-deoxy analog, 9,11-azo-prosta-5,13-dienoic acid, inhibited platelet aggregation and was found to be a selective thromboxane synthase inhibitor (83,102,104). In the corpus luteum, however, this compound was almost equipotent in blocking thromboxane synthase and prostacyclin synthase (325). Another 9,11-azo analog of PGH$_2$, 9,11-azo-13-oxo-15-hydroxy-prostanoic acid, has been described to be a potent thromboxane synthase inhibitor with an IC$_{50}$ of 1 μM (170). This compound also exhibited PGH$_2$/TXA$_2$ receptor blocking properties.

An additional thromboxane synthase inhibitor with selective effect is 9,11-iminoepoxyprosta-5,13-dienoic acid (39,85), while 9,11-epoxyiminoprosta-5,13-dienoic acid was shown to be a TXA$_2$ antagonist which inhibited neither thromboxane synthase nor fatty acid cyclooxygenase (81). The 9,11-iminomethano analog of PGH$_2$ turned out to be a more potent inhibitor than 9,11-azoprosta-5,13-dienoic acid (58).

Recently a number of stable analogs of TXA$_2$ have been synthesized (220,258, 259,268). Pinane-thromboxane A$_2$ was shown to be a selective inhibitor of coronary artery constriction, platelet aggregation, and thromboxane formation (259). Carbocyclic thromboxane A$_2$, on the other hand, exhibited extremely potent vasoconstricting activity, behaved as a TXA$_2$ antagonist on platelet aggregation induced by various stimuli, and inhibited the biosynthesis of thromboxanes without interfering with PGI$_2$ production (194,258). Thus, in contrast to TXA$_2$, carbocyclic thromboxane A$_2$ separates coronary vasoconstriction from platelet aggregating activity (194).

Several articles have been published on screening and evaluation of thromboxane synthase inhibitors; there are also a number of articles of review character (101, 117,118,144,351).

Potentiation of Thromboxane Biosynthesis

Patients with Prinzmetal's variant angina had detectable levels of TXB$_2$ in their peripheral blood, whereas in normal subjects no TXB$_2$ was detectable (196). Administration of heparin markedly increased both free plasma fatty acid and TXB$_2$ levels in patients with angina. However, there was no correlation between the plasma levels of free fatty acids and TXB$_2$, suggesting that the cause of increase in TXB$_2$ levels was indirect (195,196,197). Also, heparin was found to potentiate TXA$_2$ synthesis in citrated human platelet rich plasma (19).

It has been established that the toad urinary bladder is capable of synthesizing TXB$_2$ from endogenous precursors (45). It was found that vosopressin significantly increased thromboxane synthesis in this tissue and that the increase was markedly reduced by thromboxane synthase inhibitors. This led the authors to suggest that TXA$_2$ may act as a positive modulator of the vasopressin-stimulated water flow (45).

Cholesterol was reported to enhance conversion of released arachidonic acid into TXB$_2$ (322). This enhancement was believed to occur primarily at the level of the cyclooxygenase rather than thromboxane synthase, since this is the rate-limiting step in this reaction sequence (322).

Calcium ionophores stimulated thromboxane formation by platelets (180). The ionophores A23187 and X537A mobilized calcium from intracellular storage sites. This increased concentration of cytosolic calcium led to increased free arachidonic acid which was rapidly oxygenated to prostaglandins and thromboxanes (180).

An altered balance of platelet prostaglandin and thromboxane synthesis was observed in oral contraceptive users (300). Platelet microsomes from oral contraceptive users generated more platelet-aggregating activity than controls upon incubation with arachidonic acid. This may contribute to their increased incidence of thromboembolic disorders.

Endogenous formation of TXB$_2$ by brain tissue from guinea pig and rat was demonstrated by Wolfe et al. (374). These authors also found that noradrenaline stimulated thromboxane formation.

Dietary Manipulations of Thromboxane Biosynthesis

Recently, a great interest has arisen in the dietary influence on prostaglandin and thromboxane synthesis, especially since it was reported that Greenland eskimos have a low incidence of cardiovascular disorders and a bleeding tendency, probably because of reduced platelet aggregation (72). The decrease in aggregability may be due to the high eicosapentaenoic acid content in lipids and phospholipids of the eskimos who depend on their fish diet.

A group of white men were given a mackerel diet and the change in their plasma and platelet lipid composition as well as changes in platelet aggregation and thromboxane synthesis were investigated (306). The ratio of eicosapentaenoic acid to arachidonic acid in plasma and platelet membrane phospholipids increased considerably while the volunteers were on the mackerel diet. Collagen-induced platelet aggregation and thromboxane synthesis were significantly reduced. This suggested that the increase in eicosapentaenoic acid and the concomitant decrease in arachidonic acid due to the diet led to diminished TXA$_2$ formation and, hence, reduced platelet aggregation (306).

Eicosapentaenoic acid has been shown to be a poor substrate for platelet cyclooxygenase but competes efficiently with arachidonic acid in binding to the enzyme, thereby inhibiting the conversion of arachidonic acid into the proaggregatory TXA$_2$ (252). An exchange of arachidonic acid for eicosapentaenoic acid in platelet phospholipids might, therefore, have a beneficial influence on certain cardiovascular disorders. A hypothetical combined therapy was proposed by Needleman et al. (253), who suggested that eicosapentaenoic acid supplementation together with a thromboxane synthase inhibitor could reduce TXA$_2$ synthesis and facilitate PGI$_2$ production. An alternative therapy has also been discussed, which includes dihomo-γ-linolenic acid, an inhibitor of platelet aggregation (176,253,371). Experiments in rats showed that manipulation of the linolenic acid (precursor of dihomo-γ-linolenic acid and arachidonic acid) and α-linolenic acid (precursor of eicosapentaenoic acid) intake resulted in profound changes in prostaglandin and thromboxane synthesis (155).

Dietary supplement of fish oil was given to dogs subsequently exposed to experimentally induced myocardial infarction (59). The size of the induced infarction was reduced in oil-fed dogs compared to a control group, indicating that fish oil supplement to the diet may be beneficial in reducing myocardial damage associated with coronary thrombosis.

Cholesterol-rich platelets were shown to release more arachidonic acid than cholesterol-depleted platelets upon stimulation with thrombin (322). The conversion of the released arachidonic acid into TXB_2 was also higher in cholesterol-rich platelets than in cholesterol-depleted platelets (322). TXA_2 release after cholesterol feeding in rabbit arterial blood was described (304); this might cause the edematous arterial reaction at early stages of atherosclerosis.

Onion and garlic extracts were shown to contain a heat-stable, lipid soluble substance which inhibits platelet aggregation (33,206,207). Addition of onion extract to washed platelets resulted in marked decrease in TXB_2 formation for ^{14}C arachidonic acid. When thromboxane synthesis was inhibited a new metabolite appeared. The new metabolite was isolated and subjected to gas chromatography and mass spectrometry. From its mass spectrum the metabolite was identified as 10-hydroxy-11,12-epoxy-5,8,14-eicosatrienoic acid (207). This compound appears to arise from the platelet lipoxygenase pathway. Thus, a common foodstuff contains a compound which inhibits platelet aggregation by alterations in both the platelet cyclooxygenase and lipoxygenase pathways.

ASSAY OF THROMBOXANES

Thromboxane production by a biological system can be monitored using several different approaches and a number of different types of assay methods. Volume 5 of this series, published in 1978, dealt exclusively with methodology, and most chapters covered various aspects of thromboxane measurements (108,111,112, 113,233). A few other review articles on the topic have also been published (e.g., refs. 106,107,119).

Measurement of thromboxane biosynthesis is generally done either by assay of the immediate product, TXA_2 (as such or as a derivative), or of the later formed product, TXB_2. Both approaches can be used to monitor thromboxane produced from either endogenous or exogenous precursors, but may give somewhat different information, as discussed later. When conversion of only exogenous substrate is studied, an alternative assay is the use of radiolabeled precursors and monitoring the formed labeled TXB_2 (153,317,324,360).

In certain cases neither compound may be reliable as an indicator of thromboxane formation: The best target for measurements may then instead be a metabolite.

Assay of TXA₂

Because of the extreme instability of TXA₂, bioassay is the only possible method when the compound is assayed as such. Of the various strong biological activities that TXA₂ has been shown to possess, its contractile effects on certain vascular preparations have proved most suitable for bioassay. The preferred vessels are generally the aorta, celiac artery, mesenteric artery, inferior caval vein of the rabbit (41,121,140,165,234,237,328,329), rat aorta (151), and bovine or porcine coronary artery (70,77,271,327).

Rabbit aorta was the first preparation used for this purpose and is still widely employed. However, this organ is not entirely specific for TXA₂, being contracted also by the endoperoxides. The rabbit mesenteric artery, on the other hand, seems to be specific for TXA₂. Another smooth muscle preparation, the guinea pig lung parenchymal strip (328), is highly sensitive to TXA₂ although not entirely specific.

Nonspecificity of a TXA₂ bioassay may somewhat limit its use. However, if the identity of the assayed compound is uncertain, specificity of the assay system can be considerably increased for TXA₂, for example, by insertion of a delay coil (233). This modification would reveal the presence of a highly unstable compound such as TXA₂ in the analyzed material. An alternate possibility is to use several different types of assay organs (119,233): TXA₂ has comparatively weak effects on, for example, gastrointestinal smooth muscle in contrast to other compounds in this field.

A different approach in TXA₂ assay is based on the rapid conversion of this unstable compound into a stable derivative by trapping with excess methanol or some other nucleophilic reagent (see previous section on the discovery and structure of thromboxane). If methanol is used, the formed products are the two epimers of mono-*O*-methyl TXB₂ (140). These compounds are biologically inactive and are instead suitable for assay by some method requiring chemical stability, such as gas chromatography-mass spectrometry or radioimmunoassay.

The first assay based on this trapping procedure was developed for TXA₂ formed from exogenous substrate and was a double isotope dilution method (140). Later, a radioimmunoassay was developed for the major epimer (110) which was possible to use also for assay of TXA₂ formed from endogenous precursor (e.g., ref. 88).

The differences in information obtained when TXA₂ or its stable breakdown product, TXB₂, are monitored can be seen in Fig. 7. Washed human platelets were subjected to addition of arachidonic acid. Aliquots were removed with short intervals and treated with excess methanol for later assay of TXB₂ and mono-*O*-methyl TXB₂, respectively. Aggregation was monitored continuously. The assay of mono-*O*-methyl TXB₂ showed that TXA₂ was rapidly biosynthesized from arachidonic acid, reached a maximal level within the first minute after addition of the substrate, and then rapidly disappeared. TXB₂, on the other hand, gradually accumulated, and since it is a stable product remained at the high final level. Measurement of TXA₂ thus gives information about the kinetics of formation and disappearance of the compound; however, the total amounts formed cannot be accurately estimated with this

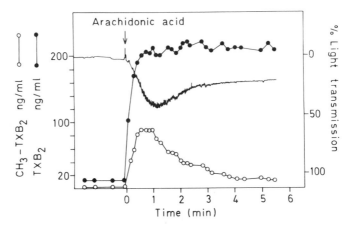

FIG. 7. Formation of TXA$_2$ during the first minute after addition of arachidonic acid to washed human platelets. The kinetics of this biosynthesis are reflected in the appearance and disappearance of mono-*O*-methyl TXB$_2$ in aliquots treated with excess methanol.

method. This is better seen when its hydrolysis product, TXB$_2$, is monitored (however, see where exceptions to this rule are discussed later); measurement of this end product, on the other hand, does not provide any information about the rapid events early during platelet aggregation.

Assay of TXB$_2$

The vast majority of quantitative studies in this field are concerned with the measurement of TXB$_2$. The first method developed for this compound was a gas chromatography-mass spectrometry method, utilizing [^{2}H$_8$]-TXB$_2$ as a carrier (139). This was later followed by others of the same type (11,113,317,374). A related gas chromatographic method was based on the electron capture technique (87); a liquid chromatographic method utilizing fluorescent derivatives of TXB$_2$ has also been described (346).

However, by far the most common method in this field is radioimmunoassay. Since the first radioimmunoassay for TXB$_2$ was published (109), a very large number of similar assays have also been described (e.g., refs. 20,86,181,276,317,338). This type of measurement has been used for detection and/or quantification of thromboxane synthesis in platelet preparations, in tissue homogenates, in various exudates or other biologic material, or to follow enzyme activity of thromboxane synthase through purification procedures.

Pitfalls in Thromboxane Assay

In addition to the various sources of error that are inherent in each type of assay method [bioassay, gas chromatography-mass spectrometry, radioimmunoassay (for discussion, e.g., see ref. 108)], certain other pitfalls also exist in the three different approaches to thromboxane measurements described above (viz., direct or indirect assay of TXA$_2$, and assay of TXB$_2$, respectively).

The most serious sources of error are probably associated with measurement of TXB$_2$ and are often overlooked because this compound is frequently regarded as a stable and reliable indicator of thromboxane biosynthesis. Generally, more precaution is taken in the experimental design when TXA$_2$ is monitored. The theoretical argument underlying measurement of TXB$_2$ as an indicator of thromboxane production is obviously that TXB$_2$ is a degradation product, in fact *the* degradation product, of all TXA$_2$ preexisting in the sample, or released into the blood stream, etc.

This concept may, however, be far from true. First, as is the well-known case with prostaglandins, artifactual thromboxane formation may occur rapidly and extensively from, e.g., blood cells during collection and processing of a blood sample. Reported TXB$_2$ levels in plasma are generally unrealistically high: Obviously they do not reflect the endogenous biological situation.

Second, even if this artifactual contribution could somehow be prevented, it is not necessarily certain that TXA$_2$ formed in the body, tissue, or other biologic material is quantitatively hydrolyzed into TXB$_2$. This hydrolysis may sometimes be a very minor pathway of TXA$_2$ degradation. It has, for example, been demonstrated that in samples containing albumin, such as platelet-rich plasma, the major part of formed TXA$_2$ is not converted into TXB$_2$ but instead covalently bound to albumin (82,204) and will thus escape detection by conventional assay methods for TXB$_2$.

In sensitized (and possibly to some extent also in normal) guinea pig lungs, an important thromboxane metabolite was found to be 15-keto-13,14-dihydro-TXB$_2$ (62): This compound gradually became the major metabolite after repeated challenge with antigen (31).

Assay of Thromboxane Metabolites

The uncertainties and practical difficulties involved in thromboxane assay when monitoring either TXA$_2$ or TXB$_2$ have prompted some groups to develop methods for further degraded metabolites instead. The major urinary metabolite of TXB$_2$, dinor-TXB$_2$ (177,288), has been monitored in the urine of the guinea pig (326) and man (265). As mentioned previously, however, it is by no means certain that the TXB$_2$ pathway reliably reflects TXA$_2$ biosynthesis. Thus, in anaphylactic guinea pigs (326), no increase in urinary dinor-TXB$_2$ was seen at all, although this condition is well known to be associated with a pronounced release of TXA$_2$ (cf. ref. 279).

The thromboxane production during pulmonary anaphylaxis could probably be better studied by measurement of 15-keto-13,14-dihydro-TXB$_2$ in the circulation (31,62), or one of the more degraded products of this pathway found in urine.

The first quantitative study monitoring 15-keto-dihydro-TXB$_2$ utilized gas chromatography-mass spectrometry of exudates of anaphylactic guinea pig lungs: The results were briefly described above (31). Later, a radioimmunoassay was developed for the same compound (22); the assay was recently improved to obtain higher sensitivity (278). This method was also used to follow thromboxane release during guinea pig anaphylaxis, in this case *in vivo*.

ROLE OF THROMBOXANES IN PLATELET FUNCTION

By three distinct functions, platelets are essential for normal hemostasis in response to vascular damage. First, there is occlusion of the injury site by adhesion and aggregation of platelets. Second, release of certain platelet constituents promote initiation of blood coagulation and propagation of platelet aggregation, and, third, release of certain substances, stored in the platelet or formed upon stimulation, affect vascular smooth muscle (366). In all of these aspects arachidonic acid metabolites seem to have important functions as modulators or effectors (97,209, 216,246,311). The second mechanism, which is characterized by secretion of one specific kind of platelet granule is commonly referred to as "the platelet release reaction."

Upon damage to the vessel wall, subendothelial tissue is exposed to platelets in the blood. Collagen in the subendothelium binds to a receptor/acceptor on the surface of the platelet (263) and subsequently induces liberation of arachidonic acid from the endogenous pool by activating a phospholipase (307). This arachidonic acid can be metabolized by two different enzymatic pathways in the platelets (294,295). With a lipoxygenase reaction 12-hydroperoxy-(HPETE) and 12-hydroxy-eicosatetraenoic acid (HETE) are formed. With the exception of a possible modulating function upon the formation of prostaglandins (305), these compounds do not seem to interfere with any physiological mechanism known, at present, in the platelets. However, the compounds exert a chemoattractant effect upon polymorphonuclear leukocytes which has been taken as evidence for a possible physiological role of platelets in the inflammatory response (347).

The alternate metabolic pathway of arachidonic acid in the platelets seems to be the physiologically more important one, viz., conversion via the cyclooxygenase pathway to form the two prostaglandin endoperoxides, PGG_2 and PGH_2 and, subsequently, the major product, TXA_2 (142,294,295). Possibly 15-hydroperoxy-TXA_2 is also formed from PGG_2 (142). Thromboxane biosynthesis in platelets from many species other than man has also been reported, for example, in the dog (51) and in the cat (215).

All these unstable intermediates (PGG_2, PGH_2, TXA_2, and 15-hydroperoxy-TXA_2) induce irreversible aggregation of human platelets (143,294,295), like platelet surface contact with collagen. Furthermore, they all induce the specific release reaction without concomitant cytoplasmic enzyme release.

At surface stimulation of platelets with collagen, TXB_2 is formed (109). If the formation of prostaglandin endoperoxides and thromboxanes is suppressed by inhibitors of the cyclooxygenase, no aggregation and no release reaction take place, although the liberation of arachidonic acid and the formation of lipoxygenase products is unimpaired (212). The final proof for the physiological role of prostaglandins and thromboxanes in platelet function was obtained by studies of some cases with a platelet disorder characterized by a pronounced tendency to bruise easily (187,212,264). Platelets from these patients did not aggregate upon exposure to collagen and, in contrast to platelets from normals, did not aggregate when arachidonic acid was administered. However, when PGG$_2$ or PGH$_2$ was added virtually normal aggregation was obtained. This bleeding disorder, which is clearly separated from other abnormalities in platelet function like thrombasthenia Glanzmann, storage pool disease, and the Bernard-Soulier syndrome (213) has been called platelet cyclooxygenase (PCO) deficiency (212).

Platelet aggregation and the release reaction can be initiated by a variety of agents in addition to collagen, arachidonic acid, and the short-lived prostaglandin endoperoxide and thromboxane intermediates. Potent in this respect are, e.g., ADP, biogenic amines like serotonin, epinephrine, and norepinephrine, proteolytic enzymes such as thrombin, trypsin, and plasmin, different kinds of particulate materials, living or dead bacteria, and viruses and endotoxins (247). In animals sensitized to endotoxins the response to endotoxins also seems to be markedly increased (37,38).

Since the ultrastructural changes produced in the platelets by all different agents are in most cases the same, and since most of the compounds cannot be taken up by the platelets, it seems logical to assume that there is a common mediator produced by the platelets in response to surface stimulation. This mediator then initiates the change in their shape, which makes aggregation possible and triggers the release reaction. In this context it is worth noting that other unsaturated fatty acids, such as 8,11,14- or 11,14-17-eicosatrienoic acid or 5,8,11,14-17-eicosapentanenoic acid, do not cause aggregation, but inhibit platelet aggregation induced by arachidonic acid and other agents. This finding suggests that they compete with arachidonic acid for some enzyme or receptor site of the platelet (308). However, an additional alternative or partly independent mechanism has been proposed for thrombin (25,302).

The aggregation of platelets can be divided into two phases. The first one corresponds to the direct effect of surface stimulation induced by the aggregating agent. The second phase corresponds to the propagation of aggregation by the release of proaggregating factors which occurs during the release reaction (247). In this aspect ADP, released from the very dense granules in the platelets, seems to be the most important factor, but also other constituents of these granules, like serotonin and Ca^{2+} might cooperate, as well as prostaglandin endoperoxides and thromboxanes. As seen in studies with platelets from cases with abnormal response to ADP (213), or in experiments where the ADP is rapidly removed under laboratory conditions (247), the response to the aggregating agent is markedly pathological if propagation by secondary ADP-stimulation cannot occur.

The formation of the stable prostaglandins PGE$_2$, PGF$_{2\alpha}$ (313), and PGD$_2$ (266), as well as of TXB$_2$ (109) occurs during platelet aggregation *in vitro* and closely parallels the release reaction (313). Neither the stable prostaglandins (209), nor TXB$_2$ (329), are able to initiate the release reaction, in contrast to the unstable PGG$_2$, PGH$_2$, TXA$_2$, and 15-hydroperoxy-TXA$_2$ (143,294,295). Since the formation of prostaglandins is restricted to the second wave of aggregation (313), and since prostaglandin synthesis inhibitors do not affect the first wave of aggregation (225,313), it has been proposed that these compounds mainly exert their effect as common initiators of the release mechanism.

The question if the prostaglandin endoperoxides must be converted into thromboxanes in order to exert their effect has been a matter in dispute. Two cases of possible thromboxane synthetase defects have been published (224,364). However, in one of these the abnormality has been shown to be a defective response to TXA_2 (and prostaglandin endoperoxides) rather than a real enzyme deficiency (191). Experiments with different inhibitors of thromboxane synthase (7,50,83, 127,194,221,259) give evidence for the hypothesis that thromboxane biosynthesis by the platelets is essential for biological activity. It also has to be stressed that TXA_2 is biologically more potent than the endoperoxides (329). Evidence for the hypothesis that conversion into thromboxane is not essential has also been presented (250), and these findings are consistent with the high biological activity of some stable endoperoxide analogs, which cannot be transformed into TXA_2 (27,57,208). A unifying hypothesis would be that the endoperoxides do have an effect per se, but that transformation into TXA_2 is essential under physiological conditions to obtain a normal biological response.

Another question of controversy is how thromboxanes and endoperoxides exert their effect in the platelets. The first aspect of this problem is the relationship to cyclic AMP. Since some inhibitors of platelet aggregation increase the cAMP level while agents that produce or augment aggregation reduce this level, it was proposed that platelet aggregation is favored by a decrease in cAMP and is inhibited by an increase in cAMP (291).

When human platelets are incubated with prostaglandin endoperoxides (52,291) or with TXA_2 (105), a decrease of cAMP accumulation can be observed. Since an inhibiting effect upon platelet adenylate cyclase activity was obtained with prostaglandin endoperoxide activity, these compounds are obviously potent in reducing the cAMP accumulation per se (226). However, under physiological conditions, the lowered cAMP level observed mainly seems to be caused by ADP liberated during the release reaction (52). Thus, the decrease of the cAMP level does not seem to be essential for the release reaction induced by TXA_2 (105), which gives further evidence for the unique properties of this compound as compared with other aggregating agents. Furthermore, it has been shown that thrombin (189) and ADP (52) both cause inhibition of cAMP accumulation, also when prostaglandin and thromboxane synthesis is inhibited. This clearly shows that prostaglandin synthesis is not a prerequisite for the cAMP-lowering effect by different aggregating agents.

On the other hand, the level of cAMP seems to interfere with the formation of prostaglandin endoperoxides and thromboxanes at different steps. The first level of interaction is the release of arachidonic acid from the phospholipids. An increase of cAMP was shown to inhibit this step (229). Secondly, an increased level of cAMP inhibits the cyclooxygenase (84,211), possibly due to lack of cell activation during aggregation (200). Thirdly, cAMP exerts a direct inhibiting effect upon the contractile mechanism of the release reaction (52,291).

Another question concerning the mode of action of thromboxanes and prostaglandin endoperoxides has been if they solely act as effectors of the release mechanism, or if they induce platelet aggregation per se. Rapid removal of ADP, released during platelet aggregation induced by PGG$_2$, clearly indicates that the main part of the aggregation under these conditions is due to ADP, and that the endoperoxide itself contributes very little (52). However, under certain conditions, when no ADP release can be obtained, aggregation has been demonstrated with endoperoxides/thromboxanes, indicating that a direct aggregating effect of these compounds also might exist (178,225). In this context it is also noteworthy that prostaglandin endoperoxides and TXA$_2$, as well as arachidonic acid, induce aggregation of washed human platelets in contrast to ADP (140).

The mechanism by which the thromboxanes exert their effect upon the release-reaction is not clearly understood. Most evidence today supports the hypothesis that they interact with intracellular calcium (160) required for the contractile process (80). Thus, prostaglandin endoperoxides have been shown to promote calcium release from a platelet membrane fraction (92) in the same way as TXA$_2$ liberates intracellular calcium in smooth muscle (15). Furthermore, the divalent ionophore A23187 initiates platelet aggregation and release. This effect is not inhibited by prostaglandin synthesis inhibitors (93,367) and gives ultrastructural changes corresponding to those seen with the endoperoxides (96).

This hypothesis also fits with the observed interrelationship with cAMP activating a cAMP-dependent protein kinase from human platelets, with an acceptor which in a phosphorylated state exhibits high calcium binding capacity (32). In addition to the inhibiting effect of cAMP upon thromboxane synthesis, there is consequently also a hypothetical balance between the Ca^{2+} binding effect induced by cAMP and the Ca^{2+} liberating effect of the thromboxanes. Using this model it is possible to explain the finding that PGG$_2$ to some extent can counteract an increase of cAMP (211,367), whereas higher concentrations of cAMP also inhibit the effect of the endoperoxide (52,367).

The interaction between platelets and the vessel wall is of particular interest for understanding the platelet aggregation and thrombus formation *in vivo*. The finding that the vessel wall forms a short-lived potent antiaggregatory intermediate from prostaglandin endoperoxides is of great importance in this respect. This 6,9-epoxy prostanoic structure is named prostacyclin or PGI$_2$ (238) and is not formed in the platelets. It has been suggested that the PGI$_2$ formation by arterial walls may explain their ability to resist platelet adhesion (124,234) and that a balance between PGI$_2$ formed in the vessel wall and TXA$_2$ formed by the platelets may be the regulatory control mechanism of thrombus formation in blood vessels (100,231,235,240,254). Although it has been demonstrated that arteries could utilize prostaglandin endoperoxides formed by platelets for the PGI$_2$ biosynthesis (121), platelets normally do not provide endoperoxides for vascular PGI$_2$ production (157). It has also been discussed whether PGI$_2$ is a physiologically important antiplatelet agent (320); a patient with platelet cyclooxygenase deficiency and no detectable formation of PGI$_2$ in the vessel wall did show prolonged bleeding time but no tendency to thrombosis (274).

The mechanism by which platelet aggregation and the release reaction is inhibited by PGI$_2$ involves binding to a specific receptor (227) and a subsequent increase of cAMP (103,342). PGI$_2$ was tenfold more potent than PGD$_2$ and 30-fold more potent than PGE$_1$ in this respect (342). 6-Keto-PGF$_{1\alpha}$, the stable product after decomposition of PGI$_2$ was at least 1,000-fold less active than PGI$_2$ itself (342).

Thromboxane Production in Pathological Conditions

After the pronounced biological activities of the thromboxanes became unraveled, and when it was realized that the thromboxane synthesizing enzymes have a widespread occurrence, a deranged thromboxane metabolism was suspected as a possible factor contributing to the symptoms of a variety of diseases.

The increased renal production of thromboxane in connection with hydronephrosis (309), renal vein constriction (381), and glycerol-induced acute renal failure (24) was briefly mentioned previously. The possible involvement of thromboxanes in asthmatic bronchoconstriction has also been discussed elsewhere.

Enhanced thromboxane production has also been found in several inflammatory conditions, such as in burns: Thromboxanes were demonstrated in burn blister fluid (166), in burned tissues (150), and in lymph from scalded limbs (167). Another inflammatory condition where thromboxane biosynthesis was demonstrated is carrageenin-induced pleurisy (173). Rheumatoid synovia was shown to synthesize TXB$_2$ (30), and the compound was found to accumulate in urate arthritis (277).

However, the majority of pathological conditions where a thromboxane involvement is suspected are of cardiovascular nature. The role of prostaglandins and thromboxanes in normal platelet and vessel functions, as well as the involvement of platelets and the vessel wall in hemostasis and thrombosis, make it of interest to attempt to correlate circulatory derangements with alterations in arachidonic acid metabolism. A number of observations provide evidence for a role of thromboxanes in some thrombotic and ischemic states, for example, the increased biosynthesis of prostaglandin endoperoxides in thrombosis (188) and the increased thromboxane production in angina pectoris with differing pathogenesis (195–198,316,334,356). Myocardial infarction has been shown to be accompanied by an increased thromboxane and prostaglandin generation (184,219,332), and inhibition or antagonism of thromboxane has been found to have a beneficial effect on ischemic myocardium (301,310). In this context, the coronary vasospastic action of TXA$_2$ in the isolated working guinea pig heart may also be mentioned (343), as well as the experimental heart attack induced by TXA$_2$ in rabbits (303). A role of TXA$_2$ in atherosclerosis has also been proposed (64,120,122). An altered balance of prostaglandin and thromboxane synthesis has, furthermore, been reported in diabetes mellitus (47,54,95,130,164,298,323,379) and during use of oral contraceptives (300), and is likely to contribute to the hyperaggregability found in these conditions.

Some of the profound hemodynamic changes seen in endotoxin-induced shock, viz., pulmonary hypertension, platelet aggregation, and systemic hypotension, have also been correlated with increases in thromboxane synthesis; however, the increased PGI$_2$ production associated with the systemic arterial hypotension is more likely the cause of the often fatal outcome of this event (36,37,55,89,148).

Finally, abnormal platelet prostaglandin or thromboxane formation, or an aberrant response to these compounds in the platelets has been reported in many other pathological conditions, such as the sudden death syndrome (154), uremia (285,286), leukemia (94,290), schizophrenia (159,169,289), and myeloproliferative disorders (56,270).

Alteration of Thromboxane—Prostacyclin Balance *In Vivo*: Approaches in Antithrombotic Therapy

A logical therapeutic approach to prevent thrombus formation and the release of vasoactive constituents involving platelets is to inhibit the platelet activity in some way (146,363). Decrease of the arachidonic acid release from the phospholipids might be obtained with hydrocortisone (152) and other agents (190,349,350). However, this approach may be doubtful since it has been shown that the concomitant inhibition of TXA$_2$ formation in the platelets and of PGI$_2$ formation in the vessel wall with hydrocortisone, in fact, leads to a shortened bleeding time (29).

The same problem, viz., difficulties in separating the effect upon TXA$_2$ and PGI$_2$ formation, arises when a cyclooxygenase inhibitor is used. Due to the well known interference of aspirin with platelet function both *in vitro* and *in vivo*, this drug has long been used clinically as an antithrombotic agent. Aspirin has even been used in various thrombosis prevention trials, for example, several aimed at lowering the mortality rate after myocardial infarction (222). However, in view of the pronounced and irreversible effect of aspirin on platelet function, the results of these clinical trials were first regarded as unexpectedly modest. The likely explanation for this lack of clinically beneficial effect was provided later when the prostacyclin pathway was discovered.

It has, however, recently been postulated that in spite of aspirin inhibiting both pathways, it may nonetheless be possible to inhibit platelet thromboxane biosynthesis selectively. Aspirin acetylates cyclooxygenase irreversibly (205). However, the platelet enzyme seems to be more sensitive than cyclooxygenase of the vessel wall in this respect (43) requiring both lower aspirin concentration and shorter exposure for inhibition. Furthermore, since this acetylation is irreversible, the inhibition of the platelet enzyme lasts for the entire life-span of these cells which have very low capacity for *de novo* protein biosynthesis. The vessel wall, on the other hand, may recover rapidly by synthesizing new cyclooxygenase (161,354). Thus, by giving aspirin in low doses and/or with long intervals it should be possible to keep the platelet cyclooxygenase continuously suppressed without undue interference with vessel wall production of prostacyclin.

During the last few years a very large number of studies have been performed with the aim of identifying such a dose or dose schedule for aspirin treatment in thrombosis prevention trials.

Bleeding time measurements reflect the balance between platelet thromboxane and vessel wall PGI$_2$ formation (cf. however ref. 314). Numerous studies on the effect of aspirin on bleeding time have been done (e.g., refs. 98,267,283,344).

The results of many of these studies are difficult to evaluate and interpret, since the drug has often been given repeatedly with short intervals or in large doses.

Others have attempted to follow the different time course of the recovery of platelet and vessel wall cyclooxygenase after aspirin, both in various animal species and in the human (e.g., 17,23,76,78,201,217,218,245,282,357). Many studies have focused on platelet function and/or thromboxane biosynthesis alone after aspirin, without simultaneous measurement of the PGI$_2$ production by the vessel wall (43,48,272,275,331). In most cases the aspirin effects on platelets and vessel walls have been estimated by various *in vitro* approaches (such as platelet aggregability, malondialdehyde formation, TXB$_2$ biosynthesis, etc.). Others have instead preferred *in vivo* models, such as thrombogenesis (175,380).

Although the results of these studies vary somewhat, in terms of definite recommendations of a clinically useful dose schedule for prevention of thrombosis, there seems to be a general agreement that low-dose aspirin given at long intervals should be beneficial in this respect. However, clinical trials using these low-dose schedules have yet to be performed.

Many recent review articles have been written on this topic (for example, refs. 231,246,273,311,312).

This area has, however, become even more complex by the recent discovery that salicylic acid (the major metabolite of aspirin *in vivo*) counteracts the inhibitory actions of aspirin (223,315,352,353). Salicylic acid has a much longer half-life in blood than aspirin and may readily accumulate to reach concentrations where this antiinhibitory effect occurs.

In this context, it is worth remembering that the case with a combined PCO-deficiency and lack of PGI$_2$ in the vessel wall—a condition which corresponds to a high-dose aspirin treatment—did not show any thrombotic tendency (274). Also other cyclooxygenase inhibitors have been investigated in this respect (12,34,46,51, 91,353).

A specific inhibition of thromboxane synthetase would be a more attractive way to inhibit the platelet activity, leaving the PGI$_2$ formation intact. Different inhibitors such as carbocyclic TXA$_2$ (194), imidazole (83), pinane-TXA$_2$ (7,259), compound L8027 (50), and 9,11-iminoepoxy prostanoic acid (85) have been investigated (see also previous discussion). Thus, pinane TXA$_2$ was shown to be effective in preservation of ischemic myocardium (301) and the same effect was observed with imidazole (310). Specific thromboxane synthetase inhibitors were also reported to maintain dermal microcirculation after burning (63). Another possible way of modulating platelet activity due to TX biosynthesis, without affecting the PGI$_2$ formation, is to inhibit the receptor for TXA$_2$/prostaglandin endoperoxides. 13-Azo prostanoic acid was shown to exert its effect by this mechanism (192).

Modulating platelet reactivity is also possible by increasing the biologically active level of PGI$_2$ (236,255,341). One such compound (EG 626) was found to be effective in prevention of stroke and heart attack induced experimentally by TXA$_2$ (303). Another possible way is, of course, intravenous infusion of PGI$_2$ (125,241,333) which, however, has the disadvantage of the short half-life of the compound. The use of stable analogs of PGI₂ thus seems to be a more suitable way (65,171,210). In this context PGI₂ and its nalogs will be a more efficient alternative to other compounds known to increase the level of cAMP, such as PGE₁ and PGD₂ (261).

Finally, manipulation of the unsaturated fatty acid pool of the phospholipids may be used in affecting platelet activity (6,155,158,162,253). Thus, essential fatty acid deficient rats are protected from elevation of thromboxane formation, probably due to lack of substrate for its formation (55,358). As mentioned previously, a diet rich in eicosapentaenoic acid, as in the salt-water fish diet of the eskimos, has been reported to decrease the thrombotic tendency by lowering thromboxane formation (73,163,306,365). The cholesterol-rich diet, on the other hand, seems to increase the formation of thromboxanes in the platelets, thus predisposing to thrombotic complications (304,322,345). Dihomo-γ-linolenic acid early drew special attention as a possible antithrombotic agent, since it both competes with arachidonic acid for transformation to thromboxanes and increases the cAMP level by formation of PGE₁ (371).

A special circulatory problem, in which thromboxane inhibition already has been proved to be of clinical importance, is the extracorporeal circulation. The increased thromboxane synthesis and platelet loss in cardiopulmonary bypass (3,4,61) can be prevented by PGI₂ (2,202,280) or PGE₁ (5). In the same way PGI₂ (375) or low-dose aspirin (149) might protect from abnormal platelet function in hemodialysis (287). In fact, there is evidence that the heparin usually used for this purpose might initiate TX synthesis under ischemic conditions (197).

REFERENCES

1. Abdel-Halim, M. S., Hamberg, M., Sjöquist, B., and Änggård, E. (1977): Identification of prostaglandin D₂ as a major prostaglandin in homogenates of rat brain. *Prostaglandins*, 14:633–643.
2. Addonizio, V. P., Macarak, J., Nicolaou, K. C., and Edmunds, L. H. (1979): Effects of prostacyclin and albumin on platelet loss during *in vitro* simulation of extracorporeal circulation. *Blood*, 53:1033–1042.
3. Addonizio, V. P., Smith, J. B., Guiod, L. R., Strauss, J. F., Colman, R. W., and Edmunds, L. H. (1979): Thromboxane synthesis and platelet protein release during simulated extracorporeal circulation. *Blood*, 54:371–376.
4. Addonizio, V. P., Smith, J. B., Strauss, F. F., Colman, R. W., and Edmunds, L. H. (1980): Thromboxane synthesis and platelet secretion during cardio-pulmonary bypass with bubble oxygenator. *J. Thorac. Cardiovasc. Surg.*, 79:91–96.
5. Addonizio, V. P., Strauss, J. F., Colman, R. W., and Edmunds, L. H. (1979): Effects of prostaglandin E₁ on platelet loss during *in vivo* and *in vitro* extracorporeal circulation with a bubble oxygenator. *J. Thorac. Cardiovasc. Surg.*, 77:119–126.
6. Agradie, E., Tremoli, E., Colombo, C., and Galli, C. (1978): Influence of short term dietary supplementation of different lipids on aggregation and arachidonic acid metabolism in rabbit platelets. *Prostaglandins*, 16:973–984.
7. Aharony, D., Smith, J. B., Smith, E. F., Lefer, A. M., Magolda, R. L., and Nicolaou, K. D. (1980): Pinane thromboxane A₂: A TXA₂ antagonist with antithrombotic properties. In: *Advances in Prostaglandin and Thromboxane Research*, Vol. 6, edited by B. Samuelsson, P. Ramwell, and R. Paoletti, pp. 489–492. Raven Press, New York.
8. Ahnfelt-Rönne, I., and Arrigoni-Martelli, E. (1979): Rabbit lung microsomes: A rapid method for assaying simultaneously drug effects on thromboxane and prostacyclin synthesis. *Agents Actions (Suppl.)*, 4:110–119.

9. Al-Ubaidi, F., and Bakhle, Y. S. (1980): Differences in biological activation of arachidonic acid in perfused lungs from guinea pig, rat and man. *Eur. J. Pharmacol.*, 62:89–96.

10. Ali, A. E., Barrett, J. C., and Eling, T. E. (1980): Prostaglandin and thromboxane production by fibroblasts and vascular endothelial cells. In: *Advances in Prostaglandin and Thromboxane Research*, Vol. 6, edited by B. Samuelsson, P. Ramwell, and R. Paoletti, pp. 533–535. Raven Press, New York.

11. Ali, M., Cerskus, A. L., Zamecnik, J., and McDonald, J. W. D. (1977): Synthesis of prostaglandin D$_2$ and thromboxane B$_2$ by human platelets. *Thromb. Res.*, 11:485–496.

12. Ali, M., Gudbranson, G. G., and McDonald, J. W. (1980): Inhibition of human platelet cyclo-oxygenase by alpha-tocopherol. *Prostaglandins Med.*, 4:79–85.

13. Ali, M., Zamecnik, J., Cerskus, A. L., Stoessl, A. J. Barnett, W. H., and McDonald, J. W. D. (1977): Synthesis of thromboxane B$_2$ and prostaglandins by bovine gastric mucosal microsomes. *Prostaglandins*, 14:819–827.

14. Allan, G., and Eakins, K. E. (1978): Burimamide is a selective inhibitor of thromboxane-A biosynthesis in human platelet microsomes. *Prostaglandins*, 15:659–661.

15. Ally, A. I., Horrobin, D. F., Manku, M. S., Morgan, R. O., Karmazyn, M., Karmali, R. A., and Cunnane, S. C. (1978): Dantrolene blocks intracellular calcium release in smooth muscle: Competitive antagonism of thromboxane A$_2$. *Can. J. Physiol. Pharmacol.*, 56:520–528.

16. Ally, A. I., Manku, M. S., Horrobin, D. F., Morgan, R. O., Karmazin, M., and Karmali, R. A. (1977): Dipyridamole: A possible potent inhibitor of thromboxane A$_2$ synthetase in vascular smooth muscle. *Prostaglandins*, 14:607–609.

17. Amezcua, J. L., O'Grady, J., Salmon, J. A., and Moncada, S. (1979): Prolonged paradoxical effect of aspirin on platelet behaviour and bleeding time in man. *Thromb. Res.*, 16:69–79.

18. Anderson, M. W., Crutchley, D. J., Tainer, B. E., and Eling, T. E. (1978): Kinetic studies on the conversion of prostaglandin endoperoxide PGH$_2$ by thromboxane synthase. *Prostaglandins*, 16:563–570.

19. Anderson, W. H., Mohammad, S. F., Chuang, H. Y., and Mason, R. G. (1980): Heparin potentiates synthesis of thromboxane A$_2$ in human platelets. In: *Advances in Prostaglandin and Thromboxane Research, Vol. 6*, edited by B. Samuelsson, P. Ramwell, and R. Paoletti, pp. 287–291. Raven Press, New York.

20. Anhut, H., Bernauer, W., and Peskar, B. A. (1977): Radioimmunological determination of thromboxane release in cardiac anaphylaxis. *Eur. J. Pharmacol.* 44:85–88.

21. Anhut, H., Jackisch, R., and Peskar, B. A. (1979): Thromboxane B$_2$ release and 3H-noradrenaline accumulation by a synaptosomal fraction of rat brain. *Pol. J. Pharmacol. Pharm.*, 31:381–386.

22. Anhut, H., Peskar, B. A., and Bernauer, W. (1978): Release of 15-keto-13,14-dihydrothromboxane B$_2$ and prostaglandin D$_2$ during anaphylaxis as measured by radioimmunoassay. *Naunyn. Schmiedebergs Arch. Pharmacol.*, 305:2247–2252.

23. Basista, M., Dobranowski, J., and Gryglewski, R. J. (1978): Prostacyclin and thromboxane generating systems in rabbits pretreated with aspirin. *Pharmacol. Res. Commun.*, 10:759–763.

24. Benabe, J. E., Klahr, S., Hoffman, M. K., and Morrison, A. R. (1980): Production of thromboxane A$_2$ by the kidney in glycerol-induced acute renal failure in the rabbit. *Prostaglandins*, 19:333–347.

25. Best, L. C., Holland, T., Jones, P. B. B., and Russell, R. G. G. (1980): The interrelationship between thromboxane biosynthesis, aggregation and 5-hydroxytryptamine secretion in human platelets *in vitro*. *Thromb. Haemost.*, 43:38–41.

26. Best, L. C., Jones, P. B., and Russell, R. G. (1979): Evidence that extracellular calcium ions inhibit thromboxane B$_2$ biosynthesis by human platelets. *Biochem. Biophys. Res. Commun.*, 90:1179–1185.

27. Best, L. C., McGuire, M. B., Martin, T. J., Preston, F. E., and Russell, R. G. (1979): Effects of epoxy-methano analogs of prostaglandin endoperoxides on aggregation, on release of 5-hydroxytryptamine and on the metabolism of 3′,5-cyclic AMP and cyclic GMP in human platelets. *Biochim. Biophys. Acta*, 583:344–351.

28. Blackwell, G. J., Flower, R. J., Russell-Smith, N., Salmon, J. A., Thorogood, P. B, and Vane, J. R. (1978): 1-*n*-Butylimidazole: A potent and selective inhibitor of thromboxane synthetase. *Br. J. Pharmacol.*, 64:435P.

29. Blajchman, M. A., Senyi, A. F., Hirsh, J., Surya, Y., Buchanan, M., and Mustard, J. F. (1979): Shortening of the bleeding time in rabbits by hydroxortisone caused by inhibition of prostacyclin generation by the vessel wall. *J. Clin. Invest.*, 63:1026–1035.

30. Blotman, F., Chaintreuil, J., Poubelle, P., Flandre, O., Crastes de Paulet, A., and Simon, L. (1980): PGE_2, $PGF_{2\alpha}$ and TXB_2 synthesis by human rheumatoid synovia. In: *Advances in Prostaglandin and Thromboxane Research*, Vol. 8, edited by B. Samuelsson, P. Ramwell, and R. Paoletti, pp. 1705–1708. Raven Press, New York.
31. Boot, J., Cockerill, A., Dawson, W., Mallen, D., and Osborne, D. (1978): Modification of prostaglandin and thromboxane release by immunological sensitisation and successive immunological challenges from guinea pig lung. *Int. Arch. Allergy Appl. Immunol.*, 57:159–164.
32. Booyse, F. M., Marr, J., Yang, D. C., Guiliani, D., and Rafelson, M. E. (1976): Adenosine cyclic $3',5'$-monophosphate-dependent protein kinase from human platelets. *Biochim. Biophys. Acta*, 422:60–72.
33. Bordia, A. (1978): Effect of garlic on human platelet aggregation *in vitro*. *Atherosclerosis*, 30:355–360.
34. Bourgain, R. H. (1978): The effect of indomethacin and ASA on *in vivo* induced white platelet arterial thrombus formation. *Thromb. Res.*, 12:1079–1086.
35. Bryant, R. W., Feinmark, S. J., Makheja, A. N., and Bailey, J. M. (1978): Lipid metabolism in cultured cells. Synthesis of vasoactive thromboxane A_2 from 14C-arachidonic acid culture lung fibroblasts. *J. Biol. Chem.*, 253:8134–8142.
36. Bult, H., Beetens, J., and Herman, A. G. (1980): Blood levels of 6-oxo-prostaglandin $F_{1\alpha}$ during endotoxin-induced hypotension in rabbits. *Eur. J. Pharmacol.*, 63:47–56.
37. Bult, H., and Herman, A. G. (1979): The role of thromboxane A_2 in endotoxin-induced aggregation of guinea-pig platelets *in vitro*. *Agents Actions (Suppl.)*, 4:147–155.
38. Bult, H., and Herman, A. G. (1979): Thromboxane A_2 biosynthesis during endotoxin induced aggregation of platelets from normal and sensitized guinea pigs. *Agents Actions*, 9:560–565.
39. Bundy, G. L., and Peterson, D. C. (1978): The synthesis of 15-deoxy-9,11-(epoxyimino)prostaglandins—potent thromboxane synthetase inhibitors. *Tetrahedron Lett.*, 1:41–44.
40. Bundy, G. L. (1975): The synthesis of prostaglandin endoperoxide analogs. *Tetrahedron Lett.*, 24:1957–1960.
41. Bunting, S., Moncada, S., and Vane, J. R. (1976): The effects of prostaglandin endoperoxides and thromboxane A_2 on strips of rabbit coeliac artery and certain other smooth muscle preparations. *Br. J. Pharmacol.*, 57:462–463.
42. Burch, J. W., Baenziger, M. L., Stanford, N., and Majerus, P. W. (1978): Sensitivity of fatty acid cyclo-oxygenase from human aorta to acetylation by aspirin. *Proc. Natl. Acad. Sci. USA*, 75:5181–5185.
43. Burch, J. W., Stanford, N., and Majerus, P. W. (1978): Inhibition of platelet prostaglandin synthetase by oral aspirin. *J. Clin. Invest.*, 61:314–319.
44. Burch, R. M., Knapp, D. R., and Halushka, P. V. (1979): Vasopressin stimulates thromboxane synthesis in the toad urinary bladder: Effects of imidazole. *J. Pharmacol. Exp. Ther.*, 210:344–348.
45. Burch, R. M., Knapp, D. R., and Halushka, P. V. (1980): Vasopressin stimulates thromboxane synthesis in the toad urinary bladder: Effects of thromboxane synthesis inhibition. In: *Advances in Prostaglandin and Thromboxane Research*, Vol. 6, edited by B. Samuelsson, P. Ramwell, and R. Paoletti, pp. 505–509. Raven Press, New York.
46. Busse, W. D., and Seuter, F. (1979): Influence on thromboxane and malondialdehyde synthesis in human thrombocytes by various inhibitors of platelet function. *Agents Actions (Suppl.)*, 4:127–137.
47. Butkus, A., Skrinska, V. A., and Shumacher, O. P. (1980): Thromboxane production and platelet aggregation in diabetic subjects with clinical complications. *Thromb. Res.*, 19:211–223.
48. Catalano, P. M., Smith, J. B., and Murphy, S. (1981): Platelet recovery from aspirin inhibition *in vivo*: Differing patterns under various assay conditions. *Blood*, 57:99–105.
49. Chanh, P. H., Sokan, I., and Chanh, A. P. (1979): Etude de l'activité du myocard de lapin sur la thromboxane synthetase. *C. R. Acad. Sci. D. (Paris)*, 288:1489–1492.
50. Chignard, M., Pruncan, A., Lefort, J., Dray, F., and Vargaftig, B. B. (1979): Arachidonate-mediated bronchoconstriction and platelet activation are inhibited by microgram doses of compound L8027 which are not selective for thromboxane synthetase. *Agents Actions (Suppl.)*, 4:184–187.
51. Chignard, M., Vargaftig, B. B., Sors, H., and Dray, F. (1978): Synthesis of thromboxane B_2 in incubates of dog platelet rich plasma with arachidonic acid and its inhibition by different drugs. *Biochem. Biophys. Res. Commun.*, 85:1631–1639.
52. Claesson, H. E., and Malmsten, C. (1977): On the interrelationship of prostaglandin endoperoxide PGG_2 and cyclic nucleotides in platelet function. *Eur. J. Biochem.*, 76:277–284.

53. Coceani, F., and Olley, P. M. (1980): Role of prostaglandins: Prostacyclin and thromboxanes in the control of prenatal potency and postnatal closure of the ductus arterious. *Semin Perinatol.*, 4:109–113.
54. Colwell, J. A., and Halushka, P. V. (1980): Platelet function in diabetes mellitus. *Br. J. Haematol.*, 44:521–526.
55. Cook, J. A., Wise, W. C., and Halushka, P. V. (1980): Elevated thromboxane levels in the rat during endotoxin shock: Protective effects of imidazole, 13-azo-prostanoic acid or essential fatty acid deficiency. *J. Clin. Invest.*, 65:227–230.
56. Cooper, B., and Ahern, D. (1979): Characterization of the platelet prostaglandin D₂ receptor. Loss of prostaglandin D₂ receptors in platelets of patients with myeloproliferative disorders. *J. Clin. Invest.*, 64:586–590.
57. Corey, E. J., Nicolaou, K. C., Machida, Y., Malmsten, C. L., and Samuelsson, B. (1975): Synthesis and biological properties of a 9,11-azo-prostanoid: Highly active biochemical mimic of prostaglandin endoperoxides. *Proc. Natl. Acad. Sci. USA*, 72:3355–3358.
58. Corey, E. J., Niwa, H., Bloom, M., and Ramwell, P. W. (1979): Synthesis of a new prostaglandin endoperoxide (PGH₂) analog and its function as an inhibitor of the biosynthesis of thromboxane A₂. *Tetrahedron Lett.*, 8:671–674.
59. Culp, B. R., Lands, W. E. M., Lucchesi, B. R., Pitt, B., and Romson, J. (1980): The effect of dietary supplementation of fish oil on experimental myocardial infarction. *Prostaglandins*, 20:1021–1031.
60. Davidson, E. M., Doig, M. V., Ford-Hutchinson, A. W., and Smith, M. J. (1980): Prostaglandin and thromboxane production by rabbit polymorphonuclear leukocytes and rat macrophages. In: *Advances in Prostaglandin and Thromboxane Research*, Vol. 8, edited by B. Samuelsson, P. Ramwell, and R. Paoletti, pp. 1661–1663. Raven Press, New York.
61. Davies, G. C., Sobel, M., and Salzman, E. W. (1980): Elevated plasma fibrinopeptide A and thromboxane B₂ levels during cardio-pulmonary by-pass. *Circulation*, 61:808–814.
62. Dawson, W., Boot, J., Cockerill, A., Mallen, D., and Osborne, D. (1976): Release of novel prostaglandins and thromboxanes after immunological challenge of guinea pig lung. *Nature*, 262:699–702.
63. Del Beccaro, E. J., Robson, M. C., Heggers, J. P., and Swaminathan, R. (1980): The use of specific thromboxane inhibitors to preserve the dermal microcirculation after burning. *Surgery*, 87:137–141.
64. Dembinska-Kiec, A., Rucker, W., and Schonhofer, P. S. (1979): Prostacyclin dependent differences in TXA₂ formation by platelets from normal and atherosclerotic rabbits. *Atherosclerosis*, 33:217–226.
65. Dembinska-Kiec, A., Rucker, W., Schonhofer, P. S., and Gandolfi, C. (1979): Prostacyclin analogs: Antiaggregatory potency and enhancement of cAMP levels in human platelet rich plasma. *Thromb. Haemost.*, 42:1340–1343.
66. Diczfalusy, U., and Hammarström, S. (1977): Inhibitors of thromboxane synthase in human platelets. *FEBS Lett.*, 82:107–110.
67. Diczfalusy, U., and Hammarström, S. (1979): A structural requirement for the conversion of prostaglandin endoperoxides to thromboxanes. *FEBS Lett.*, 105:291–295.
68. Diczfalusy, U., and Hammarström, S. (1980): Enzymatic conversion of C21 endoperoxides to thromboxanes and hydroxy acids. *Biochem. Biophys. Res. Commun.*, 94:1417–1423.
69. Diczfalusy, U., Falardeau, P., and Hammarström, S. (1977): Conversion of prostaglandin endoperoxides into C17-hydroxy acids catalyzed by human platelet thromboxane synthase. *FEBS Lett.*, 84:271–274.
70. Dusting, G. J., Moncada, S., and Vane, J. R. (1977): Prostacyclin (PGX) is the endogenous metabolite responsible for relaxation of coronary arteries induced by arachidonic acid. *Prostaglandins*, 13:3–15.
71. Dutilh, C. E., Haddeman, E., Jouvenaz, G. H., Ten Hoor, F., and Nugteren, D. H. (1979): Study of the two pathways for arachidonate oxygenation in blood platelets. *Lipids*, 14:241–246.
72. Dyerberg, J., and Bang, H. O. (1979): Haemostatic function and platelet polyunsaturated fatty acids in eskimos. *Lancet*, i:433–435.
73. Dyerberg, J., and Bang, H. O. (1979): Lipid metabolism, atherogenesis and hemostasis in eskimos: The role of the prostaglandin family. *Haemostasis*, 8:227–233.
74. Eakins, K. E., and Kulkarni, P. S. (1977): Selective inhibitory actions of sodium-*p*-benzyl-4-/1-oxo-2-(4-chlorobenzyl)-3-phenyl propyl/phenyl phosphonate (N-0164) and indometacin on the

biosynthesis of prostaglandins and thromboxanes from arachidonic acid. *Br. J. Pharmacol.*, 60:135–140.

75. Eakins, K. E., Rajadhyaksha, V., and Schroer, R. (1976): Prostaglandin antagonism by sodium *p*-benzyl-4-/1-oxo-2-(4-chlorobenzyl)-3-phenylpropyl/-phenylphosphonate (N-0164). *Br. J. Pharmacol.*, 58:333–339.

76. Ellis, E. F., Jones, P. S., Wright, K. F., Richardson, D. W., and Ellis, C. K. (1980): Effect of oral aspirin dose on platelet aggregation and arterial prostacyclin synthesis: Studies in humans and rabbits. In: *Advances in Prostaglandin and Thromboxane Research*, Vol. 6, edited by B. Samuelsson, P. Ramwell, and R. Paoletti, pp. 313–315. Raven Press, New York.

77. Ellis, E. F., Oelz, O., Roberts, L. J., II, Payne, N. A., Sweetman, B. J., Nies, A. S., and Oates, J. A. (1976): Coronary arterial smooth muscle contraction by a substance released from platelets: Evidence that it is thromboxane A$_2$. *Science*, 193:1135–1137.

78. Ellis, E. F., Wright, K. F., Jones, P. S., Richardson, D. W., and Ellis, C. K. (1980): Effect of oral aspirin dose on platelet aggregation and vascular prostacyclin (PGI$_2$) synthesis in humans and rabbits. *J. Cardiovasc. Pharmacol.*, 2:387–397.

79. Falardeau, P., Hamberg, M., and Samuelsson, B. (1976): Metabolism of 8,11,14-eicosatrienoic acid in human platelets. *Biochim. Biophys. Acta*, 441:193–200.

80. Feinstein, M. B. (1978): The role of calcium in blood platelet function. In: *Calcium in Drug Action*, edited by G. B. Weiss, pp. 197–239. Plenum Press, New York.

81. Fitzpatrick, F. A., Bundy, G. L., Gorman, R. R., and Hanahn, T. (1978): 9,11-Epoxyiminoprosta-5,13-dienoic acid is a thromboxane A$_2$ antagonist in human platelets. *Nature*, 275:764–766.

82. Fitzpatrick, F. A., and Gorman, R. R. (1977): Platelet rich plasma transforms exogenous prostaglandin endoperoxide H$_2$ into thromboxane A$_2$. *Prostaglandins*, 14:881–889.

83. Fitzpatrick, F. A., and Gorman, R. R. (1978): A comparison of imidazole and 9,11-azo-prosta-5,13-dienoic acid. Two selective thromboxane synthetase inhibitors. *Biochim. Biophys. Acta*, 539:162–172.

84. Fitzpatrick, F. A., and Gorman, R. R. (1979): Regulatory role of cyclic adenosine 3′:5′-monophosphate on the platelet cyclo-oxygenase and platelet function. *Biochim. Biophys. Acta*, 582:44–58.

85. Fitzpatrick, F. A., Gorman, R. R., Bundy, G., Hanahan, T., McGuire, J., and Sun, F. (1979): 9,11-Iminoepoxyprosta-5,13-dienoic acid is a selective thromboxane A$_2$ synthetase inhibitor. *Biochim. Biophys. Acta*, 573:238–244.

86. Fitzpatrick, F. A., Gorman, R. R., McGuire, J. C., Kelly, R. C., Wynalda, M. A., and Sun, F. F. (1977): A radioimmunoassay for thromboxane B$_2$. *Anal. Biochem.*, 82:1–7.

87. Fitzpatrick, F. A., Gorman, R. R., and Wynalda, M. A. (1977): Electron capture gas chromatographic detection of thromboxane B$_2$. *Prostaglandins*, 13:201–209.

88. Folco, G. C., Hansson, G., and Granström, E. (1981): Leukotriene C$_4$ stimulates TXA$_2$ formation in isolated sensitized guinea pig lungs. *Biochem. Pharmacol.*, 30:2491–2493.

89. Frölich, J. C., Ogletree, M., Peskar, B. A., and Brigham, K. L. (1980): Pulmonary hypertension correlated to pulmonary thromboxane synthesis. In: *Advances in Prostaglandin and Thromboxane Research*, Vol. 7, edited by B. Samuelsson, P. Ramwell, and R. Paoletti, pp. 745–750. Raven Press, New York.

90. Friedman, L. S., Fitzpatrick, T. M., Bloom, M. F., Ramwell, P. W., Rose, J. C., and Kot, P. A. (1979): Cardiovascular and pulmonary effects of thromboxane B$_2$ in the dog. *Circ. Res.*, 44:748–751.

91. Garcia Rafanell, J., Planas, J. M., and Puig-Parellada, P. (1979): Comparison of the inhibitory effects of acetyl-salicylic acid and trifusal on enzymes related to thrombosis. *Arch. Int. Pharmacodyn. Ther.*, 237:343–350.

92. Gerrard, J. M., Butler, A. M., Graff, G., Stoddard, S. F., and White, J. G. (1978): Prostaglandin endoperoxides promote calcium release from a platelet membrane fraction *in vitro*. *Prostaglandins Med.*, 1:373–385.

93. Gerrard, J., Rao, G. H. R., and White, J. G. (1974): Effects of the ionophore A27187 on blood platelets II. Influence on ultrastructure. *Am. J. Pathol.*, 77:151–166.

94. Gerrard, J. M., Stoddard, S. F., Shapiro, R. S., Coccia, P. F., Ramsay, M. K., Nesbit, M. E., Rao, G. H., Kriwit, W., and White, J. G. (1978): Platelet storage pool deficiency and prostaglandin synthesis in chronic granulocytic leukemia. *Br. J. Haematol.*, 40:597–607.

95. Gerrard, J. M., Stuart, M. J., Rao, G. H., Steffes, M. W., Mauer, S. M., Brown, D. M., and White, J. G. (1980): Alterations in the balance of prostaglandin and thromboxane synthesis in diabetic rats. *J. Lab. Clin. Med.*, 95:950–958.

96. Gerrard, J. M., and White, J. G. (1975): The influence of prostaglandin endoperoxides on ultrastructure. *Am. J. Pathol.*, 80:189–200.
97. Gerrard, J. M., and White, J. G. (1978): Prostaglandins and thromboxanes: "Middlemen" modulating platelet function in hemostasis and thrombosis. *Prog. Hemost. Thromb.*, 4:37–125.
98. Godal, H. C., Eika, C., Dybdahl, J. H., Daal, L., and Larsen, S. (1979): Aspirin and bleeding time. *Lancet*, i:1236.
99. Goldstein, I. M., Malmsten, C. L., Kindahl, H., Kaplan, H. B., Rådmark, O., Samuelsson, B., and Weissman, G. (1978): Thromboxane generation by human peripheral blood polymorphonuclear leukocytes. *J. Exp. Med.*, 148:787–792.
100. Gorman, R. R. (1979): Modulation of human platelet function by prostacyclin and thromboxane A₂. *Fed. Proc.*, 38:83–88.
101. Gorman, R. R. (1980): Biochemical and pharmacological evaluation of thromboxane synthetase inhibitors. In: *Advances in Prostaglandin and Thromboxane Research*, Vol. 6, edited by B. Samuelsson, P. Ramwell, and R. Paoletti, pp. 417–425. Raven Press, New York.
102. Gorman, R. R., Bundy, G. L., Peterson, D. C., Sun, F. F., Miller, O. V., and Fitzpatrick, F. A. (1977): Inhibition of human platelet thromboxane synthetase by 9,11-axoprostadienoic acid. *Proc. Natl. Acad. Sci. USA*, 74:4007–4011.
103. Gorman, R. R., Bunting, S., and Miller, O. V. (1977): Modulation of human platelet adenylate cyclase by prostacyclin (PGX). *Prostaglandins*, 13:377–388.
104. Gorman, R. R., Fitzpatrick, F. A., and Miller, C. V. (1977): A selective thromboxane synthetase inhibitor blocks the cAMP lowering activity of PGH₂. *Biochem. Biophys. Res. Commun.*, 79:305–313.
105. Gorman, R. R., Wieranga, W., and Miller, O. V. (1979): Independence of the cyclic AMP lowering activity of thromboxane A₂ from the platelet release reaction. *Biochim. Biophys. Acta*, 572:57–104.
106. Granström, E. (1980): Assay methods for prostaglandins and thromboxanes. In: *Advances in Prostaglandin and Thromboxane Research*, Vol. 6, edited by B. Samuelsson, R. Paoletti, and P. Ramwell, pp. 69–76. Raven Press, New York.
107. Granström, E. (1980): Assay methods for prostaglandins and thromboxanes: Gas chromatographic-mass spectometric methods and radioimmunoassay. In: *The Prostaglandin System*, edited by F. Berti and G. P. Velo, pp. 67–72. Plenum Press, New York.
108. Granström, E., and Kindahl, H. (1978): Radioimmunoassay of prostaglandins and thromboxanes. In: *Advances in Prostaglandin and Thromboxane Research*, Vol. 5, edited by J. C. Frölich, pp. 119–210. Raven Press, New York.
109. Granström, E., Kindahl, H., and Samuelsson, B. (1976): Radioimmunoassay for thromboxane B₂. *Anal. Lett.*, 9:611–627.
110. Granström, E., Kindahl, H., and Samuelsson, B. (1976): A method for measuring the unstable thromboxane A₂: Radioimmunoassay of the derived mono-O-methyl thromboxane B₂. *Prostaglandins*, 12:929–941.
111. Granström, E., and Samuelsson, B. (1978): Quantitative measurement of prostaglandins and thromboxanes: General considerations. In: *Advances in Prostaglandin and Thromboxane Research*, Vol. 5, edited by J. C. Frölich, pp. 1–13. Raven Press, New York.
112. Green, K., Hamberg, M., Samuelsson, B., and Frölich, J. C. (1978): Extraction and chromatographic procedures for purification of prostaglandins, thromboxanes, prostacyclin, and their metabolites. In: *Advances in Prostaglandin and Thromboxane Research*, Vol. 5, edited by J. C. Frölich, pp. 15–37. Raven Press, New York.
113. Green, K., Hamberg, M., Samuelsson, B., Smigel, M., and Frölich, J. C. (1978): Measurement of prostaglandins, thromboxanes, prostacyclin and their metabolites by gas-liquid chromatography-mass spectrometry. In: *Advances in Prostaglandin and Thromboxane Research*, Vol. 5, edited by J. C. Frölich, pp. 39–94. Raven Press, New York.
114. Greenwald, J. E., Wong, L. K., Alexander, M., and Bianchine, J. R. (1980): *In vivo* inhibition of thromboxane biosynthesis by hydralazine. In: *Advances in Prostaglandin and Thromboxane Research*, Vol. 6, edited by B. Samuelsson, P. Ramwell, and R. Paoletti, pp. 293–295. Raven Press, New York.
115. Greenwald, J. E., Wong, L. K., Rao, M., Bianchine, J. R., and Panganamala, R. V. (1978): A study of three vasodilating agents as selective inhibitors of thromboxane A₂ biosynthesis. *Biochem. Biophys. Res. Commun.*, 84:1112–1118.
116. Gryglewski, R. J. (1977): Prostaglandin and thromboxane biosynthesis inhibitors. *Naunyn-Schmiedebergs Arch. Pharmacol.*, 297:S85–S88.

117. Gryglewski, R. (1978): Screening for inhibitors of prostaglandin and thromboxane biosynthesis. *Adv. Lipid Res.*, 1:327–344.
118. Gryglewski, R. (1979): *In vitro* and *in vivo* models for evaluating drugs which influence arachidonic acid metabolism. *Agents Actions (Suppl.)*, 4:82–95.
119. Gryglewski, R. J. (1980): Bioassay of prostacyclin and thromboxane A$_2$. In: *The Prostaglandin System*, edited by F. Berti and G. P. Velo, pp. 73–84. Plenum Press, New York.
120. Gryglewski, R. J. (1980): Prostaglandins, platelets and arteriosclerosis. *CRC Crit. Rev. Biochem.*, 7:291–338.
121. Gryglewski, R. J., Bunting, S., Moncada, S., Flower, R. J., and Vane, J. R. (1976): Arterial walls are protected against deposition of platelet thrombi by a substance (Prostaglandin X) which they make from prostaglandin endoperoxides. *Prostaglandins*, 12:685–713.
122. Gryglewski, R. J., Dembinska-Kiec, A., and Gryglewska, T. (1978): Prostacyclin and thromboxane A$_2$ biosynthesis capacities of heart, arteries and platelets at various stages of experimental atherosclerosis in rabbits. *Atherosclerosis*, 32:385–394.
123. Gryglewski, R. J., Dembinska-Kiec, A., and Korbut, R. (1978): A possible role of thromboxane A$_2$ (TXA$_2$) and prostacyclin (PGI$_2$) in circulation. *Acta Biol. Med. Ger.*, 37:715–723.
124. Gryglewski, R., Moncada, S., and Bunting, S. (1976): Arterial walls generate from prostaglandin endoperoxides a substance (PGX) which relaxes strips of mesenteric and coeliac arteries and inhibits platelet aggregation. *Prostaglandins*, 12:897–915.
125. Gryglewski, R. J., Szczeklik, A., and Nizankowsi, R. (1978): Anti-platelet action of intravenous infusion of prostacyclin in man. *Thromb. Res.*, 13:153–163.
126. Gryglewski, R. J., and Vane, J. R. (1972): The release of prostaglandins and rabbit aorta contracting substance (RCS) from rabbit spleen and its antagonism by anti-inflammatory drugs. *Br. J. Pharmacol.*, 45:37–47.
127. Gryglewski, R. J., Zmuda, A., Dembinska-Kiec, A., and Krecioch, E. (1977): A potent inhibitor of thromboxane A$_2$ biosynthesis in aggregating human blood platelets. *Pharmacol. Res. Commun.*, 9:109–116.
128. Gryglewski, R. J., Zmuda, A., Korbut, R., Krecioch, E., and Bieron, K. (1977): Selective inhibition of thromboxane A$_2$ biosynthesis in blood platelets. *Nature*, 267:627–628.
129. Hagen, A. A., White, R. P., and Robertson, J. T. (1979): Synthesis of prostaglandins and thromboxane B$_2$ by cerebral arteries. *Stroke*, 10:306–309.
130. Halushka, P. V., Rogers, R. C., Laadholt, C. B., and Colwell, J. A. (1981): Increased platelet thromboxane synthesis in diabetes mellitus. *J. Lab. Clin. Med.*, 97:87–96.
131. Hamberg, M. (1976): On the formation of thromboxane B$_2$ and 12L-hydroxy-5,8,10,14-eicosatetraenoic acid (12 ho-20:4) in tissues from the guinea pig. *Biochim. Biophys. Acta*, 431:651–654.
132. Hamberg, M. (1980): Transformations of 5,8,11,14,17-eicosapentaenoic acid in human platelets. *Biochim. Biophys. Acta*, 618:389–398.
133. Hamberg, M., Hedqvist, P., and Rådegran, K. (1980): Identification of 15-hydroxy-5,8,11,13-eicosatetraenoic acid (15-HETE) as a major metabolite of arachidonic acid in human lung. *Acta Physiol. Scand.*, 110:219–221.
134. Hamberg, M., Hedqvist, P., Strandberg, K., Svensson, J., and Samuelsson, B. (1975): Prostaglandin endoperoxides IV. Effects on smooth muscle. *Life Sci.*, 16:451–462.
135. Hamberg, M., and Samuelsson, B. (1973): Detection and isolation of an endoperoxide intermediate in prostaglandin biosynthesis. *Proc. Natl. Acad. Sci. USA*, 70:899–903.
136. Hamberg, M., and Samuelsson, B. (1974): Novel transformations of arachidonic acid in human platelets. *Proc. Natl. Acad. Sci. USA*, 71:3400–3404.
137. Hamberg, M., and Samuelsson, B. (1974): Novel transformations of arachidonic acid in guinea pig lung. *Biochem. Biophys. Res. Commun.*, 61:942–949.
138. Hamberg, M., Svensson, J., Hedqvist, P., Strandberg, K., and Samuelsson, B. (1980): Involvement of endoperoxides and thromboxanes in anaphylactic reactions. In: *Advances in Prostaglandin and Thromboxane Research*, Vol. 1, edited by B. Samuelsson and R. Paoletti, pp. 495–501. Raven Press, New York.
139. Hamberg, M., Svensson, J., and Samuelsson, B. (1975): Prostaglandin endoperoxides. VI. A new concept concerning the mode of action and release of prostaglandins. *Proc. Natl. Acad. Sci. USA*, 71:3824–3828.
140. Hamberg, M., Svensson, J., and Samuelsson, B. (1975): Thromboxanes: A new group of biologically active compounds derived from prostaglandin endoperoxides. *Proc. Natl. Acad. Sci. USA*, 72:2994–2998.

141. Hamberg, M., Svensson, J., Wakabayashi, T., and Samuelsson, B. (1974): Isolation and structure of two prostaglandins endoperoxides which cause platelet aggregation. *Proc. Natl. Acad. Sci. USA*, 71:345–349.

142. Hammarström, S. (1980): Enzymatic synthesis of 15-hydroperoxy thromboxane A$_2$ and 12-hydroperoxy-5,8,10-heptadecatrienoic acid. *J. Biol. Chem.*, 255:518–523.

143. Hammarström, S. (1980): Biological effects of 15-hydroperoxy thromboxane A$_2$ on platelets and aorta. *Prostaglandins Med.*, 4:297–302.

144. Hammarström, S., and Diczfalusy, U. (1979): Inhibition and properties of thromboxane synthetase. In: *Advances in Inflammation Research*, Vol. 1, edited by G. Weissman, pp. 431–438. Raven Press, New York.

145. Hammarström, S., and Falardeau, P. (1977): Resolution of prostaglandin endoperoxide synthase and thromboxane synthase of human platelets. *Proc. Natl. Acad. Sci. USA*, 74:3691–3695.

146. Hardisty, R. M. (1977): Antiplatelet drugs: Rationale for use. *Bibl. Haematol.*, 44:181–187.

147 Harris, D. N., Greenberg, R., Phillips, M. B., Osman, G. H., Jr., and Antonaccio, M. J. (1980): Effect of SQ 80, 338 [1-(3-phenyl-2-propenyl)-1H-immidazole] on thromboxane synthetase activity and arachidonic acid induced platelet aggregation and bronchoconstriction. In: *Advances in Prostaglandin and Thromboxane Research*, Vol. 6, edited by B. Samuelsson, P. Ramwell, and R. Paoletti, pp. 437–441. Raven Press, New York.

148. Harris, R. H., Zmudka, M., Maddox, Y., Ramwell, P. W., and Fletcher, R. J. (1980): Relationship of TXB$_2$ and 6-keto-PGF$_{1\alpha}$ to chemodynamic changes during baboon endotoxic shock. In: *Advances in Prostaglandin and Thromboxane Research*, Vol. 7, edited by B. Samuelsson, P. Ramwell, and R. Paoletti, pp. 843–849. Raven Press, New York.

149. Harter, H. R., Burch, J. W., Majerus, P. W., Stanford, N., Delmez, J. A., Anderson, C. B., and Weerts, C. A. (1979): Prevention of thrombosis in patients on hemodialysis by low-dose aspirin. *N. Engl. J. Med.*, 301:577–579.

150. Heggers, J. P., Loy, G. L., Robson, M. C., and Del Beccaro, E. J. (1980): Histological demonstration of prostaglandins and thromboxanes in burned tissue. *J. Surg. Res.*, 28:110–117.

151. Hemker, D. P., and Aiken, J. W. (1979): Rat aortic strips as a bioassay tissue for thromboxane A$_2$ and rabbit aorta contracting substance (RCS) released from guinea pig lung by bradykinin or anaphylaxis. *Prostaglandins*, 17:239–248.

152. Herbaczynska-Cedro, K., and Staszewska-Barczak, J. (1977): Suppression of prostaglandin-like substances *in vivo*. *Prostaglandins*, 13:517–531.

153. Ho, P. P. K., Walters, P., and Sullivan, H. R. (1976): Biosynthesis of thromboxane B$_2$: Assay, isolation and properties of the enzyme system in human platelets. *Prostaglandins*, 12:951–971.

154. Hokama, Y. (1978): Platelet-endothelial prostaglandin biochemical imbalance in sudden infant death syndrome in the newborn: Capillary endothelial cell deficiency and/or lag in maturation of prostaglandin synthetase. *Med. Hypotheses*, 4:303–305.

155. ten Hoor, F., de Deckere, E. A., Haddeman, E., Hornstra, G., and Quadt, J. F. (1980): Dietary manipulation of prostaglandin and thromboxane synthesis in heart, aorta, and blood platelets on the rat. In: *Advances in Prostaglandin and Thromboxane Research*, Vol. 8, edited by B. Samuelsson, P. Ramwell, and R. Paoletti, pp. 1771–1781. Raven Press, New York.

156. Hopkins, N. K., Sun, F. F., and Gorman, R. R. (1978): Thromboxane A$_2$ biosynthesis in human lung fibroblasts WI-38. *Biochem. Biophys. Res. Commun.*, 85:827–836.

157. Hornstra, G., Haddeman, E., and Don, J. A. (1979): Blood platelets do not provide endoperoxides for vascular prostacyclin production. *Nature*, 279:66–68.

158. Hornstra, G., and Hemker, H. C. (1979): Clot-promoting effect of platelet-vessel wall interaction: Influence of dietary fats and relation to arterial thrombus formation in rats. *Haemostasis*, 8:211–226.

159. Horrobin, D. F. (1978): Dopamine supersensitivity, endorphine excess and prostaglandin E$_1$ deficiency: Three aspects of the same schizophrenic elephant. *Schizophr. Bull.*, 4:487–488.

160. Horrobin, D. F., Manku, M. S., Karmali, R. A., Oka, M., Ally, A. I., Morgan, R. O., Karmazyn, M., and Cunnane, S. O. (1978): Thromboxane A$_2$: A key regulator of prostaglandin biosynthesis and interactions between prostaglandins, calcium and cyclic nucleotides. *Med. Hypotheses*, 4:178–186.

161. Jaffe, E. A., and Weksler, B. B. (1979): Recovery of endothelial cell prostacyclin after inhibition by low doses of aspirin. *J. Clin. Invest.*, 63:532–535.

162. Jakubowski, J. A., and Ardlie, N. G. (1978): Modification of human platelet function by a diet enriched in saturated or polyunsaturated fats. *Atherosclerosis*, 31:335–344.

163. Jakubowski, J. A., and Ardlie, N. G. (1979): Evidence for the mechanism by which eicosapentaenoic acid inhibits human platelet aggregation and secretion—implications for the prevention of vascular disease. *Thromb. Res.*, 16:205–217.
164. Johnson, M., Reece, A. H., and Harrison, H. E. (1980): An imbalance in arachidonic acid metabolism in diabetes. In: *Advances in Prostaglandin and Thromboxane Research*, Vol. 8, edited by B. Samuelsson, P. Ramwell, and R. Paoletti, pp. 1283–1286. Raven Press, New York.
165. Johnson, R. A., Morton, D. R., Kinner, J. H., Gorman, R. R., McGuire, J. R., Sun, F. F., Whittaker, N., Bunting, S., Salmon, J. A., Moncada, S., and Vane, J. R. (1976): The chemical structure of prostaglandin X (prostacyclin). *Prostaglandins*, 12:915–928.
166. Jonsson, C. E., Granström, E., and Hamberg, M. (1979): Prostaglandins and thromboxanes in burn injury in man. *Scand. J. Plast. Reconstr. Surg.*, 13:45–47.
167. Jonsson, C. E., Shimizu, Y., Fredholm, B. B., Granström, E., and Oliw, E. (1979): Efflux of cyclic AMP, prostaglandin E$_2$ and F$_{2\alpha}$ and thromboxane B$_2$ in leg lymph of rabbits after scalding injury. *Acta Physiol. Scand.*, 107:377–384.
168. Kadowitz, P. J., and Hyman, A. L. (1980): Comparative effects of thromboxane B$_2$ on the canine and feline pulmonary vascular bed. *J. Pharmacol. Exp. Ther.*, 213:300–305.
169. Kafka, M. S., van Kammen, D. P., and Bunney, W. E. (1979): Reduced cAMP production in the blood platelets from schizophrenic patients. *Am. J. Psych.*, 136:685–687.
170. Kam, S., and Portoghese, P. S. (1979): 9,11-Azo-13-oxa-15-hydroxyprostanoic acid: A potent thromboxane synthetase inhibitor and a PGH$_2$/TXA$_2$ receptor antagonist. *Prostaglandins Med.*, 3:279–290.
171. Karim, S. M. M., and Adaikan, P. G. (1980): Inhibition of platelet aggregation with oral administration of a stable prostacyclin analogue (carboprostacyclin) in baboons. *IRCS. Med. Sci. Biochem.*, 8:338.
172. Kass, M. A., and Holmberg, N. J. (1979): Prostaglandin and thromboxane synthesis by microsomes of rabbit ocular tissues. *Invest. Ophthalmol. Vis. Sci.*, 18:166–171.
173. Katori, M., Harada, Y., Tanaka, K., Miyazaki, H., Ishibashi, M., and Yamashita, Y. (1980): Changes of prostaglandin and thromboxane levels in pleural fluid of rat carrageenin-induced pleurisy. In: *Advances in Prostaglandin and Thromboxane Research, Vol. 8*, edited by B. Samuelsson, P. Ramwell, and R. Paoletti, pp. 1733–1737. Raven Press, New York.
174. Kelly, R. C., Schletter, I., and Stein, S. J. (1976): Synthesis of thromboxane B$_2$. *Tetrahedron Lett.*, 37:3279–3282.
175. Kelton, J. G., Hirsch, J., Carter, C. J., and Buchanan, M. R. (1978): Thrombogenic effect of high-dose aspirin in rabbits. Relationship to inhibition of vessel wall synthesis of prostaglandin I$_2$-like activity. *J. Clin. Invest.*, 62:892–895.
176. Kernoff, P. B. A., Willis, A. L., Stone, K. J., Davies, J. A., and McNicol. G. P. (1977): Antithrombotic potential of dihomogamma-linolenic acid in man. *Br. Med. J.*, 2:1441–1444.
177. Kindahl, H. (1977): Metabolism of thromboxane B$_2$ in the cynomolgus monkey. *Prostaglandins*, 13:619–629.
178. Kinlough-Rathbone, R. L., Reimers, H. J., Mustard, J. F., and Packham, M. A. (1976): Sodium arachidonate can induce platelet shape change and aggregation which are independent of the release-reaction. *Science*, 192:1011–1012.
179. Kitchen, E. A., Boot, J. R., and Dawson, W. (1978): Chemotactic activity of thromboxane B$_2$, prostaglandins and their metabolites for polymorphonuclear leukocytes. *Prostaglandins*, 16:239–244.
180. Knapp, H. R., Oelz, O., Roberts, L. J., Sweetman, B. J., Oates, J. A., and Reed, P. W. (1977): Ionophores stimulate prostaglandin and thromboxane biosynthesis. *Proc. Natl. Acad. Sci. USA*, 74:4251–4255.
181. Koh, H., Inoue, A., Mashimo, N., Numano, F., and Maezawa, H. (1980): A radioimmunoassay of thromboxane B$_2$ with thromboxane B$_2$-^{125}I-tyramide and its application to the study on thromboxane B$_2$ formation during platelet aggregation. *Thromb. Res.*, 17:403–413.
182. Korbut, R., and Moncada, S. (1978): Prostacyclin (PGI$_2$) and thromboxane A$_2$ interaction *in vivo*. Regulation by aspirin and relationship with anti-thrombotic therapy. *Thromb. Res.*, 13:489–500.
183. Kosuge, S., Hamanaka, N., and Hayashi, M. (1976): Synthesis of thromboxane A$_2$ analog DL-(9,11), (11,12)-dideoxa-(9,11)-methylene(11,12)-epithio-thromboxane A$_2$ methyl ester. *Tetrahedron Lett.*, 22:1345–1348.
184. Kraemer, R. J., Phernetton, T. M., and Folts, J. D. (1976): Prostaglandin-like substance in coronary venous blood following myocardial ischemia. *J. Pharmacol. Exp. Ther.*, 199:611–619.

185. Kulkarni, P. S., and Eakins, K. E. (1976): N-0164 inhibits generation of thromboxane A₂-like activity from prostaglandin endoperoxides by human platelet microsomes. *Prostaglandins*, 12:465–469.

186. Ladd, N., and Lewis, G. P. (1980): Determination of specific inhibitors of thromboxane A₂ formation. *Br. J. Pharmacol.*, 69:3–5.

187. Lagarde, M., Byron, P. A., Vargaftig, B. B., and Dechavanne, M. (1978): Impairment of platelet thromboxane A₂ generation and of the platelet release reaction in two patients with congenital deficiency of platelet cyclooxygenase. *Br. J. Haematol.*, 38:251–266.

188. Lagarde, M., and Dechavanne, M. (1977): Collagen stimulates more prostaglandin endoperoxides in thrombosis. *Biomed. Express*, 27:119–123.

189. Lagarde, M., and Dechavanne, M. (1977): Thrombin decreases platelet cyclic AMP in the absence of prostaglandin synthesis. *Biomed. Express*, 27:110–112.

190. Lagarde, M., Guichardant, M., Ghazi, I., and Dechavanne, M. (1980): Nicergoline, an anti-aggregating agent which inhibits release of arachidonic acid from human platelet phospholipids. *Prostaglandins*, 19:551–557.

191. Lages, B., Malmsten, C., Weiss, H. J., and Samuelsson, B. (1981): Impaired platelet response to thromboxane A₂ and defective calcium mobilization in a patient with a bleeding disorder. *Blood*, 57:545–552.

192. Le Breton, G. C., Venton, D. L., Enke, S. E., and Halushka, P. V. (1979): 13-Azo-prostanoic acid: A specific antagonist of the human blood platelet thromboxane/endoperoxide receptor. *Proc. Natl. Acad. Sci. USA*, 76:4097–4101.

193. LeDuc, L. E., and Needleman, P. (1979): Regional localization of prostacyclin and thromboxane synthesis in dog stomach and intestinal tract. *J. Pharmacol. Exp. Ther.*, 211:181–188.

194. Lefer, A. M., Smith, E. F., III, Araki, H., Smith, J. B., Aharony, D., Claremon, D. A., Magolda, R. L., and Nicolaou, K. C. (1980): Dissociation of vasoconstrictor and platelet aggregatory activities of thromboxane by carbocyclic thromboxane A₂, a stable analog of thromboxane A₂. *Proc. Natl. Acad. Sci. USA*, 77:1706–1710.

195. Lewy, R. I. (1980): Effect of elevated plasma-free fatty acids on thromboxane release in patients with coronary artery disease. *Haemostasis*, 9:134–140.

196. Lewy, R. I., Smith, J. B., Silver, M. J., Saia, J., Walinsky, P., and Wiener, L. (1979): Detection of thromboxane B₂ in peripheral blood of patients with Prinzmetal's angina. *Prostaglandins Med.*, 5:243–248.

197. Lewy, R. I., Wiener, L., Smith, J. B., Walinsky, P., and Silver, M. J. (1979): Intravenous heparin initiates *in vivo* synthesis and release of thromboxane in angina pectoris. *Lancet*, i:97.

198. Lewy, R. I., Wiener, L., Smith, J. B., Walinsky, P., Silver, M. J., and Saia, J. (1979): Comparison of plasma concentrations of thromboxane B₂ in Prinzmetal's variant angina and classical angina pectoris. *Clin. Cardiol.*, 2:404–406.

199. Liggins, G. C., Campos, G. A., Roberts, C. M., and Skinner, S. J. (1980): Production rates of prostaglandin F, 6-keto-PGF₁ₐ and thromboxane B₂ by perfused human endometrium. *Prostaglandins*, 19:461–477.

200. Lindgren, J. Å., Claesson, H. E., Kindahl, H., and Hammarström, S. (1980): Effects of platelet aggregation and adenosine 3′:5′-monophosphate on the synthesis of thromboxane B₂ in human platelets. In: *Advances in Prostaglandin and Thromboxane Research*, Vol. 6, edited by B. Samuelsson, P. Ramwell, and R. Paoletti, pp. 275–281. Raven Press, New York.

201. Livio, M., Villa, S., and de Gaetano, G. (1978): Aspirin, thromboxane, and prostacyclin in rats: a dilemma resolved? *Lancet*, i:107.

202. Longmore, D. B., Bennett, G., Gueirrara, D., Smith, M., Bunting, S., Moncada, S., Reed, P., Read, N. G., and Vane, J. R. (1979): Prostacyclin: A solution to some problems of extracorporeal circulation. Experiments in greyhounds. *Lancet*, i:1002–1005.

203. Macintyre, D. E., and Gordon, J. L. (1977): Discrimination between platelet prostaglandin receptors with a specific antagonist of bisenoic prostaglandins. *Thromb. Res.*, 11:705–713.

204. Maclouf, J., Kindahl, H., Granström, E., and Samuelsson, B. (1980): Interactions of prostaglandin H₂ and thromboxane A₂ with human serum albumin. *Eur. J. Biochem.*, 109:561–566.

205. Majerus, P. W. (1976): Why aspirin? *Circulation*, 54:357–359.

206. Makheja, A. N., Vanderhoek, J. Y., and Bailey, J. M. (1979): Effects of onion (Allium Cepa) extract on platelet aggregation and thromboxane synthesis. *Prostaglandins Med.*, 2:413–424.

207. Makheja, A. N., Vanderhoek, J. Y., Bryant, R. W., and Bailey, J. M. (1980): Altered arachidonic acid metabolism in platelets inhibited by onion or garlic extracts. In: *Advances in Prostaglandin*

and *Thromboxane Research*, Vol. 6, edited by B. Samuelsson, P. Ramwell, and R. Paoletti, pp. 309–312. Raven Press, New York.

208. Malmsten, C. (1976): Some biological effects of prostaglandin endoperoxide analogs. *Life Sci.*, 18:169–176.

209. Malmsten, C. (1979): Prostaglandins, thromboxanes and platelets. *Br. J. Haematol.*, 41:453–458.

210. Malmsten, C., Claesson, H. E., and Fried, J. (1980): Inhibition of platelet aggregation and elevation of cAMP levels in platelets by 13,14-dehydromethyl PGI$_2$. *Prostaglandins Med.*, 4:453–463.

211. Malmsten, C., Granström, E., and Samuelsson, B. (1976): Cyclic AMP inhibits synthesis of prostaglandin endoperoxide (PGG$_2$) in human platelets. *Biochem. Biophys. Res. Commun.*, 68:569–576.

212. Malmsten, C., Hamberg, M., Svensson, J., and Samuelsson, B. (1975): Physiological role of an endoperoxide in human platelets: Hemostatic defect due to platelet cyclooxygenase deficiency. *Proc. Natl. Acad. Sci. USA*, 72:1446–1450.

213. Malmsten, C., Kindahl, H., Samuelsson, B., Levy-Toledano, S., Tobelem, G., and Caen, J. P. (1977): Thromboxane synthesis and the platelet release reaction in Bernard-Soulier syndrome, thrombasthenia Glanzmann and Hermansky-Pudlak syndrome. *Br. J. Haematol.*, 35:511–520.

214. Manku, M. S., Horrobin, D. F., Oka, M., Ally, A. I., Karmazyn, M., Cunnane, S. C., Morgan, R. O., and Karmali, R. A. (1978): Ultraviolet radiation and 8-methoxypsoralen have actions similar to those of known inhibitors of thromboxane A$_2$ synthesis in rat mesenteric blood vessels. *Prostaglandins Med.*, 1:86–95.

215. Marcinkiewicz, E., Gordzinska, L., and Gryglewski, R. J. (1978): Platelet aggregation and thromboxane A$_2$ formation in cat platelet rich plasma. *Pharmacol. Res. Commun.*, 10:1–12.

216. Marcus, A. J. (1979): The role of prostaglandins in platelet function. *Prog. Hematol.*, 11:147–171.

217. Masotti, G., Galanti, G., Poggesi, L., Abbate, R., and Neri Serneri, G. G. (1979): Differential inhibition of prostacyclin production and platelet aggregation by aspirin. *Lancet*, ii:1213–1216.

218. Masotti, G., Galanti, G., Poggesi, L., Abbate, R., and Neri Serneri, G. G. (1980): Differential inhibition of prostacyclin production and platelet aggregation by aspirin in humans. In: *Advances in Prostaglandin and Thromboxane Research*, Vol. 6, edited by B. Samuelsson, P. Ramwell, and R. Paoletti, pp. 317–320. Raven Press, New York.

219. Matthias, F. R. (1978): Soluble plasma fibrin and platelet prostaglandin endoperoxides following myocardial infarction. *Haemostasis*, 7:273–281.

220. Maxey, K. M., and Bundy, G. L. (1980): The synthesis of 11a-carba-thromboxane A$_2$. *Tetrahedron Lett.*, 2:445–448.

221. McMillan, R. M., MacIntyre, D. E., Booth, A., and Gordon, J. L. (1978): Malonaldehyde formation in intact platelets is catalyzed by thromboxane synthase. *Biochem. J.*, 176:596–598.

222. McNicol. G. P. (1980): Antiplatelet drugs in the secondary prevention of myocardial infarction. *Lancet*, ii:736–738.

223. Merino, J., Livio, M., Rajtar, G., and de Gaetano, G. (1980): Salicylate reverses *in vitro* aspirin inhibition of rat platelet and vascular prostaglandin generation. *Biochem. Pharmacol.*, 29:1093–1096.

224. Mestel, F., Oetliker, O., Beck, E., Felix, R., Imbach, P., and Wagner, H. P. (1980): Severe bleeding associated with defective thromboxane synthetase. *Lancet*, i:157.

225. Meyers, K. M., Seachard, C. L., Holmsen, H., Smith, J. B., and Prieur, D. J. (1979): A dominant role of thromboxane formation in secondary aggregation of platelets. *Nature*, 282:331–333.

226. Miller, O. V., and Gorman, R. R. (1976): Modulation of platelet cyclic nucleotide content by PGE$_1$ and the prostaglandin endoperoxide PGG$_2$. *J. Cyclic Nucleotide Res.*, 2:79–86.

227. Miller, O. V., and Gorman, R. R. (1979): Evidence for distinct prostaglandin I$_2$ and D$_2$ receptors in human platelets. *J. Pharmacol. Exp. Ther.*, 210:134–140.

228. Mills, D. C. B., and Smith, J. B. (1971): The influence on platelet aggregation of drugs that affect the accumulation of adenosine 3':5-cyclic monophosphate in platelets. *Biochem. J.*, 121:185–196.

229. Minkes, M., Stanford, N., Maggie, M.-Y. Chi, Roth, G. J., Raz, A., Needleman, P., and Majerus, P. W. (1977): Cyclic adenosine 3',5'-monophosphate inhibits the availability of arachidonate to prostaglandin synthetase in human platelet suspension. *J. Clin. Invest.*, 59:449–454.

230. Miyamoto, T., Taniguchi, K., Tanouchi, T., and Hirata, M. (1980): Selective inhibitor of thromboxane synthetase: Pyridine and its derivatives. In: *Advances in Prostaglandin and Thromboxane Research*, Vol. 6, edited by B. Samuelsson, P. Ramwell, and R. Paoletti, pp. 443–445. Raven Press, New York.

231. Moncada, S., and Amezcua, J. L. (1979): Prostacyclin, thromboxane A$_2$ interactions in haemostasis and thrombosis. *Haemostasis*, 8:252–265.
232. Moncada, S., Bunting, S., Mullane, K., Thorogood, P., Vane, J. R., Raz, A., and Needleman, P. (1977): Imidazole: A selective inhibitor of thromboxane synthetase. *Prostaglandins*, 13:611–618.
233. Moncada, S., Ferreira, S. H., and Vane, J. R. (1978): Bioassay of prostaglandins and biologically active substances derived from arachidonic acid. In: *Advances in Prostaglandin and Thromboxane Research*, Vol. 5, edited by J. C. Frölich, pp. 211–236. Raven Press, New York.
234. Moncada, S., Gryglewski, R., Bunting, S., and Vane, J. R. (1976): An enzyme isolated from arteries transforms prostaglandin endoperoxides to an unstable substance that inhibits platelet aggregation. *Nature*, 263:663–665.
235. Moncada, S., Higgs, E. A., and Vane, J. R. (1977): Human arterial and venous tissues generate prostacyclin (prostaglandin X), a potent inhibitor of platelet aggregation. *Lancet*, i:18–19.
236. Moncada, S., and Korbut, R. (1978): Dipyridamole and other phosphodiesterase inhibitors act as antithrombotic agents by potentiating endogenous prostacyclin. *Lancet*, i:1286–1289.
237. Moncada, S., Needleman, P., Bunting, S., and Vane, J. R. (1976): Prostaglandin endoperoxide and thromboxane generating systems and their selective inhibition. *Prostaglandins*, 12:323–335.
238. Moncada, S., and Vane, J. R. (1979): Arachidonic acid metabolites and the interactions between platelets and the vessel wall. *N. Engl. J. Med.*, 300:1142–1147.
239. Moncada, S., and Vane, J. R. (1979): Pharmacology and endogenous roles of prostaglandin endoperoxides, thromboxane A$_2$ and prostacyclin. *Pharmacol. Rev.*, 30:293–331.
240. Moncada, S., and Vane, J. R. (1979): The role of prostacyclin in vascular tissue. *Fed. Proc.*, 38:66–71.
241. Moncada, S., and Vane, J. R. (1980): Biological significance and therapeutic potential of prostacyclin. *J. Med. Chem.*, 23:591–593.
242. Morley, J., Bray, M. A., Jones, R. W., Nugteren, D. H., and van Dorp, D. A. (1979): Prostaglandin and thromboxane production by human and guinea-pig macrophages and leukocytes. *Prostaglandins*, 17:729–746.
243. Morrison, A. R., Nishikawa, K., and Needleman, P. (1977): Unmasking of thromboxane A$_2$ synthesis by ureteral obstruction in the rabbit kidney. *Nature*, 27:259–260.
244. Murota, S. I., Kawamura, M., and Morita, I. (1978): Transformation of arachidonic acid into thromboxane B$_2$ by the homogenates of activated macrophages. *Biochim. Biophys. Acta*, 528:507–511.
245. Musotti, G., Galanti, G., Poggesi, L., Abbate, R., and Neri Serneri, G. G. (1980): Differential inhibition of prostacyclin production and platelet aggregation by aspirin in humans. In: *Advances in Prostaglandin and Thromboxane Research*, Vol. 6, edited by B. Samuelsson, P. Ramwell, and R. Paoletti, pp. 317–320. Raven Press, New York.
246. Mustard, J. F., Kinlough-Rathbone, R. L., and Packham, M. A. (1980): Prostaglandins and platelets. *Ann. Rev. Med.*, 31:89–96.
247. Mustard, J. F., and Packham, M. A. (1970): Factors influencing platelet function: Adhesion, release and aggregation. *Pharmacol. Rev.*, 22:97–187.
248. Myers, S., Zipser, R., and Needleman, P. (1980): Exaggerated prostaglandin and thromboxane synthesis in the renal vein constricted rabbit. In: *Advances in Prostaglandin and Thromboxane Research*, Vol. 7, edited by B. Samuelsson, P. Ramwell, and R. Paoletti, pp. 1171–1173. Raven Press, New York.
249. Needleman, P., Kulkarni, O. S., and Raz, A. (1977): Coronary tone modulation. Formation and actions of prostaglandins, endoperoxides, and thromboxanes. *Science*, 195:409–412.
250. Needleman, P., Minkes, M., and Raz, A. (1976): Thromboxanes: Selective biosynthesis and distinct biological properties. *Science*, 193:163–165.
251. Needleman, P., Raz, A., Ferrendelli, J. A., and Minkes, M. (1977): Application of imidazole as a selective inhibitor of thromboxane synthetase in human platelets. *Proc. Natl. Acad. Sci. USA*, 74:1716–1720.
252. Needleman, P., Raz, A., Minkes, M. S., Ferrandelli, J. A., and Sprecher, H. (1979): Triene prostaglandins: Prostacyclin and thromboxane biosynthesis and unique biological properties. *Proc. Natl. Acad. Sci. USA*, 76:944–948.
253. Needleman, P., Whitaker, M. O., Wyche, A., Watters, K., Sprecher, H., and Raz, A. (1980): Manipulation of platelet aggregation by prostaglandins and their fatty acid precursors: Pharmacological basis for a therapeutic approach. *Prostaglandins*, 19:165–181.

254. Needleman, P., Wyche, A., and Raz, A. (1979): Platelet and blood vessel arachidonate metabolism and interactions. *J. Clin. Invest.*, 63:345–349.
255. Neichi, T., Tomisawa, S., Kubodera, N., and Uchida, Y. (1980): Enhancement of PGI_2 formation by a new vasodilator, 2-nicotin-aminoethyl nitrate in the coupled system of platelets and aortic microsomes. *Prostaglandins*, 19:577–586.
256. Nelson, N. A. (1974): Prostaglandin nomenclature. *J. Med. Chem.*, 17:911–918.
257. Nelson, N. A., and Jackson, R. W. (1976): Total synthesis of thromboxane B_2. *Tetrahedron Lett.*, 37:3275–3278.
258. Nicolaou, K. C., Magolda, R. L., and Claremon, D. A. (1980): Carbocyclic thromboxane A_2. *J. Am. Chem. Soc.*, 102:1404–1409.
259. Nicolaou, K. C., Magolda, R. L., Smith, J. B., Aharony, D., Smith, E. F., and Lefer, A. M. (1979): Synthesis and biological properties of pinane-thromboxane A_2, a selective inhibitor of coronary artery constriction, platelet aggregation, and thromboxane formation. *Proc. Natl. Acad. Sci. USA*, 76:2566–2570.
260. Nijkamp, F. P., Moncada, S., White, H. L., and Vane, J. R. (1977): Diversion of prostaglandin endoperoxide metabolism by selective inhibition of thromboxane A_2 biosynthesis in lung, spleen or platelets. *Eur. J. Pharmacol.*, 44:179–186.
261. Nishizawa, E. E., Miller, W. L., Gorman, R. R., Bundy, G. L., Svensson, J., and Hamberg, M. (1975): Prostaglandin D_2 as a potential antithrombotic agent. *Prostaglandins*, 9:109–121.
262. Nugteren, D. H., and Hazelhof, E. (1973): Isolation and properties of intermediates in prostaglandin biosynthesis. *Biochim. Biophys. Acta*, 326:448–461.
263. Nurden, A. T., and Caen, J. P. (1976): Role of surface glycoproteins in human platelet function. *Thromb. Haemost.*, 1:139–150.
264. Nyman, D., Eriksson, A. W., Lehman, W., and Blombäck, M. (1979): Inherited defective platelet aggregation with arachidonate as the main expression of a defective metabolism of arachidonic acid. *Thromb. Res.*, 14:739–746.
265. Oates, J. A., Roberts, L. J., II, Sweetman, B. J., Maas, R. N., Gerkeens, J. F., and Tabeer, D. F. (1980): Metabolism of prostaglandins and thromboxanes. In: *Advances in Prostaglandin and Thromboxane Research*, Vol. 6, edited by B. Samuelsson, P. Ramwell, and R. Paoletti, pp. 35–41. Raven Press, New York.
266. Oelz, O., Oelz, R., Knapp, H. R., Sweetman, B. J., and Oates, J. A. (1979): Biosynthesis of prostaglandin D_2. I: Formation of prostaglandin D_2 by human platelets. *Prostaglandins*, 13:225–234.
267. O'Grady, J., and Moncada, S. (1978): Aspirin: A paradoxical effect on bleeding time. *Lancet*, ii:780.
268. Ohuchida, S., Hamanaka, N., and Hayashi, M. (1979): Synthesis of thromboxane A_2 analog DL-(9,11), (11,12)-dideoxa-(9,11), (11,12)-dimetylene thromboxane A_2. *Tetrahedron Lett.*, 38:3661–3664.
269. Ohuchida, S., Hamanaka, N., and Hayashi, M. (1981): Synthesis of thromboxane A_2 analog DL-(9,11),(11,12)-dideoxa-(9,11)-epithio-(11,12)-methylene-thromboxane A_2. *Tetrahedron Lett.*, 22:1349–1352.
270. Okuma, M., and Uchino, H. (1979): Altered arachidonate metabolism by platelets in patients with myeloproliferative disorders. *Blood*, 54:1258–1271.
271. Omini, C., Moncada, S., and Vane, J. R. (1977): The effects of prostacyclin (PGI_2) on tissues which detect prostaglandins (PG's). *Prostaglandins*, 14:625–632.
272. Paccioretti, M. J., and Block, L. H. (1980): Effects of aspirin on platelet aggregation as a function of dosage and time. *Clin. Pharmacol. Ther.*, 27:803–809.
273. Packham, M. A., and Mustard, J. F. (1980): Pharmacology of platelet-affecting drugs. *Circulation*, 62 (Suppl V):V26–V40.
274. Pareti, F. I., Mannucci, P. M., D'Angelo, A., Smith, J. B., Sautebin, L., and Galli, G. (1980): Congenital deficiency of thromboxane and prostacyclin. *Lancet*, i:898–901.
275. Patrono, C., Ciabattoni, G., Pinca, E., Pugliese, F., Castrucci, G., DeSalvo, A., Satta, M. A., and Peskar, B. A. (1980): Low dose aspirin and inhibition of thromboxane B_2 production in healthy subjects. *Thromb. Res.*, 17:317–327.
276. Patrono, C., Ciabattoni, G., Pugliese, F., Pinca, E., Castrucci, G., De Salvo, A., Satta, M. A., and Parachini, M. (1980): Radioimmunoassay of serum thromboxane B_2: A simple method of assessing pharmacologic effects on platelet function. In: *Advances in Prostaglandin and Thromboxane Research*, Vol. 6, edited by B. Samuelsson, R. Paoletti, and P. Ramwell, pp. 187–191. Raven Press, New York.

277. Peskar, B. A., Glatt, M., Anhut, H., and Brune, K. (1978): Effect of imidazole on prostaglandin and thromboxane accumulation in urate arthritis. *Eur. J. Pharmacol.*, 50:437–441.

278. Peskar, B. A., and Holland, A. (1979): Plasma levels of immunoreactive 15-keto-13,14-dihydro-thromboxane B$_2$ in guinea pigs during anaphylaxis and after histamine injection. *Agents Actions (Suppl.)*, 6:51–56.

279. Piper, P. J., and Vane, J. R. (1969): Release of additional factors in anaphylaxis and its antagonism by anti-inflammatory drugs. *Nature (Lond.)*, 223:29–35.

280. Plachetka, J. R., Salomon, N. W., Larsen, D. F., and Copeland, J. G. (1980): Platelet loss during experimental cardiopulmonary by-pass and its prevention with prostacyclin. *Ann. Thorac. Surg.*, 30:58–63.

281. Prancan, A. V., Lefort, J., Chignard, M., Gerozissis, K., Dray, F., and Vargaftig, B. B. (1979): L8027 and 1-nonyl-imidazole as non-selective inhibitors of thromboxane synthesis. *Eur. J. Pharmacol.*, 60:287–297.

282. Preston, F. E., Whipps, S., Jackson, C. A., French, A. J., Wyld, P. J., and Stoddard, C. J. (1981): Inhibition of prostacyclin and platelet thromboxane A$_2$ after low-dose aspirin. *N. Engl. J. Med.*, 304:76–79.

283. Rajah, S. M., Penny, A., and Kester, R. (1978): Aspirin and bleeding time. *Lancet*, ii:1105.

284. Raz, A., Aharony, D., and Kenig-Wakshal, R. (1978): Biosynthesis of thromboxane B$_2$ and 12L-hydroxy-5,8,10-heptadecetrienoic acid in human platelets. Evidence for a common enzymatic pathway. *Eur. J. Biochem.*, 86:447–454.

285. Remuzzi, G., Livio, M., Cavenaghi, A. E., Marchesi, D., Mecca, G., Donati, M. B., and DeGaetano, G. (1978): Unbalanced prostaglandin synthesis and plasma factors in uraemic bleeding. A hypothesis. *Thromb. Res.*, 13:531–536.

286. Remuzzi, G., Marchesi, D., Livio, M., Cavenaghi, A. E., Mecca, G., Donati, M. B., and DeGaetano, G. (1978): Altered platelet and vascular prostaglandin generation in patients with renal failure and prolonged bleeding-time. *Thromb. Res.*, 13:1007–1015.

287. Remuzzi, G., Schieppati, A., and Mecca, G. (1979): Abnormal platelet function in hemodialysed patients: Current concepts. *Int. J. Artif. Organs*, 2:109–112.

288. Roberts, L. J., II, Sweetman, B. J., and Oates, J. A. (1978): Metabolism of thromboxane B$_2$ in the monkey. *J. Biol. Chem.*, 253:5305–5318.

289. Rotrosen, J., Miller, A. D., Mandio, D., Traficante, L. J., and Gershon, S. (1980): Prostaglandins, platelets and schizophrenia. *Arch. Gen. Psychiatry*, 37:1047–1054.

290. Russell, N. H., Keenan, J. P., and Bellingham, A. J. (1979): Thrombocytopathy in preleukemia: Association with a defect of thromboxane A$_2$ activity. *Br. J. Haematol.*, 41:417–425.

291. Salzman, E. W. (1977): Interrelation of prostaglandin endoperoxide (prostaglandin G$_2$) and cyclic 3′:5′-adenosine monophosphate in human blood platelets. *Biochim. Biophys. Acta*, 449:48–60.

292. Samuelsson, B. (1965): On the incorporation of oxygen in the conversion of 8,11,14-eicosatrienoic acid to prostaglandin E$_1$. *J. Am. Chem. Soc.*, 87:3011–3013.

293. Samuelsson, B. (1972): Biosynthesis of prostaglandins. *Fed. Proc.*, 31:1442–1450.

294. Samuelsson, B., Folco, G., Granström, E., Kindahl, H., and Malmsten, C. (1978): Prostaglandins and thromboxanes: Biochemical and physiological considerations. In: *Advances in Prostaglandin and Thromboxane Research*, Vol. 4, edited by F. Coceani and P. Olley, pp. 1–25. Raven Press, New York.

295. Samuelsson, B., Goldyne, M., Granström, E., Hamberg, M., Hammarström, S., and Malmsten, C. (1978): Prostaglandins and thromboxanes. *Ann. Rev. Biochem.*, 47:997–1029.

296. Samuelsson, B., and Hamberg, M. (1974): The role of endoperoxides in the biosynthesis and action of prostaglandins. In: *Prostaglandin Synthetase Inhibitors*, edited by H. J. Robinson and J. R. Vane, pp. 107–120. Raven Press, New York.

297. Samuelsson, B., Hamberg, M., Malmsten, C., and Svensson, J. (1976): Role of the prostaglandin endoperoxides and thromboxanes in platelet aggregation. In: *Advances in Prostaglandin and Thromboxane Research*, Vol. 2, edited by B. Samuelsson, and R. Paoletti, pp. 737–746. Raven Press, New York.

298. Sarji, K. E., Kleinfelder, J., Brewington, R., Gonzales, J., Hempling, H., and Colwell, J. A. (1979): Decreased platelet vitamin C in diabetes mellitus. Possible role in hyperaggregation. *Thromb. Res.*, 15:639–650.

299. Schneider, W. P., and Morge, R. A. (1976): A synthesis of crystalline thromboxane B$_2$. *Tetrahedron Lett.*, 37:3283–3286.

300. Schorer, A. E., Gerrard, J. M., White, J. G., and Krivit, W. (1978): Oral contraceptive use alters the balance of platelet prostaglandin and thromboxane synthesis. *Prostaglandins Med.*, 1:5–11.

301. Schror, K., Smith, E. F., Bickerton, M., Smith, J. B., Nicolaou, K. C., Magolda, R., and Lefer, A. M. (1980): Preservation of ischemic myocardium by pinane thromboxane A$_2$. *Am. J. Physiol.*, 238:H87–92.

302. Schuman, M. A., Botney, M., and Fenton, J. W. (1979): Thrombin-induced platelet secretion. Further evidence for a specific pathway. *J. Clin. Invest.*, 63:1212–1218.

303. Shimamoto, T. (1978): Stroke and heart attack induced experimentally by thromboxane A$_2$ in rabbits and effect of EG 626, a thromboxane A$_2$ antagonist. In: *International Symposium: State of Prevention and Therapy in Human Arteriosclerosis and in Animal Models*, edited by W. L. Hauss, R. W. Wissler, and R. Lehman, pp. 139–152. Westdeutscher Verlag, Opladen.

304. Shimamoto, T., Kobayashi, M., Takanasni, T., Takashima, Y., Sakamoto, M., and Morooka, S. (1978): An observation of thromboxane A$_2$ in arterial blood after cholesterol feeding in rabbits. *Japan Heart J.*, 19:748–753.

305. Siegel, M. I., McConnell, R. T., Abrahams, S. L., Porter, N. A., and Cuatrecasas, P. (1979): Regulation of arachidonate metabolism by 12-HPETE, the product of human platelet lipoxygenase. *Biochem. Biophys. Res. Commun.*, 89:1273–1280.

306. Siess, E., Roth, P., Scherer, B., Kurzmann, I., Bohlig, B., and Weber, P. C. (1980): Platelet-membrane fatty acids, platelet aggregation and thromboxane formation during a mackerel diet. *Lancet*, 1:441–444.

307. Silver, M. J., Bills, T. K., and Smith, J. B. (1978): Platelets and prostaglandins: The key role of platelet phospholipase A$_2$ activity. In: *Platelets: A Multidisciplinary Approach*, edited by G. DeGaetano and S. Garattini, pp. 213–225. Raven Press, New York.

308. Silver, M. J., Smith, J. B., Ingerman, C., and Kocsis, J. J. (1973): Arachidonic acid induced human platelet aggregation and prostaglandin formation. *Prostaglandins*, 4:863–875.

309. Sivakoff, M., Holmberg, S., and Needleman, P. (1980): The role of prostaglandins and thromboxanes in the modulation of perfusion pressure in the hydronephrotic rabbit kidney. In: *Advances in Prostaglandin and Thromboxane Research*, Vol. 7, edited by B. Samuelsson, P. Ramwell, and R. Paoletti, pp. 1175–1176. Raven Press, New York.

310. Smith, E. F., III, Lefer, A. M., and Smith, J. B. (1980): Influence of thromboxane inhibition on the severity of myocardial ischemia in cats. *Can. J. Physiol. Pharmacol.*, 58:294–300.

311. Smith, J. B. (1980): The prostanoids in hemostasis and thrombosis. *Am. J. Pathol.*, 99:741–804.

312. Smith, J. B., Araki, M., and Lefer, A. M. (1980): Thromboxane A$_2$, prostacyclin and aspirin: Effects on vascular tone and platelet aggregation. *Circulation*, 62 (Suppl. V):V19–V25.

313. Smith, J. B., Ingerman, C., Kocsis, J. J., and Silver, M. J. (1974): Formation of an intermediate in prostaglandin biosynthesis and its association with the platelet release reaction. *J. Clin. Invest.*, 53:1468–1472.

314. Smith, J. B., Ingerman, C. M., and Silver, M. J. (1979): Normal bleeding times in rabbits containing antibodies that bind prostacyclin (PGI$_2$). *Thromb. Haemost.*, 42:7.

315. Smith, M. J. H., Ford-Hutchinson, A. W., Walker, J. R., and Slack, A. J. (1979): Aspirin, salicylate and prostaglandins. *Agents Actions*, 9:483–487.

316. Sobel, M., Salzman, E. W., Davies, G. C., Handin, R. I., Sweeney, J., Plaetz, J., and Kurland, G. (1981): Circulating platelet products in unstable angina pectoris. *Circulation*, 63:300–306.

317. Sors, H., Pradelles, P., Dray, F., Rigaud, M., Maclouf, J., and Bernard, P. (1978): Analytical methods for thromboxane B$_2$ measurement and validation of radioimmunoassay by GLC-MS. *Prostaglandins*, 16:277–290.

318. Spagnuolo, P. J., Ellner, J. J., and Dunn, M. J. (1980): Thromboxane A$_2$ mediates augmented polymorphonuclear leukocyte adhesiveness. *J. Clin. Invest.*, 66:406–414.

319. Spagnuolo, C., Sautebin, L., Galli, G., Racagni, G., Galli, C., Mazzari, S., and Finesso, M. (1979): PGF$_{2\alpha}$, thromboxane B$_2$ and HETE levels in gerbil brain cortex after ligation of common carotid arteries and decapitation. *Prostaglandins*, 18:53–61.

320. Steer, M. L., MacIntyre, D. E., Levine, L., and Salzman, E. W. (1980): Is prostacyclin a physiological important antiplatelet agent. *Nature*, 283:194–195.

321. Steinhauer, H. B., Anhut, H., and Hertting, G. (1979): The synthesis of prostaglandins and thromboxanes in the mouse brain *in vivo*. Influence of drug induced convulsions, hypoxia and the anticonvulsants trimetadione and diazepam. *Naunyn Schmiedebergs Arch. Pharmacol.*, 310:53–58.

322. Stuart, M. J., Gerrard, J. M., and White, J. G. (1980): Effect of cholesterol on production of thromboxane B$_2$ by platelets *in vitro*. *N. Engl. J. Med.*, 302:6–10.

323. Subbich, M. T., and Dietemeyer, D. (1980): Altered synthesis of prostaglandins in platelets and aorta from spontaneously diabetic Wistar rats. *Biochem. Med.*, 23:231–235.

324. Sun, F. F. (1977): Biosynthesis of thromboxanes in human platelets. I: Characterization and assay of thromboxane synthetase. *Biochem. Biophys. Res. Commun.*, 74:1432–1440.
325. Sun, F. F., Chapman, J. P., and McGuire, J. C. (1977): Metabolism of prostaglandin endoperoxide in animal tissues. *Prostaglandins*, 14:1055–1074.
326. Svensson, J. (1979): Structure and quantitative determination of the major urinary metabolite of thromboxane B$_2$ in the guinea pig. *Prostaglandins*, 17:351–365.
327. Svensson, J., and Hamberg, M. (1976): Thromboxane A$_2$ and prostaglandin H$_2$: Potent stimulators of the swine coronary artery. *Prostaglandins*, 12:943–950.
328. Svensson, J., Hamberg, M., and Samuelsson, B. (1975): Prostaglandin endoperoxides IX. Characterization of rabbit aorta contracting substance (RCS) from guinea pig lung and human platelets. *Acta Physiol. Scand.*, 94:222–228.
329. Svensson, J., Hamberg, M., and Samuelsson, B. (1976): On the formation and effects of thromboxane A$_2$ in human platelets. *Acta Physiol. Scand.*, 98:285–294.
330. Svensson, J., Strandberg, K., Tuvemo, T., and Hamberg, M. (1977): Thromboxane A$_2$: Effects on airway and vascular smooth muscle. *Prostaglandins*, 14:425–436.
331. Szczeklik, A., Gryglewski, R. J., Grodzinska, L., Musial, J., Serwonska, M., and Marcinkiewicz, E. (1979): Platelet aggregability, thromboxane A$_2$ and malonaldehyde formation following administration of aspirin to man. *Thromb. Res.*, 15:405–413.
332. Szczeklik, A., Gryglewski, R. J., Musial, J., Grodzinska, L., Serwonska, M., and Marcinkiewicz, E. (1978): Thromboxane generation and platelet aggregation in survivals of myocardial infarction. *Thromb. Haemost.*, 40:66–74.
333. Szczeklik, A., Gryglewski, R. J., Nizankowski, R., and Musial, J. (1978): Circulatory and anti-platelet effects of intravenous prostacyclin in healthy men. *Pharmacol. Res. Commun.*, 10:545–556.
334. Tada, M., Kuznya, T., Inoue, M., Kadama, K., Fukkushima, M., and Abe, H. (1980): Significance of thromboxane A$_2$ in myocardial ischemia in patients with coronary artery disease. *Adv. Myocardiol.*, 2:397–405.
335. Tai, H. H., Lee, N., and Tai, C. L. (1980): Inhibition of thromboxane synthesis and platelet aggregation by pyridine and its derivatives. In: *Advances in Prostaglandin and Thromboxane Research*, Vol. 6, edited by B. Samuelsson, P. Ramwell, and R. Paoletti, pp. 447–452. Raven Press, New York.
336. Tai, H., Tai, C. L., and Lee, N. (1980): Selective inhibition of thromboxane synthetase by pyridine and its derivatives. *Arch. Biochem. Biophys.*, 203:758–763.
337. Tai, H., and Yuan, B. (1977): Biosynthesis of thromboxanes in sheep lung: Characterization, solubilization and resolution of the microsomal thromboxane synthetase complex. *Fed. Proc.*, 36:309.
338. Tai, H. H., and Yuan, B. (1978): Development of radioimmunoassay for thromboxane B$_2$. *Anal. Biochem.*, 87:343–349.
339. Tai, H. H., and Yuan, B. (1978): On the inhibitory potency of imidazole and its derivatives on thromboxane synthetase. *Biochem. Biophys. Res. Commun.*, 80:236–242.
340. Tai, H. H., and Yuan, B. (1978): Studies on the thromboxane synthesizing system in human platelet microsomes. *Biochim. Biophys. Acta*, 531:286–294.
341. Tanaka, K., Harada, Y., and Katori, M. (1979): EG 626: Not a thromboxane A$_2$ antagonist, but a PGI$_2$ potentiator in platelet aggregation. *Prostaglandins*, 17:235–237.
342. Tateson, J. E., Moncada, S., and Vane, J. R. (1977): Effects of prostacyclin (PGX) on cyclic AMP concentrations in human platelets. *Prostaglandins*, 13:389–397.
343. Terashita, Z., Fukkui, H., Nishikawa, K., Hirata, M., and Kikuchi, S. (1978): Coronary vasospastic action of thromboxane A$_2$ in isolated working guinea pig hearts. *Eur. J. Pharmacol.*, 53:49–56.
344. Treacher, D. T., Warlow, C., and McPherson, K. (1978): Aspirin and bleeding time. *Lancet*, ii:1378.
345. Tremoli, E., Folco, G., Agradi, E., and Galli, C. (1979): Platelet thromboxanes and serum cholesterol. *Lancet*, i:107–108.
346. Turk, J., Weiss, S. J., Davis, J. E., and Needleman, P. (1978): Fluorescent derivatives of prostaglandins and thromboxanes for liquid chromatography. *Prostaglandins*, 16:291–309.
347. Turner, S. R., Tainer, S. A., and Lynn, W. S. (1975): Biogenesis of chemotactic molecules by the arachidonate-lipoxygenase of platelets. *Nature*, 257:680–681.
348. Tuvemo, T., Strandberg, K., Hamberg, M., and Samuelsson, B. (1976): Formation and action of prostaglandin endoperoxides in the isolated human umbilical artery. *Acta Physiol. Scand.*, 96:145–149.

349. Vallee, E., Gougat, J., and Ageron, M. (1980): Inhibition of phospholipase A₂ as a mechanism for the anti-aggregatory effect of linoleic acid. *Agents Actions*, 10:57–62.
350. Vallee, E., Gougat, J., Navarro, J., and Delahayes, J. F. (1979): Anti-inflammatory and platelet anti-aggregating activity of phospholipase A₂ inhibitors. *J. Pharm. Pharmacol.*, 31:588–592.
351. Vane, J. R. (1978): Inhibitors of prostaglandin, prostacyclin, and thromboxane synthesis. In: *Advances in Prostaglandin and Thromboxane Research*, Vol. 4, edited by F. Coceani and P. Olley, pp. 27–44. Raven Press, New York.
352. Vargaftig, B. (1978): The inhibition of cyclo-oxygenase of rabbit platelets by aspirin is prevented by salicylic acid and by phenanthrolines. *Eur. J. Pharmacol.*, 50:231–241.
353. Vargaftig, B. B. (1978): Salicylic acid fails to inhibit generation of thromboxane A₂ activity in platelets after *in vivo* administration to the rat. *J. Pharm. Pharmacol.*, 30:101–104.
354. Vargaftig, B. B., and Lefort, J. (1977): Acute hypotension due to carrageenan, arachidonic acid and slow reacting substance in the rabbit: Role of platelets and nature of pharmacological antagonism. *Eur. J. Pharmacol.*, 43:125–141.
355. Vargaftig, B. B., and Zirinis, P. (1973): Platelet aggregation induced by arachidonic acid is accompanied by release of potential inflammatory mediators distinct from PGE₂ and PGF₂ₐ. *Nature New Biol.* 244:114–116.
356. Verheugt, F. W., and Serruys, P. W. (1981): Thromboxane release during pacing-induced angina. *Circulation*, 63:237.
357. Villa, S., Livio, M., and DeGaetano, G. (1979): The inhibitory effect of aspirin on platelet and vascular prostaglandins in rats cannot be completely dissociated. *Br. J. Haematol.*, 42:425–431.
358. Vincent, J. E., and Zijlstra, F. J. (1978): Formation by phospholipase A₂ of prostaglandins and endoperoxides in platelets of normal and essential fatty acid-deficient rats. In: *Advances in Prostaglandin and Thromboxane Research*, Vol. 3, edited by C. Galli, G. Galli, and G. Porcellati, pp. 147–158. Raven Press, New York.
359. Vincent, J. E., and Zijlstra, F. J. (1978): Nicotinic acid inhibits thromboxane synthesis in platelets. *Prostaglandins*, 15:629–636.
360. Vincent, J. E., Zijlstra, F. J., and van Vliet, H. (1980): Determination of the formation of thromboxane B₂ (TXB₂). 12L-hydroxy-5,8,10-heptadecatrienoic acid (HHT) and 12L-hydroxy-5,8,10,14-eicosatetraenoic acid (HETE) from arachidonic acid and of the TXB2:HHT, TXB2:HETE and (TXB2 + HHT):HETE ratio in human platelets. Possible use in diagnostic purposes. *Prostaglandins Med.*, 5:79–84.
361. Wang, H. H., Kulkarni, P. S., and Eakins, K. E. (1980): Effects of prostaglandins and thromboxane A₂ on the coronary circulation of adult dogs and puppies. *Eur. J. Pharmacol.*, 66:31–41.
362. Weidemann, M. J., Peskar, B. A., Wrogemann, K., Rietschel, E. T., Staudinger, H., and Fischer, H. (1978): Prostaglandin and thromboxane synthesis in a pure macrophage population and the inhibition, by E-type prostaglandins, of chemiluminescence. *FEBS Lett.*, 89:136–140.
363. Weiss, H. J. (1976): Antiplatelet drugs—a new approach to the prevention of thrombosis. *Am. Heart J.*, 92:86–102.
364. Weiss, H. J., and Lages, B. A. (1977): Possible congenital defect in platelet thromboxane synthetase. *Lancet*, i:760–761.
365. Whitaker, M. O., Wyche, A., Fitzpatrick, F., Sprecher, H., and Needleman, P. (1979): Triene prostaglandins: Prostaglandin D₃ and icosapentaenoic acid as potential antithrombotic substances. *Proc. Natl. Acad. Sci. USA*, 76:5919–5923.
366. White, J. G., and Gerrard, J. M. (1978): Platelet morphology and the ultrastructure of regulatory mechanisms involved in platelet activation. In: *Platelets: A Multidisciplinary Approach*, edited by G. DeGaetano and S. Garattini, pp. 17–34. Raven Press, New York.
367. White, J. G., Rao, G. H. R., and Gerrard, J. M. (1974): Effects of the ionophore A23187 on blood platelets. I. Influence on aggregation and secretion. *Am. J. Pathol.*, 77:135–149.
368. Williams, K. I., and Downing, I. (1977): Prostaglandin and thromboxane production by rat decidual microsomes. *Prostaglandins*, 14:813–817.
369. Willis, A. L. (1974): Isolation of a chemical trigger for thrombosis. *Prostaglandins*, 5:1–25.
370. Willis, A. L. (1974): An enzymatic mechanism for the antithrombotic and antihemostatic actions of aspirin. *Science*, 183:325–327.
371. Willis, A. L., Comai, K., Kuhn, D. C., and Paulsrud, J. (1974): Dihomo-γ-linolenate suppresses platelet aggregation when administered *in vitro* or *in vivo*. *Prostaglandins*, 8:509–519.
372. Willis, A. L., Vane, F. M., Kuhn, D. C., Scott, C. G., and Petrin, M. (1974): An endoperoxide aggregator (LASS) formed in platelets in response to thrombotic stimuli. *Prostaglandins*, 8:453–507.

373. Wlodawer, P., and Hammarström, S. (1978): Thromboxane synthase from bovine lung: Solubilization and partial purification. *Biochem. Biophys. Res. Commun.*, 80:525–532.
374. Wolfe, L. S., Rostworski, K., and Marion, J. (1976): Endogenous formation of the prostaglandin endoperoxide metabolite, thromboxane B$_2$, by brain tissue. *Biochem. Biophys. Res. Commun.*, 70:907–913.
375. Woods, H. F., Ash, G., Weston, M. J., Bunting, S., Moncada, S., and Vane, J. R. (1978): Prostacyclin can replace heparin in hemodialysis in dogs. *Lancet*, i:1075–1077.
376. Yarger, W. E., Schocken, D. D., and Harris, R. H. (1980): Obstructive nephropathy in the rat: Possible roles for the renin-angiotensin system, prostaglandins, and thromboxane in postobstructive renal function. *J. Clin. Invest.*, 65:400–412.
377. Yoshimoto, T., Yamamoto, S., and Hayaishi, O. (1978): Selective inhibition of prostaglandin endoperoxide thromboxane isomerase by 1-carboxyalkylimidazoles. *Prostaglandins*, 16:529–540.
378. Yoshimoto, T., Yamamoto, S., Okuma, M., and Hayaishi, O. (1977): Solubilization and resolution of thromboxane synthesizing system from microsomes of bovine blood platelets. *J. Biol. Chem.*, 252:5871–5874.
379. Ziboh, V. A., Maruta, H., Lord, J., Cagle, W. D., and Lucky, W. (1979): Increased biosynthesis of thromboxane A$_2$ by diabetic platelets. *Eur. J. Clin. Invest.*, 9:223–228.
380. Zimmerman, R., Thiessen, M., Mörl, H., and Weckesser, G. (1979): The paradoxical thrombogenic effect of aspirin in experimental thrombosis. *Thromb. Res.*, 16:843–846.
381. Zipser, R., Myers, S., and Needleman, P. (1980): Exaggerated prostaglandin and thromboxane synthesis in the rabbit with renal vein constriction. *Circ. Res.*, 47:231–237.

Prostaglandins and the Cardiovascular System,
edited by John A. Oates. Raven Press,
New York © 1982.

Prostacyclin: Its Biosynthesis, Actions, and Clinical Potential

*Gregory J. Dusting, **Salvador Moncada, and **John R. Vane

*University of Melbourne, Department of Medicine, (Austin Hospital), Heidelberg,
Victoria 3084, Australia; and **Wellcome Research Laboratories, Langley Court,
Beckenham, Kent, BR3 3BS England*

During 1975, Moncada, Gryglewski, Bunting, and Vane began to look for biosynthesis of thromboxane A_2 (TXA_2) by various tissues other than platelets. Vascular tissues did not generate TXA_2, but the cascade bioassay technique (300) showed that microsomal fractions of blood vessels converted the endoperoxide precursor enzymatically into an unknown product which was labile, and relaxed the celiac and mesenteric arteries of the rabbit (202). They called this substance PGX, and showed also that it inhibited platelet aggregation; in fact, it was the most potent inhibitor of platelet aggregation known, being 30 to 40 times more potent than prostaglandin E_1 (PGE_1) (208). In later work PGX was characterized further; it potently relaxed coronary (80) as well as splanchnic vascular strips *in vitro* (37), dilated vascular beds *in vivo* (12,13,84), and had strong antithrombotic activity *in vivo* (142,299). Furthermore, it was the major metabolite of arachidonic acid in vascular tissues (161,263). PGX was the unstable intermediate in the formation of 6-oxo-$PGF_{1\alpha}$, a compound described by Pace-Asciak as a product of prostaglandin endoperoxides in the rat stomach (239). The work which led to the elucidation of the structure of PGX was carried out as a collaborative effort between scientists from the Wellcome Research Laboratories and from the Upjohn Company (161). PGX was then renamed prostacyclin with the abbreviation of PGI_2. It has now been given the approved name of epoprostenol, but the trivial name of prostacyclin will be used throughout this review.

The discovery of prostacyclin, together with the isolation and characterization of the prostaglandin endoperoxides and TXA_2 which preceded it (130,131,132,228), have added substantially to our understanding of platelet-vessel wall interactions, and opened new lines of research in hemostasis and thrombosis. Another consequence which is also gathering momentum is a better understanding of the basis of some diseases. In this chapter we shall deal mainly with the way in which the balance between aggregatory and antiaggregatory metabolites of arachidonic acid affects the physiology and pathophysiology of hemostasis and thrombosis. We shall discuss the current view of regulation of prostacyclin biosynthesis and its pharmacological manipulation, including disturbances in its biosynthesis in some pathological conditions. Possible roles of prostacyclin in the heart will be discussed in some detail, but actions of prostacyclin in control of the general circulation and regional vascular beds are dealt with in other chapters in this volume. The therapeutic potential of prostacyclin as an antithrombotic agent will be discussed in the last section. Structures of prostacyclin and other metabolites of arachidonic acid relevant to this review are illustrated in Fig. 1.

PROSTACYCLIN BIOSYNTHESIS *IN VITRO*

Prostacyclin Synthetase

Prostacyclin is generated by blood vessel microsomes or fresh vascular tissue from the prostaglandin endoperoxide, PGH_2 (37,202). It is chemically unstable with a half-life of 2 to 3 min, breaking down to 6-oxo-$PGF_{1\alpha}$. Prostacyclin synthetase displays a broad pH optimum, and catalyzes a rapid conversion of saturating concentrations of PGH_2 at 37°C (263). Wlodawer and Hammarström (328) demonstrated

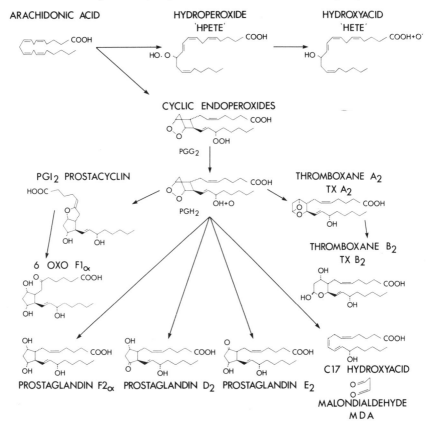

FIG. 1. Metabolic pathways of arachidonic acid.

that prostacyclin synthetase in porcine aorta microsomes was stimulated by the high-speed supernatant and that the soluble factor was nondialyzable and resistant to boiling. Unlike the formation of TXB_2 and HHT, formation of prostacyclin and 12-hydroxy,5,8,10 heptadecatrienoic acid (HHT) by porcine aortic microsomes are not coupled (328). Various tissues have been shown to generate prostacyclin or its stable breakdown product 6-oxo-$PGF_{1\alpha}$ (see Table 1).

Generation by the Vessel Wall

Prostacyclin has been shown to be the main product of arachidonic acid in all arteries and veins so far tested. Not much is known about the microcirculation but Goehlert et al. (112) have demonstrated that microvessels, mainly capillaries, isolated from rat cerebrum generate prostacyclin predominantly.

The ability of the large vessel wall to synthesize prostacyclin is greatest at the intimal surface and progressively decreases towards the adventitia (204). Production of prostacyclin by cultured cells from vessel walls also shows that endothelial cells are the most active producers of prostacyclin (186,318); moreover, this production persists after numerous subcultures *in vitro* (53).

Initially it was demonstrated that vessel microsomes in the absence of cofactors could utilize prostaglandin endoperoxides, but not arachidonic acid, to synthesize prostacyclin (202). Later it was shown that fresh vascular tissue could utilize both precursors although the endoperoxides are much better substrates (37). Moreover, vessel microsomes, fresh vascular rings, or endothelial cells treated with indomethacin could, when incubated with platelets, generate a prostacyclin-like antiaggregating activity (37,40,121). The release of this substance was inhibited by 15-hydroperoxy arachidonic acid (15-HPAA) and other fatty acid hydroperoxides known to be selective inhibitors of prostacyclin formation (121,203,263). From all these data we concluded that the vessel wall can synthesize prostacyclin from its own endogenous precursors, but also that it can utilize prostaglandin endoperoxides released by the platelets, thus suggesting a biochemical cooperation between platelet and vessel wall (208,209).

Several observations support this conclusion. Incubation of platelet-rich plasma (PRP) with fresh, indomethacin-treated arterial tissue leads to an increase in platelet cyclic AMP (24) which parallels the inhibition of the aggregation and can be abolished by previous treatment of the vascular tissue with tranylcypromine, a less active inhibitor of prostacyclin formation (121). Furthermore, Tansik et al. (291) showed that lysed aortic smooth muscle cells could be supplied with prostaglandin endoperoxides by lysed human platelets to form prostacyclin. Undisturbed endothelial cell monolayers can also readily transform PGH_2 to prostacyclin (190).

However, the hypothesis was later challenged by Needleman and associates who demonstrated that while arachidonic acid was rapidly converted to prostacyclin by perfused rabbit hearts and kidneys, PGH_2 was not readily transformed (220). They concluded that some degree of vascular damage is necessary for the endoperoxide to be utilized by prostacyclin synthetase (220).

TABLE 1. *Tissues which have been shown to generate prostacyclin or its stable breakdown product 6-oxo-PGF$_{1\alpha}$*

Tissue	Reference
Pig aortic microsomes	121,202
Rabbit microsomes	121,202
Pig mesenteric artery microsomes	121,202
Rabbit celiac and mesenteric arteries	37
Human mesenteric arteries and veins	205
Bovine coronary artery	80
Hamster aorta	141
Cultured endothelial cells; human umbilical and bovine aortic	53,318
Pig aortic endothelial cells	186
Pig post caval vein endothelium	186
Pig smooth muscle	186
Pig adventitial fibroblasts	186
Human arterial smooth muscle	16
Human skin fibroblasts	16
Mouse macrophages	152
Rabbit eye, iris, and conjunctiva	25
Bovine iris and ciliary body	174
Guinea pig perfused lung	67
Cat lung	122
Rabbit lung	206
Rabbit pleura, pericardium, and peritoneum	138
Guinea pig heart	270
Rabbit heart	68,220
Ductus arteriosus (fetal lamb)	241
Ductus arteriosus (fetal calf)	248
Fetal calf aorta	248
Rat kidney	331
Rabbit kidney	220
Human renal cortex	253
Pig kidney	294
Rabbit renal collecting tubule cells	117
Cat spleen	6
Rat stomach fundus microsomes	121
Rat stomach	239
Rat gastric mucosa	207
Rat small intestine	321
Uterus decidual tissue of pregnant rat	326
Myometrium of pregnant rat	325
Homogenates of pseudopregnant rat uterus	94
Human placenta	217
Human chorion, amnion, and decidua	201
Ram seminal vesicles	59
Rat inflammatory exudate	46
Rat cerebral microvessels and choroid plexus	112
Rat mesenteric arterial vessels	86,87

Needleman et al. (224) and Hornstra et al. (151) using vessel microsomes or fresh vascular tissue also concluded that endoperoxides from platelets cannot be utilized by other cells under their experimental conditions. However, more recently, Marcus et al. (191) showed that feeding of endoperoxides to endothelial cells suspended in PRP takes place *in vitro* but only when the platelet number is around normal blood levels. Too high a platelet concentration induces a platelet to platelet interaction which limits the platelet/endothelial cell reaction. It should be stressed, however, that the possibility of endoperoxides released from platelets being utilized by endothelial cells has not yet been tested *in vivo*. Adherence of the platelet to the vessel wall, known to be one of the first responses to injury, could well provide the close proximity that would be needed for such "cooperation."

It is also possible that formed elements of blood such as the white cells, which produce endoperoxides and TXA_2 (65,113,140), could interact with the vessel wall to promote formation of prostacyclin. Moreover, leucocytes themselves generate prostacyclin in whole blood, especially in the presence of thromboxane synthetase inhibitors (101). Thus, prostacyclin might regulate white cell behavior (143,315), and help control white cell activity during the inflammatory response. Interestingly, an artificial surface when exposed to blood *in vivo* initially becomes coated with platelets, but this is slowly replaced by a pavement of white cells. The white cell pavement is then unattractive to platelets, and this could be due to prostacyclin generation by the leucocytes.

STIMULATION OF PROSTACYCLIN BIOSYNTHESIS BY VASOACTIVE HORMONES *IN VITRO*

Bradykinin and angiotensin release prostaglandins from the kidney (5,193,194), lungs (301), and other organs *in vivo* (95). Before the discovery of prostacyclin, Gimbrone and Alexander (106) had demonstrated that angiotensin II stimulated generation of an immunoreactive, PGE-like substance by human umbilical endothelial cells in culture. Needleman and co-workers (31,219,222) had also described the release by angiotensin and bradykinin of a PGE-like substance from rabbit isolated perfused hearts and mesenteric vessels.

The PGE-like substance was characterized by bioassay on gastrointestinal tissues and chromatographic mobility on thin-layer plates. It is now clear that these techniques do not really distinguish between prostacyclin (or 6-oxo-$PGF_{1\alpha}$) and PGE_2 (208,237) and Needleman et al. (220) have now shown that bradykinin or angiotensin II release a PGI_2-like substance from Langendorff-perfused hearts of rabbits. Moreover, Dusting and Mullins (86,87) demonstrated that angiotensins I and II release much more prostacyclin than PGE_2 from perfused isolated mesenteric vasculature of rats, and prostacyclin was identified as the major prostaglandin released from the pulmonary circulation of the dog *in vivo* by angiotensin I or II (214). In contrast, the isolated perfused kidney of the rabbit converts exogenous arachidonate predominantly into prostacyclin, but PGE_2 is the main prostanoid released by bradykinin and angiotensin II into the venous effluent (220). However, perfusion of isolated kidneys with albumin-free Krebs' solution produces a large increase in glomerular filtration rate so that medullary perfusion is enhanced. Since PGE_2 is prevalent in the medulla and the effluent assayed is a mixture of venous and urinary outflow, this technique could account for the large quantities of PGE_2. In the canine kidney, *in vivo*, prostacyclin and not PGE_2 was identified as the main prostaglandin released into renal venous blood by angiotensin and bradykinin (214). Small quantities of PGE_2 (approximately 10% of those of prostacyclin) were observed in some experiments by these workers. These findings have renewed interest in the concept proposed by Vane and McGiff (302) that prostaglandins released by angiotensin and bradykinin may modulate or partly mediate the renal and vascular actions of these peptides (see following section and chapters on Prostaglandins and the Kidney, *this volume*).

The pulmonary circulation has long been recognized for its ability to transform arachidonic acid into more polar products. Indeed, all metabolites of arachidonic acid at one time or another have been proposed as major products generated by the lungs. Isolated perfused lungs of guinea pigs, rats, and rabbits release prostaglandins E_2 and $F_{2\alpha}$, TXA_2, lipoxygenase metabolites of arachidonic acid, prostacyclin, and metabolites of all these substances when they are perfused with histamine, bradykinin, 5-hydroxytryptamine, arachidonic acid, or when subjected to anaphylactic shock. These products are also generated when pulmonary tissue is subjected to mechanical trauma. Gryglewski (120) has recently reviewed evidence that isolated perfused lungs of cats, rats, rabbits, and guinea pigs release spontaneously a PGI_2-like substance, and little other arachidonate-derived material, when perfused through the pulmonary artery with Krebs' solution. Prostacyclin has been identified in the pulmonary effluent by relaxation of bovine coronary artery strips, by disaggregation of platelet clumps, and by mass spectrometric quantification of the stable degradation product of prostacyclin, 6-oxo-$PGF_{1\alpha}$. The output of prostacyclin is blocked by cyclooxygenase inhibitors and is stimulated by low concentrations of arachidonic acid (100 ng/ml), angiotensin I, angiotensin II, or bradykinin.

The release of prostacyclin induced by angiotensin I is blocked by the converting enzyme inhibitor, captopril, in guinea pig isolated lungs, rat mesenteric vasculature (86,87,118,120), and the pulmonary and renal circulation of anesthetized dogs *in vivo* (76,213). Prostacyclin release induced by angiotensin I or II is also abolished by the receptor antagonists saralasin or [Sar^1-Ile^8]-angiotensin II in both the rat and the dog (75,87,120). Thus, prostacyclin is released by activation of an angiotensin II receptor, and is not released directly by angiotensin I. Activation of the angiotensin receptor appears to be linked to a phospholipase, since angiotensin II-stimulated prostacyclin release can be abolished by dexamethasone and mepacrine (75).

Other peptides or amines tested do not release prostacyclin from perfused lungs (120). Norepinephrine and vasopressin do not release prostacyclin from rat mesenteric vessels, despite their potent vasoconstrictor effects (86,87). Moreover, prostacyclin release into the circulation of the dog was not observed with injections of epinephrine, norepinephrine, 5-hydroxytryptamine, or acetylcholine (214), despite changes in systemic blood pressure.

Therefore, the release of prostacyclin induced by angiotensin and bradykinin does not appear to be a simple consequence of the mechanical events associated with alterations in vessel diameter. These observations, together with the finding that low concentrations of prostacyclin are released from the lungs *in vivo*, prompted the proposal that the pulmonary endothelium may be regarded as an endocrine organ regulating platelet behavior (122,123,206).

EVIDENCE FOR BIOSYNTHESIS OF PROSTACYCLIN *IN VIVO*: IS IT A CIRCULATING HORMONE?

In rats and dogs, prostacyclin is a much more powerful vasodepressor agent than PGE_2, but only when the two substances are given intravenously, and not if they are given into the aorta (12,13). Using dogs, we showed by direct bioassay in circulating blood that prostacyclin escapes the pulmonary inactivation process (81), which normally removes 95% or more of PGE_2 and $PGF_{2\alpha}$ in a single circulation *in vivo*. Thus, prostacyclin can recirculate (83). Furthermore, infused arachidonic acid is converted into prostacyclin in passage across the lungs *in vivo* (79,212). Therefore, prostacyclin generated in the lung or elsewhere would not be confined to a local site of action, and is potentially a circulating hormone.

Gryglewski et al. (122) developed a technique for continuously measuring platelet aggregation in circulating blood of anesthetized cats, and showed that arterial blood contained higher concentrations of an antiaggregatory substance than mixed venous blood. They concluded that the arterial/venous difference was due to prostacyclin released from the lungs since the difference was abolished by aspirin or by incubating the blood at 37°C for 10 min, during which time prostacyclin activity disappears (81,83). Moncada et al. (206) applied this technique to anesthetized rabbits, and came to the same conclusion, since the greater disaggregatory activity present in arterial blood was abolished by an antibody raised against 5,6-dihydro PGI_2, which cross-reacts with prostacyclin. Moreover, the PGI_2-like, disaggregatory substance in arterial blood is increased during hyperventilation of the lungs, or during pulmonary embolism induced by intravenous injection of air (120). In a recent study, 6-oxo-$PGF_{1\alpha}$, measured by mass spectrometry, was found at a higher concentration in the arterial than in the venous side of the circulation of 5 patients undergoing cardiac catheterization (136). Thus, the lungs may constantly release small amounts of prostacyclin into the passing blood. This, combined with 50% overall inactivation in one circulation through peripheral tissues (83), would account for higher levels in arterial than in venous blood.

Three reservations about these results should be mentioned. Firstly, in the studies with anesthetized cats and rabbits, blood was drawn through an extracorporeal circuit with a peristaltic pump. Under such conditions, the circulating blood volume would be reduced slightly and this may lead to a stimulation of the renin-angiotensin system which, in turn, could stimulate prostacyclin release (see later). In addition, it is now well recognized that surgical procedures in anesthetized small animals can exaggerate the contribution of prostaglandins to renal homeostasis (295) and, by analogy, the same may be true for the lungs. Secondly, in these extracorporeal experiments platelet emboli dislodged from the collagen strips return to the animal in the venous blood. The trapping of platelet emboli in the lungs may be an artificial stimulus for generation of prostacyclin under these conditions (3). Platelet emboli are also generated and returned to the animal in other extracorporeal systems, particularly when venous blood is reoxygenated for bioassay on a cascade of smooth muscle strips. Thirdly, the biotransformation of prostacyclin in the human circulation is not yet fully understood, and the assumption that 6-oxo-PGF$_{1\alpha}$ determined in blood samples is a reliable index of concentrations of active prostacyclin in circulating blood may not be valid. Recent studies of human platelet aggregation performed within 3 min of withdrawal of arterial or venous blood (282) led to the conclusion that circulating levels of prostacyclin in resting man were too low to influence aggregability of platelets, but again it is important to note that these tests were performed *in vitro*. Studies in which levels of prostacyclin or its metabolites have been determined in man have failed to clarify the situation. Prostacyclin-like activity was detectable in human venous blood used to superfuse various tissues sensitive to prostacyclin (225). The level rose by several ng/ml with relief of ischemia and was reduced by pretreatment with indomethacin. However, in a study in which 6-oxo-PGF$_{1\alpha}$ in human blood samples was measured by mass spectrometry levels of 80 pg/ml in venous blood and approximately double in arterial blood were obtained (136). Although these levels are lower than those measured by bioassay they are still much higher than those obtained by measuring the daily turnover in urine of a metabolite of prostacyclin (229). Further work is necessary to establish clearly the routes of catabolism of both prostacyclin and 6-oxo-PGF$_{1\alpha}$ in the human circulation to determine if there is an effective level of circulating prostacyclin in normal man at rest or during exercise.

INTERACTIONS OF PROSTACYCLIN AND THE RENIN-ANGIOTENSIN AND KALLIKREIN-KININ SYSTEMS

There is convincing evidence that activation of the renin-angiotensin system stimulates prostacyclin release *in vivo*. In addition to the *in vitro* data discussed previously, Gryglewski (120) has demonstrated that angiotensins I and II release a PGI$_2$-like substance into arterial blood of anesthetized cats. Similar results were obtained by Dusting (75,76,86) and by Mullane and Moncada (214) in anesthetized dogs using bovine coronary strips to bioassay prostacyclin. Release of a PGI$_2$-like substance from the kidney also follows intrarenal infusion of angiotensins (120, 214,272), and it has been detected in jugular vein following intracarotid infusion of angiotensin II (120). Thus, angiotensin releases prostacyclin from at least three vascular beds *in vivo*—those of the lungs, kidneys, and the head. During intravenous infusion of angiotensin II in dogs, Dusting (76,86) found a much higher concentration of the PGI$_2$-like substance in arterial blood than in blood withdrawn from the right atrium or pulmonary artery, suggesting that at least in this species the predominant source of prostacyclin released into the circulation following activation of the systemic renin-angiotensin system is the lungs.

Interestingly, release of the PGI$_2$-like substance by angiotensin II in dogs was reduced, but not abolished, by indomethacin in doses up to 10 mg/kg, i.v. (76,86). The PGI$_2$-like substance which was released by angiotensin II from the lungs caused relaxation of bovine coronary artery and was inactivated in extravasated blood at a similar rate as prostacyclin (76,86). Its release was abolished by intravenous infusion of the antagonist [Sar^1-Ile^8]-angiotensin II (76). Catecholamines, acetylcholine, bradykinin, histamine, 5-hydroxytryptamine, adenosine, and metabolites of angiotensin were excluded as possible mediators of this effect. Moreover, Mullane et al. (212,214) noted that the arterial blood concentrations of prostacyclin induced by intravenous infusions of arachidonic acid or angiotensin, as determined by bioassay using bovine coronary artery strips, were greater than could be accounted for by radioimmunoassay of 6-oxo-PGF$_{1\alpha}$ in extracts of arterial blood. Therefore, it is possible that angiotensin II or arachidonic acid releases from the lungs, *in vivo*, prostacyclin along with another substance which has many of the properties of prostacyclin, but which is not formed via the cyclooxygenase pathway. Alternatively, if the activity is accounted for by prostacyclin, the pulmonary site of biosynthesis must be resistant to inhibition by acute intravenous indomethacin treatment.

It is interesting that kidney and brain, which appear to be rich in a local renin-angiotensin system (103), and the lung, which is the major site for angiotensin I conversion (226), can all release prostacyclin into the circulation. Indeed, stimulation of prostacyclin biosynthesis may be particularly important when the local vascular renin-angiotensin system is activated. Dusting and colleagues (75,87) suggested that the local concentration of angiotensin II at the "phospholipase receptor," which initiates prostacyclin biosynthesis, may be higher than it is at the receptor site in vascular smooth muscle. Certainly, locally formed angiotensin II is a more effective stimulus for prostacyclin biosynthesis than exogenous angiotensin II in the perfusion fluid of rat mesenteric vasculature (87).

Prostacyclin is a potent stimulator of renin release from renal tissue and it may be the obligatory endogenous mediator of renin secretion by the kidney (see chapter by Oates, Branch, and Jackson, *this volume*). It is difficult to postulate what controls the positive feedback mechanism whereby angiotensin II releases prostacyclin, which in turn stimulates renin secretion and leads to further angiotensin II formation. One possibility is that sodium balance may finely tune either angiotensin-induced prostacyclin release, or the stimulation of renin secretion by prostacyclin, or both. Perhaps Bartter's syndrome (105) represents a distortion of this regulatory mechanism (see following chapters, *this volume*). Much remains to be learned about these interrelationships.

Bradykinin is also a potent stimulus for prostacyclin release into the vascular compartment of the kidney (214). Indeed, it appears that prostacyclin is the principal mediator of renal vasodilatation elicited by bradykinin (214) since it is the major product generated in the vascular compartment, but PGE$_2$ synthesized in the medullary interstitium and collecting ducts may partly mediate the naturietic actions of this peptide (195). Furthermore, after treatment with captopril, which inhibits kininase II, the renal vasodilator action of bradykinin is potentiated, and this can be attributed to increased prostacyclin generation (213). Mullane and Moncada (213), concluded that prostacyclin, mainly of renal origin, may contribute to the antihypertensive action of captopril. Indeed, it has recently been reported that the action of captopril in patients with low-renin essential hypertension was reversed by concomitant administration of indomethacin (1). However, in another group of patients with normal or high plasma renin, administration of captopril was followed by a similar reduction in blood pressure, which was not altered by indomethacin (1). Moreover, several groups have reported that indomethacin or aspirin fail to alter the hypotensive action of captopril in spontaneously hypertensive rats which are widely studied as a model of human essential hypertension (9,71). Thus, it is possible that captopril exerts its antihypertensive action through more than one mechanism, depending not only on the form of hypertension involved, but also on the doses of captopril required to achieve reduction of blood pressure.

ACTIONS OF PROSTACYCLIN ON PLATELETS AND BLOOD VESSELS

Prostacyclin is the most potent endogenous inhibitor of platelet aggregation yet discovered. It is 30 to 40 times more potent than PGE_1 (208) and more than 1,000 times more active than adenosine (32). *In vivo*, prostacyclin applied locally in low concentrations inhibits thrombus formation due to adenosine diphosphate in the microcirculation of the hamster cheek pouch (142), and given systemically to the rabbit it prevents electrically-induced thrombus formation in the carotid artery and increases bleeding time (299). The duration of these effects *in vivo* is short; they disappear within 30 min of administration. Prostacyclin disaggregates platelets *in vitro* (203,299), in extracorporeal circuits where platelet clumps have formed on collagen strips (122,124), and in the circulation of man (287). Moreover, it inhibits thrombus formation in a coronary artery model in the dog when given locally or systemically (4) and protects against sudden death induced by intravenous arachidonic acid in rabbits (18).

Prostacyclin is unstable and its activity disappears within 15 sec on boiling or within 10 min at 22°C at neutral pH. In blood at 37°C, the activity of prostacyclin (as measured by bioassay on vascular smooth muscle) has a half-life of 3 min (81,83). It has recently been reported that prostacyclin has an extended stability in plasma or blood (107) and that this may be associated with binding to albumin or with metabolism to 6-oxo-PGE_1 (29). The relevance of these observations to the actual biological activity remains unclear. Alkaline pH increases the stability of prostacyclin (52,161) so that at pH 10.5 at 25°C, it has a half-life of 100 hr. It can be stabilized as a pharmaceutical preparation by freeze drying and can be reconstituted for use in man in an alkaline glycine buffer.

Role of Prostacyclin in Vascular Homeostasis

The generation of prostacyclin is an active mechanism by which the vessel wall could be protected from deposition of platelet aggregates. Thus, prostacyclin formation provides an explanation of the long recognized fact that contact with healthy vascular endothelium is not a stimulus for platelet clumping. An imbalance between formation of prostacyclin and TXA_2 could be of dramatic consequence.

Vascular damage leads to platelet adhesion but not necessarily to thrombus formation. When the injury is minor, platelet thrombi are formed which break away from the vessel wall and are washed away by the circulation. The degree of injury is an important determinant, and there is general agreement that for the development of thrombosis, severe damage or physical detachment of the endothelium must occur. All these observations are in accord with the differential distribution of prostacyclin synthetase across the vessel wall, decreasing in concentration from the intima to the adventitia (204). Moreover, the proaggregating elements increase from the subendothelium to the adventitia. These two opposing tendencies render the endothelial lining antiaggregatory and the outer layers of the vessel wall thrombogenic (204).

The ability of the vascular wall actively to prevent aggregation has been postulated before (261). For instance, the presence of an ADPase in the vessel wall has led to the suggestion that this enzyme, by breaking down ADP, limits platelet aggregation (139,181). We have confirmed the presence of an ADPase in the vessel wall. However, the antiaggregating activity is mainly related to the release of prostacyclin, for 15-hydroxyperoxy arachidonic acid (15-HPAA) or 13-hydroxyperoxy linoleic acid (13-HPLA), two inhibitors of prostacyclin formation which have no activity on ADPase, abolish most if not all of the antiaggregatory activity of vascular endothelial cells (40). Similar results have been obtained using an antiserum which cross-reacts with and neutralizes prostacyclin *in vitro* (39). Endothelial cells pretreated with this antiserum can no longer inhibit ADP-induced aggregation (39,53).

It is not yet clear whether prostacyclin is responsible for all the thromboresistant properties of the vascular endothelium and it would be unusual for an important biological principle to rely on a single mechanism. Prostacyclin inhibits platelet aggregation (platelet-platelet interaction) at much lower concentrations than those needed to inhibit adhesion (platelet-collagen interaction) (144). Czervionke et al. (63), using endothelial cell cultures, have demonstrated that platelet adherence to vascular endothelium in the presence of thrombin increases from 4% to 44% after treatment with 1 mM aspirin. This increase was accompanied by a decrease in 6-oxo-$PGF_{1\alpha}$ formation from 107 nM to < 3 nM and could be reversed by addition of 25 nM of exogenous prostacyclin. This work suggests that prostacyclin can allow platelets to stick to vascular tissue and to interact with it, while at the same time preventing or limiting thrombus formation. Certainly, platelets adhering to a site where prostacyclin synthetase is present could well feed the enzyme with endoperoxide, thereby producing prostacyclin and preventing other platelets from clumping on to the adhering platelets, limiting the cells to a monolayer. Weiss and Turitto (314) have observed some degree of inhibition of platelet-endothelium interactions with low concentrations of prostacyclin at high shear rates, but at none of the concentrations used could they observe total inhibition of platelet adhesion.

Mechanism of Action on Platelets

Prostacyclin inhibits platelet aggregation by stimulating adenylate cyclase, leading to an increase in cyclic AMP levels in the platelets (115,292). In this respect prostacyclin is much more potent that either PGE_1 or PGD_2 (292). 6-Oxo-$PGF_{1\alpha}$ has relatively weak antiaggregatory activity and is almost devoid of activity on platelet cyclic AMP (292).

Prostacyclin is not only more potent than PGE_1 in elevating cyclic AMP but the elevation persists longer. The elevation induced by PGE_1 in platelets *in vitro* starts falling after 30 sec, while prostacyclin stimulation is not maximal until after 30 sec and is maintained for 2 min after which it gradually wanes over 30 min (115). Prostacyclin also strongly stimulates adenylate cyclase in isolated membrane preparations (115).

Prostacyclin, PGE_1, and PGD_2 stimulate adenylate cyclase by acting on two distinct receptors on the platelet membrane (199,323). PGE_1 and prostacyclin act on one, whereas PGD_2 acts on another. This is shown by differences in activity in different species (323), and by the use of a prostaglandin antagonist (93) that selectively prevents the inhibition of platelet aggregation induced by PGD_2, but not that induced by prostacyclin or PGE_1 (323). Moreover, studies of agonist-specific sensitization of cyclic AMP accumulation in platelets show that PGE_1 or PGE_2 can desensitize for subsequent PGE_1 or prostacyclin activation, and that subthreshold concentrations of prostacyclin desensitize for PGE_1 stimulation. PGD_2, however, desensitizes to a further dose of PGD_2 but not to PGE_1 or prostacyclin (199). These results suggest (199,323) that the previously recognized PGE_1 receptor in platelets (200) is, in fact, a prostacyclin receptor, especially since there is now general acceptance that PGE_1 is unlikely to be endogenously formed in the circulatory system.

There have not been many detailed studies of the mechanism of action of prostacyclin. In contrast to TXA_2, it enhances Ca^{2+} sequestration (169). Moreover, an inhibitory effect on platelet phospholipase (177,200) and platelet cyclooxygenase have been described (188). All these activities are related to its ability to increase cyclic AMP in platelets. Moreover, prostacyclin inhibits endoperoxide-induced aggregation, which suggests additional sites of action still undefined but dependent on the cyclic AMP effect (200). These observations have extended and given important biological significance to the original observation of Vargaftig and Chignard (303), who demonstrated that substances such as PGE_1 that increase cyclic AMP in platelets inhibit the release of TXA_2 (measured as rabbit aorta contracting activity) in platelets. Prostacyclin, by inhibiting several steps in the activation of the arachidonic acid cascade, exerts an overall control of platelet aggregability *in vivo*.

Prostacyclin increases cyclic AMP levels in cells other than platelets including cultured human fibroblasts (116), human fat cell ghosts (168), and guinea pig lung homogenates (185). Thus, there is the possibility that in these cells an interaction with the thromboxane system could lead to a similar control of cell behavior to that observed in platelets, suggesting that the PGI_2/TXA_2 system has wider biological significance in cell regulation and the definition of cell receptors for prostaglandins. Recently, Hopkins and Gorman (150) have shown that prostacyclin increases cyclic AMP in the endothelial cell itself and have suggested that this may act as a negative feedback control for prostacyclin production by the endothelium.

Actions on Isolated Blood Vessels

Prostacyclin relaxes, *in vitro*, most vascular strips including rabbit celiac and mesenteric arteries (37), bovine coronary arteries (80,220), human and baboon cerebral arteries (33), and lamb ductus arteriosus (57). Exceptions to this include the porcine coronary arteries (82), some strips of rat venous tissue, and isolated human saphenous vein (179), which are weakly contracted by prostacyclin. The relevance of these contractile activities is uncertain, for prostacyclin is vasodilator *in vivo* in all vascular beds so far studied. In the human umbilical arterial strip, prostacyclin induces a dose-dependent relaxation at low concentrations ($<10^{-6}$ M) and a dose-dependent contraction at higher ones ($>10^{-5}$ M) (247). As mentioned earlier, prostacyclin, and not PGE_2, is the main metabolite of arachidonic acid in isolated vascular tissue, and this has led to intense study for reassessment of the effects and role of arachidonic acid and its metabolites in vascular tissue and the cardiovascular system. We have reviewed these aspects before (85), and they are further discussed in this chapter (under "Roles of Prostacyclin in the Heart"), and in subsequent chapters in this volume.

FACTORS AFFECTING PROSTACYCLIN FORMATION: THE ROLE OF PROSTACYCLIN IN HEMOSTASIS AND THROMBOSIS

In their early experiments, Gryglewski et al. (121) observed that a fatty acid peroxide, 15-hydroperoxy arachidonic acid (15-HPAA), strongly and selectively inhibited prostacyclin synthetase, the enzyme which forms prostacyclin from endoperoxides in vessel microsomes ($IC_{50} \simeq 0.5$ μg/ml). Other fatty acid hydroperoxides and their methyl esters also inhibit this enzyme (208,263). Tranylcypromine, which is a well known inhibitor of enzymes not related to the metabolic pathway of arachidonic acid, is a somewhat weaker inhibitor of prostacyclin synthetase ($IC_{50} \simeq 160$ μg/ml) than are the fatty acid hydroperoxides (121). Unfortunately, hydroperoxides of fatty acids are not useful tools for examining the role of endogenous prostacyclin biosynthesis *in vivo* (84), probably because they are rapidly reduced by enzymes such as glutathione peroxidase (54). Other substances which inhibit prostacyclin synthetase in blood vessel microsomes include analogs of prostaglandin endoperoxide (9,11-diaza- and 9,11-epoxyimino-prosta-5,12 dienoic acid) (100), and a hydroperoxy derivative of indole (293).

Prostaglandin endoperoxides are at the crossroads of arachidonic acid metabolism for they are precursors of substances with opposing biological properties (see Fig. 1). On the one hand, TXA_2 produced by the platelets is a strong contractor of large blood vessels and induces platelet aggregation. On the other hand, prostacyclin produced by the vessel wall is a strong vasodilator and the most potent inhibitor of platelet aggregation known. Each substance has opposing effects on cyclic AMP concentrations in platelets (209), thereby giving a balanced control mechanism which will, therefore, affect thrombus and hemostatic plug formation (see Fig. 2). Selective inhibition of the formation of TXA_2 should lead to an increased bleeding time and inhibition of thrombus formation, whereas inhibition of prostacyclin formation should be propitious for a "prothrombotic state". The amount of control exerted by this system can be tested, for selective inhibitors of each pathway have been described (see later).

Cyclooxygenase Inhibition

Until the discovery of prostacyclin, the use of aspirin as an antithrombotic agent, based on its effect on platelets, looked very clear (187,189), although the results of clinical trials were inconclusive (306). Now, however, the situation requires further clarification. Because aspirin inhibits cyclooxygenase, it can prevent production of TXA_2 and also of prostacyclin. Aspirin binds covalently to the active

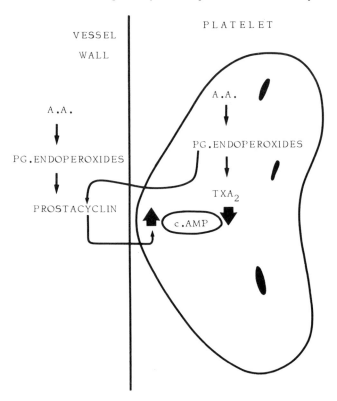

FIG. 2. Schematic representation of the relationship between prostacyclin, thromboxane A_2, and platelet cyclic AMP.

site of cyclooxygenase and, therefore, inhibits the enzyme in platelets for their entire lifespan because platelets are unable to synthesize new protein (189,283). Aspirin also has an effect on the platelet precursors in the marrow (44). Inhibition of the vascular cyclooxygenase, however, may persist for a much shorter period because of the generation of new enzyme. Also, the cyclooxygenase of human skin fibroblasts and of arterial smooth muscle cells appeared less sensitive to inhibition by aspirin than that of human platelets (16). However, Preston et al. (249) using vein samples from 5 subjects who had ingested low-dose aspirin, concluded that there is little difference in the initial (8 hr) substantial inhibition of cyclooxygenase seen in platelets or vessel wall.

In rabbits, aspirin has a biphasic effect on cutaneous bleeding time and on the formation of platelet clumps in an extracorporeal system. Low doses increase the bleeding time and are antithrombotic, but with higher doses neither effect occurs (8,172). This dose-dependent effect has been attributed to the low dose affecting only platelets and allowing prostacyclin production to continue, while both systems are inhibited by high-dose aspirin. O'Grady and Moncada (232) showed that in healthy volunteers ingestion of a single dose of aspirin of 0.3 g significantly prolonged bleeding time but a dose of 3.9 g had no significant effect on bleeding time. These results have been confirmed by some (250) but not by others (111). Godal et al. (111) measured bleeding time in healthy volunteers before and 2 hr after 0.425 or 3.875 g aspirin orally. Bleeding time increased to a similar extent after both high- and low-dose aspirin. However, the volunteers in the study by O'Grady and Moncada (232) were aged between 20 and 34 while those in the study by Godal et al. (111) were older, aged between 21 and 56. Subsequently, Jorgensen et al. (163) showed that bleeding time in man decreased with age and confirmed that higher doses of aspirin produced a significantly shorter bleeding time than low doses in the age groups 18 to 32 and 28 to 32 years, but not in the age group 66 to 70 years. These findings are consistent with a decrease in prostacyclin production with age.

Amezcua et al. (7) showed that following a single high oral dose of aspirin (3.9 g) the bleeding time is unchanged 2 hr after ingestion, although marked inhibition of platelet function and TXA_2 release is demonstrable. Twenty-four and 72 hr after aspirin, the bleeding time increased substantially, returning to normal levels 1 week after treatment. This suggests that shortly after high-dose aspirin the production of prostacyclin and TXA_2 was blocked. As the recovery of the endothelial cyclooxygenase proceeded faster than the release of new platelets, the ratio of prostacyclin to TXA_2 was changed in favor of prostacyclin at 24 and 72 hr after treatment, thus explaining the increased bleeding time and its slow recovery over 1 week. Aspirin, 0.3 g daily and 0.6 g twice daily administered for 7 days, both prolonged the bleeding time measured 2 hr after the first and last doses (296). However, at the higher dose the bleeding time was significantly shorter after the last as compared to the first aspirin dose and this could reflect inhibition of prostacyclin generation by chronic aspirin dosing. How these short-term effects relate to effects over much longer periods is unknown. However, Harter et al. (135) have shown that low-dose aspirin (160 mg/day) significantly reduced thrombus formation in arteriovenous shunts in patients on chronic hemodialysis.

Thromboxane Synthetase Inhibitors

Theoretically, a selective inhibitor of thromboxane synthetase should prove to be a superior antithrombotic agent to aspirin, by allowing prostacyclin formation by vessel walls or other cells, either from their own endoperoxides or from those released from platelets. Needleman et al. (224) observed that when platelets were treated with a thromboxane synthetase inhibitor *in vitro* then endoperoxides were available for utilization by the vessel wall. Interestingly, in the presence of a thromboxane synthetase inhibitor, arachidonic acid or collagen added to blood *in vitro* lead to the formation of 6-oxo-PGF$_{1\alpha}$ rather than TXB$_2$ (28,101). Platelets cannot synthesize prostacyclin, so some other blood cell must have done so. We have shown that injection of heterologous blood into anesthetized cats causes hypotension, respiratory distress, and frequently death and that this is accompanied by a sharp rise in blood levels of TXB$_2$ (Fig. 3). Pretreatment with either a thromboxane synthetase inhibitor (an imidazole derivative) or a cyclooxygenase inhibitor, such as aspirin, prevented death. However, after inhibition of thromboxane synthetase the blood levels of 6-oxo-PGF$_{1\alpha}$ rose about five times more than after the shock in control animals, suggesting diversion of the platelet prostaglandin endoperoxides away from TXA$_2$ production towards prostacyclin production (Fig. 3).

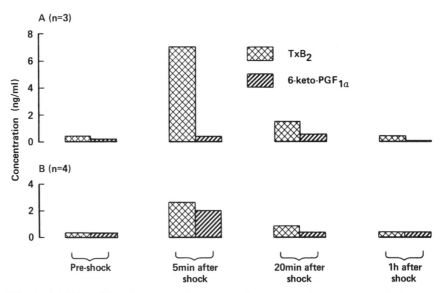

FIG. 3. Inhibition of thromboxane synthetase was demonstrated by a reduction in TXB$_2$ levels by more than 50%. Levels of 6-keto-PGF$_{1\alpha}$ in the treated group, however, were increased approximately fivefold suggesting a diversion of platelet endoperoxides towards conversion by the vessel wall to prostacyclin. **A:** Control cats. **B:** Cats given thromboxane synthetase inhibitor (6 mg/kg) 30 min before shock.

Other work on selective thromboxane synthetase inhibitors is beginning to appear (96) including the first publications on administration of one of these compounds to man (298,304).

Whether other drugs exert their antithrombotic effect by acting on the prostacyclin/thromboxane system is not yet known but studies using sulphinpyrazone in cultured endothelial cells (114) and ticlopidine given orally to rats (14) suggest that these compounds have little or no effect on prostacyclin formation at concentrations at which they affect platelet behavior. A compound which might stimulate prostacyclin formation in humans after oral ingestion has also been described (305).

Lipid Peroxides, Atherosclerosis, and Lipoproteins

High concentrations of lipid peroxides have been demonstrated in advanced atherosclerotic lesions (110). Lipid peroxidation induced by free radical formation is known to occur in vitamin E deficiency, the aging process, and perhaps also in hyperlipidemia accompanying atherosclerosis (277). Since lipid peroxides are selective inhibitors of prostacyclin generation (121,208,263), their accumulation in atheromatous plaques could predispose to thrombus formation. Moreover, platelet aggregation is induced by 15-HPAA and this aggregation is not inhibited by adenosine or PGE$_1$ (198). D'Angelo et al. (64) reported that human atheromatous plaques from 3 patients were incapable of prostacyclin production. Prostacyclin generation by atherosclerotic arterial tissue has been shown to be significantly lower than from normal arterial tissue but no difference was found between early and advanced atherosclerotic lesions (275). This suggests that the early "fatty streak" may be a biochemically critical stage of the atherosclerotic process. Bourgain et al. (34), using a model of thrombosis *in vivo* in the rat, demonstrated that application of 15-HPAA to the outside of mesenteric vessels increased the rate of thrombus formation in response to superfusion with ADP. All these results, therefore, suggest that it would be worth exploring whether attempts to reduce lipid peroxide formation by inhibiting peroxidation influence the development of atherosclerosis and arterial thrombosis. Vitamin E acts as an antioxidant and perhaps the enthusiasm for its use in arterial disease in the past (35,128,192) had, in fact, a biochemical rationale.

Raised concentrations of low density lipoprotein (LDL) are regarded as one of the risk factors associated with ischemic heart disease (166,196,284), whereas high density lipoprotein (HDL) is thought to protect against the disease (166,284). Nordoy et al. (227) were the first to show that LDL reduced the release of a prostacyclin-like substance by human endothelial cells. Beitz and Förster (19) extended these observations by showing that LDL inhibited, wherease HDL stimulated, prostacyclin synthesis. A mixture of LDL and HDL also stimulated prostacyclin synthesis. Gryglewski and Szczeklik (126) have confirmed that LDL inhibits prostacyclin synthesis. More importantly, they also discovered from an analysis of lipoproteins taken from a group of hyperlipidemics that the LDL fraction (but not the HDL) contained lipid peroxides at a concentration several times higher than those in the total serum. Thus, the interesting possibility arises that it is the lipid peroxide associated with LDL which inhibits prostacyclin synthesis and this inhibition explains the correlation between LDL and ischemic heart disease.

Cell proliferation *in vitro* is inhibited by substances which stimulate cyclic AMP formation (244). Cell growth in tissue culture (162,269), including vascular smooth muscle cell culture (154), is inhibited by PGE_1. Possibly prostacyclin has a role in the regulation of cell growth in the vascular wall. Smooth muscle proliferation in atherosclerotic plaques (21) might be a consequence of inhibition of prostacyclin generation by lipid peroxides.

Modification of Fatty Acid Precursors

Enrichment of the diet with dihomo-γ-linolenic acid, the precursor of monoenoic prostaglandins has been suggested as a means of preventing thrombosis, since PGG_1 and TXA_1 are not proaggregatory and PGE_1 is antiaggregatory (327). However, feeding rabbits with sufficient dihomo-γ-linolenic acid to elevate its content in tissues does not alter the platelet sensitivity to ADP (230). Since the discovery of prostacyclin it has become apparent that this is not the most rational approach to dietary manipulation, since PG endoperoxides of the '1' series cannot give rise to a prostacyclin. Eicosapentaenoic acid (EPA), on the other hand, gives rise to prostaglandins of the '3' series and when incubated with vascular tissue leads to the release of antiaggregating substance (125). Synthetic $\Delta 17$-prostacyclin or PGI_3 is as potent an antiaggregatory agent as prostacyclin. In contrast, TXA_3 has a weaker proaggregatory activity than TXA_2 (125,252). The fatty acid available for PG biosynthesis in Greenland Eskimos is mainly EPA, unlike that in caucasians which is mainly arachidonic acid (91). These differences may explain why Eskimos have a low incidence of acute myocardial infarction, low blood cholesterol levels, and an increased tendency to bleed (91). This prolonged bleeding time is related to a reduction in *ex vivo* platelet aggregability (89). The plasma concentrations of cholesterol, triglyceride, low and very low density lipoprotein (VLDL) are low in Eskimos, whereas that of HDL is high (17).

In a crossover experiment in which the effects on human subjects of addition of cheese or fish to a basic lacto-ovo-vegetarian diet were compared, subjects on the fish diet had lowered serum cholesterol, triglycerices, and VLDL, and elevated HDL compared with those on the cheese diet (307).

Dietary polyunsaturated fats are generally considered to be less harmful than saturated ones. However, attention should now be given to whether only those which can lead to the synthesis of prostacyclins are beneficial in preventing thrombosis and atherosclerosis. Indeed, other polyunsaturated fats may even be deleterious to the prostacyclin protective mechanism since they are easily oxidized, either spontaneously or enzymically, to the corresponding hydroperoxy acid, and fatty acid peroxides are potent inhibitors of prostacyclin synthetase (see previous section). A polyunsaturated fatty-acid-rich diet fed to pigs in the absence of vitamin E (a natural antioxidant) causes endothelial damage followed by thrombosis (218) perhaps because of inhibition of prostacyclin synthesis.

The polyunsaturated fats used in margarines are mainly oleic and linoleic (313). Linoleic acid can act as a precursor for prostacyclin but only in the cis form. However, linoleic acid in margarines is often in the trans form (313) and no information is provided on the labels as to the cis- or trans-content of different brands. γ-Linolenic acid, a vegetable oil, is converted to EPA in some species by desaturation and chain elongation, but it appears that humans have little or no capacity to metabolize γ-linolenic acid to EPA (90). Sanders and Naismith (267), however, state that man can convert linolenic acid to EPA and cite evidence from radio-tracer studies on human tissue cultures (2), tissue biopsies (70), and from a study of vegans (265) whose diets were devoid of the long-chain derivatives, and of infants reared on artificial milk formulae (266).

EPA inhibits platelet aggregation in platelet-rich plasma stimulated by ADP, collagen, arachidonic acid, and a synthetic analog of PGH_2 (125). Also, EPA inhibits aggregation in aspirin and imidazole-treated platelets (92) and inhibits thrombin-induced aggregation (156). It is clear, therefore, that both prostaglandin-dependent and -independent pathways of platelet aggregation are inhibited by EPA *in vitro*. *In vivo*, however, EPA would be incorporated into platelet phospholipids, to some extent replacing arachidonic acid and exerting an antithrombotic effect either by competing with remaining arachidonic acid for cyclooxygenase and lipoxygenase (62,223) or by being converted to the less proaggregatory PGH_3 and TXA_3 (125). Studying seven caucasians who had been on a mackerel diet for 1 week, Seiss et al. (271) showed a reduced sensitivity of platelets to collagen, associated with a reduced ability to produce TXB_2, which was dependent on the ratio of C20:5/C20:4 in platelet phospholipids. ADP-induced aggregation was significantly reduced in some subjects and platelet aggregation to exogenously added arachidonic acid was unchanged, indicating normal cyclooxygenase activity. Similarly, Sanders et al. (268) showed a significant increase in bleeding time of 40% in volunteers who had taken cod liver oil (equivalent to 1.8 g EPA) daily for 6 weeks. This was consistent with a decrease in arachidonic acid and an increase in EPA in the platelet phospholipids.

Under normal peroxide levels *in vivo* EPA is a poor substrate for the cyclooxygenase but increasing peroxide concentrations in an incubate containing purified cyclooxygenase enzyme increases the conversion of EPA considerably (62). Incubation of platelet-rich plasma with EPA does not induce the generation of a thromboxane-like material; indeed, it prevents the formation of TXA_2 induced by arachidonic acid or by collagen (125). Conversely, in human umbilical vasculature, Dyerberg and Jorgensen (92) demonstrated that EPA did not influence the conversion of arachidonic acid to prostacyclin but gave rise to additional synthesis of prostacyclin-like material. Aortic microsomes readily convert PGH_3 to Δ^{17}-6-keto-$PGF_{1\alpha}$ (278) but formation of this metabolite or Δ^{17} prostacyclin from exogenous or endogenous EPA *in vivo* has yet to be confirmed.

Fish oil fed to cats and dogs increased the amount of 20:5 ($n = 3$) fatty acids present in heart and liver of the cats and the platelets of the dogs (27,61). Brain infarct volume after experimentally induced cerebral ischemia and the neurological deficit was less in cats fed fish oil than in a corresponding control group (27). In dogs fed fish oil, coronary thrombosis and subsequent infarct size (3% compared to 25% in the control group) induced by electrical stimulation was reduced with less than 30% ectopic beats after 19 hr compared to 80% after 19 hr in the control group (61).

The prolonged bleeding time in Eskimos is reduced after aspirin ingestion (89) suggesting a decreased thromboxane synthetizing capacity coupled with a normal or possibly elevated prostacyclin production. Overall, then, the present evidence suggests that it is well worthwhile continuing to study the effects of EPA in man.

Stimulation of Prostacyclin Production

MacIntyre et al. (186) observed that prostacyclin production by cultures of vascular endothelial cells was enhanced by platelet-poor plasma. Later, Defreyn et al. (69) confirmed the presence of a factor in plasma which stimulates prostacyclin production and showed that the platelet-poor plasma from 6 out of 7 patients with chronic uremia caused more stimulation of prostacyclin production by cultured endothelial cells than the platelet-poor plasma from control volunteers. They suggested that increased levels of circulating prostacyclin could well contribute to the bleeding tendency frequently encountered in uremic patients. Conversely, deficiency of a plasma factor regulating prostacyclin has been reported in hemolytic-uremic syndrome which is associated with widespread thrombotic occlusions (255).

Thrombin, calcium ionophore A23187, and trypsin all stimulate prostacyclin production by cultured endothelial cells (316). It is interesting that all of these substances cause platelet aggregation and probably act by stimulating phospholipases which liberate free arachidonic acid from cellular phospholipids. The action of thrombin in stimulating prostacyclin production is indeed inhibited by mepacrine, a phospholipase inhibitor (317). Generation of thrombin and subsequent stimulation of prostacyclin formation at a site of vascular damage and hemostatic plug formation may be a controlling factor limiting thrombus size (316). Trypsin, but not chymotrypsin, stimulates prostacyclin production by cultured cells, an effect inhibited by soybean trypsin inhibitor (316). Release of trypsin-like enzymes by both platelets and white cells has been proposed as a mechanism by which prostacyclin production by the vessel wall might be regulated (319). Investigating the prostacyclin-stimulating activity of serum, Coughlin et al. (60) concluded that at least 80% of the activity was derived from platelets. The platelet-dependent activity was nondialyzable, stable at 56°C, and at least partially stable at 100°C. Because these properties were similar to those of platelet-derived growth factor (PDGF) and PDGF had been proposed to be the substance present in serum capable of activating phospholipase A_2 in Swiss mouse 3T3 fibroblasts (273) they tested PDGF for its ability to stimulate prostacyclin production in bovine cell cultures. PDGF reversibly stimulated prostacyclin production and at a concentration of 8.0 ng/ml stimulated synthesis by 74-fold in aortic endothelial cells, 84-fold in smooth muscle, and 15-fold in capillary endothelial cell cultures. The mitogenic activity of PDGF was only observed with smooth muscle cells indicating dissociation between the two activities (60). Control of prostacyclin production is possible, therefore, by a variety of agents acting locally at the level of the cell-vessel wall interaction but the precise mechanisms acting at any time have yet to be clarified.

Stimulation of prostacyclin release from the vessel wall by an antithrombotic compound Bay g 6575 has been reported (305) and confirmed (45). In addition, Bay g 6575 increased prostacyclin production in rats already having lowered prostacyclin synthesizing capacity as a result of streptozotocin-induced diabetes (45). Bendrofluazide used to treat patients with essential hypertension caused significant increases in circulating levels of 6-oxo-$PGF_{1\alpha}$ suggesting a possible contribution of prostacyclin to the reduction in peripheral resistance seen with thiazide treatment (312).

Other Factors Which May Regulate Prostacyclin Biosynthesis

β-Thromboglobulin is a small protein related to platelet factor IV which is stored in the α granules of platelets and released along with other granular constituents during aggregation or adherence of the platelets to a damaged vessel wall (210). Hope et al. (149) demonstrated that β-thromboglobulin inhibits formation of prostacyclin by bovine aortic endothelial cells in culture, at concentrations which are exceeded locally during platelet aggregation and release. Platelet factor IV does not have this action (149). This phenomenon may be an important component of the process of thrombosis, but the precise mechanism of inhibition has not been determined.

Finally, unidentified factors which inhibit prostacyclin formation have been found in renal cortex (294), and a microsomal fraction of rat placenta (134). Both these inhibitors appear to act at the cyclooxygenase level and they may be related to a similar endogenous cyclooxygenase inhibitor found in plasma (262). Much more work is necessary to define the significance and function of these factors.

ROLES OF PROSTACYCLIN IN THE HEART

Local injections of arachidonic acid into the coronary circulation of the dog cause vasodilatation, and because this effect was abolished by indomethacin (145) it was assumed that PGE_2 was the likely mediator. However, there were some inconsistencies with this proposal. In isolated Langendorff-perfused hearts of the rabbit, arachidonic acid dilated the coronary vasculature, but PGE_2 was inactive (30,219). Isolated strips of bovine, canine, and human coronary artery were relaxed by arachidonic acid but PGE_2 contracted them. Arachidonate-induced relaxation was abolished by indomethacin, and it was, therefore, suggested that the metabolite responsible must be the endoperoxide intermediate PGH_2 (175).

Following the discovery of prostacyclin, we showed that both prostacyclin and PGH_2 relaxed bovine coronary arteries (80), although the latter sometimes induced an initial contraction. After treatment with 15-HPAA, relaxation induced by arachidonic acid was abolished, while that induced by PGH_2 was reversed to a contraction. These experiments thus revealed that relaxation of coronary arteries induced by arachidonic acid is due to its intramural conversion to prostacyclin. This study further confirmed that the intrinsic activity of PGH_2 on isolated blood vessels is contractile (80). Similar results have been published by Needleman and associates (220,251).

In isolated, Langendorff-perfused hearts of the guinea pig and rabbit, not only is prostacyclin a potent vasodilator but it is also the predominant metabolite of arachidonic acid (270). Similarly, others have identified 6-oxo-$PGF_{1\alpha}$ as the major product released from rat and rabbit hearts during perfusion with arachidonic acid (68,220).

The Coronary Circulation

Vasodilator prostaglandins are one group of several humoral substances which have been considered as local mediators of coronary blood flow (20,85,221). We, and others, have investigated the coronary actions of prostacyclin in the intact heart of open-chest dogs (12,77,155). Local injection of prostacyclin (50–500 ng) into the coronary circulation increased coronary blood flow without systemic effects (Fig. 4), and it was a more potent coronary dilator than PGE_2. Furthermore, we found that profound and prolonged coronary vasodilatation could be elicited by applying prostacyclin (20–100 μg) topically onto the exposed surface of the left ventricle (Fig. 4), suggesting that it was rapidly absorbed through the myocardium into the coronary vasculature. Interestingly, the coronary circulation is sensitized to the vasodilator effects of exogenous prostacyclin, but not to those of PGE_2, when endogenous prostaglandin synthesis is inhibited by indomethacin or meclofenamate (77,145). These inhibitors of cyclooxygenase decrease resting coronary blood flow in anesthetized, open-chest dogs. Although this is not seen in closed-chest dogs subjected to a minimum of surgical trauma (238), it does indicate that the generation of a vasodilator metabolite of arachidonic acid increases or maintains coronary blood flow during mildly traumatic conditions.

In isolated, Langendorff-perfused hearts of rabbits, numerous diverse stimuli, such as ischemia and hypoxia, adenine nucleotides, mechanical stimulation, ace-tylcholine, adrenergic stimulation, angiotensin, and bradykinin, may all release prostacyclin or PG-like substances into the coronary venous effluent (221). A major obstacle to accepting the concept that endogenous prostacyclin regulates coronary vascular resistance was raised by the demonstration that indomethacin did not alter the response of the coronary vasculature to many of the above stimuli in open-chest dogs (145). In similar studies, Giles and Wilcken (104) showed that indomethacin did not affect the hyperemia seen after brief occlusions of coronary blood vessels, nor did it alter the adjustment of coronary blood flow which follows sudden, sustained changes in perfusion pressure (260). In contrast, reactive hyperemia following 10 min coronary occlusion is reduced by indomethacin (173). These studies suggest that prostacyclin is probably not involved in autoregulation of coronary blood flow or in "metabolic" vasodilatation resulting from short-term reduction in

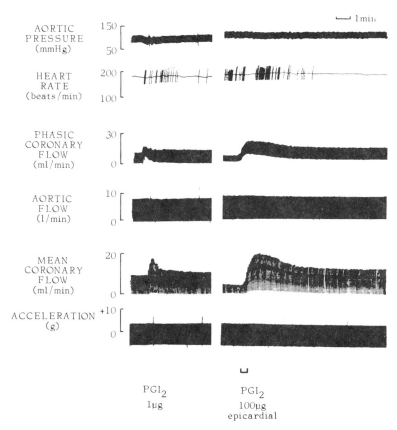

AORTIC PRESSURE (mmHg)

HEART RATE (beats/min)

PHASIC CORONARY FLOW (ml/min)

AORTIC FLOW (1/min)

MEAN CORONARY FLOW (ml/min)

ACCELERATION (g)

PGI$_2$ 1µg

PGI$_2$ 100µg epicardial

FIG. 4. Effect of prostacyclin on coronary blood flow when injected into the coronary circulation or when applied topically to the left ventricle.

myocardial oxygen tension, but leave open the question of its participation in response to more severe myocardial ischemia (20,221). Indeed, it has been reported that inhibition of prostaglandin biosynthesis by indomethacin blocked the increase in collateral flow seen an hour after coronary occlusion (164). However, in many of the above studies no attempt was made to demonstrate that indomethacin did inhibit endogenous prostacyclin formation and, as pointed out earlier, there is evidence that acute intravenous treatment with this inhibitor may not totally eliminate prostacyclin biosynthesis in lungs (75,76) or PGE formation in kidney (295).

The coronary blood vessels themselves have generally been regarded as the primary source of prostacyclin in the heart (221,276). However, serous membranes containing mesothelial cells, such as the pericardium, are also very active producers of prostacyclin *in vitro* (138). Dusting and Nolan (88) have recently demonstrated in dogs that prostacyclin is released from the epicardial surface *in vivo*. Moreover, the output of prostacyclin from the epicardium or pericardium is greatly increased when the heart is handled, and is also increased when cardiac workload is raised

(88). These findings raise the possibility that prostacyclin of pericardial origin might also influence coronary blood vessel tone. The role of prostacyclin in regulation of coronary blood flow still appears to be a fruitful area of research, and there is a particular need for studies in intact animals which ought to include measurements of myocardial, pericardial, or coronary prostacyclin formation *in vivo*.

Cardiac Reflexes Influenced by Prostacyclin

We, and others, found that bradycardia may accompany hypotension induced by prostacyclin in anesthetized dogs (12,77,146), and only transient, weak tachycardia accompanied prostacyclin infusion in anesthetized cats (178). Bradycardia induced by prostacyclin is a reflex response mediated, at least partially, by vagal pathways for it is reduced or reversed by atropine (47,48). However, the afferent arc is also subserved by vagal fibers, for vagotomy (but not atropine treatment) reduced the fall in peripheral resistance induced by prostacyclin (47,48). Intrapulmonary C-fibers are stimulated by right atrial injection of prostacyclin in the rabbit (10) and the authors propose that they contribute to the afferent arc of prostacyclin-induced bradycardia. Therefore, the hypotension induced by prostacyclin has at least two components: direct arteriolar vasodilatation and reflex, noncholinergic vasodilatation.

Hintze et al. (147) noted the similarities between the effects of prostacyclin on blood pressure and heart rate and those of veratrine, the so-called "Bezold-Jarisch" reflex (157). The receptors responsible for the Bezold-Jarisch reflex have been localized to the left ventricle, particularly in the area supplied by the circumflex coronary artery (58). However, we never observed bradycardia following injection of subhypotensive doses of prostacyclin into the circumflex artery, nor did it occur following topical application of prostacyclin to the left ventricle, although both procedures profoundly increased circumflex blood flow (77) (Fig. 4). Moreover, the Bezold-Jarisch reflex elicited by veratrine or nicotine has a very short latency, occurring within 5 to 6 sec after intracoronary or epicardial application (242,281), whereas the bradycardia elicited by prostacyclin develops more slowly, and is coincident with the fall in arterial pressure (48,147). Certainly, it appears unlikely that the concentrations of prostacyclin needed to elicit this depressor vagal reflex will be present in the circulation under any physiological or pathological conditions, but such concentrations could be attained during therapeutic use of prostacyclin or its analogs.

Whether prostacyclin induces bradycardia or tachycardia in dogs depends upon the basal heart rate, so that it produces tachycardia when the heart rate is low (<110 beats/min) but bradycardia when the basal heart rate is higher (50). Prostacyclin-induced bradycardia is reversed to tachycardia by sodium cromoglycate (50), which is known to attenuate capsaicin-induced excitation of C-fiber sensory nerve endings in canine lung (73). This work provides further evidence for the suggestion that the afferent arc of the reflex leading to bradycardia induced by prostacyclin originates in sensory C-fibers.

The opposite response, namely, an excitatory chemoreflex characterized by an increase in blood pressure and tachycardia, can be elicited by epicardial application of bradykinin (281). This response, which is mediated by afferent cardiac sympathetic nerves and an efferent sympathetic discharge to blood vessels (279,281), is potentiated by PGE_1 or PGE_2, applied epicardially, and is reduced by intravenous indomethacin (281). Since bradykinin is formed in the myocardium during ischemia (171,246), this sympathetic chemoreflex, involving both bradykinin and prostaglandins may well be the mechanism which signals the pain of ischemia. Staszewska-Barczak and Dusting (280) have recently shown that prostacyclin potentiates the sympathetic reflex when applied topically to the left ventricle in anesthetized dogs. Therefore, prostacyclin of pericardial origin, released during increased cardiac work (88), may contribute to the pain and reflex events associated with the onset of angina pectoris. In contrast, when prostacyclin was infused into the anterior descending coronary artery at rates which had negligible systemic effects, the reflex pressor effects elicited by epicardial bradykinin were reduced by 25%. Furthermore, reflex depressor effects elicited by epicardial nicotine, which are vagally mediated, were enhanced by about 40% by intracoronary prostacyclin (280). Thus, prostacyclin from the vascular compartment sensitizes vagal nerve endings which subserve depressor chemoreflexes.

The functional significance of these findings may be summarized as follows. Prostacyclin (or PGE_2) released from the ischemic myocardium (221) or from the pericardium (88) can sensitize sympathetic chemoreceptors in the epicardial surface to nociceptive stimulation by bradykinin and, thereby, contribute to the pain and tachycardia accompanying acute myocardial ischemia. These effects would tend to increase afterload and myocardial oxygen demand, and may exacerbate the ischemic damage to an already overtaxed myocardium. On the other hand, if prostacyclin is released into the coronary blood stream, either from the lungs or locally from the coronary vasculature, it can act to sensitize vagal receptors in the heart to chemical and possibly mechanical stimulation and, thereby, facilitate reflex depressor mechanisms. This action of circulating prostacyclin may be of special importance in ischemic heart disease since the predominance of vagal over sympathetically-mediated reflex activity would reduce workload and oxygen demand by the heart (26). Circulating prostacyclin, therefore, has synergistic effects on reducing myocardial ischemia by preventing platelet aggregation in the coronary circulation (4), by dilating the coronary vascular bed, and by reducing oxygen demand. These effects may explain the poorly understood "protective" effect which prostacyclin exerts in the myocardium (see later).

Cardiac Arrhythmias and Infarct Size

The effects of prostacyclin on cardiac arrhythmias and infarct size after coronary occlusion have been studied by several workers with conflicting results. Variable effects were produced on the cardiac rhythm of isolated rabbit and rat hearts depending on the dose of prostacyclin and the experimental procedure (167,197). *In vivo*, prostacyclin produced an increase in arrhythmias in the rat and cat after acute coronary artery occlusion (15,72,170). In the anesthetized dog an infusion of prostacyclin (320 ng/kg/min) for 6 hr starting 17 min after coronary occlusion did not alter infarct size (259), but infusion at 420 ng/kg/min for 6 hr in anesthetized dogs starting 3 min after occlusion reduced the infarct size (165). Prostacyclin in the rat increased arrhythmias and ventricular fibrillation following coronary occlusion but decreased infarct size in the survivors (15). Ohlendorf et al. (235) found that platelet counts in cats decreased by 30 to 35% in the first 20 min after ligation of the left anterior descending coronary artery. This decrease was reversed by intravenous prostacyclin. At the same time, prostacyclin also prevented the loss of cathepsin-D and creatine phosphokinase activities in the infarcted area and inhibited ST segment elevation. Lefer et al. (178) and Ogletree et al. (231) have also demonstrated "protective" effects of prostacyclin in acute myocardial ischemia in cats, and more recently, Ribeiro et al. (258), using dogs, have shown that intravenous infusions of prostacyclin given after coronary ligation decrease myocardial oxygen demand and maintain ischemic blood flow while reducing nonischemic blood flow. Early mortality was also greatly reduced. Further work is needed in this area to clarify the mechanism of these protective effects.

THROMBOXANE A_2 AND PROSTACYCLIN IMBALANCE IN OTHER PATHOLOGICAL STATES

A number of diseases have now been related to an imbalance in the prostacyclin-TXA_2 system. Platelets from patients with arterial thrombosis, deep venous thrombosis, or recurrent venous thrombosis produce more PG endoperoxides and TXA_2 than normal and have a shortened survival time (176). Platelets from rabbits made atherosclerotic by dietary manipulation (274) and from patients who have survived myocardial infarction (286) are abnormally sensitive to aggregating agents and produce more TXA_2 than controls. Elevated TXB_2 levels have been demonstrated in the blood of patients with Prinzmetal's angina (180). Hirsh et al. (148) also studied TXB_2 levels in coronary sinus blood of patients with unstable angina. They concluded that local TXA_2 release is associated with recent episodes of angina but were unable to distinguish whether the release was cause or effect.

Platelets from rats made diabetic display an increased release of TXA_2 whereas their blood vessels show a reduced production of prostacyclin (133,160); these effects are reversed by chronic insulin treatment (133). Prostacyclin production by blood vessels from patients with diabetes is depressed (159) and circulating levels of 6-oxo-$PGF_{1\alpha}$ are reduced in diabetic patients with proliferative retinopathy (74). Davis et al. (66) tended to confirm that vessels taken from diabetics produced less prostacyclin than normals. However, their results did not support an association between reduced prostacyclin production and diabetic retinopathy.

Thrombocytopenic purpura (TTP), like diabetes, is associated with formation of microvascular thromboemboli, and a deficiency in prostacyclin production may be responsible for the increased platelet consumption which occurs in TTP (56,255,257).

This deficiency is postulated to be secondary to a lack of a "plasma factor" which normally stimulates prostacyclin production (186). One patient with TTP had an undetectable level of 6-oxo-$PGF_{1\alpha}$ (<60 pg/ml), whereas the mean value in control subjects was 154 ± 48 pg/ml (137).

An increased prostacyclin production, resulting from an accumulation of the "plasma factor" which stimulates prostacyclin synthesis, has been suggested to explain the hemostatic defect in uremic patients (255). Patients with Bartter's syndrome excrete in the urine about four times as much 6-oxo-$PGF_{1\alpha}$ as controls (127). This has led to the suggestion that overproduction of prostacyclin mediates both the hyperreninemia and the hyporesponsiveness to pressor agents observed in these patients (127).

Pace-Asciak et al. (240) demonstrated that aortae from spontaneously hypertensive rats of the Japanese strain generate more prostacyclin than aortae from normotensive rats when incubated with exogenous arachidonic acid *in vitro*. Furthermore, Armstrong et al. (11) found that prostaglandin endoperoxide (PGH_2) has a greater hypotensive effect in genetically hypertensive rats of the New Zealand strain than in normotensive controls, whereas PGE_2 had a similar hypotensive action in the two strains. Intravenous injections of arachidonic acid also caused greater depressor effects in spontaneously hypertensive rats than in Wistar-Kyoto normotensive controls, even when allowance was made for the higher resting arterial pressure (78). Dusting et al. (78) also found similar evidence for greater conversion of arachidonate to prostacyclin in hypertensive rats of the Sprague-Dawley strain, for the vasodepressor effect of arachidonic acid was much greater in rats made hypertensive by unilateral nephrectomy and renal artery stenosis than it was in unilaterally nephrectomized controls. All these data suggest that one or more enzymes in the biosynthetic pathway for prostacyclin may be induced as an adaptive mechanism to the elevated arterial pressure. Against this, however, is the observation that chronic treatment with indomethacin or aspirin does not alter arterial pressure in spontaneously hypertensive rats (9,71), although it does markedly reduce the vasodepressor action of intravenous arachidonic acid (71). Grose et al. (119) have described a diminished excretion of 6-oxo-$PGF_{1\alpha}$ in the urine of patients with essential hypertension. This could reflect diminished prostacyclin by the kidney itself or, less likely, by the body as a whole. It is interesting that plasma exchange in patients suffering from hypertension as a complication of hemolytic uremic syndrome restored a "prostacyclin stimulating factor," and led to improved control of blood pressure (255). Moreover, others have reported that plasma exchange has an antihypertensive effect in patients with glomerular nephritis and essential hypertension (324). These observations suggest that essential hypertension in man may be associated with impairment, rather than enhancement, of prostacyclin formation in the vasculature. Clearly, much more work is necessary to define any role of prostacyclin in the experimental models of hypertension in the rat, and to confirm or deny any such parallels between development of hypertension in the rat and essential hypertension in man.

Prostacyclin production is significantly lower in umbilical and placental vessels from preeclamptic patients than in those from normally pregnant women (254). The authors suggest that in severe preeclampsia, which is characterized by hypertension, edema, proteinuria, and consumptive coagulopathy, there is a deficiency in the adaptive mechanism which normally results in elevated levels of prostacyclin in umbilical and placental vessels (256).

As yet, a clear relationship between different diseases and the PGI_2/TXA_2 balance is not established. However, it seems that conditions which favor the development of thrombosis are associated with an increase in TXA_2 and a decrease in prostacyclin formation, whereas an increased prostacyclin formation plus decreased TXA_2 is present in some conditions associated with an increased bleeding tendency.

DEVELOPMENT OF ANTITHROMBOTIC THERAPIES

Intraarterial thrombus formation and hemostatic plug formation have been described in general terms as equivalent phenomena (216). It is, however, possible that the relative importance of prostacyclin and TXA_2 in these conditions is different, for prostacyclin, at least under some conditions, is an unstable circulating hormone (122,206) as well as a locally generated one. Its role in controlling intraarterial thrombus formation might be more important than that of TXA_2 which seems to be generated only after strong interaction between aggregating platelets or by their interaction with vessel wall materials.

As far as aspirin is concerned, more information is needed on the rate of recovery of the endothelial cyclooxygenase *in vivo* after single doses of aspirin. Equally important is the assessment of any cumulative effect of a multiple-dose regime on platelet and endothelial cyclooxygenase in order to establish the optimal interval of administration. The demonstration of the ability of aspirin to prevent thromboembolism in some circumstances but not in others (158,306) may suggest a qualitative or quantitative difference in the underlying pathophysiology. Further clinical trials should be conducted in which aspirin is given at low doses either alone or in combination with phosphodiesterase inhibitors such as dipyridamole. Preferably, a selective inhibitor of thromboxane synthetase should be developed to be used alone or with a phosphodiesterase inhibitor (208).

A more direct approach to antithrombotic therapy, however, would be to stimulate formation of platelet cyclic AMP; increasing platelet cyclic AMP inhibits aggregation whether or not it is dependent on the thromboxane pathway. Since prostacyclin is the most powerful substance known in both preventing aggregation and increasing platelet cyclic AMP (115,292), prostacyclin or an analog, alone or in combination with a phosphodiesterase inhibitor, should be a more comprehensive approach to the control of platelet aggregation *in vivo*. Alternatively, drugs which stimulate endogenous prostacyclin production (305) could be developed. Several of these possibilities are, at present, being explored.

PROSTACYCLIN IN MAN

Effects on Platelets

Prostacyclin has a potent effect on platelets in man. During intravenous infusion of prostacyclin in healthy volunteers for 60 min at doses ranging from 2 to 16 ng/kg/min there was a dose-related inhibition of platelet aggregation in whole blood and in platelet-rich plasma (233,288). Inhibition of platelet aggregation at 15 or 45 min after the start of the infusion was similar. At a dose of 8 ng/kg/min partial inhibition of aggregation was demonstrable for up to 105 min after the end of infusion and this persistence of effect on platelets has been confirmed (51). Template bleeding time was not significantly increased though Szczeklik et al. (288) found an approximate doubling of bleeding time in response to prostacyclin at 20 ng/kg/min. Prostacyclin disperses circulating platelet aggregates (288). Significant inhibition of platelet aggregation was also shown by FitzGerald et al. (98) when prostacyclin was administered under double blind conditions at rates of 4 and 8 ng/kg/min. The longevity of the effects of prostacyclin on platelets, despite its short biological half-life, might be accounted for by persistent elevation of platelet cyclic AMP.

Other hematological variables such as platelet count, platelet factor 3 concentration, accelerated partial thromboplastin time, prothrombin time, euglobin clot lysis time, concentration of fibrinogen degradation products, and blood glucose were not altered by prostacyclin (233,288).

Cardiovascular Effects

It was originally suggested (288) that prostacyclin had direct positive chronotropic and inotropic effects in man. However, in a double blind controlled study of the cardiovascular effects of prostacyclin (up to 4 ng/kg/min) using noninvasive methods including systolic time intervals, which are sensitive indicators of cardiac contractile state and peripheral vascular changes, Warrington and O'Grady (309) concluded that prostacyclin caused arteriolar vasodilatation which would be expected to lower diastolic and mean blood pressure and thus reflexly increase heart rate and contractility. When heart rate was increased by more than 10% over control values during intravenous prostacyclin infusion, peripheral temperature measured at the great toe increased by 1 to 6°C (233). Increases in skin temperature as well as facial flushing were also observed by Szczeklik et al. (288) at doses of 2 to 5 ng/kg/min. Facial flushing invariably occurred at doses above 4 ng/kg/min when an increase in heart rate of more than 10% is recorded (233). This flushing limits the extent to which studies with prostacyclin can be rendered double blind.

The cardiovascular effects are shorter-lived than those on platelets and disappear within 15 min of the end of infusion (234). Plasma renin activity rose significantly during prostacyclin infusion in man (98). In the same study plasma norepinephrine and plasma aldosterone levels did not change significantly, in the latter case possibly because of the relatively short (20 min) duration of the prostacyclin infusion periods relative to the half-life of formation of aldosterone which is longer than that of renin.

Renal blood flow in man measured using ^{125}I-Hippuran increased in response to an infusion of prostacyclin (6 ng/kg/min) which caused a significant reduction in diastolic blood pressure and increase in heart rate. The glomerular filtration rate measured using ^{51}Cr-EDTA remained unchanged as did osmolar clearance, sodium and potassium excretion, urine volume, urine pH, and hydrogen ion excretion (J. Henry and J. O'Grady, *unpublished results*).

Other Effects

Headache has been reported by several subjects when doses greater than 8 ng/kg/min are administered (98,233,288). Colicky central abdominal discomfort has been less frequently experienced but was reproducible in one subject (233). The precise mechanism of these gastrointestinal effects is unclear for the effects of prostacyclin on human gastrointestinal tissue has not been studied. It may be that the gastrointestinal effects in man reflect contraction of human gastrointestinal smooth muscle by prostacyclin; they may also be vagally mediated or represent secondary effects of prostacyclin or of its metabolites.

Ill defined sensations of unease and restlessness have been experienced by subjects receiving higher doses (8–20 ng/kg/min) of prostacyclin (51,233,288). When a relatively high dose of prostacyclin (50 ng/kg/min) was administered to 2 subjects (288) both experienced sudden weakness with pallor and nausea, systolic and diastolic blood pressure fell, and bradycardia occurred. It is possible that this effect is mediated by a vagal reflex, for in dogs prostacyclin produces a vagally-dependent bradycardia (48). Whether this effect in man is inhibited by atropine is unknown. Human cardiovascular response to prostacyclin differs from that in the dog in that the latter generally responds to prostacyclin by bradycardia. This may reflect either the higher vagal tone of the dog or the fact that generally higher doses have been studied in dogs and lower doses in man, and the vagal effect may be dose-dependent.

THERAPEUTIC POTENTIAL OF PROSTACYCLIN

Extracorporeal Circulation

The circulation of blood through extracorporeal systems brings blood into contact with artificial surfaces which cannot generate prostacyclin. In the course of such procedures thrombocytopenia and loss of platelet hemostatic function occur and make an important contribution to the bleeding problems following charcoal hemoperfusion and prolonged cardiopulmonary bypass in man (102,211,320). Formation of microemboli during cardiopulmonary bypass may also contribute to cerebral complications which sometimes follow this procedure (245). In animals subjected to experimental renal dialysis (329), charcoal hemoperfusion (41), and cardiopulmonary bypass (183), infusion of prostacyclin during the procedure prevented this platelet damage and thrombocytopenia, thus increasing the biocompatibility of the procedure. Platelet aggregates in the blood returning to the animals, as measured by Swank screen filtration pressure, were also reduced by infusion of prostacyclin (Fig. 5). These findings have been confirmed in patients with fulminant hepatic failure undergoing charcoal hemoperfusion (109). Prostacyclin infusion prevented the fall in platelet count and elevation of β-thromboglobulin seen in the control patients. In addition, two of the control patients developed marked hypotension during the procedure, in one associated with a marked rise in Swank screen filtration pressure, while this did not occur in the prostacyclin-treated patients. A study of the influence of serial hemoperfusion with prostacyclin on the survival rate of patients with fulminant hepatic failure is now in progress (108). Longmore et al. (184), Bunting et al. (42), Walker et al. (308), Bennett et al. (22), and Chelly et al. (49) have published double blind clinical trials of prostacyclin in cardiopulmonary bypass. The treatment groups showed a preservation of platelet number and function, with a reduction in the blood loss in the first 18 hr after operation. In the trial by Longmore et al. (184) the blood loss was halved and the reduction was statistically significant. The heparin-sparing effect of prostacyclin was confirmed and the vasodilator effects were not troublesome.

The observation that prostacyclin potentiates the effects of heparin (41) led to further studies on this interaction. These demonstrated that prostacyclin has a small indirect anticoagulant effect. Indeed, platelets stimulated by low doses of aggregating agents accelerate clotting by providing a surface upon which coagulation factors can combine and react more efficiently (see ref. 189). Prostacyclin, by preventing platelet activation, inhibits the shortening of clotting time produced when either kaolin or collagen is incubated with platelet-rich plasma (38,43). Platelets release antiheparin activity, which reduces the anticoagulant effect of heparin *in vitro*. Prostacyclin, by inhibiting this release and by preventing the development of procoagulant activity, can enhance the action of heparin by as much as 100% (38,43).

Heparin therapy in some patients is complicated by thrombocytopenia and thromboembolic episodes (55,153) and *in vitro* can cause platelet aggregation and potentiate aggregation to other aggregating agents (264). Perhaps because the stimulus to coagulation is milder, we showed that during hemodialysis in dogs, prostacyclin could be used alone to prevent platelet loss and coagulation. Heparin was not needed. This surprising result has now been confirmed in 10 patients by Zusman et al. (331). Prostacyclin was infused intravenously for 10 min before dialysis and into the arterial line during dialysis. The rate of infusion was adjusted to prevent prostacyclin-induced hypotension. They concluded that prostacyclin can safely replace heparin as the sole antithrombotic agent during hemodialysis and that it may be more advantageous if anticoagulation is contraindicated. This work has been confirmed by Turney et al. (297) in 5 patients.

Other Applications

Clinical assessment of prostacyclin is still in its infancy with many trials in progress. Open studies and individual case reports have been described where both

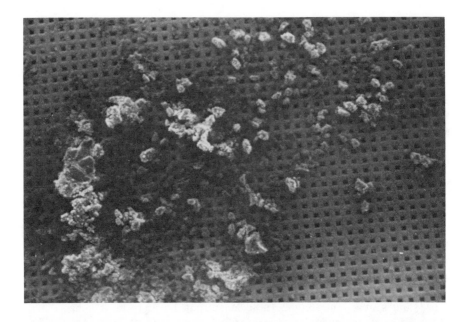

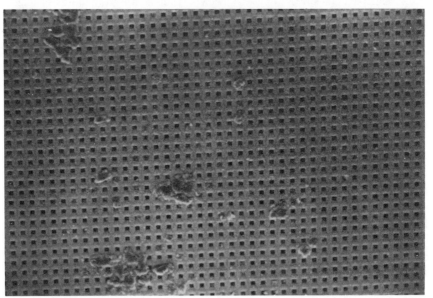

FIG. 5. Scanning electron micrograph ($\times$ 130) of stainless steel screens used in Swank screen filtration pressure apparatus. Blood samples (5 ml) were taken from the dialyzer outlines of dogs having undergone 90 min of dialysis. **Top:** heparin only; **Bottom:** heparin plus prostacyclin. Prostacyclin clearly reduced the amount of particulate material (mainly platelet aggregates) present in the blood. (We thank Dr. N. Read, Dept. of Pathology, Wellcome Research Laboratories for producing the scanning electron micrographs.) (From H. F. Woods, G. Ash, and M. J. Weston, et al., 1978, *unpublished data.*)

the platelet inhibitory activity and vasodilator properties of prostacyclin have been utilized. The results in many cases are, therefore, preliminary but, nevertheless, they point the way to conditions in which prostacyclin therapy may be useful.

Szczeklik et al. (289) reported striking and prolonged benefits following intraarterial infusion of prostacyclin in 5 patients with advanced atherosclerotic lower limb peripheral vascular disease. Rest pain disappeared, previously refractory ulcers healed, and the muscle blood flow, as measured by xenon[133] clearance, was significantly increased for at least 6 weeks after prostacyclin infusion. This group has now reported on 55 patients with advanced peripheral arterial disease of the lower extremities (285). In summary, 42% of patients treated showed a persistent, long-lasting improvement. In 40% of patients the improvement lasted no longer than 2 months, while in the remaining 18% of patients the results were virtually negative. The authors believe that these figures do not represent the true efficacy of prostacyclin therapy in advanced peripheral arterial disease and that successful treatment largely depends upon choice of patients, localization of the vascular lesions, and the advancement of the disease (285). Carefully conceived and executed trials are, therefore, required to resolve this problem. Other reports also suggest that prostacyclin may have beneficial effects in peripheral artery disease (236,243). Zygulska-Mach et al. (332) infused prostacyclin into 3 patients with sudden blockage of central retinal veins. Improvement was observed in those 2 patients who were treated within the first 48 hr.

Prostacyclin has been successfully used in cases of pulmonary hypertension. One, an 8-year-old girl with severe idiopathic pulmonary artery hypertension received a prostacyclin infusion of 8 to 44 ng/kg/min. Pulmonary vascular resistance was reduced during the period of infusion and no adverse effects were reported (310). In a group of patients with pulmonary hypertension secondary to mitral valve stenosis, prostacyclin caused a dose-dependent pulmonary vasodilatation with no observed side effects (290). In both of the above studies prostacyclin was shown to be more effective than PGE_1. Single case studies have suggested that prostacyclin may be useful in the treatment of persistent fetal circulation with pulmonary vasoconstriction (182) and preeclamptic toxemia (97).

Bergman et al. (23) gave an intravenous infusion of prostacyclin to patients with coronary artery disease and showed that doses between 2 and 8 ng/kg/min for 10 min had no deleterious effects. Heart rate and cardiac index were increased and mean blood pressure, and systemic and pulmonary resistance all fell. Mean atrial pacing time to angina rose from 142 to 241 sec. They concluded that acute administration of prostacyclin was beneficial in angina, having effects similar to short-acting nitrates. Hall and Dewar (129) concluded from their study of 5 patients with coronary artery disease that prostacyclin can safely be infused directly into diseased coronary arteries, and Szczeklik and Gryglewski (285) found a beneficial effect of intravenous prostacyclin infusions in some patients with unstable angina.

A prostacyclin deficiency has been reported in thrombotic thrombocytopenic purpura (137). However, infusion of prostacyclin into 2 patients with TTP did not produce an increase in circulating platelet count (36,137). On the other hand,

FitzGerald et al. (99) have reported an increase in platelet count and an improvement in the neurological status of one such patient during 18 days of prostacyclin infusion. They were sufficiently encouraged to conclude that the controlled evaluation of prostacyclin in TTP was warranted.

Clearly, there are many clinical conditions which may respond to prostacyclin treatment and its place in therapeutics (or that of stable analogs) will be defined in the next few years. Some of these conditions are preeclamptic toxemia (97), hemolytic uremic syndrome (311), peptic ulceration (322), and the thrombotic complications associated with transplant rejection (215). What is now clear is that our knowledge of the causes and treatment of cardiovascular diseases could well be dramatically changed during the 1980s.

REFERENCES

1. Abe, K., Itoh, T., Sato, M., Imai, Y., Haruyama, T., Sakurai, Y., Goto, T., Otsuka, Y., and Yoshinaga, K. (1980): Implication of endogenous prostaglandin system in the antihypertensive effect of captopril in low renin hypertension. *Jpn. Circ. J.*, 44:422–425.
2. Aerberhard, E. E., Corbo, L., and Menkes, J. H. (1978): Polyenoic acid metabolism in cultured human skin fibroblasts. *Lipids*, 13:758–767.
3. Aiken, J. W. (1979): Is the lung an endocrine organ that secretes prostacyclin? Gryglewski, R. J. In: *Prostacyclin*, edited by J. R. Vane and S. Bergström, p. 287. Raven Press, New York.
4. Aiken, J. W., Gorman, R. R., and Shebuski, R. J. (1979): Prevention of blockage of partially obstructed coronary arteries with prostacyclin correlates with inhibition of platelet aggregation. *Prostaglandins*, 17:483–494.
5. Aiken, J. W., and Vane, J. R. (1973): Intrarenal prostaglandin release attenuates the renal vasoconstrictor activity of angiotensin. *J. Pharmacol. Exp. Ther.*, 184:678–687.
6. Amezcua, J. -L., Higgs, E. A., Moncada, S., Salmon, J. A., and Vane, J. R. (1978): Prostacyclin (PGI₂) production in the cat spleen. *7th International Congress of Pharmacology, Paris, 1978*, Abstracts, p. 341. Pergamon Press, Oxford.
7. Amezcua, J.-L., O'Grady, J., Salmon, J. A., and Moncada, S. (1979): Prolonged paradoxical effect of aspirin on platelet behaviour and bleeding time in man. *Thromb. Res.*, 16:69–79.
8. Amezcua, J.-L., Parsons, M., and Moncada, S. (1978): Unstable metabolites of arachidonic acid, aspirin and the formation of the haemostatic plug. *Thromb. Res.*, 13:477–488.
9. Antonaccio, M. J., Harris, D., Goldenberg, H., High, J. P., and Rubin, B. (1979): The effects of captopril, propranolol and indomethacin on blood pressure and plasma renin activity in spontaneously hypertensive and normotensive rats. *Proc. Soc. Exp. Biol. Med.*, 162:429–433.
10. Armstrong, D. J., and Miller, S. A. (1981): Intrapulmonary C-fibers contribute to the afferent arm of the vagally mediated responses to right atrial injections of prostacyclin (PGI₂) into rabbits. *J. Physiol.*, 310:65P.
11. Armstrong, J. M., Boura, A. L. A., Hamberg, M., and Samuelsson, B. (1976): A comparison of the vasodepressor effects of the cyclic endoperoxides PGG₂ and PGH₂ with those of PGD₂ and PGE₂ in hypertensive and normotensive rats. *Eur. J. Pharmacol.*, 39:251–258.
12. Armstrong, J. M., Chapple, D. J., Dusting, G. J., Hughes, R., Moncada, S., and Vane, J. R. (1977): Cardiovascular actions of prostacyclin (PGI₂) in chloralose anaesthetized dogs. *Br. J. Pharmacol.*, 61:136P.
13. Armstrong, J. M., Lattimer, N., Moncada, S., and Vane, J. R. (1978): Comparison of the vasodepressor effects of prostacyclin and 6-oxo-prostaglandin F₁ₐ with those of prostaglandin E₂ in rats and rabbits. *Br. J. Pharmacol.*, 62:125–130.
14. Ashida, S.-I., and Abiko, Y. (1978): Effect of ticlopidine and acetylsalicylic acid on generation of prostaglandin I₂-like substance in rat arterial tissue. *Thromb. Res.*, 13:901–908.
15. Au, T. L. S., Collins, G. A., Harvie, C. J., and Walker, M. J. A. (1980): Actions of prostaglandins I₂ and E₂ on coronary occlusion-induced arrhythmias in the rat. In: *Advances in Prostaglandin and Thromboxane Research*, edited by P. Ramwell, B. Samuelsson, and R. Paoletti, pp. 647–649. Raven Press, New York.

16. Baenziger, N. L., Dillender, M. J., and Majerus, P. (1977): Cultured human skin fibroblasts and arterial cells produce a labile platelet-inhibitory prostaglandin. *Biochem. Biophys. Res. Commun.*, 78:294–301.
17. Bang, H. O., and Dyerberg, J. (1972): Plasma lipids and lipoproteins in Greenlandic west coast eskimos. *Acta Med. Scand.*, 192:85–94.
18. Bayer, B. L., Blass, K. E., and Förster, W. (1979): Antiaggregatory effect of prostacyclin (PGI₂) *in vivo. Br. J. Pharmacol.*, 66:10–12.
19. Beitz, J., and Förster, W. (1980): Influence of human low density and high density lipoprotein cholesterol on the *in vitro* prostaglandin I₂ synthetase activity. *Biochim. Biophys. Acta*, 620:352–355.
20. Belloni, F. T. (1979): The local control of coronary blood flow. *Cardiovasc. Res.*, 13:63–85.
21. Bendit, E. P. (1977): The origin of atherosclerosis. *Sci. Am.*, 236(2):74–85.
22. Bennett, J. G., Longmore, D. B., and O'Grady, J. (1981): Use of prostacyclin in cardiopulmonary bypass in man. In: *Clinical Pharmacology of Prostacyclin*, edited by P. J. Lewis and J. O'Grady, pp. 201–208. Raven Press, New York.
23. Bergman, G., Daly, R., Atkinson, L., Rothman, M., Richardson, P. J., Jackson, G., and Jewitt, D. E. (1981): Prostacyclin: Haemodynamic and metabolic effects in patients with coronary artery disease. *Lancet*, i:569–572.
24. Best, L. C., Martin, T. J., Russell, R. G. G., and Preston, F. E. (1977): Prostacyclin increases cyclic AMP levels and adenylate cyclase activity in platelets. *Nature*, 267:850–851.
25. Bhattacherjee, P., Kulkarni, P. S., and Eakins, K. E. (1979): The metabolism of arachidonic acid in rabbit ocular tissue. *Invest. Ophthalmol. Vis. Sci.*, 18:172–178.
26. Bishop, V. S., and Peterson, D. F. (1978): The circulatory influences of vagal afferants at rest and during coronary occlusion in conscious dogs. *Circ. Res.*, 43:840–847.
27. Black, R. L., Culp, B., Madison, D., Randall, O. S., and Lands, W. E. M. (1979): The protective effects of dietary fish oil on focal cerebral infarctions. *Prostaglandins Med.*, 3:257–268.
28. Blackwell, G. J., Flower, R. J., Russell-Smith, N., Salmon, J. A., Thorogood, P. B., and Vane, J. R. (1978): I-*n*-Butylimidazole: A potent and selective inhibitor of 'Thromboxane Synthetase'. *Br. J. Pharmacol.*, 64:436P.
29. Blasko, G., Nemesanszky, E., Szabo, G., Stadier, I., and Palos, L. A. (1980): The effects of PGI₂ and PGI₂ analogues with increased stability on platelet cAMP and aggregation. *Thromb. Res.*, 17:673–681.
30. Block, A. J., Feinberg, H., Herbaczynska-Cedro, K., and Vane, J. R. (1975): Anoxia induced release of prostaglandins in rabbit isolated heart. *Circ. Res.*, 36:34–42.
31. Blumberg, A. L., Denny, S. E., Marshall, G. R., and Needleman, P. (1977): Blood vessel hormone interactions: Angiotensin, bradykinin and prostaglandins. *Am. J. Physiol.*, 232:H303–310.
32. Born, G. V. R. (1962): Aggregation of blood platelets by adenosine diphosphate and its reversal. *Nature*, 194:927–929.
33. Boullin, D. J., Bunting, S., Blaso, W. P., Hunt, T. M., and Moncada, S. (1979): Response of human and baboon arteries to prostaglandin endoperoxides and biologically generated and synthetic prostacyclin: Their relevance to cerebral arterial spasm in man. *Br. J. Clin. Pharmacol.*, 7:139–147.
34. Bourgain, R. H., Six, F., and Andries, R. (1980): The action of cyclooxygenase and prostacyclin-synthesis inhibitors on platelet-vessel wall interaction. *Artery*, 8:96–100.
35. Boyd, A. M., and Marks, J. (1963): Treatment of intermittent claudication. A reappraisal of the value of α-tocopherol. *Angiology*, 14:198–208.
36. Budd, G. T., Bukowski, R. M., Lucas, F. V., Cato, A. E., and Cocchetto, D. M. (1980): Prostacyclin therapy of thrombotic thrombocytopenic purpura. *Lancet*, ii:915.
37. Bunting, S., Gryglewski, R., Moncada, S., and Vane, J. R. (1976): Arterial walls generate from prostaglandin endoperoxides a substance (prostaglandin X) which relaxes strips of mesenteric and coeliac arteries and inhibits platelet aggregation. *Prostaglandins*, 12:897–913.
38. Bunting, S., and Moncada, S. (1980): Prostacyclin, by preventing platelet activation, prolongs activated clotting time in blood and platelet rich plasma and potentiates the anti-coagulant effect of heparin. *Br. J. Pharmacol.*, 69:268P-269P.
39. Bunting, S., Moncada, S., Reed, P., Salmon, J. A., and Vane, J. R. (1978): An antiserum to 5,6-dihydro prostacyclin (PGI₁) which also binds prostacyclin. *Prostaglandins*, 15:565–574.
40. Bunting, S., Moncada, S., and Vane, J. R. (1977): Antithrombotic properties of vascular endothelium. *Lancet*, ii:1075–1076.

41. Bunting, S., Moncada, S., Vane, J. R., Woods, H. F., and Weston, M. J. (1979): Prostacyclin improves hemocompatability during charcoal hemoperfusion. In: *Prostacyclin*, edited by J. R. Vane and S. Bergström, pp. 361–369. Raven Press, New York.
42. Bunting, S., O'Grady, J., Fabiani, J. -N., Terrier, E., Moncada, S., Vane, J. R., and Dubost, Ch. (1981): Cardiopulmonary bypass in man: Effects of prostacyclin. In: *Clinical Pharmacology of Prostacyclin*, edited by P. J. Lewis and J. O'Grady, pp. 181–193. Raven Press, New York.
43. Bunting, S., Simmons, P. M., and Moncada, S. (1981): Inhibition of platelet activation by prostacyclin: Possible consequences in coagulation and anticoagulation. *Thromb. Res.*, 21:89–102.
44. Bye, A., Lewis, Y., and O'Grady, J. (1979): Effect of a single oral dose of aspirin on the platelet aggregation response to arachidonic acid. *Br. J. Clin. Pharmacol.*, 7:283–286.
45. Carreras, L. O., Chamone, D. A. F., Klerckx, P., and Vermylen, J. (1980): Decreased vascular prostacyclin (PGI$_2$) in diabetic rats. Stimulation of PGI$_2$ release in normal and diabetic rats by the antithrombotic compound BAY g 6575. *Thromb. Res.*, 19:663–670.
46. Chang, W.-C., Murota, S.-I., and Tsurufuji, S. (1977): Thromboxane B$_2$ transformed from arachidonic acid in carrageenin-induced granuloma. *Prostaglandins*, 13:17–24.
47. Chapple, D. J., Dusting, G. J., Hughes, R., and Vane, J. R. (1978): A vagal reflex contributes to the hypotensive effect of prostacyclin in anaesthetized dogs. *J. Physiol. (Lond.)*, 281:43–44P.
48. Chapple, D. J., Dusting, G. J., Hughes, R., and Vane, J. R. (1980): Some direct and reflex cardiovascular actions of prostacyclin (PGI$_2$) and PGE$_2$ in anaesthetized dogs. *Br. J. Pharmacol.*, 68:437–447.
49. Chelly, J., Tricot, C., Garcia, A., Boucherie, J-C., Fabiani, J-N., Passalecq, J., and Dubost, Ch. (1981): Haemodynamic effects of prostacyclin infusion after coronary bypass surgery. In: *Clinical Pharmacology of Prostacyclin*, edited by P. J. Lewis and J. O'Grady, p. 209. Raven Press, New York.
50. Chiavarelli, M., Moncada, S., and Mullane, K. (1982): Prostacyclin-induced bradycardia is dependent on the basal heart rate and is antagonised by sodium cromoglycate. *Br. J. Pharmacol. (in press)*.
51. Chierchia, S., Ciabattoni, G., Cinotti, G., Maseri, A., Patrono, C., Pugliese, F., Distante, A., Simonetti, I., and Bernini, W. (1979): Haemodynamic and antiaggregatory effects of prostacyclin (PGI$_2$) in the healthy man. *Circulation*, 59 and 60 (Suppl. II):83.
52. Cho, M. J., and Allen, M. A. (1978): Chemical stability of prostacyclin (PGI$_2$) in aqueous solutions. *Prostaglandins*, 15:943–954.
53. Christofinis, G. J., Moncada, S., Bunting, S., and Vane, J. R. (1979): Prostacyclin (PGI$_2$) release by rabbit aorta and human umbilical vein endothelial cells after prolonged subculture. In: *Prostacyclin*, edited by J. R. Vane and S. Bergström, pp. 77–84. Raven Press, New York.
54. Christopherson, B. O. (1968): Formation of monohydroxypolenic fatty acids from lipid peroxides by a glutathione peroxidase. *Biochim. Biophys. Acta*, 164:35.
55. Cimo, P. L., Moake, J. L., Weinger, R. S., Ben-Menachem, Y., and Khalil, K. G. (1979): Heparin-induced thrombocytopenia association with a platelet aggregating factor and arterial thrombosis. *Am. J. Hematol.*, 6:125–133.
56. Cocchetto, D. M., Cook, L., Cato, A. E., and Niedel, E. (1981): Rationale and proposal for use of prostacyclin in thrombotic thrombocytopenic purpura therapy. *Semin. Thromb. Hemostas.*, 7:43–51.
57. Coceani, F., Bishai, I., White, E., Bodach, E., and Olley, P. M. (1978): Action of prostaglandins, endoperoxides and thromboxanes on the lamb ductus arteriosus. *Am. J. Physiol.*, 234:H117–H122.
58. Coleridge, H. M., Coleridge, J. C. G., and Kidd, C. (1964): Cardiac receptors in the dog, with particular reference to two types of afferent ending in the ventricular wall. *J. Physiol.* 174:322–339.
59. Cottee, F., Flower, R. J., Moncada, S., Salmon, J. A., and Vane, J. R. (1977): Synthesis of 6-keto-PGF$_{1\alpha}$ by ram seminal vesicle microsomes. *Prostaglandins*, 14:413–423.
60. Coughlin, S. R., Moskowitz, M. A., Zeiter, B. R., Antoniades, H. N., and Levine, L. (1980): Platelet-dependent stimulation of prostacyclin synthesis by platelet derived growth factor. *Nature*, 288:600–602.
61. Culp, B. R., Lands, W. E. M., Luccesi, B. R., Pitt, B., and Romson, J. (1980): The effect of dietary supplementation of fish oil on experimental myocardial infarction. *Prostaglandins*, 20:1021–1031.
62. Culp, B. R., Titus, B. G., and Lands, W. E. M. (1979): Complement and leukocyte-mediated pulmonary dysfunction in hemodialysis. *Prostaglandins Med.*, 3:269–278.

63. Czervionke, R. L., Smith, J. B., Fry, G. L., and Hoak, J. C. (1979): Inhibition of prostacyclin by treatment of endothelium with aspirin. *J. Clin. Invest.*, 63:1089–1092.
64. D'Angelo, V., Villa,, S., Mysliwiec, M., Donati, M. B., and De Gaetano, G. (1978): Defective fibrinolytic and prostacyclin-like activity in human atheromatous plaques. *Thromb. Haemost.*, 39:535–536.
65. Davidson, E. M., Ford-Hutchinson, A. W., Smith, M. J.H., and Walker, J. R. (1978): The release of thromboxane B_2 by rabbit peritoneal polymorphonuclear leukocytes. *Br. J. Pharmacol.*, 63:407P.
66. Davis, T. M. E., Brown, E., Finch, D. R., Mitchell, M. D., and Turner, R. C. (1981): *In vitro* venous prostacyclin production, plasma 6-keto prostaglandin $F_{1\alpha}$ concentrations, and diabetic retinopathy. *Br. Med. J.*, 282:1259–1262.
67. Dawson, W., Boot, J. R., Cockerill, A. F., Mallen, D. N. B., and Osborne, D. J. (1976): Release of novel prostaglandins and thromboxanes after immunological challenge of guinea pig lung. *Nature*, 262:699–702.
68. De Dekere, E. A. M., Nugteren, D. H., and Ten Hoor, F. (1977): Prostacyclin is the major prostaglandin from the isolated perfused rabbit and rat heart. *Nature*, 268:160–163.
69. Defreyn, G., Vergara Dayden, M., Machin, S. J., and Vermylen, J. (1980): A plasma factor in uraemia which stimulates prostacyclin release from cultured endothelial cells. *Thromb. Res.*, 19:695–699.
70. De Gomez Dumm, I. N. T., and Brenner, R. R. (1975): Oxidative desaturation of γ-linolenic, linoleic and stearic acids by human liver microsomes. *Lipids*, 10:315–317.
71. DiNicolantonio, R., Dusting, G. J., Hutchinson, J. S., and Mendelsohn, F. A. O. (1981): Failure of aspirin to modify the hypotensive action of captopril in spontaneously hypertensive rats. *Clin. Exp. Pharmacol. Physiol.*, 8:345–352.
72. Dix, R. K., Kelliher, G. J., Jurkiewicz, N., and Lawrence, T. (1979): The influence of prostacyclin on coronary occlusion induced arrhythmia in cats. *Prostaglandins Med.*, 3:173–184.
73. Dixon, M., Jackson, D. M., and Richards, I. M. (1980): The action of sodium cromoglycate on C-fibre endings in the dog lung. *Br. J. Pharmacol.*, 70:11–13.
74. Dollery, C. T., Friedman, L. A., Hensby, C. N., Kohner, E., Lewis, P. J., Porta, M., and Webster, J. (1979): Circulating prostacyclin may be reduced in diabetes. *Lancet*, ii:1365.
75. Dusting, G. J. (1981): Prostacyclin released by angiotensins from lungs and isolated vascular tissue. In: *Adv. Physiol. Sci., Vol. 7, Cardiovascular Physiology. Microcirculation and Capillary Exchange*, edited by A. Kovach, J. Hamar, and L. Szabo, pp. 65–74. Pergamon Press, Oxford.
76. Dusting, G. J. (1981): Angiotensin-induced release of a prostacyclin (PGI₂)-like substance from the lung. *J. Cardiovasc. Pharmacol.*, 3:197–206.
77. Dusting, G. J., Chapple, D. J., Hughes, R., Moncada, S., and Vane, J. R. (1978): Prostacyclin induces coronary vasodilatation in anaesthetized dogs. *Cardiovasc. Res.*, 12:720–730.
78. Dusting, D. J., Di Nicolantonio, R., Drysdale, T., and Doyle, A. E. (1981): Vasodepressor effects of arachidonic acid and prostacyclin (PGI₂) in hypertensive rats. *Clin. Sci.*, 61:315s–318s.
79. Dusting, G. J., Moncada, S., Mullane, K. M., and Vane, J. R. (1978): Implications of prostacyclin (PGI₂) generation for modulation of vascular tone. *Clin. Sci. Mol. Med.*, 55:195s–198s.
80. Dusting, G. J., Moncada, S., and Vane, J. R. (1977): Prostacyclin (PGX) is the endogenous metabolite responsible for relaxation of coronary arteries by arachidonic acid. *Prostaglandins*, 13:3–15.
81. Dusting, G. J., Moncada, S., and Vane, J. R. (1977): Disappearance of prostacyclin in the circulation of the dog. *Br. J. Pharmacol.*, 62:414–415P.
82. Dusting, G. J., Moncada, S., and Vane, J. R. (1977): Prostacyclin is a weak contractor of coronary arteries in the pig. *Eur. J. Pharmacol.*, 45:301–304.
83. Dusting, G. J., Moncada, S., and Vane, J. R. (1978): Recirculation of prostacyclin (PGI₂) in the dog. *Br. J. Pharmacol.*, 64:315–320.
84. Dusting, G. J., Moncada, S., and Vane, J. R. (1978): Vascular actions of arachidonic acid and its metabolites in perfused mesenteric and femoral beds of the dog. *Eur. J. Pharmacol.*, 49:65–72.
85. Dusting, G. J., Moncada, S., and Vane, J. R. (1979): Prostaglandins, their intermediates and precursors: Cardiovascular roles and regulatory mechanisms in normal and abnormal circulatory systems. *Prog. Cardiovasc. Disease*, 21:405–430.
86. Dusting, G. J., and Mullins, E. M. (1980): Stimulation by angiotensin of prostacyclin biosynthesis in rats and dogs. *Clin. Exp. Pharmacol. Physiol.*, 7:545–550.
87. Dusting, G. J., Mullins, E. M., and Nolan, R. D. (1981): Prostacyclin release accompanying angiotensin conversion in rat mesenteric vasculature. *Eur. J. Pharmacol.*, 70:129–137.

88. Dusting, G. J., and Nolan, R. D. (1981): Stimulation of prostacyclin release from the epicardium of anaesthetized dogs. *Br. J. Pharmacol.*, 74:553–562.
89. Dyerberg, J., and Bang, H. O. (1979): Haemostatic function and platelet polyunsaturated fatty acids in Eskimos. *Lancet*, ii:433–435.
90. Dyerberg, J., Bang, H. O., and Aagaard, O. (1980): γ-Linolenic acid and eicosapentaenoic acid. *Lancet*, i:199.
91. Dyerberg, J., Bang, H. O., Stofferson, E., Moncada, S., and Vane, J. R. (1978): Eicosapentaenoic acid and prevention of thrombosis and atherosclerosis? *Lancet*, ii:117–119.
92. Dyerberg, J., and Jorgensen, K. A. (1980): The effect of arachidonic and eicosapentaenoic acid on the synthesis of prostacyclin-like material in human umbilical vasculature. *Artery*, 8:12–17.
93. Eakins, K. E., Rajadhyaksha, V., and Schroer, R. (1976): Prostaglandin antagonism by sodium P-benzyl-4-(1-oxo-2(4-chlorobenzyl)-3-phenylpropyl) phenyl phosphonate (N-0164). *Br. J. Pharmacol.*, 58:333–339.
94. Fenwick, L., Jones, R. L., Naylor, B., Poyser, N. L., and Wilson, N. H. (1977): Production of prostaglandins by the pseudopregnant rat uterus "in vitro" and the effect of tamofixen with the identification of 6-keto prostaglandin $F_{1\alpha}$ as a major product. *Br. J. Pharmacol.*, 59:191–196.
95. Ferreira, S. H., Moncada, S., and Vane, J. R. (1973): Prostaglandins and the mechanism of analgesia produced by aspirin-like drugs. *Br. J. Pharmacol.*, 49:86–97.
96. Feuerstein, N., and Ramwell, P. W. (1981): OKY-1581, a potential selective thromboxane synthetase inhibitor. *Eur. J. Pharmacol.*, 69:533–534.
97. Fidler, J., Bennett, M. J., Swiet, M. de., Ellis, C., and Lewis, P. J. (1980): Treatment of pregnancy hypertension with prostacyclin. *Lancet*, ii:31–32.
98. FitzGerald, G. A., Friedman, L. A., Miyamori, I., O'Grady, J., and Lewis, P. J. (1979): A double blind placebo controlled crossover study of prostacyclin in man. *Life Sci.*, 25:665–672.
99. FitzGerald, G. A., Roberts, L. J., II, Maas, D., Brash, A. R., and Oates, J. A. (1981): Intravenous prostacyclin in thrombotic thrombocytopenic purpura. In: *Clinical Pharmacology of Prostacyclin*, edited by P. J. Lewis and J. O'Grady, p. 81. Raven Press, New York.
100. Fitzpatrick, F. A., Bundy, G. L., Gorman, R. R., and Honohan, T. (1978): 9,11-Epoxyimino prosta-5,13 dienoic acid is a thromboxane A_2 antagonist in human platelets. *Nature*, 275:764–766.
101. Flower, R. J., and Cardinal, D. G. (1979): Use of a novel platelet aggregometer to study the generation by, and actions of prostacyclin in whole blood. In: *Prostacyclin*, edited by J. R. Vane and S. Bergström, pp. 211–220. Raven Press, New York.
102. Friedenberg, W. R., Myers, W. O., Plotka, E. D., Beathard, J. N., Kummer, D. J., Gatlin, P. F., Stoiber, D. L., Ray, J. F., and Sautter, R. D. (1978): Platelet dysfunction associated with cardiopulmonary bypass. *Ann. Thorac. Surg.*, 25:298–305.
103. Ganten, D., and Speck, G. (1978): The brain renin-angiotensin systems: A model for synthesis of peptides in the brain. *Biochem. Pharmacol.*, 27:2379–2389.
104. Giles, R. W., and Wilcken, D. E. L. (1977): Reactive hyperemia in the dog heart: Inter-relation between adenosine, ATP and aminophylline and the effect of indomethacin. *Cardiovasc. Res.*, 11:111–121.
105. Gill, J. R., Frolich, J. C., Bowden, R. E., Raylor, A. A., Keiser, H. R., Seyberth, H. W., Oates, J. A., and Bartter, F. C. (1976): Bartter's syndrome: A disorder characterized by high urinary prostaglandins and a dependence of hyperreninemia on prostaglandin synthesis. *Am. J. Med.*, 61:43–51.
106. Gimbrone, M. A., and Alexander, R. W. (1975): Angiotensin II stimulation of prostaglandin production in cultured human vascular endothelium. *Science*, 189:219–220.
107. Gimeno, M. F., Sterin-Borda, L., Borda, E. S., Lazzari, M. A., and Gimeno, A. L. (1980): Human plasma transforms prostacyclin (PGI_2) into a platelet antiaggregatory substance which contracts isolated bovine coronary arteries. *Prostaglandins*, 19:907–916.
108. Gimson, A. E. S., Canalese, J., Hughes, R. D., Langley, P. G., Mellon, P. J., and Williams, R. (1981): Charcoal haemoperfusion with prostacyclin in the treatment of fulminant hepatic failure. In: *Clinical Pharmacology of Prostacyclin*, edited by P. J. Lewis and J. O'Grady, pp. 211–218. Raven Press, New York.
109. Gimson, A. E. S., Hughes, R. D., Mellon, P. J., Woods, H. F., Langley, P. G., Canalese, J., Williams, R., and Weston, M. J. (1980): Prostacyclin to prevent platelet activation during charcoal haemoperfusion in fulminant hepatic failure. *Lancet*, i:173–175.
110. Glavind, J., Hartmann, S., Clemmesen, J., Jessen, K. E., and Dam, H. (1952): Studies on the role of lipoperoxides in human pathology. II. The presence of peroxidized lipids in the atherosclerotic aorta. *Acta Pathol. Microbiol. Scand.*, 30:1.

111. Godal, H. C., Eika, C., Dybdahl, J. H., Daae, L., and Larsen, S. (1979): Aspirin and bleeding time. *Lancet*, i:1236.
112. Goehlert, U. G., Ng Ying Kin, N. M. K., and Wolfe, L. S. (1981): Biosynthesis of prostacyclin in rat cerebral microvessels and the choroid plexus. *J. Neurochem.*, 36:1192–1201.
113. Goldstein, I. M., Malmsten, C. L., Kaplan, H. B., Kindahl, H., Samuelsson, B., and Weissman, G. (1977): Thromboxane generation by stimulated human granulocytes: Inhibition by glucocorticoids and superoxide dismutase. *Clin. Res.*, 25:518A.
114. Gordon, J. L., and Pearson, J. D. (1978): Effects of sulphinpyrazone and aspirin on prostaglandin I₂ (prostacyclin) synthesis by endothelial cells. *Br. J. Pharmacol.*, 64:481–483.
115. Gorman, R. R., Bunting, S., and Miller, O. V. (1977): Modulation of human platelet adenylate cyclase by prostacyclin (PGX). *Prostaglandins*, 13:377–388.
116. Gorman, R. R., Hamilton, R. D., and Hopkins, N. K. (1979): Stimulation of human foreskin fibroblast adenosine 3′5′-cyclic monophosphate levels by prostacyclin (prostaglandin I₂). *J. Biol. Chem.*, 254:1671–1676.
117. Grenier, F. C., and Smith, W. L. (1978): Formation of 6-keto-PGF₁ₐ by collecting tubule cells isolated from rabbit renal papillae. *Prostaglandins*, 16:759–772.
118. Grodzinska, L., and Gryglewski, R. J. (1980): Angiotensin-induced release of prostacyclin from perfused organs. *Pharmacol. Res. Commun.*, 12:339–347.
119. Grose, J. H., Lebel, M., and Gbeassor, F. M. (1980): Diminished urinary prostacyclin metabolite in essential hypertension. *Clin. Sci.*, 59:121s–123s.
120. Gryglewski, R. J. (1979): Prostacyclin as a circulating hormone. *Biochem. Pharmacol.*, 28:3161–3166.
121. Gryglewski, R. J., Bunting, S., Moncada, S., Flower, R. J., and Vane, J. R. (1976): Arterial walls are protected against deposition of platelet thrombi by a substance (prostaglandin X) which they make from prostaglandin endoperoxides. *Prostaglandins*, 12:685–714.
122. Gryglewski, R. J., Korbut, R., and Ocetkiewicz, A. C. (1978): Generation of prostacyclin by lungs *in vivo* and its release into the arterial circulation. *Nature*, 273:765–767.
123. Gryglewski, R. J., Korbut, R., Ocetkiewicz, A., Splawinski, J., Wojtaszek, B., and Swiens, J. (1978): Lungs as a generator of prostacyclin. Hypothesis on physiological significance. *Naunyn Schmiedebergs Arch. Pharmacol.*, 304:45–50.
124. Gryglewski, R. J., Korbut, R., Ocetkiewicz, A. C., and Stachura, T. (1978): *In vivo* method for quantitation of anti-platelet potency of drugs. *Naunyn Schmiedebergs Arch. Pharmacol.*, 302:25–30.
125. Gryglewski, R. J., Salmon, J. A., Ubatuba, F. B., Weatherley, B. C., Moncada, S., and Vane, J. R. (1979): Effects of all *cis*-5,8,11,14,17 eicosapentaenoic acid and PGH₃ on platelet aggregation. *Prostaglandins*, 18:453–478.
126. Gryglewski, R. J., and Szczeklik, A. (1981): Prostacyclin and atherosclerosis. In: *Clinical Pharmacology of Prostacyclin*, edited by P. J. Lewis and J. O'Grady, pp. 89–95. Raven Press, New York.
127. Gullner, H-G., Cerletti, C., Bartter, F. C., Smith, J. B., and Gill, J. R., Jr. (1979): Prostacyclin overproduction in Bartter's syndrome. *Lancet*, ii:767–768.
128. Haeger, K. (1968): The treatment of peripheral occlusive arterial disease with alpha-tocopherol as compared with vasodilator agents and antiprothrombin. *Vasc. Dis.*, 5:199–213.
129. Hall, R. J. C., and Dewar, H. A. (1981): Safety of coronary arterial prostacyclin infusion. *Lancet*, i:949.
130. Hamberg, M., and Samuelsson, B. (1973): Detection and isolation of an endoperoxide intermediate in prostaglandin biosynthesis. *Proc. Natl. Acad. Sci. USA*, 70:899–903.
131. Hamberg, M., Svensson, J., and Samuelsson, B. (1975): Thromboxanes: A new group of biologically active compounds derived from prostaglandin endoperoxides. *Proc. Natl. Acad. Sci. USA*, 72:2994–2998.
132. Hamberg, M., Svensson, J., Wakabayashi, T., and Samuelsson, B. (1974): Isolation and structure of two prostaglandin endoperoxides that cause platelet aggregation. *Proc. Natl. Acad. Sci. USA*, 71:345–349.
133. Harrison, H. E., Reece, A. H., and Johnson, M. (1978): Decreased vascular prostacyclin in experimental diabetes. *Life Sci.*, 23:351–356.
134. Harrowing, P. D., and Williams, K. I. (1979): Homogenates of rat placenta contain a factor(s) which inhibits uterine arachidonic acid metabolism. *Br. J. Pharmacol.*, 67:428P.
135. Harter, H. R., Burch, J. W., Majerus, P. W., Stanford, N., Pelmes, J. A., Anderson, C. B., and Weerts, C. A. (1979): Prevention of thromboembolism in patients of haemodialysis by low dose aspirin. *N. Engl. J. Med.*, 301:577–579.

136. Hensby, C. N., Barnes, P. J., Dollery, C. T., and Dargie, H. (1979): Production of 6-oxo-$PGF_{1\alpha}$ by human lung *in vivo. Lancet*, ii:1162–1163.
137. Hensby, C. N., Lewis, P. J., Hilgard, P., Mufti, G. J., Hows, J., and Webster, J. (1979): Prostacyclin deficiency in thrombotic thrombocytopenic purpura. *Lancet*, ii:748.
138. Herman, A. G., Claeys, M., Moncada, S., and Vane, J. R. (1978): Prostacyclin production by rabbit aorta, pericardium, pleura, peritoneum and dura mater. *Arch. Int. Pharmacodyn. Ther.*, 236:303–304.
139. Heyns, A. du P., van den Berg, D. J., Potgieter, G. M., and Retief, F. P. (1974): The inhibition of platelet aggregation by an aorta intima extract. *Thromb. Diath. Haemorrh.*, 32:417–431.
140. Higgs, G. A., Bunting, S., Moncada, S., and Vane, J. R. (1976): Polymorphonuclear leukocytes produce thromboxane A_2-like activity during phagocytosis. *Prostaglandins*, 12:749–757.
141. Higgs, E. A., Higgs, G. A., Moncada, S., and Vane, J. R. (1978): Prostacyclin (PGI_2) inhibits the formation of platelet thrombi in arterioles and venules of the hamster cheek pouch. *Br. J. Pharmacol.*, 63:535–539.
142. Higgs, G. A., Moncada, S., and Vane, J. R. (1977): Prostacyclin (PGI_2) inhibits the formation of platelet thrombi induced by adenosine diphosphate (ADP) *in vivo. Br. J. Pharmacol.*, 61:137P.
143. Higgs, G. A., Moncada, S., and Vane, J. R. (1978): Prostacyclin reduces the number of 'slow moving' leucocytes in hamster pouch cheek venules. *J. Physiol.*, 280:55P–56P.
144. Higgs, E. A., Moncada, S., Vane, J. R., Caen, J. P., Michel, H., and Tobelem, G. (1978): Effect of prostacyclin (PGI_2) on platelet adhesion to rabbit arterial subendothelium. *Prostaglandins*, 16:17–22.
145. Hintze, T. H., and Kaley, G. (1977): Prostaglandins and the control of blood flow in the canine myocardium. *Circ. Res.*, 40:313–320.
146. Hintze, T. H., Martin, E. G., Baez, A., Messina, E. J., and Kaley, G. (1978): PGI_2 induces bradycardia in the dog. *Circulation*, 58:67.
147. Hintze, T. H., Martin, E. G., Messina, E. J., and Kaley, G. (1979): Prostacyclin elicits bradycardia in dogs: Evidence for vagal mediation. *Proc. Soc. Exp. Biol. Med.*, 162:96–100.
148. Hirsh, P. D., Hillis, L. D., Campbell, W. D., Firth, B. G., and Willerson, J. T. (1981): Release of prostaglandins and thromboxane into the coronary circulation in patients with ischemic heart disease. *N. Engl. J. Med.*, 304:685–691.
149. Hope, W., Martin, I. J., Chesterman, C. N., and Morgan, F. J. (1979): Human β-thromboglobulin inhibits PGI_2 production and binds to a specific site in bovine aortic endothelial cells. *Nature*, 228:210–212.
150. Hopkins, N. K., and Gorman, R. R. (1981): Regulation of endothelial cell cyclic nucleotide metabolism by prostacyclin. *J. Clin. Invest.*, 67:540–546.
151. Hornstra, G., Haddeman, E., and Don, J. A. (1979): Blood platelets do not provide endoperoxides for vascular prostacyclin production. *Nature*, 279:66–68.
152. Humes, J. L., Bonney, R. J., Pelus, L., Dahlgren, M. E., Sadowski, S. J., Kuehl, F. A., and Davis, P. (1977): Macrophages synthesise and release prostaglandins in response to inflammatory stimuli. *Nature*, 269:149–151.
153. Hussey, C. V., Bernhard, V. M., McLean, M. R., and Fobian, J. E. (1979): Heparin-induced platelet aggregation: *In vitro* confirmation of thrombotic complications associated with heparin therapy. *Ann. Clin. Lab. Sci.*, 9:487–493.
154. Huttner, J. J., Gwebu, E. T., Panganamala, R. V., Milo, G. E., Cornwell, D. G., Sharma, H. M., and Geer, J. C. (1977): Fatty acids and their prostaglandin derivatives: Inhibitors of proliferation in aortic smooth muscle cells. *Science*, 197:289–291.
155. Hyman, A. L., Kadowitz, P. J., Lands, W. E. M., Crawford, C. G., Fried, J., and Barton, J. (1978): Coronary vasodilator activity of 13,14-dihydro prostacyclin methyl ester: Comparison with prostacyclin and other prostanoids. *Proc. Natl. Acad. Sci. USA*, 75:3522–3526.
156. Jakubowski, J. A., and Ardlie, N. G. (1979): Evidence for the mechanism by which eicosapentaenoic acid inhibits human platelet aggregation and secretion—implications for the prevention of vascular disease. *Thromb. Res.*, 16:205–217.
157. Jarisch, A., and Richter, W. (1939): Die Afferent in Bahnen des Veratrine effekts in den Herznerven. *Arch. Exp. Pathol. Pharmacol.*, 193:355–371.
158. Jobin, F. (1978): *Sem. Thromb. Hemost.*, 4:199–240.
159. Johnson, M., Harrison, H. E., Raftery, A. T., and Elder, J. B. (1979): Vascular prostacyclin may be reduced in diabetes in man. *Lancet*, i:325–326.
160. Johnson, M., Reece, A. H., and Harrison, H. E. (1978): Decreased vascular prostacyclin in experimental diabetes. *7th International Congress of Pharmacology, Paris*, Abstract, p. 342. Pergamon Press, Oxford.

161. Johnson, R. A., Morton, D. R., Kinner, J. H., Gorman, R. R., McGuire, J. C., Sun, F. F., Whittaker, N., Bunting, S., Salmon, J., Moncada, S., and Vane, J. R. (1976): The chemical structure of prostaglandin X (prostacyclin). *Prostaglandins*, 12:915–928.

162. Johnson, G. S., Pastan, I., Peery, C. V., Otten, J., and Willingham, M. C. (1972): The role of prostaglandins in the regulation of growth and morphology of transformed fibroblasts. In: *Prostaglandins in Cellular Biology and the Inflammatory Process*, edited by P. W. Ramwell and B. B. Pharriss, pp. 195–205. Plenum Press, New York.

163. Jorgensen, K. A., Dyerberg, J., Anders, S., Olesen, A. S., and Stoffersen, E. (1980): Acetylsalicylic acid, bleeding time and age. *Thromb. Res.*, 19:799–805.

164. Jugdutt, B., Becker, L., and Pitt, B. (1977): Effect of prostaglandin inhibition on collateral blood flow after coronary artery occlusion in conscious dogs. *Circulation*, 55/56(Suppl. 3):111–122.

165. Judgutt, B. F., Hutchins, G. M., Bulkley, B. H., and Becker, L. C. (1979): Infarct size reduction by prostacyclin after coronary occlusion in conscious dogs. *Clin. Res.*, 27:177a.

166. Kannel, W. B., Castelli, W. P., and Gordon, T. (1979): Cholesterol in the prediction of atherosclerotic disease. *Ann. Intern. Med.*, 90:85–91.

167. Karmazyn, M., Horrobin, D. F., Manku, N. J., Cunnane, S. C., Karmali, R. A., Ally, A. I., Morgan, R. O., Nicolaou, K. C., and Barnette, W. E. (1978): Effects of prostacyclin on perfusion pressure, electrical activity, rate and force of contraction in isolated rat and rabbit hearts. *Life Sci.*, 22:2079–2086.

168. Kather, H., and Simon, B. (1979): Effects of some naturally occurring prostaglandins of the D,E, and I-type and synthetic analogues on adenylate cyclase of human fat cell ghosts. *Res. Exp. Med.*, 176:25–29.

169. Kazer-Glanzman, R., Jakabova, M., George, J., and Luscher, E. (1977): Stimulation of calcium uptake in platelet membrane vesicles by adenosine 3′,5′-cyclic monophosphate and protein kinase. *Biochim. Biophys. Acta*, 446:429–440.

170. Kelliher, G. J., Lawrence, L. T., Jurkiewicz, N., and Dix, R. F. (1979): Comparison of the effects of prostaglandins E_1 and A_1 on coronary occlusion induced arrhythmia. *Prostaglandins*, 17:163–177.

171. Kimura, E., Hashimoto, K., and Furukawa, S. (1973): Changes in bradykinin level in coronary sinus blood after the experimental occlusion of a coronary artery. *Am. Heart J.*, 85:635–647.

172. Korbut, R., and Moncada, S. (1978): Prostacyclin (PGI_2) and thromboxane A_2 interaction *in vivo*. Regulation by aspirin and relationship with antithrombotic therapy. *Thromb. Res.*, 13:489–500.

173. Kraemer, R. J., Phernetton, T. M., and Folts, J. D. (1976): Prostaglandin-like substances in coronary venous blood following myocardial ischaemia. *J. Pharmacol. Exp. Ther.*, 199:611–619.

174. Kulkarni, P. S., Eakins, H. M. T., Saber, W. L., and Eakins, W. E. (1977): Microsomal preparations of hormonal bovine iris—ciliary body generate prostacyclin-like but not thromboxane A_2-like activity. *Prostaglandins*, 14:689–700.

175. Kulkarni, P. S., Roberts, R., and Needleman, P. (1976): Paradoxical endogenous synthesis of a coronary dilating substance from arachidonate. *Prostaglandins*, 12:337–353.

176. Lagarde, M., and Dechavanne, M. (1977): Increase of platelet prostaglandin cyclic endoperoxides in thrombosis. *Lancet*, i:88.

177. Lapetina, E. G., Schmitges, G. J., Chandrabose, K., and Cuatrecasas, P. (1977): Cyclic adenosine 3′,5′-monophosphate and prostacyclin inhibit membrane phospholipase activity in platelets. *Biochem. Biophys. Res. Commun.*, 76:828–835.

178. Lefer, A. M., Ogletree, M. L., Smith, J. B., Silver, M. J., Nicolaou, K. C., Barnette, W. E., and Gasic, G. P. (1978): Prostacyclin: A potentially valuable agent for preserving myocardial tissues in acute myocardial ischaemia. *Science*, 220:52–54.

179. Levy, S. V. (1978): Contractile responses to prostacyclin (PGI_2) of isolated human saphenous and rat venous tissue. *Prostaglandins*, 16:93–97.

180. Lewy, R. I., Smith, J. B., Silver, M. J., Wiener, L., and Walinsky, P. (1979): Detection of thromboxane A_2 in peripheral blood of patients with Prinzmetal's angina. *Prostaglandins Med.*, 2:243–248.

181. Lieberman, G. E., Lewis, G. P., and Peters, T. J. (1977): A membrane-bound enzyme in rabbit aorta capable of inhibiting adenosine-diphosphate-induced platelet aggregation. *Lancet*, ii:330–332.

182. Lock, J. E., Olley, P. M., Coceani, F., Swyer, P. R., and Rowe, R. D. (1979): Use of prostacyclin in persistent foetal circulation. *Lancet*, i:1343.

183. Longmore, D. B., Bennett, G., Gueirrara, S., Smith, M., Bunting, S., Reed, P., Moncada, S., Read, N. G., and Vane, J. R. (1979): Prostacyclin: A solution to some problems of extracorporeal circulation. *Lancet*, i:1002–1005.

184. Longmore, D. B., Bennett, J. G., Hoyle, P. M., Smith, M. A., Gregory, A., Osivand, T., and Jones, W. A. (1981): Prostacyclin administration during cardiopulmonary bypass in man. *Lancet*, i:800–804.

185. Macdermot, J., and Barnes, P. J. (1980): Activation of guinea pig pulmonary adenylate cyclase by prostacyclin. *Eur. J. Pharmacol.*, 67:419–425.

186. MacIntyre, D. E., Pearson, J. D., and Gordon, J. L. (1978): Localisation and stimulation of prostacyclin production in vascular cells. *Nature*, 271:549–551.

187. Majerus, P. (1976): Why aspirin? *Circulation*, 54:357–359.

188. Malmsten, C., Granstrom, E., and Samuelsson, B. (1976): Cyclic AMP inhibits synthesis of prostaglandin endoperoxide (PGG_2) in human platelets. *Biochem. Biophys. Res. Commun.*, 68:569–576.

189. Marcus, A. J. (1978): The role of lipids in platelet function with particular reference to the arachidonic acid pathway. *J. Lipid Res.*, 19:793–826.

190. Marcus, A. J., Weksler, B. B., and Jaffe, E. A. (1978): Enzymatic conversion of prostaglandin endoperoxide H_2 and arachidonic acid to prostacyclin by cultured human endothelial cells. *J. Biol. Chem.*, 253:7138–7141.

191. Marcus, A. J., Weksler, B. B., Jaffe, E. A., and Broekman, M. J. (1979): Synthesis of prostacyclin (PGI_2) from platelet-derived endoperoxides by cultured human endothelial cells. *Blood*, 54(Suppl. 1):290a (Abstract 803).

192. Marks, J. (1962): Critical appraisal of the therapeutic value of α-tocopherol. *Vitam. Horm.*, 20:573–598.

193. McGiff, J. C., Crowshaw, K., Terragno, N. A., and Lonigro, A. J. (1970): Release of a prostaglandin E-like substance into renal venous blood in response to angiotensin II. *Circ. Res.*, 26,27 (Suppl. 1):1–121–1–130.

194. McGiff, J. C., Terragno, N. A., Malik, K. U., and Lonigro, A. J. (1972): Release of a prostaglandin E-like substance from canine kidney by bradykinin. Comparison with eledoisin. *Circ. Res.*, 31:36–43.

195. McGiff, J. C., and Wong, P. Y. K. (1979): Compartmentalization of prostaglandins and prostacyclin with the kidney: Implications for renal function. *Fed. Proc.*, 38:89–93.

196. Medalie, J. H., Kahn, H. A., Naufeld, H. N., Riss, E., and Gouldbourt, U. (1973): Five year myocardial infarction incidence. II. Association of single variables to age and birth place. *J. Chronic Dis.*, 26:329–349.

197. Mest, H. J., and Forster, W. (1978): The antiarrhythmic action of prostacyclin (PG_2) on aconitine-induced arrhythmias in rats. *Acta Biol. Med. Ger.*, 37:827–828.

198. Mickel, H. S., and Horbar, J. (1974): The effect of peroxidized arachidonic acid upon human platelet aggregation. *Lipids*, 9:68–71.

199. Miller, O. V., and Gorman, R. R. (1979): Evidence for distinct PGI_2 and PGD_2 receptors in human platelets. *J. Pharmacol. Exp. Ther.*, 210:134–140.

200. Minkes, S., Stanford, M., Chi, M., Roth, G., Raz, A., Needleman, P., and Majerus, P. (1977): Cyclic adenosine 3'5'-monophosphate inhibits the availability of arachidonate to prostaglandin synthetase in human platelet suspensions. *J. Clin. Invest.*, 59:449–454.

201. Mitchell, M. D., Bibby, J. G., Hicks, B. R., and Turnbull, A. C. (1978): Possible role for prostacyclin in human parturition. *Prostaglandins*, 16:931–937.

202. Moncada, S., Gryglewski, R. J., Bunting, S., and Vane, J. R. (1976): An enzyme isolated from arteries transforms prostaglandin endoperoxides to an unstable substance that inhibits platelet aggregation. *Nature*, 263:663–665.

203. Moncada, S., Gryglewski, R. J., Bunting, S., and Vane, J. R. (1976): A lipid peroxide inhibits the enzyme in blood vessel microsomes that generates from prostaglandin endoperoxides the substance (prostaglandin X) which prevents platelet aggregation. *Prostaglandins*, 12:715–733.

204. Moncada, S., Herman, A. G., Higgs, E. A., and Vane, J. R. (1977): Differential formation of prostacyclin (PGX or PGI_2) by layers of the arterial wall. An explanation for the anti-thrombotic properties of vascular endothelium. *Thromb. Res.*, 11:323–324.

205. Moncada, S., Higgs, E. A., and Vane, J. R. (1977): Human arterial and venous tissues generate prostacyclin (prostaglandin X) a potent inhibitor of platelet aggregation. *Lancet*, i:18–21.

206. Moncada, S., Korbut, R., Bunting, S., and Vane, J. R. (1978): Prostacyclin is a circulating hormone. *Nature*, 273:767–768.

207. Moncada, S., Salmon, J. A., Vane, J. R., and Whittle, B. J. R. (1977): Formation of prostacyclin (PGI_2) and its product 6-oxo-$PGF_{1\alpha}$ by the gastric mucosa of several species. *J. Physiol.*, 275:4P–5P.

208. Moncada, S., and Vane, J. R. (1978): Unstable metabolites of arachidonic acid and their role in haemostasis and thrombosis. *Br. Med. Bull.*, 34:129–135.
209. Moncada, S., and Vane, J. R. (1979): The role of prostacyclin in vascular tissue. *Fed. Proc.*, 38:62–66.
210. Moore, S., Pepper, D. S., and Cash, J. D. (1975): The isolation and characterization of a platelet-specific beta-globulin (β-thromboglobulin). *Biochim. Biophys. Acta*, 379:360–369.
211. Moriau, M., Masure, R., Hurlet, A., Debeys, C., Chalant, C., Ponlot, R., Jaumain, P., Servaye-Kestens, Y., Ravaux, A., Louis, A., and Goenen, M. (1977): Haemostasis disorders in open heart surgery with extracorporeal circulation. *Vox Sang.*, 32:41–51.
212. Mullane, K. M., Dusting, G. J., Salmon, J. A., Moncada, S., and Vane, J. R. (1979): Biotransformation and cardiovascular effects of arachidonic acid in the dog. *Eur. J. Pharmacol.*, 54:217–228.
213. Mullane, K. M., and Moncada, S. (1980): Prostacyclin mediates the potentiated hypotensive effect of bradykinin following captopril treatment. *Eur. J. Pharmacol.*, 66:355–365.
214. Mullane, K. M., and Moncada, S. (1980): Prostacyclin release and the modulation of some vasoactive hormones. *Prostaglandins*, 20:25–49.
215. Munday, B. R., Bewick, M., Moncada, S., and Vane, J. R. (1980): Suppression of hyperacute renal allograft rejection in presensitized dogs with prostacyclin. *Prostaglandins*, 19:595–603.
216. Mustard, J. F., and Packham, M. A. (1975): Platelets, thrombosis and drugs. *Drugs*, 9:19–76.
217. Myatt, L., and Elder, M. G. (1977): Inhibition of platelet aggregation by a placental substance with prostacyclin-like activity. *Nature*, 268:159–160.
218. Nafstad, I. (1974): Endothelial damage and platelet thrombosis associated with PUFA-rich vitamin E deficient diet fed to pig. *Thromb. Res.*, 5:25–28.
219. Needleman, P. (1976): The synthesis and function of prostaglandins in the heart. *Fed. Proc.*, 35:2376–2381.
220. Needleman, P., Bronson, S. D., Wyche, A., Sivakoff, M., and Nicolaou, K. (1978): Cardiac and renal prostaglandin I₂. *J. Clin. Invest.*, 61:839–849.
221. Needleman, P., and Kaley, G. (1978): Cardiac and coronary prostaglandin synthesis and function. *N. Engl. J. Med.*, 298:1122–1128.
222. Needleman, P., Marshall, G. R., and Sobel, B. E. (1975): Hormone interactions in the isolated rabbit heart: Synthesis and coronary vasomotor effects of prostaglandins, angiotensin and bradykinin. *Circ. Res.*, 37:802–808.
223. Needleman, P., Raz, A., Minkes, M. S., Ferrendelli, J. A., and Sprecher, H. (1979): Triene prostaglandins: Prostacyclin and thromboxane biosynthesis and unique biological properties. *Proc. Natl. Acad. Sci. USA*, 79:944–948.
224. Needleman, P., Wyche, A., and Raz, A. (1979): Platelet and blood vessel arachidonate metabolism and interactions. *J. Clin. Invest.*, 63:345–349.
225. Neri Serneri, G. G., Masotti, G., Poggesi, L., and Galante, G. (1980): Release of prostacyclin into the bloodstream and its exhaustion in humans after local blood flow changes (ischaemia and venous stasis). *Thromb. Res.*, 17:197–208.
226. Ng, K. K. F., and Vane, J. R. (1967): Conversion of angiotensin I to angiotensin II. *Nature*, 21:762–766.
227. Nordoy, A., Svensson, B., Wiebe, D., and Hoak, J. C. (1978): Lipoproteins and the inhibitory effect of human endothelial cells on platelet function. *Circ. Res.*, 43:527–534.
228. Nugteren, D. H., and Hazelhof, E. (1973): Isolation and properties of intermediates in prostaglandin biosynthesis. *Biochim. Biophys. Acta*, 326:448–461.
229. Oates, J. A., Falardeau, P., FitzGerald, G. A., Branch, R. A., and Brash, A. R. (1981): Quantification of urinary prostacyclin metabolites in man: Estimates of the rate of secretion of prostacyclin into the general circulation. In: *The Clinical Pharmacology of Prostacyclin*, edited by P. J. Lewis and J. O'Grady, pp. 21–24. Raven Press, New York.
230. Oelz, O., Seyberth, H. W., Knapp, H. R., Sweetman, B. J., and Oates, J. A. (1976): Effects of feeding ethyl-dihomo-γ-linolenate on prostaglandin biosynthesis and platelet aggregation in the rabbit. *Biochim. Biophys. Acta*, 431:268–277.
231. Ogletree, M. L., Lefer, A. M., Smith, J. B., and Nicolaou, K. 2C. (1979): Studies on the protective effect of prostacyclin in acute myocardial ischaemia. *Eur. J. Pharmacol.*, 56:95–103.
232. O'Grady, J., and Moncada, S. (1978): Aspirin: A paradoxical effect on bleeding time. *Lancet*, ii:780.
233. O'Grady, J., Warrington, S., Moti, M. J., Bunting, S., Flower, R. J., Fowle, A. S. E., Higgs, E. A., and Moncada, S. (1979): Effects of intravenous prostacyclin infusions in healthy volun-

teers—some preliminary observations. In: *Prostacyclin*, edited by J. R. Vane and S. Bergström, pp. 409–417. Raven Press, New York.

234. O'Grady, J., Warrington, S., Moti, M. J., Bunting, S., Flower, R., Fowle, A. S. E., Higgs, E. A., and Moncada, S. (1980): Effects of intravenous infusion of prostacyclin (PGI₂) in man. *Prostaglandins*, 19:319–332.

235. Ohlendorf, R., Perzborn, E., and Schror, K. (1980): Prevention of infarction-induced decrease in circulating platelet count by prostacyclin. *Thromb. Res.*, 19:447–453.

236. Olsson, A. G. (1980): Intravenous prostacyclin for ischaemic ulcers in peripheral artery disease. *Lancet*, ii:1076.

237. Omini, C., Moncada, S., and Vane, J. R. (1977): The effects of prostacyclin (PGI₂) on tissues which detect prostaglandins (PG's). *Prostaglandins*, 14:625–632.

238. Owen, T. L., Ehrhart, I. C., Weidner, W. J., Scott, J. B., and Haddy, F. J. (1975): Effects of indomethacin on local blood flow regulation in canine heart and kidney. *Proc. Soc. Exp. Biol. Med.*, 149:871–876.

239. Pace-Asciak, C. (1976): Isolation, structure and biosynthesis of 6-keto prostaglandin $F_{1\alpha}$ in the rat stomach. *J. Am. Chem. Soc.*, 98:2348–2349.

240. Pace-Asciak, C. R., Carrara, M. C., Rangaraj, G., and Nicolaou, K. G. (1978): Enhanced formation of PGI₂, a potent hypotensive substance, by aortic rings and homogenates of the spontaneously hypertensive rat. *Prostaglandins*, 15:1005–1012.

241. Pace-Asciak, C., and Rangaraj, G. (1977): The 6-keto prostaglandin $F_{1\alpha}$ pathway in the lamb ductus arteriosus. *Biochim. Biophys. Acta*, 486:583–585.

242. Paintal, A. S. (1973): Vagal sensory receptors and their reflex effects. *Physiol. Rev.*, 53:159–227.

243. Pardy, B. J., Lewis, J. D., and Eastcott, H. H. G. (1980): Preliminary experience with prostaglandins E₁ and I₂ in peripheral vascular disease. *Surgery*, 88:826–832.

244. Pastan, I. H., Johnson, G. S., and Anderson, W. B. (1975): Role of cyclic nuleotides in growth control. *Ann. Rev. Biochem.*, 44:491–522.

245. Patterson, R. H., and Kessler, J. (1969): A filter for microemboli in cardiopulmonary bypass. *Circulation*, 40 (Suppl. 3):160.

246. Pitt, B., Mason, J., and Conti, C. R. (1970): Activation of the plasma kallikrein system during myocardial ischaemia. *Adv. Exp. Med. Biol.*, 8:403–410.

247. Pomerantz, K., Sintetos, A., and Ramwell, P. (1978): The effect of prostacyclin on the human umbilical artery. *Prostaglandins*, 15:1035–1044.

248. Powell, W. S., and Solomon, S. (1977): Formation of 6-oxo-prostaglandin $F_{1\alpha}$ by arteries of the fetal calf. *Biochem. Biophys. Res. Commun.*, 75:815–822.

249. Preston, F. E., Whipps, S., Jackson, C. A., French, A. J., Wyld, P. J., and Stoddard, C. J. (1981): Inhibition of prostacyclin and platelet thromboxane A₂ after low dose aspirin. *N. Engl. J. Med.*, 304:76–79.

250. Rajah, S. M., Penny, S., and Kester, R. (1978): Aspirin and bleeding time. *Lancet*, ii:1104.

251. Raz, A., Isakson, P. C., Minkes, M. S., and Needleman, P. (1977): Characterization of a novel pathway of arachidonate in coronary arteries which generates a potent endogenous coronary vasodilator. *J. Biol. Chem.*, 252:1123–1126.

252. Raz, A., Minkes, M. S., and Needleman, P. (1977): Endoperoxides and thromboxanes. Structural determinants for platelet aggregation and vasoconstriction. *Biochim. Biophys. Acta*, 488:305–311.

253. Remuzzi, G., Cavenaghi, A. E., Mecca, G., Donati, M. B., and De Gaetano, G. (1978): Human renal cortex generates prostacyclin-like activity. *Thromb. Res.*, 12:363–366.

254. Remuzzi, G., Marchesi, D., Zoja, C., Muratore, D., Mecca, G., Misiani, R., Rossi, E., Barbato, M., Capetta, P., Donati, M. B., and De Gaetano, G. (1980): Reduced umbilical and placental vascular prostacyclin in severe preeclampsia. *Prostaglandins*, 20:105–110.

255. Remuzzi, G., Misiani, R., Marchesi, D., Livio, M., Mecca, G., De Gaetano, G., and Donati, M. B. (1978): Haemolytic-uraemic syndrome: Deficiency of plasma factor(s) regulating prostacyclin activity. *Lancet*, ii:871–872.

256. Remuzzi, G. R., Misiani, D., Muratore, D., Marchesi, M., Livio, A., Schieppati, A., Mecca, G., De Gaetano, G., and Donati, M. B. (1979): Prostacyclin and human foetal circulation. *Prostaglandins*, 18:341–348.

257. Remuzzi, G., Rossi, E. C., Misiani, R., Marchesi, D., Mecca, G., de Gaetano, G., and Donati, M. B. (1980): Prostacyclin and thrombotic microangiopathy. *Sem. Thromb. Hemost.*, 6:391–394.

258. Ribeiro, L. G. T., Brandon, T. A., Hopkins, D. G., Reduto, L. A., Taylor, A. A., and Miller, R. R. (1981): Prostacyclin in experimental myocardial ischemia: Effects on hemodynamics, regional myocardial blood flow, infarct size and mortality. *Am. J. Cardiol.*, 47:835–840.

259. Ribeiro, L. G. T., Reduto, L. A., Brandon, T. A., Taylor, A. A., Hopkins, D. G., and Miller, R. R. (1979): Effects of prostacyclin on hemodynamics, regional myocardial blood flow, infarct size and mortality in experimental infarction. *Clin. Res.*, 27:199A.
260. Rubio, R., and Berne, R. M. (1975): Regulation of coronary blood flow. *Prog. Cardiovasc. Dis.*, 18:105–122.
261. Saba, S. R., and Mason, R. G. (1974): Studies of an activity from endothelial cells that inhibits platelet aggregation, serotonin release and clot retraction. *Thromb. Res.*, 5:747–757.
262. Saeed, S. A., McDonald-Gibson, W. J., Cuthbert, J., Copas, J. L., Schneider, C., Gardiner, P. J., Butt, N. M., and Collier, H. O. J. (1977): Endogenous inhibitor of prostaglandin synthetase. *Nature*, 270:32–33.
263. Salmon, J. A., Smith, D. R., Flower, R. J., Moncada, S., and Vane, J. R. (1978): Further studies on the enzymatic conversion of prostaglandin endoperoxide into prostacyclin by porcine aorta microsomes. *Biochim. Biophys. Acta*, 523:250–262.
264. Salzman, E. W., Rosenberg, R. D., Smith, M. H., Lindon, J. N., and Favreau, L. (1980): Effect of heparin and heparin fractions on platelet aggregation. *J. Clin. Invest.*, 65:64–73.
265. Sanders, T. A. B., Ellis, F. R. and Dickerson, J. W. T. (1978): Studies of vegans. *Am. J. Clin. Nutr.*, 31:805–813.
266. Sanders, T. A. B., and Naismith, J. (1979): A comparison of the influence of breast feeding and bottle feeding on the fatty acid composition of the erythrocytes. *Br. J. Nutr.*, 41:619.
267. Sanders, T. A. B., and Naismith, J. (1980): Conflicting roles of polyunsaturated fatty acids. *Lancet*, i:654–655.
268. Sanders, T. A. B., Naismith, D. J., Haines, A. P., and Vickers, M. (1980): Cod liver oil, platelet fatty acids, and bleeding time. *Lancet*, i:1189.
269. Santoro, M. G., Philpott, G. W., and Jaffe, B. M. (1976): Inhibition of tumour growth *in vivo* and *in vitro* by prostaglandin E. *Nature*, 263:777–779.
270. Schrör, K., Moncada, S., Ubatuba, F. B., and Vane, J. R. (1978): Transformation of arachidonic acid and prostaglandin endoperoxides by the guinea pig heart. Formation of RCS and prostacyclin. *Eur. J. Pharmacol.*, 47:103–114.
271. Seiss, W., Roth, P., Scherer, B., Kurzmann, I., Bohlig, B., and Weber, P. C. (1980): Platelet-membrane fatty acids, platelet aggregation, and thromboxane formation during a mackerel diet. *Lancet*, i:441–444.
272. Shebuski, R. J., and Aiken, J. W. (1980): Angiotensin II-induced renal prostacyclin release suppresses platelet aggregation in the anesthetized dog. In: *Advances in Prostaglandin and Thromboxane Research*, Vol. 7, edited by B. Samuelsson, P. W. Ramwell, and R. Paoletti, pp. 1149–1152. Raven Press, New York.
273. Shier, W. T. (1980): Serum stimulation of phospholipase A_2 and prostaglandin release in 3T3 cells is associated with platelet-derived growth-promoting activity. *Proc. Natl. Acad. Sci. USA*, 77:137–141.
274. Shimamoto, T., Kobayashi, M., Takahashi, T., Takashima, Y., Sakamoto, M., and Morooka, S. (1978): An observation of thromboxane A_2 in arterial blood after cholesterol feeding in rabbits. *Jpn. Heart J.*, 19:748–753.
275. Sinzinger, H., Feigl, W., and Silberbauer, K. (1979): Prostacyclin generation in atherosclerotic arteries. *Lancet*, ii:469.
276. Sivakoff, M., Pure, E., Hsueh, W., and Needleman, P. (1979): Prostaglandins and the heart. *Fed. Proc.*, 38:78–82.
277. Slater, T. F. (1972): *Free Radical Mechanisms in Tissue Injury.* Pion Ltd., London.
278. Smith, D. R., Weatherly, B. C., Salmon, J. A., Ubatuba, F. B., Gryglewski, R. J., and Moncada, S. (1979): Preparation and biochemical properties of PGH_3. *Prostaglandins*, 18:423–438.
279. Staszewska-Barczak, J., and Dusting, G. J. (1977): Sympathetic cardiovascular reflex initiated by bradykinin-induced stimulation of cardiac pain receptors in the dog. *Clin. Exp. Pharmacol. Physiol.*, 4:443–452.
280. Staszewska-Barczak, J., and Dusting, G. J. (1981): Effect of prostacyclin on the sympathetically-mediated nociceptive cardiovascular reflex. In: *Adv. Physiol. Sci.*, Vol. 7, *Cardiovascular Physiology. Microcirculation and Capillary Exchange*, edited by A. Kovach, J. Hamar, and L. Szabo, pp. 75–82. Pergamon Press, Oxford.
281. Staszewska-Barczak, J., Ferreira, S. H., and Vane, J. R. (1976): An excitatory nociceptive cardiac reflex elicited by bradykinin and potentiated by prostaglandins and myocardial ischaemia. *Cardiovasc. Res.*, 10:314–327.

282. Steer, M. L., MacIntyre, D. E., Levine, L., and Salzman, E. W. (1980): Is prostacyclin a physiologically important circulating antiplatelet agent? *Nature*, 283:124–125.

283. Steiner, M. (1970): Platelet protein synthesis studied in a cell-free system. *Experientia*, 26:786–789.

284. Streja, D., Steiner, G., and Kwiterovich, P. O. (1978): Plasma high-density lipoproteins and ischemic heart disease. *Ann. Intern. Med.*, 89:871–880.

285. Szczeklik, A., and Gryglewski, R. J. (1981): Treatment of vascular disease with prostacyclin. In: *Clinical Pharmacology of Prostacyclin*, edited by P. J. Lewis and J. O'Grady, pp. 159–167. Raven Press, New York.

286. Szczeklik, A., Gryglewski, R. J., Musial, J., Grodzinska, L., Serwonska, M., and Marcinkiewicz, E. (1978): Thromboxane generation and platelet aggregation in survivals of myocardial infarction. *Thromb. Diath. Haemorrh.*, 40:66–74.

287. Szczeklik, A., Gryglewski, R. J., Nizankowski, R., and Musial, J. (1978): Pulmonary and antiplatelet effects of intravenous and inhaled prostacyclin in man. *Prostaglandins*, 16:654–660.

288. Szczeklik, A., Gryglewski, R. J., Nizankowski, R., Musial, J., Pieton, R., and Mruk, J. (1978): Circulatory and antiplatelet effects of intravenous prostacyclin in healthy man. *Pharmacol. Res. Commun.*, 10:545–556.

289. Szczeklik, A., Nizankowski, R., Skawinski, S., Szczeklik, J., Gluszko, P., and Gryglewski, R. J. (1979): Successful therapy of advanced arteriosclerosis obliterans with prostacyclin. *Lancet*, i:1111–1114.

290. Szczeklik, J., Szczeklik, A., and Nizankowski, R. (1980): Prostacyclin for pulmonary hypertension. *Lancet*, ii:1076.

291. Tansik, R. L., Namm, D. H., and White, H. L. (1978): Synthesis of prostaglandin 6-keto $F_{1\alpha}$ by cultured aortic smooth muscle cells and stimulation of its formation in a coupled system with platelet lysates. *Prostaglandins*, 15:399–408.

292. Tateson, J. E., Moncada, S., and Vane, J. R. (1977): Effects of prostacyclin (PGX) on cyclic AMP concentrations in human platelets. *Prostaglandins*, 13:389–399.

293. Terashita, Z., Nishikawa, K., Terao, S., Nakagawa, M., and Hino, T. (1979): A specific prostaglandin I_2 synthetase inhibitor, 3-hydroperoxy 3-methyl-2 phenyl-3H Indole. *Biochem. Biophys. Res. Commun.*, 91:72–78.

294. Terragno, N. A., Terragno, D. A., Early, J. A., Roberts, M. A., and McGiff, J. C. (1978): Endogenous prostaglandin synthesis inhibitor in the renal cortex. Effects on production of prostacyclin by renal blood vessels. *Clin. Sci. Mol. Med.*, 55:199s–202s.

295. Terragno, N. A., Terragno, D. A., and McGiff, J. C. (1977): Contribution of prostaglandins to the renal circulation in conscious anaesthetized and laparatomized dogs. *Circ. Res.*, 40:590–595.

296. Treacher, D., Warlow, C., and McPherson, K. (1978): Aspirin and bleeding-time. *Lancet*, ii:1378.

297. Turney, J. H., Dodd, N. J., and Weston, M. J. (1981): Prostacyclin in extracorporeal circulations. *Lancet*, i:1101.

298. Tyler, H. M., Saxton, C. A. P. D., and Parry, M. J. (1981): Administration to man of UK-37,248-01, a selective inhibitor of thromboxane synthetase. *Lancet*, i:629–632.

299. Ubatuba, F. B., Moncada, S., and Vane, J. R. (1979): The effect of prostacyclin (PGI_2) on platelet behaviour, thrombosis formation *in vivo* and bleeding time. *Thromb. Diath. Haemorrh.*, 41:425–434.

300. Vane, J. R. (1964): The use of isolated organs for detecting active substances in the circulating blood. *Br. J. Pharmacol. and Chemother.*, 23:360–373.

301. Vane, J. R., and Ferreira, S. H. (1976): Interactions between bradykinin and prostaglandins. In: *Chemistry and Biology of the Kallikrein-kinin System in Health and Disease*, Fogarty International Center Proceedings, No. 27, edited by J. J. Pisano and K. F. Austen, pp. 255–266. U.S. Government Printing Office, Washington, D.C.

302. Vane, J. R., and McGiff, J. C. (1975): Possible contributions of endogenous prostaglandins to the control of blood pressure. *Circ. Res.*, 36 and 37 (Suppl. 1):I-68–I-75.

303. Vargaftig, B. B., and Chignard, M. (1975): Substances that increase the cyclic AMP content prevent platelet aggregation and concurrent release of pharmacologically active substances evoked by arachidonic acid. *Agents Actions*, 5:137–144.

304. Vermylen, J., Carreras, L. O., Schaeren, J. V., Defreyn, G., Machin, S. J., and Verstraete, M. (1981): Thromboxane synthetase inhibition as antithrombotic strategy. Lancet, i:1073–1075.

305. Vermylen, J., Chamone, D. A. F., and Verstraete, M. (1979): Stimulation of prostacyclin release from vessel wall by BAYg6575, an antithrombotic compound. *Lancet*, i:518–520.

306. Verstraete, M. (1976): Are agents affecting platelet functions clinically useful? *Am. J. Med.*, 81:897–914.
307. Von Lossonczy, T. O., Ruiter, A., Bronsgeest-Schoute, H. C., Van Gent, C. M., and Hermus, R. J. J. (1978): The effect of a fish diet on serum lipids in healthy human subjects. *Am. J. Clin. Nutr.*, 31:1340–1345.
308. Walker, I. D., Davidson, J. F., Faichney, A., Wheatley, D., and Davidson, K. (1981): Prostacyclin in cardiopulmonary bypass surgery. In: *Clinical Pharmacology of Prostacyclin*, edited by P. J. Lewis and J. O'Grady, pp. 195–199. Raven Press, New York.
309. Warrington, S., and O'Grady, J. (1980): Cardiovascular effects of prostacyclin (PGI_2) in man. In: *Advances in Prostaglandin and Thromboxane Research*, Vol. 7, edited by B. Samuelsson, P. W. Ramwell, and R. Paoletti, pp. 619–624. Raven Press, New York.
310. Watkins, W. D., Peterson, M. B., Crone, R. K., Shannon, D. C., and Levine, L. (1980): Prostacyclin and prostaglandin E_1 for severe idiopathic pulmonary artery hypertension. *Lancet*, i:1083.
311. Webster, J., Borysiewicz, L. K., Rees, A. J., and Lewis, P. J. (1981): Prostacyclin therapy for haemolytic uremic syndrome. In: *Clinical Pharmacology of Prostacyclin*, edited by P. J. Lewis and J. O'Grady, pp. 77–80. Raven Press, New York.
312. Webster, J., Dollery, C. T., and Hensby, C. N. (1980): Circulating prostacyclin concentrations may be increased by bendrofluazide in patients with essential hypertension. *Clin. Sci.*, 59:125s–128s.
313. Weihrauch, J. L., Brignoli, C. A., Reeves, J. B., and Iverson, J. L. (1977): Fatty acid composition of margarines, processed fats and oils. *Food Technol.*, 31:80.
314. Weiss, H. J., and Turitto, V. T. (1979): Prostacyclin (prostaglandin I_2, PGI_2) inhibits platelet adhesion and thrombus formation on subendothelium. *Blood*, 53:244–250.
315. Weksler, B. B., Knapp, J. M., and Jaffe, E. A. (1977): Prostacyclin synthesized by cultured endothelial cells modulates polymorphonuclear leukocyte function. *Blood*, 50:287.
316. Weksler, B. B., Ley, C. W., and Jaffe, E. W. (1978): Stimulation of endothelial cell prostacyclin production by thrombin, trypsin, and the ionophore A23187. *J. Clin. Invest.*, 62:923–930.
317. Weksler, B. B., Ley, C. W., and Jaffe, E. A. (1978): Phospholipase activity regulates prostacyclin (PGI_2) synthesis by human endothelial cells. *Clin. Res.*, 26:619A.
318. Weksler, B. B., Marcus, A. J., and Jaffe, E. A. (1977): Synthesis of prostaglandin I_2 (prostacyclin) by cultured human and bovine endothelial cells. *Proc. Natl. Acad. Sci. USA*, 74:3922–3926.
319. Weksler, B. B., Reinus, J., and Eldor, A. (1981): Interactions between platelets and prostaglandins: Modulation of prostacyclin production and action in platelets. In: *Prostaglandins and Cardiovascular Disease*, edited by R. Johnsson Hegyeli, pp. 125–138. Raven Press, New York.
320. Weston, M. J., Rubin, M., Hanid, A., Langley, P. G., Westaby, S., and Williams, R. (1977): Platelet function regulating agents—experimental data relevant to hepatic disease. In: *Thromboembolism—A New Approach to Therapy*, edited by J. R. A. Mitchell and J. G. Domenet, pp. 76–82. Academic Press, London.
321. Whittle, B. J. R. (1978): Inhibition of prostacyclin (PGI_2) formation to the rat small intestine and gastric mucosa by the ulcerogen, indomethacin. *Br. J. Pharmacol.*, 63:438P.
322. Whittle, B. J. R. (1981): Antisecretory actions of prostacyclin and its analogues on the gastric mucosa. In: *Clinical Pharmacology of Prostacyclin*, edited by P. J. Lewis and J. O'Grady, pp. 219–232. Raven Press, New York.
323. Whittle, B. J. R., Moncada, S., and Vane, J. R. (1978): Comparison of the effects of prostacyclin (PGI_2), prostaglandin E_1 and D_2 on platelet aggregation in different species. *Prostaglandins*, 16:373–388.
324. Whitworth, J. A., D'Apice, A. J. F., Kincaid-Smith, P., Shulkes, A. A., and Skinner, S. L. (1978): Antihypertensive effect of plasma exchange. *Lancet*, i:1205.
325. Williams, K. I., Dembinska-Kiec, A., Zmuda, A., and Gryglewski, R. J. (1978): Prostacyclin production by myometrial and decidual fractions of the pregnant rat uterus. *Prostaglandins*, 15:343–350.
326. Williams, K. I., and Downing, I. I. (1977): Prostaglandin and thromboxane production by rat decidual microsomes. *Prostaglandins*, 14:813–817.
327. Willis, A. L., Comai, K., Kuhn, D. C., and Paulsrud, J. (1974): Dihomo-γ-linolenate suppresses platelet aggregation when administered *in vitro* or *in vivo*. *Prostaglandins*, 8:509–519.
328. Wlodawer, P., and Hammerström, S. (1979): Some properties of prostacyclin synthase from pig aorta. *FEBS Lett.*, 97(1):32–36.
329. Woods, H. F., Ash, G., Weston, M. J., Bunting, S., Moncada, S., and Vane, . R. (1978): Prostacyclin can replace heparin in haemodialysis in dogs. *Lancet*, ii:1075–1077.

330. Zenser, T. V., Herman, C. A., Gorman, R. R., and Davis, B. B. (1977): Metabolism and action of the prostaglandin endoperoxide PGH_2 in rat kidney. *Biochem. Biophys. Res. Commun.*, 79:357–363.

331. Zusman, R. M., Rubin, R. H., Cato, A. E., Cocchetto, D. M., Crow, J. W., and Tolkoff-Rubin, N. (1981): Hemodialysis using prostacyclin instead of heparin as the sole antithrombotic agent. *N. Engl. J. Med.*, 304:934–939.

332. Zygulska-Mach, H., Kostka-Trabka, E., Niton, A., and Gryglewski, R. J. (1980): Prostacyclin in central retinal vein occlusion. *Lancet*, ii:1075–1076.

Prostaglandins and the Cardiovascular System,
edited by John A. Oates. Raven Press,
New York © 1982.

Pharmacology and Pharmacokinetics of Platelet-Active Drugs Under Current Clinical Investigation

*G. A. FitzGerald and **Sol Sherry

*Department of Pharmacology, Vanderbilt University School of Medicine, Nashville, Tennessee 37232; and **Department of Medicine, Temple University School of Medicine, Philadelphia, Pennsylvania 19140*

In recent years, the commonly available drugs—aspirin, dipyridamole, and sulfinpyrazone—have been shown to be active in suppressing thrombus formation in experimental animals, presumably by inhibiting the ability of platelets to aggregate at sites of vascular injury. Accordingly, there has been considerable interest in evaluating their effects in situations where platelet phenomena and thrombus formation may play an important role in the pathogenesis of certain important clinical disorders, e.g., stroke, myocardial infarction, etc. Since these particular drugs are in an advanced stage of clinical evaluation, this and the following chapter are designed to review current information; this chapter deals with the pharmacology and pharmacokinetics of aspirin, dipyridamole, and sulfinpyrazone, and the subsequent one describes the status of their clinical evaluation in preventing presumed platelet-mediated phenomena.

ASPIRIN

Introduction

Although the early interest in aspirin-like drugs was fueled by an increasing scarcity of quinine at the turn of the century, salicylates remain the topic of hundreds of articles each year (134). The reasons for this are probably multiple. Certainly, being cheap and effective analgesics and antipyretics, salicylates are widely consumed, both as over-the-counter and as prescribed drugs. Secondly, they represent a convenient research tool, being representative organic acids that can be isolated easily and detected by fluorescent or chromatographic means, can be radiolabeled inexpensively, are of low toxicity suitable for human experimentation, and exhibit a variety of metabolic pathways. Finally and of most importance recently, the recognition that many of the actions of aspirin-like drugs were linked to inhibition of prostaglandin (PG) synthesis (463) has provided a further stimulus to research involving these compounds.

Copious amounts of aspirin are consumed throughout the world. It has been estimated that 10 to 20 thousand tons of the drug are ingested in the United States annually (213). Despite such widespread use, it is the prospect of further broadening the therapeutic application of salicylates that engenders fascination in the 1980s.

Salicylic acid derivatives comprise two large classes. These are esters of salicylic acid (orthohydroxybenzoic acid) that may be obtained by substitution in the carboxyl group, and salicylate esters of organic acids in which the carboxyl group of salicylic acid is retained and substitution is made in the hydroxyl group (Fig. 1). The most important representative of the latter group is aspirin, an ester of acetic acid. Several salts of salicylic acid also are used because of their greater solubility, palatability, and possibly lower toxicity. Aluminum and calcium salts of aspirin are also used in medicine; however, the more soluble sodium and potassium salts are not pharmaceutically stable (110). Substitution of the carboxyl or hydroxyl groups change the potency or toxicity of the compound. The ortho position for the OH group is an important feature for the action of salicylate.

Inhibition of Prostaglandin Synthesis

The association between aspirin-like drugs and prostaglandins became clear in 1971. Aspirin and indomethacin were shown to inhibit prostaglandin release from human platelets (430), the perfused dog spleen (137), and to prevent prostaglandin

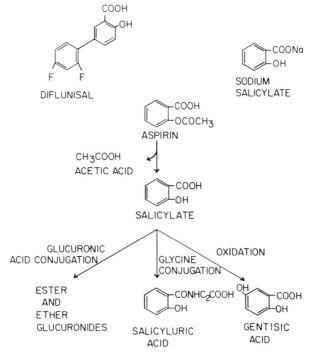

FIG. 1. Structures of several aspirin metabolites and of Diflunisal.

synthesis in cell free preparations of guinea pig lung (213). These observations had been preceded by the demonstration by Piper and Vane (354) that aspirin inhibited the release of an unknown compound, "rabbit aorta constricting substance" [later identified as thromboxane A_2 (TXA_2)] from guinea pig lungs during anaphylaxis. Inhibition of prostaglandin synthesis by aspirin-like compounds since has been demonstrated in some 30 different systems (144).

Microsomal preparations have been studied widely as models of prostaglandin synthesis inhibition since the synthesizing enzymes are located in the precipitated fraction while the most important inactivating enzymes are in the soluble fraction. Examples of preparations that have been employed are dog spleen and rabbit kidney microsomes and homogenates of rabbit brain and guinea pig lung. These preparations also have the advantage of relatively high specific activity. Assay techniques have included radiometric (146), spectrophotometric (451), polarographic (429), and immunochemical (71,248) techniques as well as gas chromatography-mass spectrometry (181). The basic findings are, however, independent of the system of assay used. Published drug concentrations necessary to inhibit enzyme activity by 50% in such systems (ID 50) suggest the following order of decreasing potency: meclofenamic acid > indomethacin > mefenamic acid > flufenamic acid > naproxen > phenylbutazone > aspirin or ibuprofen (144). Two salicylic isomers that have no therapeutic effect, m- and p-hydroxybenzoic acid, are almost devoid of activity.

Prostaglandin synthesis inhibition also has been studied in isolated tissues. Although cellular prostaglandin release appears generally equivalent to *de novo* synthesis (355), the necessity of relying upon this assumption introduces a potential error of quantitation in cellular systems. An additional problem concerns intracellular prostaglandin metabolism. Smith and Willis found that indomethacin was approximately 10 times more potent than aspirin in inhibiting prostaglandin synthesis by human platelets *in vitro* (430) and that aspirin was approximately 10 times more potent than salicylate. Inhibition of prostaglandin synthesis by aspirin or indomethacin also has been demonstrated in rabbit spleen (137), guinea pig lung (354), cultured fibrosarcoma (248), bovine thyroid cells (71), rabbit polymorphonuclear leukocytes (274), and toad bladders (488).

Finally, the inhibition of prostaglandin synthesis by aspirin-like compounds has been studied in intact animals and man. Although the primary prostaglandins disappear rapidly from the circulation, metabolite concentrations in urine may be used as an index of total body prostaglandin synthesis. Prostaglandins of the E and F series undergo rapid dehydrogenation of the 15-hydroxyl group by the lung followed by reduction of the 13,14-double bond to yield 15-keto-13,14,-dihydro prostaglandins (16). These undergo further *in vivo* β- and w-oxidation to yield a number of metabolites (171,180). Hamberg (180) utilized the 16 carbon dicarboxylic acid, 7 α-hydroxy-5,11-diketo tetranorprostane 1, 16-dioic acid, the major urinary metabolite of PGE_1 and PGE_2, to study the effects of aspirin on whole body prostaglandin synthesis in man. When a dose of 750 mg aspirin was administered four times a day, almost maximal inhibition (63–92%) occurred in females after the first day's treatment. The decline was more gradual in male subjects over 3 days. Metabolite concentrations attained pretreatment levels 2 to 3 days after stopping aspirin. Indomethacin appeared approximately 15 times more potent by weight than aspirin, whereas salicylate was approximately equipotent in this system. Aspirin has been demonstrated to reduce the E and F prostaglandin content of human semen (93) and to virtually abolish prostaglandin synthesis by human platelets (430). Aspirin or other nonsteroidal, antiinflammatory compounds have been shown to reduce prostaglandin release provoked by hemorrhage, endotoxin, angiotensin II, and scalding in dogs, cats, and rabbits (313). Aspirin treatment also markedly reduces the elevated renal content of PGE_2 and PGA_2 in Goldblatt hypertensive rats (438).

Although the rank order of inhibitory potency of aspirin-like drugs is strikingly similar when the same tissue from several species is studied, there is great variability between tissues within a species (144). This is evident in the sixfold difference in the inhibitory potency of aspirin on $PGF_{2\alpha}$ release from human platelets and synovial tissue (ID50; 29 vs 172 μM respectively). Both systems are equally sensitive to indomethacin (ID50; 1.33 and 1.08 μM respectively). In concentrations that nearly completely inhibit dog spleen synthetase, aspirin is ineffective against the synthetase of canine myocardium (259,338). This has led to the suggestion (464) that prostaglandin synthetase, or at least one of its component proteins, may exist in several forms.

Although aspirin inhibits a variety of other enzyme systems, this usually occurs at concentrations much greater than that required to inhibit prostaglandin synthesis (144). The concentration of aspirin necessary for this purpose ranges from 1.5 μM to 1.5 mM; although the inhibition of protein synthesis (for example) may occur at 0.15 to 0.6 mM, concentrations of 5 mM or greater are required for other enzyme effects (428). It since has been demonstrated that prostaglandin biosynthesis is inhibited at normal therapeutic doses of aspirin and salicylic acid (209).

Acidic nonsteroidal antiinflammatory drugs, particularly aryl acids, form the predominant group of prostaglandin synthetase inhibitors in man. Most inhibit the cyclooxygenase enzyme by competing with the substrate arachidonic acid at the active site. Aspirin inhibits prostaglandin synthesis by quantitatively and selectively acetylating cyclooxygenase at its functional site. Following the observation that aspirin labeled with ^{14}C in the acetyl but not the carboxyl position irreversibly binds to platelets in platelet-rich plasma (11), Roth and Majerus (386), using acetyl-^{3}H-aspirin of high specific activity, demonstrated permanent acetylation of a particulate platelet protein with a molecular weight in the range of 85,000 daltons. The acetylation reaction reached saturation at a low aspirin concentration (30 μM) which correlates with its effect on human platelets *in vivo* and *in vitro*. Two other platelet protein fractions were also acetylated, but the reaction was not saturated. When acetyl-^{3}H-aspirin was incubated with sheep and bovine seminal vesicles, a single protein with a molecular weight of 85,000 daltons was acetylated (388). Since acetylation of the protein was associated with loss of cyclooxygenase activity and since arachidonic acid, a natural substrate of cyclooxygenase, inhibited acetylation by aspirin, it was assumed that aspirin inhibited cyclooxygenase by acetylating its active site. Subsequently, Roth and Siok (387) showed that aspirin caused formation of N-acetyl serine and suggested that aspirin acetylated the NH_2 group of the N-terminal serine of the oxygenase portion of the enzyme. These studies also demonstrated that cyclooxygenase is a dimer consisting of two subunits of 63,000 daltons each. It was postulated (387) that one subunit contains the oxygenase activity, while the other contains the peroxidase activity and is not acetylated by aspirin. Optimal acetylation seems dependent upon the presence of hemoprotein activators that lend actual enzyme activity to the oxygenase. The acetylation also is blocked partially by preincubation with indomethacin which presumably alters the active site (381,388). Recently, Van der Oudera et al. (328) have demonstrated that alanine, not serine, is the N-terminal residue of the enzyme. Although radioactive N-acetylserine is obtained after proteolysis of ^{3}H-acetyl-protein with pronase, the hydroxyl group of an internal serine residue in the chain is acetylated and the formation of N-acetyl-serine can be explained by a rapid O–N acetyl shift as soon as the NH_2 group of serine is liberated (329).

The structural specificity of salicylates has been examined using substituents at the 3, 4, and 5 positions. All are inactive as inhibitors of prostaglandin synthetase in sheep seminal vehicles and are also inactive in assay models of inflammation *in vivo*. Replacement of the phenolic OH by SH or OCH_3 completely abolishes inhibitory activity in the same system, and the methyl ester of aspirin demonstrates considerably reduced activity (49).

Interesting exceptions are analogues with 5-fluorinated phenyl and certain 5-heteroaryl substituents such as diflunisal and the 5-(1-pyrryl) derivative of salicylic acid (Fig. 1) Neither the inhibition of prostaglandin synthetase nor the antiinflammatory action of these compounds appears to be significantly affected by the presence or absence of an O-acetyl group. Although diflunisal reduces the excretion of 7-hydroxy-5, 11, diketoteranor-prostane-1,16-dioic acid concomitant with its analgesic and antiinflammatory effects, its effect on platelet aggregability at therapeutic doses is much more variable than is seen with aspirin (290,440). Modification of the salicylic acid structure by the addition of OH at C-5 or C-6 to form gentisic or γ-resorcylic acid increases the antisynthetase activity almost 30-fold (49). However gentisic acid also has the hydroquinone structure that may inhibit the enzyme by a different mechanism.

Aspirin inhibits prostaglandin synthesis *in vitro* approximately four times more potently than does salicylic acid. Nevertheless, approximately one-third of an orally administered dose of aspirin is hydrolyzed to salicylic acid before it reaches systemic circulation. Plasma levels of aspirin are approximately 4 times lower than that of salicylic acid 30 min after oral administration of 650 mg aspirin to normal subjects (148).

Although when administered orally to rats (197,484) salicylic acid is as active as aspirin in reducing the content of prostaglandins in inflammatory exudates, it shows little activity *in vitro* (49,463). For this reason, it has been suggested that metabolic transformation is necessary for full activity of the compound (147,463,484). Gentisic acid (2,5-dihydroxybenzoic acid) is a metabolite of salicylic acid, and a conversion rate of 10% would be necessary to account for the activity of salicylic acid *in vivo* (8). Estimated conversion rates in man vary from 4 to 8% (21,36,219,398). Salicyluric acid, by contrast, does not possess antisynthetic activity (144).

An alternative view is that the salicylate ion, being only weakly bound to circulating proteins in the rat, is able to accumulate so rapidly in developing inflammatory exudates that it attains concentrations sufficient to inhibit prostaglandin synthesis *in vivo* (426). These explanations suggest a biphasic action of aspirin on prostaglandin synthesis, a rapid and irreversible inhibition due to acetylation, and a later action due to the metabolic generation of either salicylic acid or gentisic acid.

Recently Smith et al. (433) have shown that whereas sodium salicylate and aspirin are equipotent in the carrageenin-induced paw edema rat model of inflammation, gentisic acid has no effect. Similar results were obtained when the accumulation of total leukocytes, the content of prostaglandin-like material, and the concentration of salicylic acid were studied in the exudates provoked by implanting inert sponges in the rat. Whereas gentisic acid produced no effect, aspirin and salicylate produced identical inhibitions of prostaglandin-like activity and leukocyte accumulation.

Despite the poor activity of salicylate as an inhibitor of platelet function *in vitro*, aspirin-induced inhibition of rabbit platelet cyclooxygenase can be prevented by salicylate (465). Salicylate also has been shown to inhibit and reverse the effects of 1-min incubation with aspirin on malondialdehyde (MDA) generation produced from arachidonic acid in rat platelets (286). Similarly, salicylate reversed the *in vitro* inhibitory effect of aspirin on vascular prostacyclin-like activity. Thus, the early inhibitory action of aspirin in this system was reversible and not dependent upon irreversible acetylation of cyclooxygenase. These studies have suggested that the acetyl residue might make the salicylic acid moiety more acceptable to, and/or more effective on, the cyclooxygenase. Fast, reversible binding by aspirin might be made subsequently irreversible by slower acetylation.

Aspirin also may interact with prostaglandins by interfering with their catabolism. Gibson et al. (165) have demonstrated a small but significant (approximately 10%) decrease in the pulmonary extraction of $PGF_{2\alpha}$ in dogs treated with aspirin (50 mg/kg/hr). However, aspirin was inactive when the experiment was repeated in sheep, and although salicylates are known to inhibit several dehydrogenases (428), the concentrations required are considerably greater than those required to inhibit the synthetase.

Summary

Aspirin irreversibly acetylates the cyclooxygenase enzyme at its active site and thereby inhibits prostaglandin synthesis. This is how the drug acts *in vitro* and may act *in vivo* if it is in direct contact with the target tissue and is not removed too rapidly by hydrolysis. The subsequent generation of salicylic and gentisic acids also may contribute to prostaglandin synthesis inhibition by independent mechanisms.

Effect of Aspirin on Platelets

Biological Properties and Reactions of Platelets

Circulating platelets appear as smooth, colorless discs with a diameter of 2 to 4 μm and a thickness of 0.5 μm. They are anuclear and distinct from the nucleated thrombocytes of lower vertebrates (14,48).

In the course of maturation, the megakaryocyte (210,446,490) is demarcated into cytoplasmic zones by the development of a membrane system (261). This system is formed by invagination of the megakaryocyte cell membrane (455). Subsequently, megakaryocytes, located in the subendothelial region of the vascular sinuses (415), penetrate the endothelium to the vascular lumen (37). The cytoplasmic protrusions that enter the lumen (known as proplatelets) are further fragmented, probably outside the marrow, to form platelets. This may occur in the pulmonary circulation where proplatelets could be trapped (455). Megakaryocytes also can move into the bloodstream where they are transported to the pulmonary circulation and then trapped and fragmented into platelets (347). Platelets themselves contain a complex cannalicular structure, the surface-connected cannalicular system (SCCS). The dense tubular system associated with this serves as a calcium reservoir (89).

Although platelets do not usually adhere to each other or to normal endothelium, they can adhere and spread on nonendothelial surfaces and be induced to aggregate by agents such as epinephrine, thrombin, and ADP (39). When platelets have been activated either via adhesion or by incubation with thrombin (89), they undergo a shape change and secrete (the "release reaction") various substances into the surrounding medium (206). The shape change involves a transformation from a discoid to a spherical structure together with pseudopod formation. This appears to result from calcium-sensitive actin–myosin interaction (90) and is associated with the approximation of platelet storage granules to the SCCS (477). Platelets contain at least three types of granules: (a) α granules that contain fibrinogen, platelet factors 4 and 5, and mitogenic factors, (b) dense granules where ADP, serotonin, calcium, and pyrophosphate are stored, and (c) lysosomal granules (205,206). Some agents such as ADP only cause secretion from the dense granules. Others (such as thrombin and collagen cause secretion from dense and α granules. Thrombin (420) stimulates platelet secretion at concentrations generated physiologically (1–2 nM). In contrast to most other agents that induce secretion, thrombin does not require the formation of prostaglandin endoperoxides, TXA_2, or the release of ADP (85,333) and appears to act via a distinct pathway (160,421). In addition to its potential physiological role as a proaggregant, thrombin has been shown to stimulate prostacyclin production by cultured human endothelial cells, a response likely to localize thrombus formation (473).

Platelet aggregation is dependent on external calcium and occurs when activated platelets attach to each other. This process probably reflects a change in the external platelet proteins or lipids and readily can be evaluated photometrically in platelet-rich plasma at 37°C.

When arachidonic acid is incubated with platelets, the "oxygen burst" aggregation response and release reactions that normally occur are inhibited by preincubation of the platelets with aspirin (60). In contrast, both the prostaglandin endoperoxide PGH_2 and TXA_2 aggregate "aspirinized" platelets and induce normal release (163,267,402). Thus, arachidonic acid must be cyclooxygenated to induce platelet aggregation. Although platelet aggregation induced by TXA_2 and PGH_2 in platelet-rich plasma seems largely dependent upon prior release of ADP from platelets, they also may act directly (84). Thrombin-degranulated platelets that cannot undergo a release reaction aggregate normally to arachidonic acid (225).

Antiplatelet Drugs

Weiss (470) has suggested that the term "antiplatelet drug" be applied to compounds possessing any of the following features: (a) That it inhibits a measurable property of platelets. This might be a modification of the response to inducers of aggregation, of the "spontaneous" tendency of platelets to aggregate (59), of platelet retention on glass beads, or of platelet adhesion to surfaces such as glass, collagen, or subendothelium (470). Recently, interest has focused on *in vivo* measures of platelet aggregability such as circulating platelet aggregates (14), platelet factors 4 (63) and 5 (467), β-thromboglobulin (108,114), and the urinary thromboxane metabolite, 2,3-dinor-TXB_2 (143). (b) Antiplatelet drugs may inhibit platelet-induced thrombus formation. (c) Antiplatelet drugs may prolong the survival of radioactive-labeled platelets. This approach is especially useful for study in clinical conditions such as rheumatic mitral valve disease (312) and coronary atherosclerosis (399), in which platelet survival is often shortened. In this setting, a drug might lengthen survival by suppressing platelet reactivity or by diminishing the process that activated the platelet.

The Antiplatelet Effect of Aspirin

Neither aspirin nor indomethacin substantially influence platelet shape change, primary aggregation, or the release reaction induced by thrombin. Therefore, it seems unlikely that these effects are mediated by prostaglandin formation. On the other hand, aspirin does inhibit "irreversible" or second wave aggregation and the associated release reaction induced by agents such as collagen, ADP, and epinephrine (60,331,446). Thus it seems likely that these effects are dependent upon prostaglandin formation.

Prolongation of the bleeding time following ingestion of aspirin is well documented (333,470). Platelets taken from subjects taking single doses of aspirin demonstrate impaired aggregation responses to epinephrine (319), ADP, and collagen (318). The aggregation response to ADP and epinephrine is limited to a single wave of "reversible" aggregation and both the "oxygen burst" and the release of 5-HT, ADP, and TXA_2 is abolished. Due to the irreversible acetylation of platelet cyclooxygenase by aspirin, it has been proposed that the recovery of platelet thromboxane formation after a single dose of aspirin might provide a simple, nonisotopic, method for determining platelet lifespan (267). However, it recently has been appreciated that aspirin also may act on the megakaryocyte. *N*-ethylmaleimide (NEM) augments platelet prostaglandin production *in vitro* (194,431). Demers et al. (112) have demonstrated that isolated megakaryocytes exposed to NEM are capable of significant prostaglandin production which is inhibited by preincubation with aspirin. Thus, the time required for recovery of platelet function after aspirin inhibition cannot be calculated on the basis of platelet lifespan alone.

The dose of aspirin required to inhibit platelet cyclooxygenase in man is of obvious clinical interest. Burch et al. (70) studied the ability of ^{3}H acetyl aspirin to acetylate washed platelets periodically obtained from volunteers. These radioligand binding studies suggested that more than 50% inhibition was obtained by daily doses of 20 mg aspirin. An effect on megakaryocytes seemed to occur as no unacetylated platelet enzyme was evident in the circulation for 2 days following aspirin ingestion.

The appreciation that prostacyclin, a potent inhibitor of platelet aggregation (293), was synthesized by isolated arterial and venous endothelium and cultured human and bovine endothelial cells (292) led to speculation that a dose of aspirin that inhibited cyclooxygenase in vascular tissues would be potentially undesirable, as platelet aggregation could still proceed by mechanisms independent of cyclooxygenase. Two pieces of evidence suggested that a critical dose of aspirin might selectively inhibit thromboxane formation. Burch et al. (70) found that platelet cyclooxygenase was 31-fold more sensitive to aspirin inhibition than sheep seminal vesicle preparations. Subsequently the same workers found that aortic and coronary artery microsomes were 1/250th as sensitive to aspirin as the enzyme in intact platelets and 1/60th as sensitive as a platelet microsomal preparation (69). Baenziger et al. (29) found that cyclooxygenase in vascular tissues in culture was 20- to 40-fold less sensitive to aspirin inactivation than is the cyclooxygenase of platelets. The cyclooxygenase of human cultured fibroblasts and arterial smooth muscle cells was inactivated by 9 to 12%, whereas platelet cyclooxygenase was inhibited by 92% at corresponding doses of aspirin.

However, the situation may not be so straightforward. Jaffe and Weksler (215) found endothelial cell cyclooxygenase to be as sensitive to aspirin as the enzyme in platelets. Whereas platelets were unable to synthesize a new cyclooxygenase, the enzyme turnover in endothelial cell culture was very high and therefore its acetylated form was rapidly replaced. These observations suggested that the rapid resynthesis of vascular cyclooxygenase might render a thrombogenic effect of aspirin unlikely in clinical practice.

An alternative mechanism by which aspirin might reduce prostacyclin is based on the proposal (67,68,298) that prostacyclin synthase activity in the vessel wall is, in large part, dependent on the provision of platelet endoperoxide substrate released during aggregation or adhesion. Using high endothelial cell/platelet ratios in stirred suspensions, Marcus et al. (268) have shown that thrombin stimulated 6-keto-PGF$_{1\alpha}$ production by endothelial cells is more than doubled by the addition of platelets. However, Needleman et al. (313) have been unable to demonstrate endoperoxide release from platelets during aggregation or adhesion with endogenous or exogenous arachidonate as a substrate. Furthermore, prostacyclin synthesis from platelet endoperoxides by cultured endothelial cells pretreated with aspirin occurs only when thromboxane synthesis is inhibited selectively and amounts to only 10 to 20% of the prostacyclin production by endothelium in the absence of aspirin (30). These observations and the demonstration that endogenous and exogenous arachidonate, but not exogenous PGH_2, stimulate prostacyclin synthesis by the perfused rabbit mesenteric vascular bed (361), make it unlikely that aspirin might indirectly reduce prostacyclin generation by inhibiting platelet activation. Finally, recent studies (479) of cultured vascular smooth muscle cells indicate that resting cells can rapidly resynthesize cyclooxygenase but that aspirin inactivated another component of the prostacyclin biosynthetic system that can only be replaced by cellular division.

Does high-dose aspirin constitute a potential risk of thrombosis? Czervionke et al. (103) have shown that aspirin treatment of cultured endothelial cells from the umbilical vein increased the adherence of ^{51}Cr platelets in the presence of thrombin. Thrombin-stimulated prostacyclin release was inversely related to thrombin-stimulated platelet adherence to the endothelial monolayer. *In vivo*, Reyers et al. (372) failed to identify a beneficial or harmful effect of high (50–200 mg/kg) or low (2.5–10 mg/kg) dose aspirin on arterial and venous models of experimental thrombosis. However, high-dose aspirin therapy (200 mg/kg) significantly augmented experimentally induced thrombus size in rabbits compared to animals treated with low-dose (10 mg/kg) aspirin, sodium salicylate (200 mg/kg), and untreated controls (223). The thrombogenic effect of high-dose aspirin was lost if the interval between thrombus induction and drug administration was greater than 2.5 hr, presumably reflecting the high turnover of vascular cyclooxygenase. Recently, Rosenblum et al. (384) have noted that aspirin (100 mg/kg ip) and indomethacin (5 mg/kg ip) enhanced platelet aggregation in mouse mesenteric vessels, supporting observations that the same drugs enhance platelet aggregation in transected rabbit mesenteric vessels.

These and similar observations (294), were supplemented by the studies of Amezcua et al. (12) on the effects of aspirin on bleeding time in rabbits. Low-dose (10 mg/kg) aspirin prolonged bleeding time (252s vs 157s controls) more than high dose (100 mg/kg) aspirin (214s). In addition to its antiaggregatory properties, other hemostatic influences of prostacyclin independent of platelets may be lost during high-dose aspirin therapy. Thus, Buchanan et al. (64) have shown that aspirin, in doses that inhibited vascular prostacyclin-like activity, shortened bleeding time in severely thrombocytopenic rabbits. O'Grady and Moncada (321) gave normal volunteers 300 mg and 3.9 g aspirin 14 days apart. Bleeding times measured 2 hr after dosing were significantly longer after the lower dose. Consistent observations were obtained by Amezcua et al. (13). Rajah et al. (364) found that 1-g doses of aspirin lengthened bleeding time while 3.9 g failed to do so. Others (457) have studied bleeding time at 2 hr and 1 week after daily dosing of 300 and 600 mg aspirin. Bleeding time was prolonged at both time points after both doses, and there was no evidence of a differential dose-dependent effect. Differences in technique (362) and confounding of bleeding time response to aspirin by age (18) and sex (491) may have contributed to apparent discrepancies in these results. In normal volunteers, maximal inhibition of collagen-induced aggregation, adhesion to glass beads, and platelet factor 4 availability was produced by ingestion of a single dose of 300 mg aspirin in a study in which doses ranging from 60 mg to 1 g were administered in random order at fortnightly intervals (365). Significant antiplatelet effects were obtained with 180 mg and 240 mg aspirin. More recently platelet aggregability has been shown to be significantly impaired by 81 mg aspirin in normal subjects. More direct attempts have been made to study the differential effects of aspirin dosage on thromboxane and prostacyclin synthesis *in vivo*. Cerskus et al. (82) infused rabbits intravenously with collagen or arachidonic acid. Pretreatment with aspirin (25 and 250 mg/kg) and sulfinpyrazone (30 mg/kg) provided total protection from the hypotension and thrombocytopenia caused by arachidonic acid but only partial protection from that caused by collagen. Although TXA_2 synthesis was blocked in protected rabbits, basal and arachidonate induced elevation of 6-keto-$PGF_{1\alpha}$ in plasma were unaffected.

Patrono et al. (339) have studied time and dose dependence of the inhibitory effect of oral aspirin on the production of thromboxane by human platelets stimulated by thrombin *in vitro*. A single 100-mg aspirin dose reduced TXB_2 by 98% within 1 hr in 45 human volunteers. Doses of 100 to 400 mg reduced TXB_2 by 94 to 98% after 24 and 48 hr and 90 to 92% after 72 hr. More than 90% inhibition could be maintained over one month by giving a 200 mg dose every 72 hr. Masotti et al. (271) studied platelet aggregation, MDA formation and prostacyclin production in 25 volunteers. Prostacyclin-like activity was measured by a superfusion technique (138) in venous blood after 3 min of forearm ischemia. MDA production was assayed (323) following thrombin stimulation of platelets *in vitro*. The doses that inhibited 50% of platelet aggregation (ID50) for epinephrine, ADP, and collagen ranged from 3.2 to 3.4 mg/kg. The ID50 for prostacyclin production was 4.9 mg/kg and increased linearly to 8 mg/kg. Whereas prostacyclin production had returned to normal in all subjects by 24 hr after 2, 3.5, and 5 mg/kg and in 6 of 9 subjects who received 8 and 10 mg/kg, MDA production was still inhibited 72 hr after dosing (41% after 2 mg/kg and 85% after 10 mg/kg). Recently it has been suggested (337) that a single daily dose of aspirin as low as 20 mg may result in suppression of platelet thromboxane formation, raising the possibility that there might be a dose of aspirin which blocked platelet thromboxane biosynthesis without altering production of PGI_2 by the endothelium. However, currently available data do not permit the designation of a dose of aspirin that is selective for the platelet cyclooxygenase. In one study of four volunteers, both circulating TXB_2 and the 6-keto-$PGF_{1\alpha}$ content of forearm vein homogenates were markedly reduced 2 hr after both 300 and 1,500 mg aspirin (335). More recently, two groups have studied prostacyclin production by human venous biopsies following aspirin ingestion. Preston et al. (360) found that 6-keto-$PGF_{1\alpha}$ production was substantially depressed 2 hr after acute doses of 150 mg and 300 mg aspirin. Prostacyclin synthesis appeared cumulative during chronic administration of 40 mg aspirin per day (359). Platelet thromboxane production remained depressed 48 hr after these doses. Hanley et al. (183) found that 81 mg aspirin resulted in approximately 60% depression of release of prostacyclin-like activity from venous biopsies and that suppression was still present 48 hr after a 300 mg dose. Platelet thromboxane production was assayed indirectly by MDA formation, and remained depressed at least 96 hr after only 40 mg aspirin.

We recently measured the excretion of 2,3-dinor thromboxane and 2,3-dinor-6-keto-PGF$_{1\alpha}$, urinary thromboxane (TX-M), and urinary prostacyclin (PGI-M) metabolites, during chronic dose ranging in normal volunteers (143). The measurement of urinary metabolites represents a validated approach to the estimation of endogenous prostaglandin biosynthesis. Doses were administered orally, daily for 7 days in sequential weeks. Aspirin, 20 mg/day resulted in a reduction of TX-M excretion to $33.1 \pm 15.7\%$ of the control values of 245 ± 52.3 pg/mg creatinine and of PGI-M to $65.2 \pm 14.2\%$ of the control values of 32.8 ± 95.5 pg/mg/creatinine. Chronic dosing is the range of 20 mg/day to 325 mg/day resulted in a dose-dependent reduction in the excretion of TX-M and PGI-M. In doses of 325 mg/day to 2,600 mg/day, aspirin reduced mean TX-M to 4.7 to 3.3% of control, while PGI-M remained at 40 to 23% of control values. Three days after the last dose of aspirin (2,600 mg/day), TX-M excretion had returned to $86.7 \pm 12.3\%$ of control values, whereas PGI-M excretion remained at $29.6 \pm 6.8\%$ of control, the converse of what was expected from turnover studies of cyclooxygenase in endothelial cells and platelets *in vitro* (10,215). Further observations have suggested that PGI-M excretion may remain below control values for up to 1 week after dosing. Recent studies by other groups have suggested that prostacyclin formation may remain depressed for longer periods than one would expect from enzyme kinetics. In the investigation of Buchanan et al. (65), aspirin inhibition of prostacyclin synthesis by rabbit carotid arteries persisted at least 20 hr. Chronic dosing may have a cumulative effect on prostacyclin synthesis. Persistence of inhibition of prostacyclin generation by cultured endothelial cells appears to increase with aspirin dosage (215). Recovery of prostaglandin biosynthesis after chronic dosing with aspirin, as in this study, may have differed from what may occur after acute doses *in vivo*. One possible explanation for the discordance with the enzyme kinetic data has been provided recently. In a study of the capacity of cultured rat aortic endothelial cells to generate prostacyclin in response to thrombin, prostacyclin generation was only 25% of pretreatment values four days after aspirin treatment. However, when the endothelial cells were subcultured and stimulated to divide by trypsinization, the prostacyclin response to thrombin returned to approximately 60% of pretreatment values by 24 hr after aspirin (479). This suggested that although resting vascular cells could rapidly resynthesize new cyclooxygenase, aspirin had destroyed additional components of the prostacyclin synthetic system that only could be replaced by cell division.

Our investigation demonstrated a more rapid recovery of endogenous thromboxane production in man than expected from studies of platelet cyclooxygenase *in vitro*. However, these data do not necessarily imply that the inhibitory effect of aspirin on platelets is not as long as previously indicated. Although prostacyclin is unlikely to act as a circulating antiplatelet agent (142), it is probably of importance in inhibiting the release of thromboxane from platelets at local sites of interaction with endothelium. Thus a 60 to 70% inhibition of prostacyclin synthesis post aspirin may have rendered newly released platelets more readily activatable. Replacement of about 10% of affected platelets restores near normal function (83). Thus, increased production of thromboxane by newly released platelets may have been reflected by an increase in total thromboxane production that does not directly correlate with turnover of the inhibitory effects of aspirin on platelet cyclooxygenase *in vivo*. This phenomenon may have been facilitated by inhibition of acetylation of megakaryocyte cyclooxygenase by the high levels of salicylic acid in plasma at the end of this study.

Summary

The most appropriate antithrombotic dosage of aspirin remains unestablished. First, methodological difficulties are associated with much of the published data. Superfusion techniques may greatly overestimate prostacyclin-like activity in the circulation (294). MDA production is an indirect method of quantitating TXA_2 generation, and sampling artifacts may contribute to estimates of TXB_2 in plasma. Quantitation of PGI-M and TX-M in healthy volunteers suggests that although generation of thromboxane is more inhibited than generation of prostacyclin over a wide dose range of aspirin, no chronically administered dose is likely to be completely selective of thromboxane synthesis inhibition.

Finally, most human studies have been performed in small numbers of healthy volunteers. Substantial interindividual differences in platelet responses to aspirin may exist in such subjects (320) and may limit the extrapolation of results to a larger population. Diseased individuals may respond anomalously to aspirin. Lipid peroxides in atheromatous blood vessels already may have inhibited prostacyclin generation prior to administration of aspirin. There is considerable evidence (10) that blood vessels have the capacity to synthesize and release thromboxane, which may continue following inhibition of platelet cyclooxygenase by low-dose aspirin. Thus, in these individuals the risks of prostacyclin inhibition by high-dose aspirin may be outweighed by the necessity to inhibit thromboxane production from all sources. Finally the possibility that aspirin therapy might influence atherogenesis (352) requires further elucidation. The development of selective inhibitors of thromboxane synthesis for use in man (461,466) seems a more logical direction for research in antiplatelet therapy than the search for a critical dose of aspirin.

Other Pharmacological Properties

Aspirin belongs to a chemically diverse class of nonsteroidal antiinflammatory drugs that have in common antiinflammatory, analgesic, and antipyretic activity, pK_a values in the region of 4, and the ability to bind to albumin. Although they differ in some respects (26), they all inhibit prostaglandin biosynthesis, which is presumed relevant to their antiinflammatory effect. The antiinflammatory (54,136,139,167,198,275,307,327), analgesic (38,86,92,125,369,485), and anti-pyretic (135,144,145) aspects of aspirin and its effects on endocrine function (184,220,221,287,377,450) have been reviewed elsewhere.

Pharmacokinetics and Metabolism

Absorption

Salicylates are characterized by a relatively low aqueous and high lipid solubility in their unionized forms (91). Aspirin is soluble in water at approximately 3.3 g/l, salicylic acid and salicylamide at approximately 2 g/l and methylsalicylate at 0.6 g/l. Tablets containing several hundred milligrams of these substances consequently will not dissolve immediately if taken with a small volume of water. Aspirin (pK$_a$ 3.5) and salicylic acid (pK$_a$ 3.0) are moderately strong organic acids and readily form highly soluble salts in which form they are often administered. Both salicylate and aspirin are absorbed extensively at acidic pH as the fraction of unionized drug rises (190,249). However a rise in pH enhances the aqueous solubility of aspirin, increasing its dissolution rate and facilitating its absorption. *In vivo*, aspirin is absorbed rapidly, partly from the stomach but mostly from the small intestine. Contrary to the pH-partition theory, aspirin is absorbed much more slowly from the stomach than from the small intestine: The rate of gastric emptying is enhanced by a fall in pH, and aspirin in solution passes rapidly from the stomach to the small intestine, where the greater surface area favors rapid absorption (425). Thus, within 20 min, 94% of a buffered solution of aspirin has left the stomach (97). Absorption half-lives for unbuffered and buffered aspirin are about 30 and 20 min, respectively, and somewhat less for a solution (110). A peak plasma value is obtained in approximately 2 hr.

Rectal absorption of salicylates is slow, incomplete, and unreliable (317). Salicylic acid is rapidly absorbed from the skin. Application of methylsalicylate ointment equivalent to 6 g aspirin to the backs of volunteers resulted in plasma levels similar to those resulting from 325 mg aspirin taken orally (305).

Distribution and Protein Binding

Rowland et al. (390) have demonstrated that 28 to 35% of an oral dose of 650 mg aspirin in aqueous solution is hydrolyzed during absorption in man. As this hydrolysis is an enzymatic process, the "first-pass" hydrolysis may be capacity-limited and absorption site-dependent.

There seem to be marked interindividual differences in the presystemic hydrolysis of orally administered aspirin (203,250). In man, administration of aspirin with food reduces maximum aspirin concentrations to about 50% of that when aspirin is taken with 250 ml water on an empty stomach (111,270). Food does not alter the amount of aspirin absorbed intact (232). Following single oral doses, aspirin pharmacokinetics may vary with age (299).

Thirty minutes after an oral dose of 650 mg aspirin, only 27% of total plasma salicylate is in the acetylated form. The ester is rapidly hydrolyzed to salicylic acid in plasma, liver, erythrocytes, and more slowly in synovial fluid (110). The synovial fluid concentration of aspirin and salicylate rise more slowly and reach a lower level than in plasma (439). Studies in patients with rheumatoid arthritis showed that maximum concentration of aspirin attained in synovial fluid is about half the peak concentration in plasma (419). However, the concentration of free salicylate [apparently identical in the two fluids (385)] essentially is due to decreased affinity of primary protein binding sites in synovial fluid (456).

Aspirin covalently binds to serum albumin although less strongly than salicylic acid (211,301,305). Salicylate anion competes with aspirin at its binding site on albumin (1) similar to its competition at the cyclooxygenase site (348). Aspirin also acetylates hemoglobin and erythrocyte membrane peptides (172).

Protein binding partially protects aspirin from spontaneous hydrolysis, the half-life for hydrolysis being about twice that for unbound aspirin. Albumin actually activates enzyme catalyzed hydrolysis (1). It has been demonstrated by various workers that salicylate competes for the binding of penicillin, thyroxine, trilodothyronine, thiopental, sulfinpyrazone, tryptophan, uric acid, naproxen, phenytoin, and possibly steroids to plasma proteins *(vide infra)*. Displacement of phenytoin recently has been shown not to result in an increase in free drug concentration and pharmacologic activity (342). This may be because an increase in total phenytoin clearance during aspirin therapy compensates for displacement of the anticonvulsant from protein binding sites (153). Prostaglandins are carried in the blood in non-covalent linkage to serum proteins (174). Interestingly, aspirin, salicylic acid, and indomethacin recently have been shown to inhibit reversibly prostaglandin binding to human serum proteins (27). Binding of salicylates to plasma proteins is dose-dependent; thus the relationship of free fraction to dose is not linear (489). The free fraction is 15 to 20% when the plasma salicylate is 100 to 200 pg/ml, but for concentrations over 400 pg/ml, the free fraction may be as high as 50% (266).

Many analytical procedures have been used to quantify salicylates in biological fluids. The older colorimetric and fluorimetric assays (190,225) are now being replaced with gas liquid chromatography (7) and high-pressure liquid chromatography (25,50). Administration of aspirin in doses ranging from 325 to 650 mg, sufficient for mild analgesic and antipyretic actions, usually result in plasma levels of 3 to 6 mg/dl. Doses sufficient for arthritic conditions usually result in a therapeutic range of approximately 15 to 39 mg/dl. Above this range, toxicity occurs, the optimal plasma level being generally only a little below toxic levels (191,253). A linear correlation recently has been described between salivary salicylic acid and the free fraction in plasma (175), although considerable intra- and intersubject variations in the saliva:serum drug concentration ratio limit the clinical usefulness of the procedure (254). Large variations occur in maximum plasma salicylate concentrations in patients with rheumatoid arthritis who have received the same daily dose of aspirin (176,452). When high doses (3.9 g/day) of aspirin were administered chronically (36 days) to patients with rheumatoid arthritis, plasma levels had declined by 25% on day 36 from the peak levels obtained from days 3 to 10. Salivary concentrations declined even more rapidly, resulting in a decrease in the saliva: plasma ratio for salicylate (397). This decline may be due to induction of glycine synthetase, resulting in an increased formation of the salicylurate metabolite (157). Alternative explanations have included altered disposition or elimination due to concurrent medication (164), hypoalbuminemia or altered protein binding due to uremia (158,481), genetic variability in metabolism (391), and concentration dependence of protein binding (266).

Salicylic acid but not aspirin accumulates in plasma during repeated administration of aspirin. Although peak plasma salicylate concentrations increase gradually after each dose until steady-state is attained, aspirin concentrations decline essentially to zero during the usual dosing interval due to its short half-life. Although plasma concentrations of aspirin do not persist, it is likely that cumulative acetylation of cyclooxygenase occurs *in vivo*. Preliminary reports indicate a cumulative inhibition of prostacylin synthesis by venous biopsies *ex vivo* during chronic dosing of volunteers with 40 mg/day aspirin (359).

Both aspirin and salicylate have volumes of distribution that average approximately 150 ml/kg, although higher values (400 ml/kg) have been calculated when high doses (10 g/day) of aspirin have been administered (110,391). Although the volume of distribution approximates to extracellular space, salicylates are distributed unevenly throughout the body. Brain concentrations are approximately 1/10th those in plasma, but this fraction may be increased in the presence of hypercapnia (110). The smaller volume of distribution in patients with connective tissue diseases may result from altered kinetics, long term drug ingestion, and variation in protein binding (170).

Biotransformation and Excretion

Following hydrolysis of aspirin, salicylic acid is eliminated by formation of its glycine conjugate, salicyluric acid, salicylphenolic glucoronide, salicylacyl glucuronide, gentisic acid, and by renal excretion of unchanged salicylic acid (250). Salicyluric acid and salicylphenolic glucuronide are formed by capacity limited processes (Michaelis Menten kinetics) with *in vivo* K_m values well below the therapeutic concentrations of the drug (253). Consequently, steady-state plasma salicylate levels increase much more than proportionately with increasing daily dose of the drug, and the time required to reach steady-state increases as a function of dose (252). This phenomenon is most pronounced with regard to free (unbound) salicylate as protein binding decreases with increasing plasma concentrations.

The liver is the principal site of biotransformation of salicylates in man. The area under the time–concentration curve for aspirin after intravenous administration exceeds that after oral administration by about one third, (389) indicating a substantial first pass effect *(vide supra)*. The three chief metabolic products are salicylic acid (approximately 80% in urine), the ether or phenolic glucuronide (approximately 10%), and the ester of acylglucuronide (approximately 5%). A small fraction is metabolized to gentisic acid, trihydroxyderivatives, and to the glycine conjugate of gentisic acid, gentisuric acid (110).

Renal excretion of unaltered salicylate occurs by glomerular filtration of the unbound drug plus both active tubular secretion and passive tubular reabsorption. The renal clearance of free salicylate is markedly pH-dependent. Following aspirin dosage, whereas only a small percentage of the total urinary salicylate excretion at pH 5 is free salicylate, this increases to over 80% when the urinary pH is raised to 8 (434). Water diuresis may promote further salicylate excretion by lowering the concentration in renal tubules and thus reducing the opportunity for passive resorption. Although the elimination half-life of salicylates correlate with creatinine clearance in patients with renal failure, the rate of transformation of salicylates into salicylurates and the clearance of salicylurates remains unchanged (392). In normal man, the half-life of aspirin is approximately 15 min and for salicylates, 2 to 3 hr at low doses and 15 to 30 hr at high doses. The change to zero order kinetics at high doses may result from a limited ability to form salicylurate (vide supra). Salicylamide is excreted much more rapidly than salicylate with a half-life of about 1 hr (251).

The influence of salicylates on uric acid excretion is markedly dose-dependent. Whereas low doses (1–2 g/day) of aspirin may decrease urate excretion and intermediate doses (2–3 g/day) may have little effect, high doses (> 5 g/day) induce uricosuria and lower plasma urate level. Because such doses are usually poorly tolerated and because more rational forms of therapy are now available, salicylates are rarely used in the therapy of diseases such as gout. Even large doses can result in urate retention when combined with a uricosuric agent such as probenecid (427), sulfinpyrazone (453), or phenylbutazone (453). Conversely, hyperuricemia resulting from pyrazinamide may be reduced by concomitant therapy with aspirin (34). Aspirin may increase urinary potassium excretion by direct effect on the renal tubule (378).

Aspirin can increase displacement of warfarin, tolbutamide, phenytoin, and steroids from serum proteins (19,120,153,326,486). Corticosteroids themselves may lower plasma salicylate by increasing the glomerular filtration rate and decreasing tubular reabsorption of water (129,231). Conversely, both ascorbic acid and ammonium chloride reduce renal clearance of salicylates by increasing urine acidity. Aspirin also may be involved in a variety of miscellaneous drug interactions. Aspirin may inhibit the natriuresis produced by spironolactone, perhaps by competing at the site of the aldosterone receptor (459), although in a double-blind crossover trial, aspirin failed to antagonize the antihypertensive effect of spironolactone in low-renin essential hypertensives (202). Aspirin also blunts the natriuresis and diuresis induced by furosemide (35,195), possibly by competing for proximal tubular secretion. Acute administration of aspirin does not alter salt or free water clearance by the kidney (45). Diflunisal interacts with furosemide in a similar, albeit less pronounced, manner (196). Finally, aspirin may precipitate hemolysis in patients with G-6PD deficiency (144) and para amino benzoic acid (PABA), an ingredient of many proprietary analgesic mixtures, may increase salicylate blood levels by inhibiting metabolic conversion to salicyluric acid (427). Aspirin may interfere with a variety of clinical laboratory tests (184).

Adverse Effects and Hypersensitivity

Gastrointestinal

Aspirin ingestion may cause nausea and vomiting by acting locally or at higher doses, centrally, probably at the medullary chemoreceptor trigger zone. The damaging effect of aspirin on gastric mucosa has been well documented by endoscopy (123,241,242,247,368) and by studies of fecal blood loss (353). Ingestion of 4 to 5 g aspirin/day for 26 days resulted in an average fecal blood loss of 3 to 8 ml/day compared to 0.6 ml/day in untreated subjects (246). Alcohol enhances gastrointestinal blood loss in patients taking aspirin (169). However many of the studies that incriminate aspirin use the ^{51}Cr-tagged red cell technique. This assumes that when tagged erythrocytes leak into the alimentary tract, the radioisotope is not significantly reabsorbed and may be detected in the stool where it indicates blood loss. This technique does not distinguish gastric bleeding from blood loss elsewhere in the gut, and the biliary contribution to stool radioactivity may be substantial (441). Salicylates stimulate biliary secretion (404) and thus stool ^{51}Cr radioactivity may prove an unreliable index of aspirin-induced gastric bleeding.

The association of aspirin ingestion with major gastrointestinal bleeding is more tenuous. Levy (255) reported that 16% of 88 patients with major gastrointestinal bleeding had taken aspirin 4 or more days per week compared to 6.9% of 14,000 controls. No association was observed when aspirin was taken less frequently, and the overall risk was 15 per 100,000 aspirin takers per annum.

Patients may take aspirin for the symptoms of gastrointestinal bleeding, thus confounding retrospective studies (240). When such patients are excluded, a significant difference in the rates of aspirin ingestion persists between patients with gastric ulcer and controls (445). It is not currently known whether peptic ulcer patients bleed more readily on aspirin (356), but ulcer recurrence rates seem unaffected (370).

The mechanism by which aspirin causes gastric damage may involve the cytoprotective effect of prostaglandins (375). Salicylates break down the normal gastric mucosal barrier to back diffusion of hydrogen ion resulting in injury to the submucosal capillaries with subsequent necrosis and bleeding. Ultrastructural studies in rats indicate that the first structural damage to occur after aspirin is damage to the basement membrane of the endothelial cell of the capillary and postcapillary venule (379). Gastric mucous secretion is reduced and its biochemistry altered by aspirin (224,284). Aspirin also may reduce the alkaline component of mucosal defence (483) via its inhibition of prostaglandin synthesis (370). Aspirin causes a dramatic reduction in gastric PGE_2-like activity followed by gastric mucosal injury in healthy subjects and patients with duodenal ulceration (234). Prostacyclin appears important in the regulation of gastric mucosal blood flow, and its inhibition by aspirin may result in focal ischemia (480). Damage may also occur in relatively ischemic areas where the dissipation of aspirin is retarded (215). Another factor that may contribute to these effects of aspirin is a reduction in platelet aggregability resulting in a bleeding tendency.

Enteric coated aspirin results in comparable cyclooxygenase inhibition as does plain aspirin, although the effect is delayed, reflecting the slower appearance of aspirin in plasma (6). Although parenteral as well as oral administration of salicylates cause gastric erosions (289), recent studies have demonstrated that aspirin-induced gastroduodenal erosions are reduced by enteric coating despite similar circulating salicylate levels. This suggests that topical rather than systemic effects are of greater importance in the production of gastroduodenal damage by aspirin (200,423). Recent results (480) suggest that it may be possible to develop aspirin-like drugs which, while selectively inhibiting prostaglandin formation in the inflammatory zones, do not affect the enzyme in the gastric mucosa, thereby reducing the risk of topical irritation.

Aspirin–antacid combinations seem impractical, since large amounts of antacid must be frequently ingested to keep the gastric pH above 3.5 (151). A compound containing more antacid than most commercially available preparations (3.9 g aspirin + 300 mg MgA10H) recently has been shown to cause more mucosal damage than enteric coated aspirin (243). Nonacetylated products such as choline salicylate and choline magnesium salicylate are expensive and no more effective than buffered aspirin (88,212). Esters of benorylate and the triglyceride ester of aspirin fail to readily release the active drug after absorption (237,367). However, rapid hydrolysis occurs after absorption of the carbonate and methyl esters of aspirin, and the latter recently has been shown in the rat to be almost devoid of gastric ulcerogenic activity (478). Diflunisal, a difluorphenyl derivative of salicylic acid does not covalently acetylate cyclooxygenase (265). In healthy subjects, diflunisal (750 mg) causes a slower and less pronounced inhibitory effect than aspirin (400 mg) on plasma TXB_2 levels. In arthritic patients, aspirin (1 g) caused significantly greater reduction of gastric PGE_2 output than a therapeutically equivalent dose of diflunisal (500 mg) (46). Diflunisal causes a lower incidence of gastric erosion than aspirin (10% vs 50%) when given at equally effective antiinflammatory doses (80).

The effects of aspirin on the intestinal tract have been reviewed elsewhere (74,133,140,285,366,424).

Hepatic and Renal Effects

Although liver damage has been related to therapy with salicylates, it remains unclear whether these compounds are primarily hepatotoxic or merely tend to exacerbate underlying liver dysfunction (178). Thus, although aspirin therapy results in an increased frequency of abnormal liver function tests in rheumatic fever and several connective tissue diseases (373,412), high-dose (40 mg/kg) therapy of healthy volunteers gave normal results (156). Up to 40% of children receiving salicylate therapy for rheumatoid arthritis develop liver dysfunction. Generally, the amount of damage is slight and reversible, and patients with preexisting liver damage or hypoalbuminemia seem predisposed to its development. A transient, asymptomatic increase in transaminases recently have been documented in children with rheumatoid arthritis receiving aspirin (122). Sodium salicylate has been shown to inhibit factor VII synthesis in the perfused rat liver (330).

Although aspirin therapy may cause a decline in renal blood flow and glomerular filtration rate (228), this is usually transient and most pronounced in the presence of preexisting renal impairment. Glomerular filtration rate did not alter significantly in nine normal volunteers following aspirin (2,400 mg/day) therapy for 1 week (311). The greater susceptibility of patients with preexisting renal impairment may reflect their increased dependence on prostaglandins for the maintenance of renal blood flow (94,126). Recently, Brooks et al. (62) have demonstrated a rebound rise in plasma–renin concentration following suppression by aspirin therapy (3.9 g/day) for 2 and 5 weeks. The rebound effect was maximal 2 weeks after stopping aspirin and probably reflected the removal of suppression of prostaglandin production. Prostaglandins may critically regulate the renin-angiotensin system under certain conditions (2).

Although the renal capillary necrosis of chronic analgesic consumption is usually associated with mixtures of aspirin, caffeine, and phenacetin (309,407), most epidemiological studies implicate phenacetin as the nephrotoxic component of such combinations (442).

Miscellaneous Effects

When administered during pregnancy, salicylates may reach substantial levels in the fetus. Although the incidence of birth defects does not appear to be increased, smaller babies are born to habitual users of aspirin (96). Administration of aspirin at term may delay the onset of labor and lead to bruising of the neonate (257). The incidence of ante- and post-partum hemorrhage and complications of delivery appears to be increased by chronic maternal consumption of salicylates (95). Although beneficial effects of aspirin have been reported in the treatment of preeclamptic toxemia (217), further evidence is required to establish its role in the management of this condition.

Ordinary therapeutic doses of salicylates have no important direct cardiovascular actions. Large doses may have a deleterious effect on a compromised circulation by increasing plasma volume, and toxic doses may cause hypotension by acting centrally or directly on vascular smooth muscle. Anesthetized rats treated with intravenous lysine acetylsalicylate (200 mg/kg) developed markedly potentiated pressor responses to norepinephrine (141). By contrast, patients with migraine who have increased platelet aggregability may respond to aspirin prophylaxis (325).

Drug Interactions

Aspirin may enhance the action of oral anticoagulants (233). Although antiplatelet drugs ought to be given cautiously with anticoagulants, this combination has been successfully employed in certain thromboembolic disorders (105).

In a study of 148 patients with aortic half valve prostheses, 2 patients received either aspirin (1 g/day) or placebo with anticoagulant (thrombotest 10% normal) therapy. Only two embolic episodes occurred in the combined group as compared with 12 episodes in the placebo group. Bleeding episodes were more common in the aspirin (15) than in the placebo (6) group, and the intensity of anticoagulation correlated with the occurrence of bleeding. The authors suggested that although the risk of bleeding seemed acceptable, less intensive anticoagulation might attain an antithrombotic affect at lower risk.

Toxic Effects and Hypersensitivity

Although the measurement of salicylates in plasma may be used to devise dosing regimens (53) and to monitor patient compliance (405), its most critical value is in the management of salicylate overdosage. The time after drug ingestion is of great importance and a nomogram has been prepared on the basis of the elimination of salicylate and the observed relationship between the theoretical extrapolated salicylate level at zero time and the severity of intoxication (121).

Salicylism

Mild chronic intoxication, termed "salicylism," is characterized by tinnitus, dizziness, headache, confusion, lassitude, nausea, and hyperpnea. These symptoms usually correspond to plasma salicylate levels in the range 30 to 80 mg%. Blood levels in excess of this usually result in major intoxication characterized by fever, acid-base imbalance, restlessness, tremors, vertigo, diplopia, hallucinations, and coma. An acneform eruption may occur if aspirin has been continued longer than 1 week, and uremia or hemorrhagic phenomena may further complicate the picture. Hyperglycemia may occur in adults, although children may develop serious hypoglycemia. The management of acute aspirin overdose has been reviewed elsewhere (256).

Aspirin Intolerance

"Aspirin intolerance" has been described as acute urticaria–angioedema, bronchospasm, severe rhinitis, or shock occurring within 3 hr of aspirin ingestion (276,400,401). Based on patients' histories, it occurs most commonly in individuals with chronic urticaria (23%) in whom it is usually of the urticarial variety, and in asthmatics (4%) in whom it is usually of the bronchospastic type (414). The asthmatic syndrome occurs classically in middle aged females and is rare in children. Reports on the frequency of aspirin intolerance vary from 2 to 16% of adult asthmatics (400,401,413,448).

Specific IgE (antiaspiryl) and other antibodies have been found inconsistently in the sera of intolerant patients (474). Positive skin tests to aspirylpolylysine are probably nonspecific urticarial reactions. Crossreactivity to structurally unrelated azo dyes of benzoates occurs in 8 to 44% of aspirin-sensitive individuals, but sensitivity to salts of salicylic acid, used as food preservatives and flavoring agents, does not occur (104). The crossreactivity with acetaminophen is low (approximately 5%). This drug has been suggested as an aspirin substitute in sensitive individuals (414).

Because there are no reliable *in vitro* tests that identify individuals with aspirin intolerance, oral challenge with aspirin has been used for this purpose (273). Attacks occur within minutes to 4 hr after aspirin ingestion and may be associated with an increase in circulating levels of histamine, reflecting mast cell degranulation (443). Wojnar et al. (487) have demonstrated that aspirin and sodium salicylate, like other nonsteroidal antiinflammatory agents, augment histamine release from human leukocytes in response to allergens. It recently has been reported (444) that following oral challenge with aspirin, two such subjects became refractory to further adverse effects of aspirin and could tolerate sustained and increased dosages of the drug. Ketotifen, an antihistamine with mast cell stabilizing properties, has been reported to protect aspirin-sensitive asthmatics from bronchoconstriction in response to aspirin challenge (449).

Drugs that provoke an asthmatic reaction in patients with aspirin-sensitive asthma have in common the ability to inhibit cyclooxygenase, but the precise role of prostaglandins in this disease remains unestablished (447). One possible mechanism of this reaction is via the loss of a prostaglandin-mediated inhibitory feedback mechanism of acetylcholine release in response to nerve stimulation (214). Cyclooxygenase inhibitors also enhance the immunological release of SRS-A from the lungs of man and other species (72,468). Cyclooxygenase inhibition may thus divert arachidonate metabolism into the lipoxygenase pathway, a product of which could account for aspirin-induced asthma (73,258).

DIPYRIDAMOLE

Introduction

The interest evoked by the therapeutic potential of dipyridamole has been matched by speculation as to its mechanism of action. Shortly after the first reports (218,432) of its administration to animals and man, it was recognized that dipyridamole retarded the breakdown of adenosine, a potent coronary vasodilator. More recently, the inhibitory effects of dipyridamole on platelet aggregation have prompted research into its involvement in the formation of prostacyclin and thromboxane. Parallel to these efforts, the initial therapeutic potential of dipyridamole purely as a vasodilator has been overshadowed somewhat by its evaluation in clinical trials as an antithrombotic agent (350,363).

Chemistry

Dipyridamole (2,6-*bis*-diethylamino-4,8-dipiperidinopyrimido-5,4-d-pyrimidine) is a pyrimidopyrimidine derivative (Fig. 2) that has both vasodilating and antiplatelet properties. The hemodynamic and antiplatelet effects are not structurally interdependent, although *in vivo*, the increase in blood flow resulting from vasodilatation may facilitate its antithrombotic effect (115). Didisheim and Owen (116) studied the effects of various pyrimidopyrimidines in a rat model in which thrombi were induced by crush-injury in a femoral arteriovenous Teflon shunt. They found that 2,4,6-trimorpholinopyrimido-5,4-d-pyrimidine (RA433) was more effective than dipyridamole or 2,6-*bis*-(diethanolamino)-4-piperidino-pyrimide-5,4-3-pyrimidine (RA233) in inhibiting thrombosis and platelet stickiness. These authors suggested that the presence of the morpholino groups in RA433 may have accounted for the discrepancy between these derivatives. However, Horch et al. (207) demonstrated that the structure–activity relationships of pyrimidopyrimidines are probably more complex than this. When dipyrimidole was compared with RA233, RA433, and the thienopyrimidine, VK744, (2- (2-amino-ethyl)amino-4-morpholinothieno 3,2-d-pyrimidine-dihydrochloride), RA433 most potently prolonged the bleeding time. However, RA233 impaired the velocity of platelet aggregation most effectively, and VK744 was significantly more effective than the other compounds at impairing platelet adhesion to glass beads. Dipyridamole, perhaps in part because of its vasodilator effect, was the most potent inhibitor of electrically induced platelet thrombi in rat mesenteric veins. However, the antithrombotic effect of dipyridamole is independent of its hemodynamic action as it is demonstrable in rigid synthetic tubing models of thrombosis (116). Dipyridamole subsequently was shown to be generally less effective than the other derivatives at inhibiting adenosine diphosphate (ADP), collagen, and thrombin-induced aggregation (393). However, the entire group appeared to have a stronger effect on the release reaction than on ADP-induced aggregation. All of these pyrimido–pyrimidine derivatives inhibit platelet

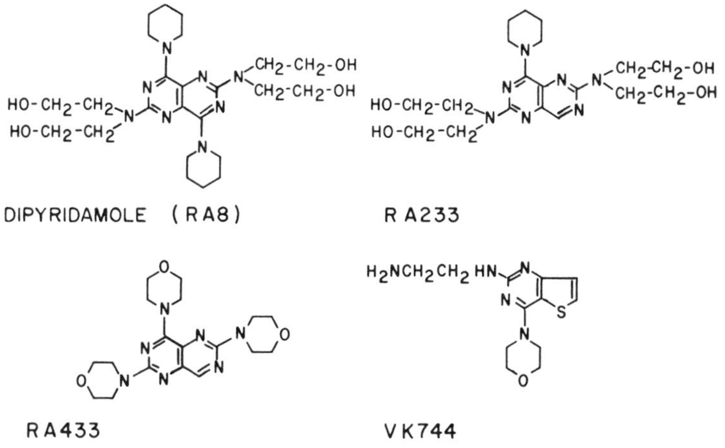

FIG. 2. Dipyridamole and its analogues.

phosphiodiesterase, the enzyme responsible for conversion of cyclic AMP to 5'-AMP. The platelet release reaction is inhibited by compounds that elevate platelet cAMP (291,393).

Interaction with Adenosine

Born et al. (56) observed that systemic administration of adenosine and 2-chloradenosine modified the behavior of platelet thrombi in injured arteries of the rabbit cerebral cortex. Adenosine, proved to be a powerful systemic vasodilator (291) which undergoes rapid cellular uptake (280) and subsequent deamination of phosphorylation (57). Although more resistant to deamination (55), 2-chloradenosine produced respiratory arrest when administered to rabbits (56).

West et al. (475) first observed that dipyridamole caused coronary vasodilation in the dog without an associated increase in cardiac work. Gerlach and Deuticke (162) demonstrated that dipyridamole enhanced the accumulation of adenosine in ischemic rat heart. Additionally, dipyridamole was shown to increase the myocardial content of ATP (55) and potentiate adenosine-induced coronary vasodilation in anesthetized dogs (61).

The mechanism by which dipyridamole interacted with adenosine was studied by Bunag et al. (66). Dipyridamole markedly retarded the disappearance of adenosine from both a suspension of washed canine erythrocytes and from dog whole blood *in vitro* (230). This effect was again observed in whole, but not hemolyzed human blood. Although dipyridamole appeared to inhibit adenosine deaminase in this system, it also delayed the disappearance of adenosine at doses at which enzyme inhibition was unlikely. An alternative explanation was that dipyridamole first prevented the uptake of adenosine by erythrocytes and thereby its consequent deamination.

The kinetics of adenosine uptake by erythrocytes were characterized by Roos and Pfleger (382). Two mechanisms were involved. One, which was saturable at high substrate concentrations, was inhibited by dipyridamole and could be described by Michaelis-Menten kinetics. The second corresponded to the laws of simple diffusion; it was not saturable, could not be inhibited, and had the characteristics of diffusion across lipophylic areas of the membrane. These, and studies in human erythrocyte ghosts (406), demonstrated that whereas simple diffusion predominated at unphysiologically high extracellular concentrations of adenosine, saturable, facilitated diffusion was the major mechanism of uptake at extracellular concentrations within the physiological range. Although dipyridamole significantly reduced adenosine uptake by intact erythrocyte ghosts, it did not inhibit adenosine deaminase or kinase in solubilized ghost cells. Phosphorylation appeared to predominate once adenosine had undergone cellular uptake, as the K_m for adenosine kinase was significantly lower than that of adenosine deaminase.

These properties of dipyridamole may be related to its ability to cause coronary vasodilation. Diminished cardiac blood flow or increased myocardial oxygen utilization would result in a decline in myocardial oxygen tension with a consequent breakdown of adenine nucleotides to adenosine (324). The adenosine thus formed would diffuse out of the cell and, via the interstitial fluid, reach the coronary arterioles and produce vasodilatation (394).

Vasodilatation might result from adenosine reducing intracellular calcium influx (437), increasing intracellular cAMP, thus decreasing calcium availability (357), acting centrally (322), or binding to a specific receptor on vascular smooth muscle cells. Although the mechanism is not precisely elucidated and phosphodiesterase inhibitors may mobilize intracellular ionized calcium independently of the increase in cAMP, a role for cAMP or neural factors in the adenosine-induced relaxation of vascular smooth muscle seems unlikely (281,408). The identification of adenosine binding sites on a crude plasma membrane isolated from canine carotid and coronary arteries (127) suggests that dipyridamole may facilitate vasodilatation by inhibiting the intracellular uptake of adenosine, thereby increasing its concentration at these receptor sites. Although inhibition of adenosine uptake by erythrocytes and platelets also may be important in the antiplatelet action of dipyridamole (99), it appears to be exerted primarily via inhibition of platelet cAMP phosphodiesterase (291). Potentiation of the platelet inhibitory effect of adenosine also may contribute to the antithrombotic activity of dipyridamole (58).

Interaction with Prostaglandins

Following the observation that the inhibition of ADP-induced platelet aggregation caused by both PGE_1 and isoprenaline was potentiated by theophylline, a cAMP phosphodiesterase inhibitor, Mills and Smith (291) established that dipyridamole and its RA233 derivative possessed properties similar to those of theophylline. Sufficient concentrations of PGE_1 in the presence of RA233 caused a dose-dependent increase in the degree of inhibition of aggregation which correlated with increased accumulation of radioactive cAMP.

The antiaggregatory effects of prostacyclin are also closely related to the stimulation of platelet adenylate cyclase (168,454) and are enhanced by phosphodiesterase inhibitors. Theophylline, a weak inhibitor of phosphodiesterase, has been shown to enhance the deaggregatory action of prostacyclin in anesthetized, heparinized cats (173). Moncada and Korbut (295) have suggested that dipyridamole and other phosphodiesterase inhibitors might act as antithrombotic agents by potentiating the antiplatelet effect of endogenous prostacyclin. Prostacyclin is not extensively metabolized by the lung and has been postulated as a circulating hormone (297), activating platelet adenylate cyclase and increasing platelet cAMP, thereby decreasing aggregability. These workers observed that the antiplatelet action of dipyridamole was more pronounced in arterial than venous blood, consistent with its dependence upon adenylate cyclase activation by prostacyclin. Moreover, antiprostacyclin antiserum and high-dose aspirin antagonized the action of dipyridamole, whereas it was enhanced by a low-dose of aspirin such as might selectively inhibit TXA_2 synthesis, sparing endogenous prostacyclin. Studies in healthy volunteers suggest that prostacyclin is unlikely to act as a circulating antiplatelet hormone in man (142). However, it is of probable local importance in the regulation of platelet blood vessel wall and platelet–platelet interactions, and dipyridamole might interact with endogenous prostacyclin at this level.

Although prostacyclin may not act as a circulating antiaggregatory agent (142,432) and others have found that dipyridamole reduced, rather than potentiated the antiaggregatory effect of prostacyclin in human platelet-rich plasma (119), Masotti et al. (272) found that an infusion of dipyridamole (8 μg/kg/min for 2 hr) resulted in an increase in prostacyclin-like activity. Incubation of rabbit aortic rings with dipyridamole produced a dose-dependent increase in prostacyclin-like activity suggesting that prostacyclin generation was increased rather than its activity merely potentiated. This accords with the observations of Blass et al. (51) who have noted that dipyridamole caused a dose-dependent increase in prostacyclin biosynthesis from tritiated arachidonic acid in rat stomach fundus and stimulated the transformation of PGH_2 to prostacyclin by pig aortic microsomes. This suggested that dipyridamole acts at the second step of prostacyclin biosynthesis.

In addition to an effect on prostacyclin biosynthesis, dipyridamole may influence the generation of TXA_2 (8). Best et al. (43) found that preincubation of human platelet-rich plasma with dipyridamole resulted in inhibition of collagen and arachidonate induced aggregation without any alteration in platelet cAMP. Dipyridamole also reduced collagen and arachidonate induced release of TXB_2 from platelet-rich plasma. TXA_2 may promote release of calcium from intracellular or membrane-bound stores (9,163). Prostacyclin appears to inhibit release of intracellular calcium. Inhibition of TXA_2 release by dipyridamole would leave this effect unopposed, potentiating the antiaggregatory effect of prostacyclin (208).

However, others have failed to show an effect of dipyridamole in concentrations up to 100 μg/ml upon the conversion of PGH_2 to TXA_2 by rabbit, horse, and human platelets (343). Although dipyridamole inhibits ADP-induced aggregation and thromboxane synthesis at 50 μM or more (344), blood levels *in vivo* rarely exceed 10 μM (363). The observation that concentrations of 2 μM can inhibit platelet phosphodiesterase (44) supports the hypothesis of Moncada and Korbut.

An additional mechanism of action has been suggested by recent studies of the ability of cultured endothelial and smooth muscle cells from bovine pulmonary artery to metabolize 8-^{14}C ADP (99). Cellular uptake of radioactivity was almost completely inhibited by 10 μM dipyridamole, and inosine (an adenosine metabolite) was largely replaced in the medium by adenosine. This was accompanied by an increased antiaggregatory activity of the conditioned medium that could be matched by authentic adenosine at the same concentrations. Thus, in addition to its effects on prostacyclin and thromboxane, dipyridamole may inhibit platelet aggregation by increasing local concentrations of adenosine via inhibition of erythrocyte and platelet uptake mechanisms. Finally, it has been suggested (17) that dipyridamole has an inhibitory effect on platelet aggregation dependent on albumin but independent of prostacyclin and thromboxane.

Platelet Effects

The effects of dipyridamole on platelets have been extensively investigated in animals and man. In contrast to aspirin, dipyridamole inhibits the first and second phase of ADP-induced platelet aggregation (296,493). Inhibition of the second phase alone requires much lower drug concentrations (100). These studies indicate that dipyridamole does not prolong bleeding time in man (288). Recently, however, Cunningham et al. (102) reported a patient with a prolonged Ivy bleeding time and hematuria on dipyridamole (150 mg/day). Hemorrhage stopped and the bleeding time shortened from greater than 30 min to 4 min within 48 hr of stopping dipyridamole. Others have failed to demonstrate an effect of dipyridamole on platelet aggregation *ex vivo* (100,128).

Dipyridamole powerfully inhibited thrombus formation in injured vessels on rabbit cerebral cortex (130). When given intravenously, it produced a transient decrease in the platelet clumping response to ADP. Topical application of dipyridamole to the injured arteries was also effective. The same authors further investigated the antiplatelet effect in man (131). Dipyridamole at 10^{-4}M (50 μg per ml) but not at 10^{-5}M, diminished ADP-induced aggregation and enhanced the subsequent disaggregation of human platelets *in vitro*. The aggregatory response to epinephrine was unaffected. Intravenous dipyridamole (30–50 mg) produced plasma levels of 3 to 5 μg/ml. Both intravenous and oral (200–600 mg for 3 to 20 weeks giving plasma levels ranging from 0.9–7.0 μg/ml) dipyridamole also reduced "spontaneous" platelet clumping.

Oral dipyridamole prolonged platelet survival in patients with increased platelet consumption in association with arterial thromboembolism, arteriovenous prosthetic cannulas, vasculitis, and prosthetic aortic grafts (181). However, dipyridamole did not significantly alter the combined consumption of platelets and fibrinogen in patients with venous thrombosis. Dipyridamole may, in high doses, inhibit thrombus formation in extracorporeal shunts (100,329). Rittenhous et al. (374) reported that microaggregate formation in canine blood circulated in pump oxygenators was reduced by dipyridamole.

Failure to demonstrate the antiplatelet effects of dipyridamole may result from inadequate blood levels. Rajah et al. (363) have observed that platelet aggregation and platelet factor 4 availability inversely correlated with circulating concentrations of dipyridamole achieved in man. Others have noted that concentrations of dipyridamole that have an antithrombotic effect *in vivo* have no effect *in vitro*. Dipyridamole is far more effective against collagen-induced aggregation *in vivo* than *in vitro* (100). Moncada and Korbut (295) suggest that this agrees with the hypothesis that dipyridamole acts by potentiating endogenous prostacyclin. Due to the instability of prostacyclin, its effects on platelets *in vivo* may have disappeared by the time a blood sample has been processed for aggregation studies *in vitro*. However, others have observed a prolonged stability of prostacyclin in plasma at room temperature (343). Weiss et al. (472) have recently studied the effects of aspirin (650 mg twice a day), dipyridamole (100 mg four times a day), or placebo on the interaction of human platelets with rabbit aortic subendothelium. Although aspirin markedly reduced platelet thrombi in titrated blood, neither aspirin nor dipyridamole markedly inhibited platelet thrombus formation in directly sampled human blood.

Other Pharmacological Properties

Cardiac Actions

Dipyridamole is a potent coronary vasodilator in dogs, achieving this effect without an increase in cardiac work or contractility (218). This results in an increase in the coronary venous oxygen content and an increase in coronary flow. Dipyridamole appears to act predominantly on the small resistance vessels of the coronary bed, and it alters transcapillary exchange in the same way as does severe hypoxemia. In therapeutic doses, dipyridamole produces only slight alterations in systemic blood pressure and peripheral blood flow (314).

In view of the coronary vasodilating properties of dipyridamole and the controversy that surrounds its mechanism of action, two recent publications concerning the interaction of prostacyclin and adenosine in the coronary vasculature are of interest. Blass et al. (52) examined the influence of prostacyclin on adenosine release in rabbit heart perfused by the Langendorf method. Prostacyclin increased both coronary flow and the myocardial release of adenosine in a dose-dependent manner. Low concentrations of aminophyline which antagonize the circulatory effects of adenosine (281) and had no intrinsic effect on basal coronary flow and prostacyclin release suppressed prostacyclin-induced enhancement of coronary flow. Thus, it seemed that in this model, the coronary vasodilator effects of dipyridamole were mediated, at least in part, by prostacyclin. By contrast, Shrör et al. (409) found that coronary vasodilating doses of prostacyclin in the Langendorf perfused rat heart were associated with a decline rather than an increase in adenosine release and were not inhibited by isobutylmethylxanthine.

Although the vasodilating properties of dipyridamole may thus involve its interaction with prostacyclin or adenosine or both, it has been uncertain whether the increase in coronary flow (227) which it produces would actually benefit ischemic myocardium or result in further deterioration via a "coronary steal" (279) phenomenon. Convincing evidence is lacking that either acute or chronic dosing with dipyridamole reduces the frequency or severity of anginal attacks in man (314). Roberts et al. (376) have now demonstrated that infusion of dipyridamole limited infarct size following coronary artery ligation in the dog. Both radionuclide uptake *in vivo* and infarct weight were reduced by approximately one-half in the dipyridamole treated group. These changes were associated with functional improvement: The anterior wall regional ejection fraction decreased less and the posterior wall ejection fraction increased more in the dipyridamole treated dogs. Finally, dipyridamole has been shown to increase glucose consumption and reduce lactic acid formation in the hypoxic canine heart (238) in agreement with its capacity for mitochondrial fixation, stimulation of oxidative phosphorylation, and reduction of critical oxygen pressure in tissue culture studies (155).

Miscellaneous Actions

Dipyridamole has been claimed to increase the rate and depth of respiration and produce bronchodilation (218). A recent trial of dipyridamole in migraine (193) was stopped because of an increase in migraine attack frequency in all patients. It has been suggested that benefit might be obtained by restricting dipyridamole to those patients with a demonstrable platelet defect (106).

Pharmacokinetics and Metabolism

Early studies suggested that dipyridamole is rapidly absorbed from the stomach and small intestine in man. Peak blood levels occur within 60 min of oral dosing (40). Absorption is hastened and peak blood levels are higher when dipyridamole is administered as a crushed tablet (282). Ben et al. (41) noted a marked difference in LD_{50} values obtained in the mouse following oral (>7.0 g/kg) and intravenous (0.225 g/kg) administration, suggesting poor oral utilization or absorption in this species.

Mellinger and Bohorfoush (283) studied tissue distribution of dipyridamole in the guinea pig, rabbit, rat and mouse. They found that the drug was rapidly absorbed and found in all organs except the brain. High concentrations were noted in liver and kidney. Peak tissue levels occurred within 3 to 4 hr, and these concentrations had halved 12 hr after dosing.

von Beisenherz et al. (40) described the hepatic transformation of dipyridamole to monoglucuronide, a compound that underwent partial enterohepatic circulation and subsequent fecal extraction. These investigators found only 1 to 3% of the glucuronide and none of the unchanged drug in the urine. Following oral and intravenous administration to rats, approximately 50% of the dose was recovered in the feces within 72 hr.

More recently, Nielsen-Kudsk and Pedersen (315) have studied the pharmacokinetics of dipyridamole in man. Circulating drug concentrations were measured by a highly specific HPLC-method (344). The serum concentration curve after intravenous dipyridamole approximated to an open two-compartment model with first-order, linear disposition kinetics and elimination occurring from the first compartment. Oral administration produced results consistent with a model with two consecutive first order input steps representing the dissolution and absorption processes. The absorption rate constant was about 0.07 min^{-1} and the biological half lives ranged from 83 to 145 min. This is consistent with a value in man of 95 min calculated from the data of Rajah et al. (363) and 75 min in rats (492). The systemic bioavailability of an oral 100 mg dose ranged from only 37 to 66%, probably reflecting both poor gastrointestinal absorption and an unknown degree of first-pass metabolism.

A recent study (316) suggests that rabbit myocardium behaves as a two-compartment system with half lives of 1.4 min (α) and 6.3 min (β). Myocardial accumulation of dipyridamole in these studies coincided with a progressive decrease in contractility, while oxygen consumption remained unchanged. Coronary vasodilatation was not observed. Previous studies (41) have shown that oral, intravenous, and intracoronary administration of dipyridamole resulted in coronary vasodilation which coincided with an increase in myocardial contractile force.

Drug Interactions

Dipyridamole may interact with other agents that interfere with hemostasis. Although the combination of heparin therapy with dipyridamole must be treated gingerly (28), the combined antiplatelet effects of aspirin and dipyridamole are currently under clinical investigation. The combination of aspirin with dipyridamole increased the plasma concentration of dipyridamole in studies in humans, dogs, and pigs (460). Rajah et al. (365) suggested that a combination of either dipyridamole 50 mg three times daily and aspirin 180 mg, or dipyridamole 75 mg three times daily and 120 mg aspirin achieved maximal platelet inhibiting effects in healthy volunteers. These doses did not prolong bleeding time.

Toxic Effects

Dipyridamole is usually unassociated with adverse effects at normal therapeutic doses. Gastrointestinal upset accompanied by nausea, vomiting, and diarrhea occurs occasionally as do rashes, headache, and vertigo (266). Excessive doses produce hypotension. A "coronary steal" phenomenon was suggested as the mechanism by which acute myocardial ischemia was provoked by intravenous dipyridamole in three patients with coronary artery disease (480). Acute psychiatric disturbance has been reported in two patients with acute myocardial infarction who received dipyridamole (161). A recent preliminary report (113) suggests that dipyridamole, despite an antiplatelet effect, may enhance atherosclerotic plaque formation in rabbits fed an atherogenic diet.

SULFINPYRAZONE

Introduction

Although sulfinpyrazone shares a platelet inhibitory effect in common with aspirin and dipyridamole, it is unique within this class of compounds. The uniqueness of sulfinpyrazone becomes particularly obvious with a study of its pharmacology, for the action *in vivo* not only differs in several respects from the other drugs discussed here, but is dependent in part on the effects of several of its metabolites. In the following discussion of the pharmacology and biotransformation of sulfinpyrazone, the differences as well as similarities in the action of these drugs will be noted.

Chemistry

Sulfinpyrazone is a phenylbutazone analogue with the chemical name 1,2 di-phenyl-4-(2-phenylsulfinyl-ethyl)-3,5-pyrazolidinedione. A description of the chemical synthesis of sulfinpyrazone and of several of its metabolites has been described fully by Pfister and Hafliger (351). Early interest in this substance was generated because of marked metabolic conversion to the sulfoxide, which is a more potent uricosuric agent than the parent compound. Subsequently, other metabolites have been identified and are known to be pharmacologically active. Figure 3 illustrates the structure of the parent compound, its three known major metabolites (the sulfone, the sulfide, and the para-hydroxy sulfide derivative), and three minor metabolites.

Inhibition of Prostaglandin Synthesis

Sulfinpyrazone, like aspirin, inhibits platelet release reaction and interferes with prostaglandin synthesis in the platelet. However, the mechanism (or mechanisms) by which this occurs differs somewhat from that of aspirin. Moreover, prostacyclin synthesis by endothelial cells appears to be much less affected by sulfinpyrazone than by aspirin.

McDonald et al. (277,278) and others (3,4) have elucidated the influence of sulfinpyrazone on the various stages of prostaglandin synthesis. Their data have provided evidence of an inhibitory effect on the cyclooxygenase step of prosta-glandin synthesis (Fig. 4).

The cyclooxygenase acts as a catalyst in the biochemical conversion of arachi-donic acid to the unstable prostaglandins PGG_2 and PGH_2. Another enzyme, throm-boxane synthase, catalyzes the further conversion of PGH_2 to TXA_2. All three of these substances (PGG_2, PGH_2, and TXA_2) contribute to aggregation and platelet release. PGH_2 also is converted to various stable prostaglandins, of which PGD_2 is of particular importance since it is an inhibitor of platelet aggregation.

In *in vitro* experiments, Ali et al. (3) incubated human platelet lysates with ^{14}C-arachidonic acid following a 2-min preincubation with either saline or various

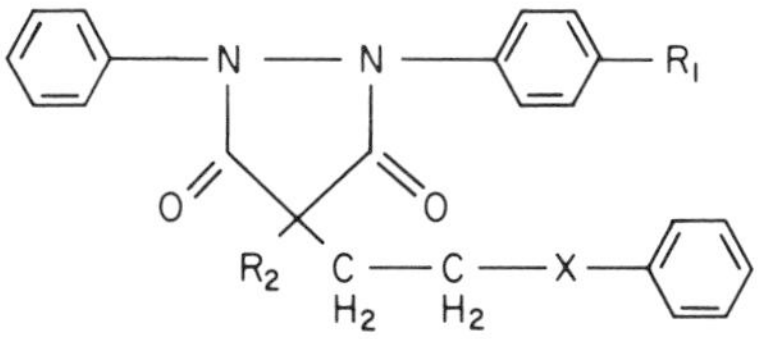

COMPOUND	R_1	R_2	X
SULFINPYRAZONE	H	H	SO
SULFIDE	H	H	S
SULFONE	H	H	SO₂
p–OH–SULFIDE	OH	H	S
p–OH–SULFONE	OH	H	SO₂
p–OH–SULFINPYRAZONE	OH	H	SO
4–OH–SULFINPYRAZONE	H	OH	SO

FIG. 3. Sulfinpyrazone and its metabolites.

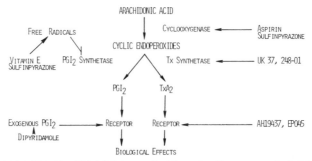

FIG. 4. Sites of action of antiplatelet drugs. Aspirin and sulfinpyrazone both inhibit cyclooxygenase. Like vitamin E, sulfinpyrazone may also act as a free radical scavenger. Dipyridamole may enhance endogenous PGI$_2$ production, thromboxane synthase inhibitors such as UK37, 248-01, and thromboxane receptor antagonists such as AH 19437 and EPO45 are under preliminary investigation.

concentrations of sulfinpyrazone. The reaction products were chromatographed to separate the prostaglandins and to measure the amount of precursor that was converted in the presence or absence of the drug. With low arachidonic acid concentrations, sulfinpyrazone proved to be a competitive inhibitor of platelet prostaglandin synthesis. In fact, significant inhibition was achieved with drug concentrations as low as 2.5 and 5 μM as long as the concentration of arachidonic acid remained between 2 and 10 μM. The result of this inhibitory effect on cyclooxygenase activity was a block or partial block of PGG$_2$, PGH$_2$ and TXA$_2$ production. If the arachidonic acid concentration was elevated, the inhibitory effect of sulfinpyrazone was overwhelmed and moreover, platelet aggregation could be triggered by a nonprostaglandin pathway.

From consideration of the various pathways involved in prostaglandin synthesis, one could theorize that sulfinpyrazone inhibited not only cyclooxygenase activity but also thromboxane synthetase activity. However, other *in vitro* experiments by Ali et al. (5) eliminated this possibility. First, they showed that PGD$_2$ and TXB$_2$ production were equally inhibited by sulfinpyrazone. This could only occur if there was interference with the production of PGG$_2$, the common precursor to PGD$_2$ and TXB$_2$. Moreover, PGG$_2$ is produced early in the synthesis from arachidonic acid.

The authors then were able to confirm the location of sulfinpyrazone interference even more precisely and at the same time, demonstrated that sulfinpyrazone antagonizes the irreversible inhibition of platelet cyclooxygenase activity caused by aspirin (278). First, they prepared suspensions of washed intact platelets and preincubated them with aspirin, sulfinpyrazone, or combinations of the two drugs for 10 min before adding ^{14}C-arachidonic acid (10 μM). Not only did aspirin or sulfinpyrazone inhibit cyclooxygenase activity, but with aspirin and sulfinpyrazone combinations, the level of inhibition was identical to that achieved with sulfinpyrazone alone. Thus, it was demonstrated that sulfinpyrazone antagonized the action of aspirin and probably did so by preferentially occupying the site on the cyclooxygenase enzyme that otherwise would have been acetylated by aspirin.

That sulfinpyrazone acts at the cyclooxygenase level of prostaglandin synthesis also has been demonstrated in the animal model. In rabbits, intravenous infusions of arachidonic acid produce increased plasma levels of PGD_2, TXB_2, and the prostacyclin metabolite 6-keto-$PGF_{1\alpha}$, as measured by radioimmunoassay (4,81,422). The increases were blocked totally by large doses of aspirin (250 mg/kg) and by relatively low doses of sulfinpyrazone (30 mg/kg), as were the physical symptoms from arachidonic acid infusions—intense, intravascular platelet aggregation as measured by a decrease in the peripheral blood platelet count, respiratory distress, profound hypotension, and death (278). In untreated animals, death was almost invariably associated with thromboxane levels greater than 10 ng/ml and a drop in the peripheral platelet count of more than 60%.

Rabbits also have been subjected to intravenous infusions of collagen that produced intravascular platelet aggregation and thromboxane formation (278). Aspirin and sulfinpyrazone again protected the animals from hypotension and death, but the effect on intravascular platelet aggregation was less dramatic than in the arachidonic acid experiment.

The observation that inhibition of cyclooxygenase activity by aspirin not only inhibits the formation of platelet TXA_2 but of endothelial cell prostacyclin would suggest that sulfinpyrazone also would inhibit endothelial cell prostacyclin production. Surprisingly, while this could be demonstrated in cultured endothelial cells (166), the concentrations of sulfinpyrazone required were 50 to 100 times greater than those of aspirin. This lack of effect of sulfinpyrazone on prostacyclin production requires further study since it may provide a better understanding of the differences in action between these two compounds as well as having important therapeutic implications.

Platelet Effects

The action of sulfinpyrazone on platelets was first reported by Smythe et al. (435), after they observed that the drug prolonged shortened platelet survival and decreased platelet turnover in patients suffering from both gout and thromboembolic disorders. This effect on platelets, first observed clinically, soon stimulated pharmacological investigations designed to define the mechanism of this effect and to determine whether it could occur independently of the uricosuric action of the drug.

The latter problem was solved first by Mustard et al. in 1967 (310). They selected the rabbit for study since uric acid is absent in the plasma. Using ^{32}p-diisopropyl-fluorophosphonate as the platelet label, Mustard and associates administered sulfinpyrazone in a dose of approximately 20 mg/kg s.c. daily for a minimum of 4 weeks. During this treatment period, platelet survival time nearly doubled when computed on an exponential model, and platelet turnover was correspondingly reduced. These results were later corroborated in a study in which 50 mg/kg/day sulfinpyrazone was administered intravenously at the same time as ^{51}Cr-labeled platelets (476). Having established the mutual autonomy of the drug's uricosuric and platelet inhibitory effects, pharmacology research subsequently concentrated on its platelet effects, principally its interference with platelet aggregation.

Under normal conditions, platelets will not adhere to each other or to the walls of the blood vessels. However, if the vascular wall is injured or denuded, the platelets come into contact with subendothelial elements including collagen, microfibrils, and basement membrane (31,32). This contact triggers a "release reaction" wherein platelets secrete ADP and TXA_2. TXA_2, a product of prostaglandin synthesis, strikingly promotes platelet aggregation. ADP also stimulates platelet adherence and stimulates the formation of a platelet–fibrin thrombus, but independently of the prostaglandin pathway (204). However, there is also evidence that sulfinpyrazone acts via other pathways to inhibit the release reaction and platelet aggregation.

Packham et al. (332) looked for an interaction between sulfinpyrazone and ADP. They induced aggregation in platelet-rich plasma using collagen, an agonist which acts independently of the arachidonate pathway (226). Sulfinpyrazone inhibited this collagen-induced aggregation in a relatively weak but generally dose-dependent manner, but without inhibiting the action of ADP or thrombin. These results were later confirmed by Renaud and Lecompte (371) in rats, Muirhead (306), and Rosenberg and Sell (383). Thus, the mechanism of drug action was independent of ADP, and the inhibition noted in these studies may have been a result of reduced platelet adherence or possibly a reduced response to surface stimuli.

Indeed, sulfinpyrazone has been shown to be highly effective as a platelet inhibitor in *in vitro* studies using such agonists as globulin-coated latex (332), Ag/Ab complexes (332), Newcastle disease virus (458), epinephrine (306), and collagen (4). The latter study was of particular importance since it revealed that if the concentration of collagen is kept low so that only 10 to 35% of serotonin is secreted, then 160 μg/ml sulfinpyrazone can produce 30 to 70% inhibition of the release reaction in platelet-rich plasma. This "low-dose collagen" technique also has been found to be very effective *ex vivo* in normal human subjects.

Over the past decade, several animal models have been employed to demonstrate the platelet inhibitory and antithrombotic effects of sulfinpyrazone. Platelet aggregates have been induced by various methods and using many types of stimuli. One of the best ways devised for examining the effect of the drug against mural thrombus formation utilizes the exposed microcirculation of the hamster cheek pouch (31,42). In one such study (256), mural platelet thrombi were produced on the vessel walls of the cheek pouch arterioles by positive square wave DC pulses. The number of white thrombi increased in proportion with the length of time the animals were exposed to the stimulation. Following the oral administration of 3, 10, 20, and 60 mg/kg sulfinpyrazone 18 hr and 1 hr prior to stimulation, there was a reduction in thrombus formation that was significant with doses of 20 mg/kg and 60 mg/kg. The plasma concentrations corresponding to this effect were 60 μg/ml and 83 μg/ml, respectively.

In another variation, Wiedeman (481) studied the effect of the drug on thrombi produced in the wing vasculature of the bat. The animals were premedicated with a 50 mg/kg intravenous injection of sulfinpyrazone. Then, instead of using an electrical stimulus, she produced platelet thrombi with a single-pulse ruby-red laser (the heat from the laser lysed the red blood cells, releasing ADP, and causing the platelets to aggregate). When the bats were tested immediately after stimulation, there was only an 18% decrease in adherence, but after 1 hr, there was a 58.5% reduction in platelet activity. This study showed that although sulfinpyrazone is not particularly active against the action of ADP as previously discussed, it is able to interfere with platelet adherence to the endothelial lining and to one another. Wiedeman (481) also demonstrated the same principle in hamsters after mechanically injuring the wall of an arterial vessel that produced collagen-induced platelet aggregation. One hour after a 50 mg/kg intravenous injection of sulfinpyrazone, the duration of platelet activity decreased by 44.9%.

The platelet suppressant effect of sulfinpyrazone also has been demonstrated in experiments utilizing sheep that had been cannulated for venovenous perfusion so that blood flowed either through a membrane oxygenator or through a shunt (47). Transient thrombocytopenia was produced by the oxygenator or shunt, and pulmonary vascular responses were measured in control animals and in animals treated with 35 to 50 mg/kg sulfinpyrazone administered intravenously. In the treated animals, thrombocytopenia due to platelet aggregation was almost totally inhibited as were simultaneous increases in pulmonary vascular resistance and pulmonary artery pressure. Using similar techniques, Cooper et al. (98) measured the platelet response to ADP stimulation in cannulated sheep that had been treated with sulfinpyrazone. During the first 2 hr of the oxygenator perfusion, platelet aggregation decreased markedly in the sulfinpyrazone-treated animals. After 2 hr, however, platelet aggregation in the treated animals were significantly greater than in the controls. These and subsequent experiments also revealed that exposure of blood to dialyzer membranes activates the complement system which results in peripheral leukopenia, pulmonary leukostasis and an increase in pulmonary artery pressure. On the basis of these findings, Cooper repeated the sheep experiment infusing complement-activated plasma. Seven sheep served as controls and another 7 received 2 g sulfinpyrazone intravenously at least 30 min prior to the infusion. No significant changes in platelet count occurred in either group. However, animals pretreated with sulfinpyrazone were protected against the rise in pulmonary artery pressure and pulmonary vascular pressure, and cardiac output remained stable. The mechanism for this activity has not been identified.

Another suitable model for testing platelet inhibition by sulfinpyrazone involves the measurement of intravascular platelet aggregation formed in the acute phase of the Arthus reaction in rabbit (75) and guinea pig (76). In both species, the extent of aggregation could be obtained by direct counting of the platelets in the plasma since a transient thrombocytopenia was accomplished by a sequestration of platelet aggregates in liver, lungs, and spleen. When the animals were pretreated with 50 to 100 mg/kg sulfinpyrazone intravenously, the platelet response was significantly blocked. Heparin did not inhibit this response (77), indicating that coagulation processes were not involved.

Sulfinpyrazone also has been shown to protect animals from thrombus formation induced by the intravenous injection of an endotoxin such as *S. typhosa* lipopolysaccharide. Hyperlipidemic rats were given 1,000 mg/kg sulfinpyrazone p.o. 2 hr prior to the endotoxin and then sacrificed (371). The average size of the hepatic infarcts found in the treated animals was 66% smaller than that of the controls. Similarly, when premedicated with 100 mg/kg sulfinpyrazone at various times up to 1 min prior to the endotoxin injection, rabbits were protected from its lethal effect, and the number of platelet aggregates in the microcirculation was reduced (132). The drug was ineffective when given after the endotoxin. So far, the drug has not been effective in inhibiting endotoxin shock in dogs (101).

In 1979, Butler and White (78) reported on the effects of sulfinpyrazone in guinea pigs challenged with intravenous injections of the Forssman antibody. This antibody induces a rapid antigen antibody reaction in the lungs (as bronchospasm) and also produces subendothelial vascular lesions to which platelets readily adhere. Several test drugs, including sulfinpyrazone, aspirin, indomethacin, phenylbutazone, and three sulfinpyrazone metabolites were administered intravenously, 30 or 60 min prior to the Forssman antiserum. In a 100-mg/kg dosage, sulfinpyrazone totally inhibited thrombocytopenia when given 60 min prior to challenge. Aspirin, indomethacin, and phenylbutazone had no effect. Sulfinpyrazone metabolites were active, but less so than the parent compound. The significance of these findings lies in the fact that the platelet response to the Forssman challenge apparently occurred independently of the prostaglandin pathway, as otherwise, aspirin and indomethacin would have inhibited the fall in platelet count. Again this provides evidence for a very specific and distinctive effect of sulfinpyrazone that is not shared with other platelet-active drugs and not even with its own phenylbutazone analogue. So far, there has been no adequate explanation for these differences. In this regard, it is interesting to note that the major *in vivo* metabolite of sulfinpyrazone, the sulfide (thioether), recently has been shown to inhibit thrombin-induced platelet aggregation (411), an action not shared by aspirin, dipyridamole, or sulfinpyrazone itself.

Other Pharmacological Properties

Other than for its potent uricosuric action (the mechanism for which remains unclear), its mild antiinflammatory properties, and its platelet effects, several other interesting pharmacological actions of sulfinpyrazone (or its metabolites) recently have been described.

Endothelial Cell Protection

In the previous section it was shown that sulfinpyrazone possesses only a weak effect against ADP- and collagen-induced platelet aggregation following various types of stimulation. Nevertheless, the drug still can inhibit platelet aggregation by protecting the damaged endothelial wall, even when ADP and collagen are used as the agonists. This endothelial protective effect is unique among the known platelet suppressant drugs (187) and merits special attention.

There are many ways of inducing endothelial desquamation for the purpose of studying the possible protective effect of a drug against such damage: It can be accomplished mechanically, nutritionally, immunologically, or chemically. Harker and colleagues (186,188) chose to induce endothelial damage by infusing 12 baboons with homocysteine for 3 months. Besides endothelial desquamation, these infusions also produced a 3-fold increase in platelet consumption and arteriosclerotic intimal lesions. Sulfinpyrazone (250 mg/kg/day) was administered to 6 of the 12 baboons throughout the 3-month period. As compared to the control animals, the sulfin-pyrazone-treated animals showed a significant reduction ($p < 0.001$) in endothelial desquamation (as measured by ^{111}In-platelet imaging); the drug also normalized platelet turnover and significantly reduced the intimal lesion score ($p < 0.001$). By contrast, dipyridamole (30 mg/kg/day) reduced the intimal lesion score ($p < 0.001$) but had no effect on endothelial cell loss as compared to the controls. A similar effect also was observed in hyperlipidemic monkeys who had sustained mechani-cally-induced endothelial injury in one iliac artery and in the abdominal aorta (189). When these monkeys were treated with 250 mg/kg/day sulfinpyrazone, they showed far less lesion formation than the untreated hyperlipidemic controls.

Sulfinpyrazone protection of endothelial cells also has been demonstrated *in vitro* using a cytotoxicity assay of cultured ^{51}Cr-labeled endothelial cells derived from human umbilical veins (189). Release of the label from uninjured cells was induced either by rabbit antibody, in which there was a clear dose–response relationship, or by homocysteine. Sulfinpyrazone (10^{-4} to 10^{-6} M) reduced the release of ^{51}Cr caused by both immunological and sulphydryl-mediated endothelial injury. This response was dose-dependent. Neither dipyridamole nor aspirin has a notable effect on ^{51}Cr release.

A similar *in vitro* experiment was conducted on endothelial cells from pig aorta (308). A ^{3}H-adenine uptake assay was used in place of the ^{51}Cr label since the latter was not found to be suitable in this system. In concentrations of 5×10^{-5} or 5×10^{-4} M, sulfinpyrazone provided no protection against homocysteine-induced cell damage in pig aorta, although the degree of homocysteine-induced cell damage in this study was comparable to that reported by Harker and Ross (188) in the human umbilical vein. The reason for the discrepancy in the effect of sulfinpyrazone in the two experiments could not be explained with certainty, although the authors suggested that species differences may have been responsible, and that for reasons still unknown, porcine endothelial cells were insensitive to the drug. It was further conjectured that the cytotoxicity tests were not strictly comparable methods for measuring endothelial injury. On the other hand, the argument favoring species differences has gained support in a recent study by Clopath et al. (87) who also found the porcine model responded quite differently to the drug than did the rabbit and rat models. As will be discussed under Pharmacokinetics, these discrepancies may have their basis in the differences in biotransformation of sulfinpyrazone in different species.

Free Radical Scavenger

Phenylbutazone is a known superoxide and free OH scavenger (235,403). Its analogue, sulfinpyrazone, also apparently possesses a similar attribute (236), a property not shared by aspirin or dipyridamole. Considering that free radicals are formed during the oxidative steps involved in the elaboration of the various prostaglandins, this pharmacological activity may account for its protection effects on endothelial cells *(vide supra)* and for other pharmacological differences between it and the other platelet suppressant drugs.

Arrhythmia Inhibitory Effect

Several drugs which modify the effects of prostacyclin and/or thromboxane A_2 have been shown to influence myocardial ischemia in a variety of models (245,410). Kelliher et al. (222) studied the effect of sulfinpyrazone in preventing ventricular fibrillation and ventricular arrhythmias in vagotomized and intact anesthetized cats following coronary artery occlusion. Sulfinpyrazone was administered intravenously in a dose of 100 mg/kg. One hour later, coronary occlusion was produced by abruptly tying the left anterior descending (LAD) coronary artery. Prior to occlusion, sulfinpyrazone did not alter cardiac rhythm. Coronary occlusion produced ECG signs of ischemia and ventricular arrhythmias including premature ventricular contractions (PVCs) and ventricular tachycardia which persisted for approximately 30 min. Ventricular arrhythmias occurred earlier in the vagotomized cats (1 ± 1 sec) than in cats with intact vagus nerves (5 ± 2 sec). Sulfinpyrazone did not alter time of onset of the arrhythmias in the intact cats, but lengthened time of onset to 4 ± 1 sec in the vagotomized animals.

In the intact control cats, the number of PVCs in the first 30 sec after occlusion ranged from 50 to 500. This range was reduced to 7 to 102 in the sulfinpyrazone-treated intact cats ($p < 0.02$). The survival rate among vagotomized cats was too low to permit this comparison. Again, in the intact control animals, ventricular tachycardia occurred in 71% of the survivors; this is in contrast to 17% in the sulfinpyrazone-treated cats ($p < 0.05$). The duration of ventricular tachycardia in both the intact and vagotomized animals was also reduced by 60% and 40%, respectively, when pretreated with sulfinpyrazone. Finally, the drug also reduced the incidence of ventricular fibrillation in intact and vagotomized cats from 30 to 14% in the former and from 47 to 17% in the latter. These results demonstrated a potent and very prompt inhibitory action on both the incidence and severity of ventricular arrhythmias; however, infarct size following occlusion was not affected. On the basis of his observations, Kelliher et al. (222) have proposed that the arrhythmia-sparing effect of sulfinpyrazone is probably attributable to an inhibition of the release of certain cardiac prostaglandins that can facilitate an arrhythmia in an acutely ischemic myocardium.

Povalski et al. (358) also observed a cardioprotective effect in conscious dogs with symptoms of myocardial ischemia induced by coronary occlusion. These investigators have given 30 mg/kg sulfinpyrazone orally twice daily for 4 days and once on the 5th day prior to surgical occlusion of the left circumflex coronary artery. ECG manifestations of myocardial ischemia (e.g., ST-T wave elevation) were slightly reduced in the treated dogs as compared to the placebo controls.

Again, infarct sizes were not affected by the drug, but the incidence of abnormal or ectopic beats was more than halved during the first 3 hr postoperatively. These investigators also monitored a group of dogs after they had undergone occlusion of the LAD coronary artery. In this experiment, sulfinpyrazone (30 mg/kg) or aspirin (30 mg/kg) or placebo were given orally for 3 days. The occlusion was performed on the second day of therapy. Abnormal ventricular ectopic beats occurred in 90% of the placebo-treated animals. Sulfinpyrazone significantly reduced this incidence to about 75% ($p < 0.05$). Heart rate was not affected by sulfinpyrazone except for a very slight bradycardia after acute drug administration. Aspirin also caused a significant ($p < 0.05$) decrease in the incidence of arrhythmias, but the effect was more transient than that of sulfinpyrazone.

Within the same series of experiments, Povalski et al. (358) studied the effects of sulfinpyrazone and aspirin in dogs who were temporarily reperfused following LAD coronary artery occlusion. This technique reliably produces ventricular fibrillation. Four groups of dogs were pretreated for 7 days with placebo, sulfinpyrazone (30 mg/kg p.o.), or aspirin (30 mg/kg p.o.; 10 mg/kg p.o.). The final dose was given 1.5 hr preoperatively. Sulfinpyrazone therapy markedly reduced the incidence of ventricular fibrillation from 58% (controls) to 17%, but neither dose of aspirin afforded any protection. The mortality rate also was greatly reduced in the sulfinpyrazone group, but actually increased among the aspirin-treated animals. ST-T segment elevation was reduced in the sulfinpyrazone group but remained essentially unchanged in both aspirin groups. The absence of a cardioprotective effect on the part of aspirin was an unexpected result, and the authors had no immediate explanation. However, reports in the literature have been inconsistent on this point (245,302).

Moschos et al. (303,304) also studied ventricular function in dogs who had been subjected to coronary occlusion. Some of the dogs had been pretreated daily for 7 days with 300 mg/kg sulfinpyrazone by mouth, while other received 300 mg sulfinpyrazone i.v. on the day the occlusion was performed. Arrhythmia inhibitory effects were studied in the former group immediately after occlusion was completed. For 4 hr after occlusion, no ventricular fibrillation occurred in any of the treated animals but was seen in 39% of the controls. Again, in the dogs treated for 7 days, a significantly lower ($p < 0.01$) aortic pressure was found as well as a significant reduction in ST-segment elevations ($p < 0.02$) as compared to the controls and a zero mortality rate. By contrast, the mortality rate increased to 3/9 in the group of dogs that received only the one i.v. dose and to 3/11 in a group of dogs in which occlusion was delayed for 24 hr after the last dose of oral sulfinpyrazone. This suggests that plasma sulfinpyrazone levels are not the sole determining factor in this arrhythmia-inhibiting effect.

Another dimension to the subject of the arrhythmia-inhibiting effects of sulfinpyrazone has been provided by Folts and Beck (150). They reasoned that since platelet aggregation in stenosed coronary arteries is implicated as a mechanism leading to acute ischemia and fatal arrhythmias, sulfinpyrazone might be effective in improving blood flow in stenosed, narrowed coronary arteries. They tested this theory in dogs with 70% stenosis of the left circumflex artery and attendant cyclical reductions in blood flow. With a single dose of 30 mg/kg i.v., sulfinpyrazone abolished the cyclical flow disruption, significantly reduced heart rate, caused a reappearance of the hyperemic response, and significantly reduced epinephrine-exacerbated platelet plugging. While other agents including aspirin can be shown to prevent the onset of the process of platelet plugging of a stenosed vessel (149,150), sulfinpyrazone is the only agent that has been shown to restore coronary flow to normal after it had been progressively obstructed by platelet plugs in the narrowed lumen. This effect may be attributable not only to the drug's direct action on platelet aggregation, but may also be related to its protection of the vessel wall or to its capacity to reduce platelet adherence. This positive action on blood flow has been corroborated in one other study (107) where the antiarrhythmic effect of sulfin-pyrazone was at least partially attributed to increased collateral blood flow to the myocardial tissue.

Effect on ECG and Cardiovascular Functions

As preliminary work on her studies on the effects of sulfinpyrazone on the microcirculation of the hamster cheek pouch and the bat wing, Wiedeman (481) performed several measurements to establish whether the drug possesses any vaso-active properties that might influence the vascular or cellular responses. Measurement of arterial diameters in the vessels of the hamster cheek pouch revealed no significant changes following a single intravenous injection of 50 mg/kg sulfin-pyrazone; likewise, no changes occurred in the vessels of the bat wing after an intraarterial injection of the same dose. Normal mongrel dogs were then treated with an intravenous injection of 50 mg/kg and this too failed to produce any changes in the ECG, systemic blood pressure, heart rate, or cardiac function. However, other studies suggest that there may be some effect on the cardiovascular function. In dogs with stenosed coronary arteries, Folts and Beck (150) conducted a number of hemodynamic studies. In the presence of the induced pathological condition, sulfinpyrazone produce significant changes in the form of reduced heart rate, increased diastolic–systolic flow ratio and increased reactive hyperemia. Also Forfar et al. (152) have recently reported that the administration of sulfinpyrazone to normal human volunteers significantly alters pulse rate–blood pressure response to exercise.

Effect on Atherogenesis

Recent studies in several animal models have linked the development of athero-sclerosis with increased platelet function (124,154,159,300,352). Furthermore, some of the studies have demonstrated that a reduction in platelet count or a suppression of platelet function can, in large measure, protect animals from atherosclerotic lesions.

Using the experimental homocystinemic baboon as a model for studying endo-thelial cell injury and platelet response in the pathogenesis of atherosclerosis (186), Harker et al. (188) observed that daily sulfinpyrazone administration effectively prevents the lesion. Also hyperlipidemic monkeys treated with sulfinpyrazone (250 mg/kg/day) have shown markedly reduced lesion formation compared with hyperlipidemic untreated controls (189).

Clopath et al. (87) tested the possible effect of sulfinpyrazine on atherogenesis in the rat and miniature swine. The rats were treated for nearly 8 weeks with sulfinpyrazone at a dose of 160 mg/kg/day p.o. The atherosclerotic lesions were produced in the aorta by immunological injury and cholesterol feeding. None of the treated animals showed any aortic lesions, although 5 of 9 control rats showed early intimal changes. The drug did not affect the serum cholesterol levels.

In the miniature swine, the abdominal aorta was repeatedly injured with a balloon catheter during oral treatment with 30 mg/kg sulfinpyrazone twice daily. The drug exerted no preventive effect against the intimal lesions that had been produced, nor did it have any effect on the vascular concentrations of collagen, elastin, or cholesterol.

The effect of sulfinpyrazone on intimal lesions in rabbits more closely resembled that observed in rats (33). After treatment with either sulfinpyrazone, aspirin or dipyridamole, the iliac artery of the rabbits was injured using a balloon catheter. Sulfinpyrazone was very effective in reducing the volume of the neointima, but neither aspirin nor dipyridamole showed any such effect.

Inhibition of the Humoral Immune Response

Organ graft rejection can occur either by leukocyte infiltration into the graft or by antibody-related development of arteriosclerosis. The former manifestation is commonly treated with azathioprine, steroids, or antithymocyte globulin. There is no known treatment for arteriosclerosis in organ transplants, but sulfinpyrazone, aspirin, dipyridamole, and several nonsteroidal, antiinflammatory agents have been tested because of their platelet activity. Some of the results have been encouraging.

Hyperacute rejection of kidney (416) and heart (417,462) transplants in dogs and cats have appeared to be susceptible to suppression by sulfinpyrazone. Platelet aggregation and vascular injury were absent in the transplanted kidneys of most of the treated dogs for up to 24 hr. In a few dogs in which early graft rejection occurred, platelet aggregates were found in some peritubular capillaries. However, these aggregates were loose, with less tendency toward pseudopod formation and degranulation than those found in the control animals.

In a more recent development, combinations of platelet-inhibiting drugs with azathioprine were used to treat rats subjected to heart transplants (216). Survival times were extended after treatment with combinations of azathioprine with either aspirin, sodium salicylate, sulfinpyrazone, or promethazine. However, the aspirin and sodium salicylate combinations had to be abandoned because they produced severe bone marrow depression leading to leukopenia and death.

In animals treated with azathioprine–sulfinpyrazone, cytotoxic antibody was determined in order to determine if sulfinpyrazone depressed circulating antibody levels. The results of the analysis revealed that there was no inhibition of cytotoxic antibody formation in the treated rats, and the their antibody levels conformed to those of the untreated rats throughout a 12-day observation period.

Fibrinolytic Effect

Euglobulin clot lysis time (ECLT) is more than three times longer in rats with kaolin paw edema than in normal rats. Following the oral administration of 3 to 30 mg/kg sulfinpyrazone, ECLT was reduced in a dose-related manner that was significant with the higher dose group (395). In another study (396), a dose of 40 mg/kg p.o. completely normalized prolonged ECLT in the rats.

Induction of Drug Metabolizing Enzymes

A study of human volunteers by Walter et al. (469) has demonstrated an increase in serum y-glutamyltranspeptidase, urinary D-glucaic acid excretion, and antipyrine clearance, suggesting *in vivo* hepatic enzyme induction.

Pharmacokinetics and Metabolism

Metabolic Studies in Various Animal Species

As previously noted, the pharmacological behavior of sulfinpyrazone varies between different animal species. These unexpected discrepancies have been attributed to a variety of factors including species and metabolic differences and indeed, recent pharmacokinetic and metabolic studies have lent credence to this notion.

Recent studies have identified several potential active metabolites of sulfinpyrazone (Fig. 3). Buchanan et al. (64) first noted a prolonged and biphasic effect of sulfinpyrazone on platelet function in the rabbit. A delayed depression of platelet function followed an immediate concentration-related platelet inhibition. The same pattern was later observed in guinea pigs and man (79,262). Livio et al. (260) demonstrated a prolonged effect of sulfinpyrazone on rat platelet MDA production but not on release of prostacyclin-like activity from rat aorta or vena cava. Recently, a reductive metabolic pathway was demonstrated in the rabbit in which the maximum concentrations of the sulfide (Thioether) and p-OH-sulfide correlated with the delayed depression of platelet function (346). The sulfide was at least 3 times as potent, and the p-OH-sulfide was at least as potent as sulfinpyrazone in inhibition of collagen-induced platelet aggregation *in vitro*.

Clopath et al. (87) have described the results of their extensive biotransformation studies in several animal species. Following intravenous administration of 100 mg/kg ^{14}C-sulfinpyrazone to rabbits, the total radioactivity in plasma was found to decrease slowly from 552 μg/ml (19 min) to 223 μg/ml (6 hr) and then increase again to 260 μg/ml after 8 hr. From 8 to 24 hr, there was a steady decrease to 41 μg/ml. By contrast, the concentration of unchanged sulfinpyrazone declined to a regular linear manner with an initial half-life of 2 hr. From the areas under the concentration–time curves (AUC, 0–24 hr), sulfinpyrazone, the sulfone metabolite, and the p-hydroxy sulfinpyrazone metabolite accounted for 42.6%, 5.0%, and 1.8% respectively of the total ^{14}C. A 4-hydroxy metabolite and the p-hydroxy-sulfone accounted for only 0.4% and 0.2% of the total radioactivity. Fifty percent of the plasma radioactivity remained unidentified.

Within 3 days, 96.3% of the total radioactivity was recovered: 70.7% was in the urine and 26.3% in the feces. Analysis of the pooled urine samples (up to 48 hr) revealed the excretion patterns shown in Table 1.

Plasma levels and excretion patterns in miniature pigs (82) were found to be quite different from those just decribed in rabbits. Following the same 100 mg/kg i.v. dose of ^{14}C-sulfinpyrazone, the total radioactivity declined in a more linear manner from 622 μg/ml to 8.4 μg/ml over 24 hr. The concentration of intact sulfinpyrazone declined very rapidly to 1.2 μg/ml after 24 hr with an apparent half-life of 3 hr. The decline, except for the p-hydroxy compound, was delayed. The AUCs for sulfinpyrazone and the sulfone derivative accounted for 65.8% and 16.9% of the total plasma ^{14}C, respectively; the AUCs of the other three metabolites totalled 8.2% of the radioactivity present. In this species, all but 9.1% of the radioactive compounds present in the plasma were identified.

Within 4 days, 93.8% of the dose administered to the swine was recovered. Unlike the rabbits where renal excretion predominated, biliary excretion was responsible for 68.6% of the total elimination in the pigs. Only 25.1% of the drug was excreted in the urine. Analysis of the pooled urine samples (up to 48 hr) revealed the excretion patterns shown in Table 2.

From these results, Clopath et al. (87) suggested that the effectiveness of sulfinpyrazone in rabbits may have been due to its particular biotransformation in that species. Moreover, since sulfinpyrazone and its known metabolites accounted for only 50% of the plasma radioactivity in the rabbit, it was conjectured that it was the unidentified metabolites that were responsible for the preventive effect of sulfinpyrazone against atherogenesis and for its prolonged effect.

The identity of at least one of the major metabolites responsible for prolonged platelet inhibition was revealed in guinea pigs by Butler et al. (78). During the course of their studies of the Arthus reaction, these investigators found that the effect was maximal 4 to 6 hr after oral administration of 100 mg/kg sulfinpyrazone.

TABLE 1. *Urine excretion pattern 3 days following i.v. administration of 100 mg/kg ^{14}C-sulfinpyrazone to rabbits*

Moiety	%
Unchanged sulfinpyrazone	65.0
Sulfone	6.9
p-Hydroxy sulfinpyrazone	3.4
p-Hydroxy sulfone	1.5
4-Hydroxy sulfinpyrazone	0.2
Unidentified	23.0
	100.0%

TABLE 2. *Urine excretion pattern 4 days
following i.v. administration of 100 mg/kg
^{14}C-sulfinpyrazone to miniature pigs*

Moiety	%
Unchanged sulfinpyrazone	27.1
Sulfone	9.7
p-Hydroxy sulfinpyrazone	13.3
p-Hydroxy sulfone	14.6
4-Hydroxy sulfinpyrazone	0.7
Unidentified	34.6
	100.0%

Only high doses (up to 200 mg/kg p.o.) were inhibitory after only 1 hr, but doses as low as 30 mg/kg were still inhibitory 4 to 18 hr after ingestion. Metabolic studies of ^{14}C-sulfinpyrazone, similar to those in rabbits and swine, were performed in guinea pigs following an intravenous dose of 100 mg/kg. The plasma concentrations revealed peak radioactivity levels of 269 μg/ml at 6 hr. Intact sulfinpyrazone and the sulfone derivative accounted for 8.2% and 11.3% of total radioactivity, while the p-hydroxy sulfinpyrazone, 4-hydroxy sulfinpyrazone, and p-hydroxy-sulfone derivatives together accounted for a total to only 0.6% of the ^{14}C present. In this species, 80% of the total plasma radioactivity remained unidentified. Since the majority of this unidentified material was present between 3 and 24 hr, Butler pooled the plasma samples from this time period and was able to extract approximately 80% of it. Liquid chromatography and mass spectrometry identified the major component as the sulfide (thioether) of sulfinpyrazone (see Fig. 3), which therefore assumed the role of the major circulating metabolite in the guinea pig.

Pay et al. (341) found that the sulfide (Thioether) metabolite was 8 to 13 times more potent than the parent compound as a comparative inhibitor of human, guinea pig, and rabbit platelet aggregation induced by sodium arachidonate. After intravenous administration of the sulfide to guinea pigs, the inhibitory effect on sodium arachidonate-induced platelet aggregation *ex vivo* was prolonged up to 24 hr.

Pharmacokinetic Studies in Man

The biotransformation of sulfinpyrazone in animals may explain some of its behavior in man. Indeed, numerous investigators have reported prolonged effects with sulfinpyrazone clinically (78,118,244,263,264). Butler, for example, reported that healthy volunteers were protected for more than 72 hr against arachidonic-induced platelet aggregation *ex vivo* (78).

The pharmacokinetics of sulfinpyrazone following oral and intravenous administration in man have been investigated (118,244). Following a single oral dose of 200 mg to two healthy volunteers, the drug was rapidly and completely absorbed from the gastrointestinal tract. Maximum plasma concentrations of 22.67 and 13.04 μg/ml, respectively, were reached after 1 to 2 hr (118). The elimination half-life, calculated between 3 and 8 hr, was 2.7 and 2.2 hr respectively for the two volunteers. Most of the radioactivity in the plasma was identified as intact sulfinpyrazone. Nearly 80% of the ingested oral dose was recovered in the urine and feces in 24 hr; 95% was recovered within 4 days. In both volunteers, urinary excretion accounted for 85% of the recovered ^{14}C-substances; of this amount 51 to 54% was identified as intact sulfinpyrazone. The p-hydroxy, sulfone, and 4-hydroxy metabolites were recovered in amounts corresponding to 8.2 to 8.8%, 2.7 to 3.0%, and 0.6 to 0.8% respectively of the total radioactivity. All identified substances, therefore, accounted for 62 to 66% of urinary radioactivity. Dieterle et al (118) reported that 28% of the remaining material was the C-β-glucuronide of the sulfone. As far as is known, this direct attachment of the pyrazolidine ring to glucuronic acid is unique among all drugs to sulfinpyrazone.

Pedersen and Jakobsen (345) recently have studied sulfinpyrazone metabolism in eight insulin-dependent diabetics who received the drug for at least 2½ years. Two hours after receiving sulfinpyrazone, the mean plasma concentrations of the parent compound was 7.1 to 16.0 μg/ml. The most abundant metabolites were the sulfide (2.8 to 4.3 μg/ml) and the sulfone (1.7 to 4.8 μg/ml). The plasma concentration of sulfinpyrazone correlated significantly with that of the sulfide and the p-hydroxy sulfide metabolites. *In vivo*, sulfinpyrazone was excreted in amounts corresponding to 1 to 30% of the ingested dose. Up to 3% was excreted as the sulfone. Concentrations of all compounds in urine increased after treatment with β-glucuronidase indicating 0-conjugation with glucuronic acid. Maguire et al. (262) noted that the inhibitory effect on sodium arachidonate-induced platelet aggregation observed in volunteers receiving sulfinpyrazone (200 mg four times a day or 400 mg twice a day for 5 days) correlated with the plasma concentration of the sulfide but not the sulfone or the parent compound.

The sulfide is approximately 10 times as active as the sulfone and approximately 5 times as active as sulfinpyrazone as an inhibitor of arachidonic acid-induced platelet aggregation. Considering their relative abundance, it is probable that these metabolites, rather than sulfinpyrazone itself, account for the major antiplatelet effect of this compound *in vivo*.

Experimental studies using an equilibrium dialysis method have shown that sulfinpyrazone is strongly and almost totally bound to plasma proteins (178,239,361). In the body, the distribution of the drug has been described by a 3-compartment open model (244), whereby approximately one-half the drug is in the plasma or interstitial fluids and approximately 45% is in an extravascular compartment from which it readily diffuses back to the plasma. Approximately 3% of the dose is still in the body in a deep compartment 24 hr after ingestion. This deep compartment may permit a limited amount of accumulation in the body.

Drug Interactions

Sulfinpyrazone may potentiate the action of coumarin-type anticoagulants by a mechanism that does not involve the prostaglandins and presumably is related to its protein binding (109). It may also potentiate some of the sulfonamides such as sulfadiazine and sulfisoxisole. Although not confirmed, sulfinpyrazone may potentiate the hypoglycemic effects of insulin and the sulfonylureas in diabetic patients. On the other hand, a recent report has denied that insulin requirements must be changed significantly in diabetics receiving concomitant sulfinpyrazone (334).

Toxic Effects

Like aspirin, sulfinpyrazone is a gastric irritant and therefore should be avoided in patients with active peptic ulcer. There is some indication that the ulcerative effect of sulfinpyrazone is weaker than that of aspirin and the nonsteroidal antiinflammatory drugs. This trait may be attributable to the fact that sulfinpyrazone itself is a weak inhibitor of prostaglandin synthetase in the stomach as compared to aspirin and indomethacin (269).

Generally, sulfinpyrazone is well tolerated in therapeutic doses, even over protracted periods (20). Allergic reactions and episodes of transient renal failure have been reported, but only rarely. Blood dyscrasias including anemia, leukopenia, agranulocytosis, thrombocytopenia, and aplastic anemia also have been observed clinically, but the incidence of such complications is low.

CONCLUSION

It should be recognized that information on the pharmacology and pharmacokinetics of aspirin, dipyridamole, and sulfinpyrazone continues to expand rapidly because of the lively interest in these drugs as antithrombotic agents (44,117, 192,380,418). While this review has attempted to incorporate much of this new information, it is equally apparent that much more needs to be learned before a clear picture emerges of the details of the biochemical mechanisms by which these compounds produce their various pharmacological effects *in vivo*.

ACKNOWLEDGMENT

The authors are indebted to Stacy Miller, Karen Grigsby, Susan Britt, and Sue Wehner for their assistance in the preparation of this chapter.

REFERENCES

1. Aaron, S. L., Clifton, P., Fleming, G., and Rowland, M. (1980): Aspirin binding and the effect of albumin on spontaneous and enzyme-catalysed hydrolysis. *J. Pharm. Pharmacol.*, 32:537–543.
2. Aiken, J. W., and Vane, J. R. (1971): Blockade of angiotensin release for dog kidney by indomethacin. *Pharmacologist*, 13:293.
3. Ali, M., Cerskus, A. L., Zamecnik, J., and McDonald, J. W. D. (1977): Synthesis of prostaglandin D_2 and thromboxane B_2 by human platelets. *Thromb. Res.*, 11:485–496.
4. Ali, M., and McDonald, J. W. D. (1977): Effects of sulfinpyrazone on platelet release of serotonin. *J. Lab. Clin. Med.*, 89:868–875.
5. Ali, M., Zamecnik, J., Cerskus, A. L., Stoessl, A. J., Barnett, W. H., and McDonald, J. W. D. (1977): Synthesis of thromboxane B_2 and prostaglandin by bovine gastric mucosal microsomes. *Prostaglandins*, 14:819–827.

6. Ali, M., McDonald, J. W. D., Thiessen, J. J., and Coates, P. F. (1980): Plasma acetylsalicylate and salicylate and platelet cyclooxygenase activity following plain and enteric-coated aspirin. *Stroke*, 11:9–13.
7. Ali Laik, S. (1975): A comparative study of the derivitization of salicylic acid and acetylsalicylic acid with BSTFA, MSTFA and methyliodide in presence of potassium carbonate prior to GLC determination. *Chromatografia*, 8:33–34.
8. Ally, A. I., Manku, M. S., Horrobin, D. F., Morgan, R. O., Karmazyn, M., and Karmali, R. A. (1977): Dipyridamole: a possible potent inhibitor of thromboxane A_2 synthetase in vascular smooth muscle. *Prostaglandins*, 14:607–609.
9. Ally, A. I., Barnette, W. E., Cunnane, S. C., Horrobin, D. F., Karmali, R. A., Karmazyn, M., Manku, M. S., Morgan, R. O., and Nicolaou, K. C. (1978): Prostaglandin I_2 (prostacyclin) inhibits intracellular calcium release. *J. Physiol.*, 276:40p.
10. Ally, A. I., and Horrobin, D. F. (1980): Thromboxane A_2 in blood vessel walls and its physiological significance: relevance to thrombosis and hypertension. *Prostaglandins Med.*, 4:431–438.
11. Al-Mondhiry, H., Marcus, A. J., and Spaet, T. H. (1970): On the mechanism of platelet function inhibition by acetysalicylic acid. *Proc. Soc. Exp. Biol. Med.*, 133:632–636.
12. Amezcua, J. L., Parsons, M., and Moncada, S. (1978): Unstable metabolites of arachidonic acid: aspirin and the formation of the haemostatic plug. *Thromb. Res.*, 13:477–488.
13. Amezcua, J. L., O'Grady, J., Salman, J. A., and Moncada, S. (1979): Prolonged paradoxical effect of aspirin on platelet behavior and bleeding time in man. *Thromb. Res.*, 16:69–79.
14. Amodeo, P., Angelico, F., Arca, M., and Ricci, G. (1980): Circulating platelet aggregates in an adult population sample. *Atherosclerosis*, 35:375–381.
15. Andrew, W. (1965): Comparative aspects of blood in vertebrates. In: *Comparative Haematology*. Grune and Stratton, New York.
16. Änggård, E., and Samuelsson, B. (1964): Prostaglandins and related factors. 28. Metabolism of prostaglandin E_1 in guinea pig lung: the structures of two metabolites. *J. Biol. Chem.*, 239:4097–4102.
17. Anker Jørgensen, K., and Stoffersen, E. (1978): Dipyridamole and platelet function. *Lancet*, ii:1258.
18. Anker Jørgensen, K., Dyerberg, J., Olesen, A. S., and Stoffersen, E. (1980): Acetylsalcylic acid, bleeding time and age. *Thromb. Res.*, 19:799–805.
19. Anton, A. H. (1968): The effect of disease, drugs and dilution on the binding of sulfonamides in human plasma. *Clin. Pharmacol. Ther.*, 9:561–567.
20. Anturane Reinfarction Trial Research Group (1978): Sulfinpyrazone in the prevention of cardiac death after myocardial infarction. *N. Engl. J. Med.*, 298:289–295.
21. Arata, L., and Mongola, S. (1962): Richerche sul metabolismo dell' acido salicilico nell 'uomo. *Prog. Med.*, 18:229–234.
22. Arfors, K. E., Bergqvist, D., Bygdeman, S., McKenzie, N., and Svensjo, E. (1972): The effect of inhibition of the platelet release reaction on platelet behavior in vitro and in vivo. *Scand. J. Haematol.*, 9:322–332.
23. Arfors, K. E., Arturson, G., Bergqvist, D., and Svensjo, E. (1976): The effect of inhibition of prostaglandin synthesis on microvascular haemostasis and macromolecular leakage. *Thromb. Res.*, 8:393–402.
24. Arfors, K. E., and Bergqvist, D. (1978): Platelet aggregability in microvascular haemostasis and the effect of local inflammation. *Haemostasis*, 7:46–53.
25. Ascione, P. P., and Cherekian, G. P. (1979): Automated high-pressure liquid chromatographic analysis of aspirin, phenacetin and caffeine. *J. Pharm. Sci.*, 64:1029–1033.
26. Atkinson, D. C. (1980): Nonsteroidal acidic anti-inflammatory agents: do they constitute a single drug class? *Agents Actions*, 9:480–482.
27. Altallah, A. A., and Lee, J. B. (1980): Indomethacin, salicylates and prostaglandin binding. *Prostaglandins*, 19:311–318.
28. Azarnoff, D. L., and Horwitz, A. (1970): Drug interactions. *Pharmacol. Physicians*, 4:1–6.
29. Baenziger, N. L., Dillender, M. J., and Majerus, P. W. (1977): Cultured human skin fibroblasts and arterial cells produce a labile platelet inhibitory prostaglandin. *Biochem. Biophys. Res. Comm.*, 78:294–301.
30. Baenziger, N. L., Becherer, P. R., and Majerus, P. W. (1979): PGI_2 production in cultured human arterial smooth muscle cells, venous endothelial cells and skin fibroblasts. *Cell*, 16:967–974.
31. Baumgartner, H. R. (1972): Platelet interaction with vascular structures. *Thromb. Diath. Haemorrh.*, 51:161.

32. Baumgartner, H. R., Muggli, R., Tschopp, T. B., and Turitto, V. T. (1976): Platelet adhesion, release and aggregation in flowing blood: Effects of surface properties and platelet function. *Thromb. Haemostas.* (Stuttg.), 35:124–138.
33. Baumgartner, H. R., and Studer, A. (1977): Platelet factors and the proliferation of vascular smooth muscle cells. In: *Atherosclerosis.* IV. Proc. 4th Int. Symp. Atheroscl., Tokyo, 1976, edited by G. Gots, Y. Klose, pp. 605–609. Springer Verlag, Berlin.
34. Bardare, M., Chislaghi, G. U., Mandrelli, M., and Sereni, F. (1978): Value of monitoring plasma salicylate levels in treating juvenile rheumatoid arthritis: observations in 42 cases. *Arch. Dis. Child.*, 53:381–385.
35. Bartoli, E., Arras, S., Faedda, R., Saggia, G., Satta, A., and Lema, N. A. (1980): Blunting of furosemide diuresis by aspirin in man. *J. Clin. Pharmacol.*, 20:452–458.
36. Batterman, R. C., and Sommer, E. M. (1953): Fate of gentesic acid in man as influenced by alkalinization and acidification. *Proc. Soc. Exp. Biol.*, 82:376–379.
37. Becker, R. P., and DeBruyn, P. P. H. (1976): The transmural passage of blood cells into myeloid sinusoids and the entry of platelets into sinusoidal circulation. *Am. J. Anat.*, 145:183–206.
38. Beecher, H. K. (1957): The measurement of pain. Prototype for the quantitative study of subjective responses. *Pharmacol. Rev.*, 9:59–209.
39. Begent, N., and Born, G. V. R. (1970): Growth rate *in vivo* of platelet thrombi, produced by iontophoresis of ADP, as a function of mean blood flow velocity. *Nature (Lond.)*, 227:926–930.
40. Beisenherz von, G. F., Koss, W., Schüle, A., Gelbauer, B. I., Bärisch, R., and Fröde, R. (1960): Das Schicksal des 2,6-Bis (diäethanolamino)-4,8-dipiperidino-pyrimido (4,5-d) pyrimidin im menschlichen und tierischen Organismus. *Arzneim. Forsch.*, 10:307–312.
41. Ben, M., Boxill, G. C., Scott, C. C., and Warren, M. R. (1963): Cardiovascular actions of 2,6-Bis (Bis(2-hydroxyethyl)amino)-4,8-dipiperidinopyrimido (5,4-D) pyrimidine. *Arch. Int. Pharmacodyn.*, 143:228–236.
42. Berman, H. J. (1961): Anticoagulant-induced alterations in haemostasis, platelet thrombosis and vascular fragility in the peripheral vessels of the hamster cheek pouch. In: *Anticoagulants and Fibrinolysins*, edited by R. L. MacMillan and J. F. Mustard, pp. 95–107. Lea and Febiger, Philadelphia.
43. Best, L. C., Martin, T. J., McGuire, M. B., Preston, F. E., Russel, R. G. G., and Segal, D. S. (1978): Dipyridamole and platelet function. *Lancet*, ii:846.
44. Best, L. C., McGuire, M. B., Jones, P. B. B., Holland, T. K., Martin, T. J., Preston, F. E., Segal, D. S., and Russell, R. G. G. (1979): Mode of action of dipyridamole on human platelets. *Thromb. Res.*, 16:367–379.
45. Bhattacherjee, P., and Eakins, K. (1973): Inhibition of PG-synthetase systems in ocular tissues by indomethacin. *Pharmacologist*, 15:209.
46. Bianchi Porro, G., Caruso, I., Ciabattoni, G., Patrignani, P., Patrono, C., and Pugliese, F. (1980): Comparative effects of aspirin and diflunisal on platelet and gastric prostaglandin-synthetase in humans. *Br. J. Clin. Pharmacol.*, 40–41.
47. Birek, A., Duffin, J., Glynn, M. F. Y., and Cooper, J. D. (1976): The effect of sulfinpyrazone on platelet and pulmonary responses to onset of membrane oxygenator perfusion. *Trans. Am. Soc. Artificial Int. Organs*, 22:94–100.
48. Bizzozero, G. (1882): Uber einen neuen Formbestandteil des Blutes und dessen Rolle bei der Thrombose und der Blutgerinnung. *Virchow's Arch. Pathol. Anat. Physiol.*, 90:267–270.
49. Blackwell, G. J., Flower, R. J., and Vane, J. R. (1975): Some characteristics of the prostaglandin synthesizing system in rabbit kidney microsomes. *Biochem. Biophys. Acta*, 398:178–190.
50. Blair, D., Rumback, B. H., and Peterson, R. G. (1978): Analysis for salicylic acid in serum by high performance liquid chromatography. *Clin. Chem.*, 24:1543–1544.
51. Blass, K. E., Block, H.-U., Förster, W., and Pönicke, K. (1980): Dipyridamole: a potent stimulator of prostacyclin (PGI_2) biosynthesis. *Br. J. Pharm.*, 68:71–73.
52. Blass, K.-E., Förster, W., and Zehl, U. (1980): Coronary vasodilatation: interactions between prostacyclin and adenosine. *Br. J. Pharmacol.*, 69:555–559.
53. Bluestone, R., Kippen, I., and Klinenberg, J. R. (1969): Effect of drugs on urate binding to plasma proteins. *Br. Med. J.*, 4:590–593.
54. Borgeat, P., and Samuelsson, B. (1979): Metabolism of arachidonic acid in polymorphonuclear leukocytes: structure analysis of novel hydroxylated compounds. *J. Biol. Chem.*, 254:7865–7869.
55. Born, G. V. R. (1964): Strong inhibition by 2-chloroadenosine of blood platelets by adenosine diphosphate. *Nature*, 202:95–96.

56. Born, G. V. R., Honour, A. J., and Mitchell, J. R. A. (1964): Inhibition by adenosine and by 2-chloroadenosine of the formation and embolization of platelet thrombi. *Nature*, 202:761–765.
57. Born, G. V. R., Haslam, R. J., and Lowe, R. D. (1965): Comparative effectiveness of adenosine analogues as inhibitors of blood-platelet aggregation and as vasodilators in man. *Nature*, 205:678–680.
58. Born, G. V. R., and Mills, D. C. B. (1969): Potentiation of the inhibitory effect of adenosine on platelet aggregation by drugs that prevent its uptake. *J. Physiol. (Lond.)*, 202:41p.
59. Breddin, K., Gruhn, H., Krazywanek, H. J., and Schremmer, W. P. (1976): On the measurement of spontaneous platelet aggregation. The platelet aggregation test III. *Thromb. Haemostas.*, (Stutt.), 35:669–691.
60. Bressler, N. M., Broekman, M. J., and Marcus, A. J. (1979): Concurrent studies of oxygen consumption and aggregation in stimulated human platelets. *Blood*, 53:167–178.
61. Bretschneider, H. J., Frank, A., Bernard, U., Kochsiek, K., and Scheler, F. (1959): Die Wirkung eines Pyrimidopyrimidin-Derivates auf die Sauerstoff versorgung des Herz-muskels. *Arzneim. Forsch.*, 9:49–54.
62. Brooks, P. M., Cossum, P. A., and Boyd, G. W. (1980): Rebound rise in renin concentrations after cessation of salicylates. *N. Engl. J. Med.*, 303:562–564.
63. Brown, T. R., Ho, T. T. S., and Walz, D. A. (1980): Improved radioimmunoassay of platelet factor 4 and β-thromboglobulin in plasma. *Clin. Chem. Acta*, 101:225–233.
64. Buchanan, M. R., Rosenfield, J., and Hirsh, J. (1978): The prolonged effect of sulfinpyrazone on collagen induced platelet aggregation in vivo. *Thromb. Res.*, 13:883–892.
65. Buchanan, M. R., Blajchman, M. A., Dejana, E., Mustard, J. F., Senyi, A. F., and Hirsch, J. (1979): Shortening of the bleeding time in thrombocytopenic rabbits after exposure of the jugular vein to high aspirin concentration. *Prostaglandins Med.*, 3:333–342.
66. Bunag, R. D., Douglas, C. R., Imai, S., and Berne, R. M. (1964): Influence of a pyridimidio pyrimidine derivative on deamination of adenosine by blood. *Drug Res.*, 15:83–88.
67. Bunting, S. R., Gryglewski, R., Moncada, S., and Vane, J. R. (1976): Arterial walls generate from prostaglandin endoperoxides or substance (prostaglandin X) which relaxes strips of mesenteric and coeliac arteritis and inhibits platelet aggregation. *Prostaglandins*, 12:897–915.
68. Bunting, S., Moncada, S., and Vane, J. R. (1977): Antithrombotic properties of vascular endothelium. *Lancet*, ii:1075–1076.
69. Burch, J. W., Baenziger, N. L., Stanford, N., and Majerus, P. W. (1978): Sensitivity of fatty acid cyclooxygenase from human aorta to acetylation by aspirin. *Proc. Natl. Acad. Sci. USA*, 75:5181–5184.
70. Burch, J. W., Stanford, N., and Majerus, P. W. (1978): Inhibition of platelet prostaglandin synthetase by oral aspirin. *J. Clin. Invest.*, 61:314–319.
71. Burke, G. (1972): Aspirin and indomethacin abolish thyrotropin-induced increase in thyroid cell prostaglandins. *Prostaglandins*, 2:413–415.
72. Burka, J. F., and Eyre, P. (1975): Modulation of the formation and release of bovine SRS-A in vitro by several anti-anaphylactic drugs. *Int. Archs. Allergy Appl. Immunol.*, 49:774–780.
73. Burka, J. F., and Patterson, N. A. M. (1980): Evidence for lipoxygenase pathway involvement in allergic tracheal contraction. *Prostaglandins*, 19:499–515.
74. Burke, V., Suharyono, Gracey, M., and Sunoto (1980): Reduction by aspirin of intestinal fluid-loss in acute childhood gastroenteritis. *Lancet*, i:1329–1330.
75. Butler, K. D., and White, A. M. (1975): The effect of sulfinpyrazone on the thrombocytopenia occurring in the arthus reaction. *Br. J. Pharmacol.*, 55:256.
76. Butler, K. D., Pay, G. F., and White, A. M. (1976): A comparison between sulfinpyrazone and other drugs on the thrombocytopenia of the Arthus reaction in the guinea pig. *Br. J. Pharmacol.*, 57:441.
77. Butler, K. D., and White, A. M. (1977): Basic problems in the search for antithrombotic therapy. In: *Thromboembolism—A New Approach to Therapy*, edited by J. R. A. Mitchell and J. G. Domenet, pp. 29–39. Academic Press, London.
78. Butler, K. D., and White, A. M. (1979): Inhibition of platelet involvement in the sublethal Forssman reaction of sulfinpyrazone. In: *Cardiovascular Actions of Sulfinpyrazone—Basic and Clinical Research*, edited by M. McGregor, J. F. Mustard, M. Oliver, and S. Sherry, pp. 3–18. Symposium Specialists Inc., Miami.
79. Butler, K. D., Pay, G. F., Wallis, R. B., and White, A. N. (1979): Biphasic prolonged inhibition of platelet prostaglandin biosynthesis induced by sulfinpyrozone. *Thromb. Haemostas.*, 42:101.

80. Caruso, I., and Biachi Porro, G. (1980): Gastroscopic evaluation of antiinflammatory drugs. *Br. Med. J.*, 1:75–78.
81. Cerskus, A. L., Ali, M., Zamecnik, J., and McDonald, J. W. D. (1978): Effects of indomethacin and sulfinpyrazone on *in vivo* formation of thromboxane B_2 and prostaglandin D_2 during arachidonate infusion in rabbits. *Thromb. Res.*, 12:549–553.
82. Cerskus, A. L., Ali, M., and McDonald, J. W. D. (1980): Thromboxane B_2 and 6-keto-prostaglandin $F_{1\alpha}$ synthesis during infusion of collagen and arachidonic acid in rabbits: inhibition by aspirin and sulfinpyrazone. *Thromb. Res.*, 18:693–705.
83. Cerskus, A. L., Ali, M., Davies, B. J., and McDonald, J. W. D. (1980): Possible significance of small numbers of functional platelets in a population of aspirin treated platelets in vitro and in vivo. *Thromb. Res.*, 18:389–397.
84. Charo, I. F., Feinman, R. D., and Detwiler, T. C. (1977): Prostaglandin endoperoxides and thromboxane A_2 can induce platelet aggregation in the absence of secretion. *Nature*, 269:66–69.
85. Charo, I. F., Feinman, R. D., and Detwiler, T. C. (1977): Interrelations of platelet aggregation and secretion. *J. Clin. Invest.*, 60:866–873.
86. Chen, A. G. N., and Chapman, C. R. (1980): Aspirin analgesia evaluated by event-related potentials in man: possible central action in brain. *Exp. Brain Res.*, 39:359–364.
87. Clopath, P., Horsch, A. K., and Dieterle, W. (1979): Effect of sulfinpyrazone on development of atherosclerosis in various animal models. In: *Cardiovascular Actions of Sulfinpyrazone—Basic and Clinical Research*, edited by M. McGregor, J. F. Mustard, M. Oliver, and S. Sherry, pp. 121–138. Symposium Specialists Inc., Miami.
88. Cohen, A., and Garber, H. E. (1978): Comparison of choline magnesium trisalicylate and acetylsalicylic acid in relation to faecal blood loss. *Curr. Ther. Res.*, 23:187–193.
89. Cohen, I. (1980): Platelet structure and function: role of prostaglandins. *Ann. Clin. Lab. Sci.*, 10:187–194.
90. Cohen, I., and Cohen, C. (1972): A tropomyosin-like protein from human platelets. *J. Mol. Biol.*, 68:383–387.
91. Cohen, L. S. (1976): The clinical pharmacology of acetylsalicylic acid. *Sem. Thromb. Haematol.*, 2:146–175.
92. Collier, H. O. J., and Schneider, C. (1972): Nociceptive response to prostaglandins and analgesic actions of aspirin and morphine. *Nature (New Biol.)*, 236:141–143.
93. Collier, J. G., and Flower, R. J. (1971): Effect of aspirin on human seminal prostaglandins. *Lancet*, ii:852–853.
94. Collier, J. G., Herman, A. G., and Vane, J. R. (1973): Appearance of prostaglandins in renal venous blood of dogs in response to acute systemic hypotension produced by bleeding or endotoxin. *J. Physiol. (Lond.)*, 230:19–20p.
95. Collins, G., and Turner, E. (1975): Maternal effects of regular salicylate ingestion in pregnancy. *Lancet*, ii:335–338.
96. Collins, G., and Turner, E. (1975): Fetal effects of regular salicylate ingestion in pregnancy. *Lancet*, ii:338–339.
97. Cooke, A. R., and Hunt, I. N. (1970): Absorption of acetylsalicylic acid from unbuffered and buffered gastric contents. *Am. J. Dig. Dis.*, 15:95–102.
98. Cooper, J. D., Fountain, S. W., Menkes, E., and Martin, B. A. (1979): Effect of sulfinpyrazone on complement-mediated pulmonary dysfunction in sheep. In: *Cardiovascular Actions of Sulfinpyrazone—Basic and Clinical Research*, edited by M. McGregor, J. F. Mustard, M. Oliver, and S. Sherry, pp. 55–68. Symposium Specialists, Inc. Miami.
99. Crutchly, D. J., Ryan, U. S., and Ryan, J. W. (1980): Effects of aspirin and dipyridamole on the degranulation of adenosine diphosphate by cultured cells derived from bovine pulmonary artery. *J. Clin. Invest.*, 66:29–35.
100. Cucuianu, M. P., Nishizawa, E. E., and Mustard, J. F. (1971): Effect of pyrimido-pyrimidine compounds on platelet function. *J. Lab. Clin. Med.*, 77:958–974.
101. Culp, J. R., Erdos, E. G., and Hinshaw, L. B. (1971): Effects of anti-inflammatory drugs in shock caused by injection of living E. coli cells (35548). *Proc. Ioc. Exper. Biol.*, 137:219–223.
102. Cunningham, R. J., Brouhard, B. H., Travis, L. B., Berger, M., and Petrusick, T. (1979): Haemorrhage as a complication of dipyridamole therapy. *South. Med. J.*, 72:498–499.
103. Czervionke, R. L., Smith, J. B., Fry, G. L., Hoak, J. C., and Haycroft, D. L. (1979): Inhibition of prostacyclin by treatment of endothelium with aspirin. *J. Clin. Invest.*, 63:1089–1092.
104. Dahl, R. (1980): Sodium salicylate and aspirin disease. *Allergy*, 35:155–156.

105. Dale, J., Myhre, E., and Loew, D. (1980): Bleeding during acetylsalicylic acid and anticoagulant therapy in patients with reduced platelet reactivity after aortic value replacement. *Am. Ht. J.*, 99:746–751.
106. Damasio, H. (1978): Success or failure of dipyridamole in migraine. *Lancet*, ii:478–479.
107. Davenport, N., Goldstein, R. E., Capurro, N. L., Shulman, R., and Epstein, S. E. (1979): Sulfinpyrazone increases collateral blood flow following acute coronary occlusion. *Am. J. Cardiol.*, 43:396.
108. Davies, J., Smith, R. C., and Pepper, D. S. (1978): The release, distribution and clearance of human β-thromboglobulin and platelet factor 4. *Thromb. Res.*, 12:851–861.
109. Davis, J. W., and Johns, L. E. (1978): Possible interaction of sulfinpyrazone with coumarins. *N. Engl. J. Med.*, 299:955.
110. Davison, C. (1971): Salicylate metabolism in man. *Ann. N. Y. Acad. Sci.*, 179:249–268.
111. Davison, C., and Mandel, H. G. (1971): Nonnarcotic analgesics and antipyretics. I. Salicylates. In: *Drill's Pharmacology in Medicine*, edited by C. DiPalma, pp. 379–403. McGraw-Hill, New York.
112. Delmers, L. M., Budin, R. E., and Shaikh, B. S. (1980): The effects of aspirin on megakaryocyte prostaglandin production. *Proc. Soc. Exp. Biol. Med.*, 163:24–29.
113. Dembinska-Kiec, A., Rücker, W., and Schönhöfer, P. S. (1980): Effects of dipyridamole in experimental atherosclerosis. Action on PGI$_2$, platelet aggregation and atherosclerotic plaque formation. *Stroke*, II:117.
114. Dewar, H. A., Marshall, T., Weightman, D., Prakash, V., and Boon, P. J. (1979): β-thromboglobulin in antecubital vein blood—the influence of age, sex and blood group. *Thromb. Haemostas. (Stuttg.)*, 42:1159–1163.
115. Didisheim, P. (1968): Inhibition by dipyridamole of arterial thrombosis in rats. *Thromb. Diath. Haemorrh. (Stuttg.)*, 20:257–266.
116. Didisheim, P., and Owen, C. A. (1969): Effect of dipyridamole (persantin) and its derivatives on thrombosis and platelet function. *Throm. Diath. Haemorrh. (Stuttg.)*, Suppl. 42:267–275.
117. Didisheim, P., and Fuster, V. (1978): Actions and clinical status of platelet-suppressive agents. *Sem. Hematol.*, 15:55–72.
118. Dieterle, W., Faigle, J. W., Mory, H., Richter, W. J., and Theobald, W. (1975): Biotransformation and pharmacokinetics of sulfinpyrazone (Anturan®) in man. *Eur. J. Clin. Pharmacol.*, 9:135–145.
119. DiMinno, G., Silver, M. J., and DeGaetano, G. (1979): Ingestion of dipyridamole reduces inhibitory effect of prostacyclin on human platelets. *Lancet*, ii:701–702.
120. Dixon, R. L., Henderson, E. S., and Rall, D. P. (1965): Plasma protein binding of methotrexate and its displacement by various drugs. *Fed. Proc.*, 24:454.
121. Done, A. K. (1960): Significance of measurements of salicylate in blood in a case of acute ingestion. *Paedratics*, 26:800–807.
122. Doughty, R. A, Gresecke, I., and Athreya, B. (1979): Prospective study of salicylate therapy in juvenile rheumatoid arthritis. Dosage serum salicylate levels and clinical/biochemical toxicity. *Clin. Pharmacol. Ther.*, 25:221–227.
123. Douthwaite, A. H., and Linott, G. A. M. (1938): Gastroscopic observation of effect of aspirin and certain other substances on the stomach. *Lancet*, ii:1222–1225.
124. Duguid, J. B. (1976): *The Dynamics of Atherosclerosis*, pp. 64–113. Aberdeen University Press, Aberdeen.
125. Dubas, T. S., and Parker, J. M. (1971): A central component in the analgesic action of sodium salicylate. *Arch. Int. Pharmacodyn Ther.*, 194:117–122.
126. Dunn, M. J., and Hood, V. L. (1977): Prostaglandins and the kidney. *Am. J. Physiol.*, 233:F169–F184.
127. Dutta, P., and Mustafa, S. J. (1980): Binding of adenosine to the crude plasma membrane fraction isolated from dog coronary and carotid arteries. *J. Pharmacol. Exp. Ther.*, 214:496–502.
128. Eliasson, R., Bygdeman, S. (1969): Effects of dipyridamole and two pyrimido pyrimidine derivatives on the kinetics of human platelet aggregation and on platelet adhesiveness. *Scand. J. Clin. Lab.*, 24:145–151.
129. Elliot, H. C. (1962): Reduced adrenocortical steroid excretion rates in man following aspirin administration. *Metabolism*, 11:1015–1018.
130. Emmons, P. R., Harrison, M. J. G., Honour, A. J., and Mitchell, J. R. A. (1965): Effect of pyrimidopyrimidine derivative on thrombus formation in the rabbit. *Nature*, 208:255–257.

131. Emmons, P. R., Harrison, M. J. G., Honour, A. J., and Mitchell, J. R. A. (1965): Effect of dipyridamole on human platelet behavior. *Lancet*, ii:603–606.
132. Evans, G., and Mustard, J. F. (1968): Inhibition of the platelet surface reaction in endotoxic shock and the generalized Schwartzman reaction. *J. Clin. Invest.*, 47:319.
133. Farris, R. K., Tapper, E. J., Powell, D. W., and Smith, S. M. (1976): Effect of aspirin on normal and cholera toxin-stimulated intestinal electrolyte transport. *J. Clin. Invest.*, 57:916–924.
134. Fehlmann, H. R. (1980): Aspirin. *Pharmacy Int.*, 1:89–90.
135. Feldberg, W., and Gupta, K. P. (1973): Pyrogen fever and prostaglandin like activity in cerebrospinal fluid. *J. Physiol. (Lond.)*, 228:41–53.
136. Ferreira, S. H. (1972): Prostaglandins, aspirin-like drugs and analgesia. *Nature (New Biol.)*, 240:200–203.
137. Ferreira, S. H., Moncada, S., and Vane, J. R. (1971): Indomethacin and aspirin abolish prostaglandin release from the spleen. *Nature (New Biol.)*, 231:237–239.
138. Ferreira, S. H., and DeSouza Costa, F. (1976): A laminar flow superfusion technique with much increased sensitivity for the detection of smooth muscle stimulating substance. *Eur. J. Pharmacol.*, 39:379–381.
139. Ferreira, S. H., and Vane, J. R. (1979): Mode of action of anti-inflammatory agents which are prostaglandin synthetase inhibitors. In: *Antiinflammatory Drugs*, edited by J. R. Vane and S. H. Ferreira, pp. 348–398, Springer-Verlag, Berlin.
140. Finck, A. D., and Katz, R. L. (1972): Prevention of cholera induced intestinal secretion in the cat by aspirin. *Nature*, 238:273–274.
141. Fischetti, B., Carmignani, M., Marchetti, P., Reinelletti, F. O., and Caprino, L. (1980): Prostacyclin reversal of aspirin and indomethacin effects on blood pressure responses to norepinephrine. *Pharm. Res. Comm.*, 12:319–328.
142. FitzGerald, G. A., Brash, A. R., Falardeau, P., and Oates, J. A. (1982): Estimated rate of prostacyclin secretion into the circulation of normal man. *J. Clin. Invest.*, 68:1272–1276.
143. FitzGerald, G. A., Brash, A. R., Maas, R. L., Oates, J. A., and Roberts, L. J. II (1981): The relation of the dose of aspirin to inhibition of thromboxane and prostacyclin biosynthesis during chronic administration to healthy volunteers. *Circulation (abstr.)*, 64:55.
144. Flower, R. J. (1974): Drugs which inhibit prostaglandin biosynthesis. *Pharm. Rev.*, 26:33–67.
145. Flower, R. J., and Vane, J. R. (1972): Inhibition of prostaglandin synthetase in brain explains the anti-pyretic activity of paracetemol (4-acetamidophenol). *Nature*, 240:410–411.
146. Flower, R. J., Chung, H. S., and Cushman, D. W. (1973): Quantitative determination of prostaglandins and malonyldialdehyde formed by the arachidonate oxygenase system of bovine seminal vesicles. *Prostaglandins*, 4:325–341.
147. Flower, R. J., and Vane, J. R. (1974): Some pharmacologic and biochemical aspects of prostaglandin biosynthesis and its inhibition. In: *Prostaglandin Synthetase Inhibitors*, edited by H. J. Robinson and J. R. Vane, pp. 9–18. Raven Press, New York.
148. Flower, R. J., Moncada, S., and Vane, J. R. (1980): Drug therapy of inflammation. In: *The Pharmacological Basis of Therapeutics*, edited by A. Goodman Gilman, L. S. Goodman and A. Gilman. Macmillan, New York.
149. Folts, J. D., Crowell, E. B., and Rowe, G. G. (1976): Platelet aggregation in partially obstructed vessels and its elimination with aspirin. *Circulation*, 54:365–370.
150. Folts, J. D., and Beck, R. A. (1979): Inhibition of platelet plugging in stenosed dog coronary arteries with sulfinpyrazone. In: *Cardiovascular Actions of Sulfinpyrazone: Basic and Clinical Research*, edited by M. McGregor, J. F. Mustard, M. F. Oliver, and S. Sherry, pp. 211–225. Symposium Specialists Inc., Miami.
151. Fordtran, J. S., Morawski, S. G., and Richardson, C. F. (1973): In vivo and in vitro evaluation of liquid antacids. *N. Engl. J. Med.*, 288:923–928.
152. Forfar, J. C., Russell, D. C., and Oliver, M. F. (1980): Haemodynamic effects of sulphinpyrazone in exercise responses in normal subjects. *Lancet*, ii:718–720.
153. Fraser, D. G., Ludden, T. M., Evans, R. P., and Sutherland, E. W. (1980): Displacement of phenytoin from plasma binding sites by salicylate. *Clin. Pharmacol. Ther.*, 27:165–169.
154. Friedman, R. J., Stemerman, M. B., Wenz, B., Morre, S., Gandie, J., Gent, M., Tiell, M. C., and Spaet, T. H. (1977): The effect of thrombocytopenia on experimental arteriosclerotic lesion formation in rabbits. *J. Clin. Invest.*, 60:1191–1201.
155. Frimmer, M., Hegner, D., and Winkelman, W. (1963): Die Wirkung von 2,6-bis (Diaethanolamino)-4,8-Dipiperidino-Pyrimido-(5,4-d)-Pyrimidin (Persantin) auf die Atmung von Mitochondrien bei niederen O_2-Drucken. *Klin. Wochenschr.*, 41:715–716.

156. Furst, D. E., Kar, N. C., Sarkissian, E. S., Gupta, N., and Paulus, H. E. (1976): Effects of salicylate on liver enzymes in normal young adults. *Arthritis Rheum.*, 19:267–268.
157. Furst, D. E., Gupta, N., and Paulus, H. E. (1977): Salicylate metabolism in twins: evidence suggesting a genetic influence and induction of salicylurate formation. *J. Clin. Invest.*, 60:32–42.
158. Furst, D. E., Tozer, T. N., and Melmon, K. L. (1979): Salicylate clearance, the resultant of protein binding and metabolism. *Clin. Pharmacol. Ther.*, 26:380–389.
159. Fuster, V., Bowie, E. J. W., Lewis, J. C., Foss, D. N., Owen, C. A., and Brown, A. L. (1978): Resistance to arteriosclerosis in pigs with von Willebrand's disease. *J. Clin. Invest.*, 61:722–730.
160. Ganguly, P. (1974): Binding of thrombin to human platelets. *Nature (Lond.)*, 247:306–307.
161. Geraga, W., Gwozdz, E., and Mroszczyk, M. (1971): Mozliwosci wystepowania zaburzen psychicznych w przebiegu podawania persantyny. *Wiad. Lek*, 24:855–858.
162. Gerlach, E., and Deuticke, B. (1972): Bildung und Bedeutung von Adenosin in dem durch Sauerstoffmangel geschädigten Herzmuskel unter dem Einfluss von 2,6-Bis(diaethanolamino)-4,8-dipiperidino-pyrimidol(5,4d) pyrimidine. *Arzneim. Forsch.*, 12:48–50.
163. Gerrard, J. M., Townsend, D., Stoddard, S., and Witkop, C. J. (1977): The influence of prostaglandin G$_2$ on platelet ultrastructure and platelet secretion. *Am. J. Pathol.*, 86:99–110.
164. Gibaldi, M., Grendhofer, B., and Levy, G. (1975): Time course and dose dependence of antacid effect on urine pH. *J. Pharm. Sci.*, 64:2003–2004.
165. Gibson, E. L., Hodge, R. L., Jackson, H. R., Katic, F. P., and Stevens, A. M. (1972): The effect of aspirin on pulmonary removal of prostaglandin F$_{2\alpha}$ in dogs and sheep. *Proc. Aust. Physiological Soc.*, Adelaide.
166. Gordon, J. L., and Pearson, J. D. (1978): Effects of sulphinpyrazone and aspirin on prostaglandin I$_2$ prostacyclin) synthesis by endothelial cells. *Br. J. Pharmacol.*, 64:481–483.
167. Goetzel, E. J. (1980): Mediators of immediate hypersensitivity derived from arachidonic acid. *N. Engl. J. Med.*, 303:822–825.
168. Gorman, R., Bunting, S., and Miller, O. V. (1977): Modulation of human platelet adenylate cyclase by prostacyclin (PGX). *Prostaglandins*, 13:377–388.
169. Goulsten, K., and Cook, A. R. (1968): Alcohol, aspirin and gastrointestinal bleeding. *Br. Med. J.*, 4:664–668.
170. Graham, G. G., Champion, G. D., Day, R. O., and Paull, P. D. (1977): Patterns of plasma concentrations and urinary excretion of salicylate in rheumatoid arthritis. *Clin. Pharmacol. Ther.*, 22:410–420.
171. Granström, E., and Samuelsson, B. (1971): On the metabolism of prostaglandin F$_{2\alpha}$ in female subjects. *J. Biol. Chem.*, 246:5254–5263.
172. Green, F. A., Jung, C. Y. (1981): Acetylation of erythrocyte membrane peptides by aspirin. *Transfusion*, 21:55–58.
173. Gryglewski, R., Korbut, R., and Ocetlziewicz, A. (1978): De-aggregatory action of prostacyclin *in vivo* and its enchancement by theophyline. *Prostaglandins*, 15:637–644.
174. Gueniguian, J. L. (1976): Prostaglandin-Macromolecule interactions. I. Noncovalent binding of prostaglandins A$_1$, E$_1$, F$_{2\alpha}$ and E$_2$ by human and bovine serum albumins. *J. Pharmacol. Exp. Ther.*, 197:391–401.
175. Gunsberg, M., Cham, B. I. Imhoff, D. M., Parsons, G., Bochner, F., and Johnson, F. I. (1980): Correlation of aspirin dose with concentrations of salicylic acid in plasma, plasma water and saliva and chemical response in patients with rheumatoid disease. *Aust. N. Z. J. Med.*, 10:268–278.
176. Gupta, N., Sarkissian, E., and Paulus, H. E. (1975): Correlation of plateau serum salicylate level with the rate of salicylate metabolism. *Clin. Pharmacol. Ther.*, 18:350–355.
177. Hacam, L. E., and Burns, J. J. (1960): A study of the inverse relationship between p$_{Ka}$ and rate of renal excretion of phenylbutazone analogs in man and dog. *Am. J. Med.*, 29:1017–1033.
178. Halla, J. T. (1976): Aspirin:liver and rheumatic diseases. *J. Med. Assoc. State Ala.*, 46:23–25.
179. Hamberg, M. (1972): Inhibition of prostaglandin synthesis in man. *Biochem. Biophys. Res. Comm.*, A9:720–726.
180. Hamberg, M., and Samuelsson, B. (1971): On the metabolism of prostaglandin E$_1$ and E$_2$ in man. *J. Biol. Chem.*, 246:6713–6721.
181. Hamberg, M., and Samuelsson, B. (1972): On the metabolism of prostaglandins E$_1$ and E$_2$ in the guinea pig. *J. Biol. Chem.*, 247:3495–3502.
182. Hamberg, M., Svensson, J., and Samuelsson, B. (1974): Mechanism of the antiaggregative effect of aspirin on human platelets. *Lancet*, ii:223–224.

183. Hanley, S. P., Bevan, J., Cockbill, S. R., and Hepinstall, S. (1981): Differential inhibition by low dose aspirin of human venous prostacyclin synthesis and platelet thromboxane synthesis. *Lancet*, ii:969–972.
184. Hansten, P. D. (1973): In: *Drug Interactions*. Lea and Febiger, Philadelphia.
185. Harker, L. A., and Slichter, S. J. (1972): Platelet and fibrinogen consumption in man. *N. Engl. J. Med.*, 287:999–1005.
186. Harker, L., Ross, R., Slichter, S., and Scott, C. (1976): Homocystine-induced arteriosclerosis: the role of endothelial cell injury and platelet response in its genesis. *J. Clin. Invest.*, 58:731–741.
187. Harker, L. A., Wall, R. T., Harlan, J. M., and Ross, R. (1978): Sulfinpyrazone-prevention of homocysteine-induced endothelial cell injury and arteriosclerosis. *Proc. 35th Ann. Meet. Am. Fed. Clin. Res.*, San Francisco.
188. Harker, L. A., and Ross, R. (1978): Prevention of homocysteine-induced arteriosclerosis: sulphinpyrazone endothelial protection. In: *A New Approach to Reduction in Cardiac Death*, edited by T. Abe and S. Sherry, pp. 59–72. Hans Huber Publishers, Vienna.
189. Harker, L. A. (1979): Sulfinpyrazone in primate models of vascular disease. In: *Cardiovascular Action of Sulfinpyrazone: Basic and Clinical Research*, edited by M. McGregor, J. F. Mustard, J. M. F. Oliver, and S. Sherry, pp. 81–95. Symposium Specialists Inc., Miami.
190. Harris, P. A., and Riegelman, S. (1967): Acetylsalicylic acid hydrolysis in human blood and plasma. I. Methodology and in vitro studies. *J. Pharm. Sci.*, 56:713–716.
191. Hart, F. D., Huskisson, E. C., and Ansell, B. M. (1978): Nonsteroidal antiinflammatory analgesics. In: *Drug Treatment of Rheumatoid Diseases*, edited by F. D. Hart, pp. 8–43. ADIS Press, Sydney, Australia.
192. Harter, H. R., Burch, J. W., Majerus, P. W., Stanford, N., Delmez, J. A., Anderson, C. B., and Weerts, C. A. (1979): Prevention of thrombosis in patients on haemodialysis by low dose aspirin. *N. Engl. J. Med.*, 301:577–579.
193. Hawkes, C. H. (1978): Dipyridamole in migraine. *Lancet*, ii:153.
194. Helmer, M. E., Crawford, C. G., and Lands, W. E. M. (1978): Lipoxygenation activity of purified prostaglandin-forming cyclooxygenase. *Biochemistry*, 17:1772–1779.
195. Henry, J. A. (1980): Salicylate furosemide interactions. *Br. J. Clin. Pharmacol.*, 158p–159p.
196. Herlihy, J. T., Bockman, E. L., Berne, R. M., and Rubio, R. (1976): Adenosine relaxation of isolated vascular smooth muscle. *Am. J. Physiol.*, 1293–1243.
197. Higgs, G. A., Harvey, E. A., Ferreira, S. H., and Vane, J. R. (1976): The effects of antiinflammatory drugs on the production of prostaglandins in vivo. In: *Advances in Prostaglandin and Thromboxane Research, Vol. 1*, edited by B. Samuelsson and R. Paoleti, pp. 105–110. Raven Press, New York.
198. Higgs, G. A., Moncada, S., and Vane, J. R. (1979): The role of arachidonic acid metabolites in inflammation. In: *Advances in Inflammation Research, Vol. 1*, edited by G. Weissman, B. Samuelsson, and R. Paoletti, pp. 413–418. Raven Press, New York.
199. Hockerts, T. H., and Bögelmann, G. (1959): Untersuhungen Über die Wirkung von 2,6-Bis-(diaethanolamino)-4, 8-dipiperidino-pyrimido-(5,4-d) pyrimidin auf Herz und Kreislauf. *Arzneim. Forsch.*, 9:39–41.
200. Hoftiezer, J. W., Burks, M., Silvoso, G. R., and Ivey, K. J. (1980): Comparison of the effects of regular and enteric coated aspirin on gastroduodenal mucosa of man. *Lancet*, ii:609–612.
201. Hogben, C. A. M., Schanker, L. S., Tocco, D. J., and Brodie, B. B. (1957): Absorption of drugs from the stomach. II. The human. *J. Pharmacol. Exp. Ther.*, 120:540–545.
202. Hollifeld, J. W. (1976): Failure of aspirin to antagonize the antihypertensive effect of spironolactone in low renin hypertension. *South Med. J.*, 69:1034–1036.
203. Hollister, L. E. (1972): Measuring Measurin: Problems of oral prolonged action medications. *Clin. Pharmacol. Ther.*, 13:1–5.
204. Holmsen, H. (1972): The platelet: its membrane, physiology and biochemistry. In: *Clinics in Haematology, Vol. 1*, edited by J. R. O'Brien, p. 235. W. B. Saunders Company Ltd., London.
205. Holmsen, H. (1976): Platelet secretion—current concepts and methodological aspects. Platelet Function Testing Day, pp. 112–132, edited by H. J. Holmsen, and M. B. Zucker. DHEW Publ. No. (NIH) 78–1087.
206. Holmsen, H., and Weiss, H. J. (1979): Secretable storage pools in platelets. *Ann. Rev. Med.*, 30:119–134.
207. Horch, U., Kadatz, R., Kopitar, Z., Ritschard, J., and Weisenberger, H. (1969): Pharmacology of dipyridamole and its derivatives. *Throm. Diath. Haemorrh. (Stuttg.)(Suppl.)*, 42:253–266.

208. Horrobin, D. F., Ally, A. I., and Manku, M. S. (1978): Dipyridamole and platelet aggregation. *Lancet*, ii:270.
209. Horton, E. W., Jones, R. L., and Marr, G. C. (1973): Effects of aspirin on prostaglandin and fructose levels in human semen. *J. Reprod. Fertil.*, 33:385–392.
210. Howell, W. W. (1890): Observations upon the occurrence, structure and function of the giant cells of the marrow. *J. Morphol.*, 4:117–119.
211. Hucker, H. B., Stauffer, S. C., and White, J. E. (1972): Effect of Halofenate on binding of various drugs to human plasma proteins and on plasma half-life of antipyrine in monkeys. *J. Pharm. Sci.*, 61:1490–1492.
212. Huskisson, E. C. (1977): Antiinflammatory drugs. *Sem. Arthritis Rheum.*, 7:1–20.
213. Ingelfinger, F. (1974): The side effects of aspirin. *N. Engl. J. Med.*, 290:1196–1197.
214. Ito, Y., and Tajima, K. (1981): Spontaneous activity in the trachea of dogs treated with indomethacin: An experimental model for aspirin-related asthma. *Br. J. Pharmacol.*, 73:563–571.
215. Jaffe, E. A., and Weksler, B. B. (1979): Recovery of endothelial cell prostacyclin production after inhibition by low doses of aspirin. *J. Clin. Invest.*, 63:532–535.
216. Jamieson, S. W., Burton, U. A., and Reitz, B. A. (1979): Platelets, sulfinpyrazone and organ graft rejection. In: *Cardiovascular Actions of Sulfinpyrazone: Basic and Clinical Research*, edited by M. McGregor, J. F. Mustard, M. F. Oliver, and S. Sherry, pp. 229–247. Symposium Specialists Inc., Miami.
217. Jespersen, J. (1980): Disseminated intransvascular coagulation in toxaemia of pregnancy. Correction of the decreased platelet counts and raised levels of serum uric acid and fibrin (ogen) degradation products by aspirin. *Thromb. Res.*, 17:743–746.
218. Kadatz, R. (1959): Die pharmakologischen Eigenschaften der neuen coronarerwerternden Substanz 2, 6-Bis-(diaethanolamino)-4, 8-dipiperidino-pyrimido-(5,4-d) pyrimidin. *Arzneim Forsch.*, 9:39–45.
219. Kapp, E. M., and Coburn, A. F. (1942): Urinary metabolites of sodium salicylate. *J. Biol. Chem.*, 145:549–565.
220. Kawashima, H., Hayashi, M., Kurozumi, S., and Hashimoto, Y. (1978): Inhibitory effect of aspirin on bone resorption by 1_α-hydroxyvitamin D_3 and parathyroid hormone in rats. *Jpn. J. Pharm., (Suppl.)*, 28:121p.
221. Kawashima, H., Monji, N., and Castro, A. (1980): Effect of calcium chloride on aspirin induced hypoinsulinaemia in rats. *Biochem. Pharm.*, 29:1627–1630.
222. Kelliher, G. J., Dix, R. K., Jurkiewicz, N., and Lawrence, T. L. (1979): Effects of sulfinpyrazone on arrhythmia and death following coronary occlusion in cats. In: *Cardiovascular Actions of Sulfinpyrazone—Basic and Clinical Research*, edited by M. McGregor, J. F. Mustard, M. Oliver, and S. Sherry, pp. 193–209. Symposium Specialists, Inc., Miami.
223. Kelton, J. G., Hirsh, J., Carter, C. J., and Buchanan, M. R. (1978): Thrombogenic effect of high-dose aspirin in rabbits. *J. Clin. Invest.*, 62:892–895.
224. Kent, P. W., and Allen, A. (1968): The biosynthesis of intestinal mucus. The effect of salicylates on glycoprotein biosynthesis by sheep colonic and human gastric mucosal tissue in vitro. *Biochem. J.*, 106:645–658.
225. Kinlough-Rathbone, R. L., Reimers, H. J., Mustard, J. F., and Packham, M. A. (1976): Sodium arachidonate can induce platelet shape change and aggregation which are independent of the release reaction. *Science*, 192:1011–1012.
226. Kinlough-Rathbone, R. L., Packham, M. A., Reimers, H. J., Cazenave, J.-P., and Mustard, J. F. (1977): Mechanism of platelet shape change, aggregation and release induced by collagen, thrombin or A23,187. *J. Lab. Clin. Med.*, 90:707–719.
227. Kinsella, D., Troup, W., and McGregor, M. (1962): Studies with a new vasodilator drug: Persantin. *Am. Heart J.*, 63:146–151.
228. Kimberly, R. P., and Plotz, P. H. (1977): Aspirin-induced depression of renal function. *N. Engl. J. Med.*, 296:418–424.
229. Kivilaakso, E., and Silen, W. (1979): Pathogenesis of experimental gastric mucosal injury. *N. Engl. J. Med.*, 301:364–369.
230. Klabunde, R. E., and Althouse, D. G. (1981): Adenosine metabolism in dog whole blood: Effects of dipyridamole. *Life Sci.*, 28:2631–2641.
231. Klinenberg, J. R., and Miller, F. (1965): Effect of corticosteroids on blood salicylate concentration. *JAMA*, 194:601–604.
232. Koch, P. A., Schultz, C. A., Wills, R. J., Halliquist, S. L., and Welling, P. G. (1978): Influence of food and fluid ingestion on aspirin bioavailability. *J. Pharm. Sci.*, 67:1533–1535.

233. Koch-Weser, J., and Sellers, E. M. (1971): Drug interactions with coumarin anticoagulants. *N. Engl. J. Med.*, 285:487–498.
234. Konturek, S. T., Obtulowicz, W., Sito, E., Oleksky, J., Wilkon, S., and Dembinska-Kiec, A. (1981): Distribution of prostaglandins in gastric and duodenal mucosa of healthy subjects and duodenal ulcer patients: Effects of aspirin and paracetemol. *Gut*, 22:283–289.
235. Kuehl, F. A., Jr., Humes, J. L., and Torchiana, M. L. (1979): Oxygen-centered radicals in inflammatory processes. In: *Advances in Inflammation Research*, edited by G. Weissman et al., pp. 419–430. Raven Press, New York.
236. Kuehl, F. A., Jr. (1981): *(personal communication).*
237. Kumar, R., and Billimeria, J. D. (1978): Gastric ulceration and the concentration of salicylate in plasma in rats after administration of ^{14}C-labeled aspirin and its synthetic triglyceride, 1,3-dipalmitoyl-2(2′-acetoxy-^{14}C carboxylbenzoyl) glycerol. *J. Pharm. Pharmacol.*, 30:754–758.
238. Kunz, V. W., Schmid, W., and Siess, M. (1961): Untersuchungen zur Wirkung von 2,6-Bis(diaethanolamino)-4,8-dipiperidino pyrimido (5,4-d) pyrimidin auf dem Herzstoffwechsel. *Arzeim. Forsch.*, 11:1098–1109.
239. Kurz, H., and Friemel, G. (1967): Artspezifische Unterschiede der Buidung an Plasmaproteine. *Nauyn-Schmiedeberg Arch. Exp. Pathol. Pharmakol.*, 257:35–36.
240. Lange, H. F. (1957): Salicylates and gastric haemorrhage. II. Manifest bleeding. *Gastroenterology*, 33:778–788.
241. Lanza, F., Royer, G., and Nelson, R. (1975): An endoscopic evaluation of the effects of nonsteroidal antiinflammatory drugs on the gastric mucosa. *Gastrointes. Endosc.*, 21:103–105.
242. Lanza, F. L., Royer, Jr., G. L. Nelson, R. S., Chen, T. F., Seckman, C. E., and Raek, M. F. (1979): The effects of ibuprofen, indomethacin, aspirin, naproxen, and placebo on the gastric mucosa of normal volunteers: a gastroscopic and photographic study. *Dig. Dis. Sci.*, 24:823–828.
243. Lanza, F. L., Royer, G. L., and Nelson, R. S. (1980): Endoscopic evaluation of the effects of aspirin, buffered aspirin and enteric coated aspirin on gastric and duodenal mucosa. *N. Engl. J. Med.*, 303:136–138.
244. Lecaillon, J. B., Souppart, C., Schoeller, J. P., Humbert, G., and Massias, P. (1979): Sulfinpyrazone kinetics after intravenous and oral administration. *Clin. Pharmacol. Ther.*, 26:611–617.
245. Lefer, A. M., and Ogeltree, M. L. (1976): Influence of non-steroidal anti-inflammatory agents on myocardial ischemia in the cat. *J. Pharmacol. Exp. Ther.*, 197:582–593.
246. Leonards, J. R. (1963): The influence of solubility on the rate of gastric absorption of aspirin. *Clin. Pharmacol. Ther.*, 4:476–479.
247. Leonards, J. R. (1963): Gastrointestinal blood loss during prolonged aspirin administration. *N. Engl. J. Med.*, 289:1020–1022.
248. Levine, L. (1972): Prostaglandin production by mouse fibrosarcoma cells in culture: Inhibition by indomethacin and aspirin. *Biochem. Biophys. Res. Comm.*, 47:888–896.
249. Levy, G. (1978): Chemical pharmacokinetics of aspirin. *Paediatrics*, 62:867–872.
250. Levy, G. (1980): Clinical pharmacokinetics of salicylates: A reassessment. *Br. J. Clin. Pharmacol.*, 10:2862–2908.
251. Levy, G., and Matsuzawa, T. (1966): Pharmacokinetics of salicylamide elimination in man. *J. Pharmacol. Exp. Ther.*, 156:285–293.
252. Levy, G., and Tsuchiya, T. (1972): Salicylate accumulation kinetics in man. *N. Engl. J. Med.*, 287:430–432.
253. Levy, G., Tsuchiya, T., and Amsel, L. P. (1972): Limited capacity of salicylic phenolic glucuronide formation and its effect on the kinetics of salicylate elimination in man. *Clin. Pharmacol. Ther.*, 13:258–268.
254. Levy, G., Procknal, J. A., Olufs, B. A. R., and Pachman, I. M. (1980): Relationship between serum salicylate concentration and free as total salicylate concentration in serum of children with juvenile arthritis. *Clin. Pharmacol. Ther.*, 27:619–627.
255. Levy, M. (1974): Aspirin use in patients with major upper gastrointestinal bleeding. *N. Engl. J. Med.*, 290:1158–1162.
256. Lewis, G. P., and Westwick, J. (1977): An *in vivo* model for studying arterial thrombosis. In: *Thromboembolism—A New Approach to Therapy*, edited by J. R. A. Mitchell and T. G. Domenet, pp. 40–54. Academic Press, London.
257. Lewis, R. B., and Schulman, J. D. (1973): Influence of acetylsalicylic acid, an inhibitor of prostaglandin synthesis on the duration of human gestation and labor. *Lancet*, ii:1159–1161.
258. Lewis, R. A., Austen, K. F., Drazen, J. M., Clark, D. A., Marafat, A., and Corey, E. J. (1980): Slow reacting substances of anaphylaxis: Identification of leukotrienes C and D from human and rat sources. *Proc. Natl. Acad. Sci. USA*, 77:3710–3714.

259. Lima, S. C. J., and Cohn, J. N. (1973): Isolation and properties of myocardial prostaglandin synthetase. *Cardiovasc. Res.*, 7:623–638.
260. Livio, M., Villa, S., and deGaetano, G. (1980): Long lasting inhibition of platelet prostaglandin but normal vascular prostacyclin generation following sulfinpyrazone administration to rats. *J. Pharm. Pharmacol.*, 32:718–719.
261. MacPherson, G. C. (1971): Development of megakaryocytes in bone marrow of the rat: an analysis by electron microscopy and high resolution autoradiography. *Proc. Roy. Soc. Lond. (Biol.)*, 177:265–274.
262. Maguire, E. D., Pay, G. F., Turney, J., Wallis, R. B., Weston, M. J., White, A. M., Williams, L., and Wood, H. F. (1979): Inhibition of human platelet function induced by sulfinpyrazone. *Thromb. Hemostat.*, 42:101.
263. Maguire, E. D., Pay, G. F., Turney, J., Wallis, R. B., Weston, M. J., White, A. M., Williams, L., and Woods, H. F. (1981): The effects of two different dosage regimens of sulfinpyrazone on platelet function *ex vivo* and blood chemistry in man. *Hemostasis*, 10:153–164.
264. Maguire, E. D., Pay, G. F., Wallis, R. B., White, A. M. (1981): Prolonged inhibition of ex vivo sodium arachidonate induced platelet aggregation and malondialdehyde production by sulfinpyrazone in man. *Thromb. Res.*, 21:321–327.
265. Majerus, P. W., and Stanford, N. (1977): Comparative effects of aspirin and diflunisal on prostaglandin synthetase from human platelets and sheep seminal vesicles. *Br. J. Clin. Pharmacol.*, 4:155–188.
266. Mandelli, M., and Tagnoni, G. (1980): Monitoring plasma concentrations of salicylate. *Clin. Pharmacokin.*, 5:424–440.
267. Marcus, A. J. (1978): The role of lipids in platelet function with particular reference to the arachidonic acid pathway. *J. Lipid Res.*, 19:793–826.
268. Marcus, A. J., Weksler, R. B., Jaffe, E. A., and Broekman, M. J. (1980): Synthesis of prostacyclin from platelet-observed endoperoxides by cultured human endothelial cells. *J. Clin. Invest.*, 66:979–986.
269. Margulies, E. H., White, A. M., and Sherry, S. (1980): Sulfinpyrazone: A review of its pharmacological properties and therapeutic use. *Drugs*, 20:179–197.
270. Mason, W. B., and Winer, N. (1981): Kinetics of aspirin, salicylic acid and salicyluric acid following oral administration of aspirin as a tablet and two buffered solutions. *J. Pharm. Sci.*, 70:262–265.
271. Masotti, G., Poggesi, L., Galanti, G., Abbate, R., and Neri Serneri, G. G. (1979): Differential inhibition of prostacyclin production and platelet aggregation by aspirin. *Lancet*, ii:1213–1216.
272. Masotti, G., Poggesi, L., Galanti, G., and Neri Serneri, G. G. (1979): Stimulation of prostacyclin by dipyridamole. *Lancet*, i:1412.
273. Mathison, G. A., and Stevenson, D. D. (1979): Hypersensitivity to nonsteroidal antiinflammatory drugs: indications and methods for oral challenge. *J. Allergy Clin. Immunol.*, 64:669–674.
274. McCall, E., and Youlten, L. J. F. (1973): Prostaglandin E$_1$ synthesis by phagocytosing rabbit polymorphonuclear leucocytes: its inhibition by indomethacin and its role in chemotaxis. *J. Physiol. (Lond.)*, 234:98–100p.
275. McCord, J. M., and Fridovich, I. (1978): The biology and pathology of oxygen radicals. *Ann. Intern. Med.*, 89:122–127.
276. McDonald, J. R., Mathison, D. A., and Stevenson, D. D. (1972): Aspirin intolerance in asthma. Detection by oral challenge. *J. Allergy Clin. Immunol.*, 4:198–206.
277. McDonald, J. W. D., Ali, M., Barnett, W. H., Nagai, G. R., and Barnett, H. J. M. (1976): Effects of sulfinpyrazone on platelet release reaction and prostaglandin synthesis. *Stroke*, 7:11.
278. McDonald, J. W. D., Ali, M., and Cerskus, A. L. (1979): Effects of sulfinpyrazone on synthesis of prostaglandins and thromboxanes by platelets *in vitro* and *in vivo*. In: *Cardiovascular Actions of Sulfinpyrazone—Basic and Clinical Research*, edited by M. McGregor, J. F. Mustard, M. F. Oliver, and S. Sherry, pp. 37–54. Symposium Specialists Inc., Miami.
279. McGregor, M., and Fam, W. M. (1966): Regulation of coronary blood flow. *Bull. NY Acad. Med.*, 42:940–950.
280. McKenzie, S. G., Frew, R., and Hans-Peter, B. (1977): Effects of adenosine on adenylate cyclase and cyclic AMP levels in smooth muscle. *Eur. J. Pharmacol.*, 41:193–203.
281. Meisel, M., and Meisel, P. (1974): 1st Adenosin der Mediator für die Regulation des koronaren Blutstroms und für die Wirkung der Koronar dilatatoren? *Pharmazie*, 29:561–568.
282. Mellinger, T. J., and Bohorfoush, J. G. (1962): Blood levels of dipyridamole (Persantin) in humans. *Arch. Int. Pharmacodyn.*, 163:471–480.

283. Mellinger, T. J., and Bohorfoush, J. G. (1965): Pathways and tissue distribution of dipyridamole (Persantin). *Arch. Int. Pharmacodyn.*, 156:380–388.
284. Menguy, R., and Masters, Y. F. (1965): Effects of aspirin on gastric mucus secretion. *Surg. Gynaecol. Obstet.*, 120:920–998.
285. Mennie, A. T., Dalley, V. M., Dinneen, L. C., and Collier, H. O. J. (1975): Treatment of radiation-induced gastrointestinal distress with acetylsalicylate. *Lancet*, ii:942–943.
286. Merino, J., Livio, M., Rajtar, G., and de Gaetano, G. (1980): Salicylate reverses in vitro aspirin inhibition of rat platelet and vascular prostaglandin generation. *Biochem. Pharmacol.*, 29:1093–1096.
287. Metz, S., Halter, J., and Robertson, R. P. (1980): Sodium salicylate potentiates neurohumoral responses to insulin-induced hypoglycaemia. *J. Clin. Endocrin. Metab.*, 51:93–100.
288. Mieke, C. H., Kaneshiro, M. M., and Maher, I. A. (1969): The standardized normal Ivy bleeding time and its prolongation by aspirin. *Blood*, 34:204–215.
289. Mielants, H., Veys, E. M., Verbruggen, G., and Schelstraete, K. (1979): Salicylate-induced gastrointestinal bleeding: comparison between soluble buffered enteric coated and intravenous administration. *J. Rheumatol.*, 6:210–218.
290. Mikhailidis, D. P., Freedman, D. B., and Dandona, P. (1980): Effect of diflunisal on in vitro platelet aggregation. *Lancet*, ii:215.
291. Mills, D. C. B., and Smith, J. B. (1971): The influence on platelet aggregation of drugs that affect the accumulation of adenosine 3':5'-cyclic monophosphate in platelets. *Biochem. J.*, 121:185–196.
292. Moncada, S. R., Gryglewski, R. J., Bunting, S., and Vane, J. R. (1975): An enzyme isolated from arteries transforms prostaglandin endoperoxides to an unstable substance that inhibits platelet aggregation. *Nature*, 263:663–665.
293. Moncada, S., Gryglewski, R., Bunting, S., and Vane, J. R. (1976): A lipid peroxide inhibits the enzyme in blood vessel microsomes that generates from prostaglandin endoperoxide the substance (prostaglandin X) which prevents platelet aggregation. *Prostaglandins*, 12:715–738.
Moncada, S., Herman, A. G., Higgs, E. A., and Vane, J. R. (1977): Differential formation of prostacyclin (PGX or PGI₂) by layers of the arterial wall. An explanation for the antithrombotic properties of vascular endothelium. *Thromb. Res.*, 11:323–344.
Moncada, S., and Korbut, R. (1978): Dipyridamole and other phosphodiesterase inhibitors act as antithrombotic agents by potentiating endogenous prostacyclin. *Lancet*, i:1286–1289.
Moncada, S., Flower, R. J., and Russel-Smith, N. (1978): Dipyridamole and platelet function. *Lancet*, ii:1257–1258.
Moncada, S., Korbut, R., Bunting, S., and Vane, J. R. (1978): Prostacyclin is a circulating hormone. *Nature*, 273:767–768.
Moncada, S., and Vane, J. R. (1978): Unstable metabolites of arachidonic acid and their role in haemostasis and thrombosis. *Br. Med. Bull.*, 34:129–135.
R., Sitar, D. S., and Mitenko, P. A. (1980): Effect of age on the pharmakokinetic acetylsalicylic acid (ASA) after a single dose. *Clin. Res.*, 28:665A.
R. J., Snigal, D. P., Gouldie, J., and Blajchman, M. A. (1976): Inhibition atherosclerotic lesions by anti-platelet serum in rabbits. *Thromb. Hae-*
W. H. C. (1968): The binding of salicylate to human semen. *Biochem.*
De La Cruz, C., Lyons, M. M., and Regan, T. J. (1978): Antiaring non-thrombotic coronary occlusion. *Circulation*, 57:681–684.
303. Mo.. A. J., and Jorgensen, O. B. (1979): Effects of sulfinpyrazone on ischemic myocardial diovascular Actions of Sulfinpyrazone—Basic and Clinical Research, edited by M. M r, J. F. Mustard, M. Oliver, and S. Sherry, pp. 175–191. Symposium Specialists Inc.,
304. Moschos, C. B., Escobina ., and Jorgensen, O. B. (1979): Effect of sulfinpyrazone on survival following experime. n-thrombogenic coronary occlusion. *Am. J. Cardiol.*, 43:372.
305. Muirden, K. D., Deutschman. nd Phillips, M. (1974): Competition between salicylate and other drugs in binding to hum. m protein in vitro. *Aust. N. Z. J. Med.*, 4:149–153.
306. Muirhead, C. R. (1973): The fi. p technique as a method of measuring platelet aggregation in the following blood of the rat, hibitory activity of 5-oxo-1-cyclopentene-1-heptanoic acid (AY-16,804) on platelet aggregati. hromb. Diath. Haemorrh. (Stuttg.), 30:138–147.

307. Mullane, K. M., and Moncada, S. (1980): Prostacyclin release and the modulation of some vasoactive hormones. *Prostaglandins*, 20:25–50.
308. Muller, K. R. (1979): Lack of protective effect of sulfinpyrazone on endothelial cells from pig aorta in culture. In: *Cardiovascular Actions of Sulfinpyrazone: Basic and Clinical Research*, edited by M. McGregor, J. F. Mustard, M. F. Oliver, and S. Sherry, pp. 113–120. Symposium Specialists Inc., Miami.
309. Murray, T., and Golbury, M. (1975): Analgesic abuse and renal disease. *Annu. Rev. Med.*, 26:537–550.
310. Mustard, J. F., Rowsell, H. C., Smythe, M. A., Senyi, A., and Murphy, E. A. (1967): The effect of sulfinpyrazone on platelet economy and thrombus formation in rabbits. *Blood*, 29:859–866.
311. Muther, R. S., and Bennet, W. M. (1980): Effects of aspirin and glomerular filtration rate in normal humans. *Ann. Intern. Med.*, 92:386–387.
312. Najean, Y., Dassin, E., and Vigneron, N., and Wacquet, M. (1979): Platelet survival studies in patients with vascular disease. *Eur. J. Clin. Inves.*, 9:461–464.
313. Needleman, P., Wyche, A., and Raz, A. (1978): Platelet and blood vessel arachidonate metabolism and interaction. *J. Clin. Invest.*, 63:345–349.
314. Needleman, P., and Johnston, Jr., E. M. (1980): Vasodilators and the treatment of angina. In: *The Pharmacological Basis of Therapeutics*, edited by A. Goodman Gillman, L. S. Gillman, and A. Goodman, pp. 819–833. Macmillan, New York.
315. Nielsen-Kudsk, F., and Pedersen, A. K. (1979): Pharmacokinetics of dipyridamole, *Acta Pharmacol. Toxicol. (Copenh).*, 44:391–399.
316. Nielsen-Kudsk, F., and Ashkolt, J. (1980): Myocardial pharmacokinetics and pharmacodynamics of dipyridamole in the isolated rabbit heart. *Acta Pharmacol. Toxicol. (Copenh.)*, 7:195–201.
317. Nowak, M. M., Brundhofer, B., and Gilbaldi, M. (1974): Rectal absorption from aspirin suppositories in children and adults. *Paediatrics*, 54:23–26.
318. O'Brien, J. R. (1968): Aspirin and platelet aggregation. *Lancet*, i:204–205.
319. O'Brien, J. R. (1968): Effects of salicylates on human platelets. *Lancet*, i:779–783.
320. O'Brien, J. R. (1980): Platelets and the vessel wall: How much aspirin? *Lancet*, ii:372–373.
321. O'Grady, J., and Moncada, S. (1978): Aspirin: paradoxical effect on bleeding-time. *Lancet*, ii:780.
322. Okwuasaba, F. K., Hamilton, J. T., and Cook, M. A. (1976): Relaxation of guinea pig fundic strip by adenosine adenine nucleotides and electrical stimulation: Antagonism by theophylline and desensitization to adenosine and its derivatives. *Eur. J. Pharmacol.*, 46:181–198.
323. Okuma, M., Steiner, M., and Baldin, M. (1970): Studies on lipid peroxides in platelets. I. Method of assay and effect storage. *J. Lab. Clin. Med.*, 75:283–296.
324. Olssen, R. A. (1969): Adenosine metabolism during myocardial reactive hyperaemia. *Fed. Proc.*, 28:779.
325. O'Neill, B. F., and Mann, J. D. (1978): Aspirin prophylaxis in migraine. *Lancet*, ii:1179–1181.
326. O'Reilly, R. A. (1980): Anticoagulant, antithrombotic and thrombolytic drugs. In: *The Pharmacological Basis of Therapeutics*, edited by A. Goodman Gillman, L. S. Goodman, and A. Gillman, pp. 1345–1366. Macmillan, New York.
327. Örning, L., Hammarström, S., and Samuelsson, B. (1980): Leukotriene D: a slow reacting substance from rat basophillic leukaemia cells. *Proc. Natl. Acad. Sci. USA*, 77:2014–2017.
328. Ouderaa van der, F. J., van der Buytenhek, M., Nugteren, D. H., and Van Dorp, D. A. (1977): *Biochem. Biophys. Acta*, 487:315–331.
329. Ouderaa van der, F. J., van der Buytenhek, M., Nugteren, D. H., and Van Dorp, D. (1980): Acetylation of prostaglandin endoperoxide synthetase with acetylsalicylic acid. *Eur. J. Biochem.*, 109:1–8.
330. Owens, M. R., and Cimino, C. D. (1980): The inhibitory effects of sodium salicylate on synthesis of factor VII by the perfused rat liver. *Thromb. Res.*, 18:839–845.
331. Paccioretti, M. J., and Block, L. H. (1980): Effect of aspirin on platelet aggregation as a function of dosage and time. *Clin. Pharmacol. Ther.*, 27:803–809.
332. Packham, M. A., Warrior, E. S., Glynn, M. F., Senyi, A. S., and Mustard, J. F. (1967): Alteration of the response of platelets to surface stimuli by pyrazole compounds. *J. Exp. Med.*, 126:171–188.
333. Packham, M. A., Guccione, M. A., Greenborg, R. L., Kinlough-Rathbone, R. L., and Mustard, J. F. (1977): Release of ¹⁴C-serotonin during initial platelet changes induced by thrombin, collagen or A23187. *Blood*, 50:915–926.
334. Pannebakker, M. A. G., Den Octolander, G. J. H., and ten Pas, J. G. (1979): Insulin requirements in diabetic patients treated with sulfinpyrazone. *J. Int. Med. Res.*, 7:328–331.

335. Pareti, F. I., D'Angelo, A., Mannucci, P. M., and Smith, J. B. (1980): Platelets and the vessel wall: How much aspirin? *Lancet*, i:371–372.
336. Parratt, J. R., and Wadsworth, R. M. (1972): The effects of dipyridamole on coronary post-occlusion hyperaemia and on myocardial vasodilatation induced by systemic hypoxia. *Br. J. Pharmacol.*, 46:594–601.
337. Patrignani, P., Caltani, P., Minuz, P., and Patrono, C. (1980): Low dose aspirin: how low, how often? *Clin. Res.*, 28:636A.
338. Patrono, C., Ciabottoni, G., Greco, F., and Grossi-Belloni, D. (1976): Comparative evaluation of the inhibitory effects of aspirin-like drugs on prostaglandin production by human platelets and synovial tissue. In: *Advances in Prostaglandin and Thromboxane Research, Vol. 1*, edited by B. Samuelsson and R. Paoletti, pp. 125–131. Raven Press, New York.
339. Patrono, C., Ciabattoni, G., Pinca, E., Pugliese, F., Castrucci, G., De Salvo, A., Satta, M. A., and Peskar, B. A. (1980): Low dose aspirin and inhibition of thromboxane B_2 production in healthy subjects. *Thromb. Res.*, 17:317–327.
340. Paulus, H. E., Siegel, M., Morgan, E., Okun, R., and Calabro, J. J. (1971): Variations of serum concentrations and half life of salicylate in patients with rheumatoid arthritis. *Arthritis Rheum.*, 14:527–532.
341. Pay, G. F., Wallis, R. B., and Zelaschi, D. (1981): The effect of sulfinpyrazone and its metabolites on platelet function in vitro and ex vivo. *Haemostasis*, 10:165–175.
342. Paxton, J. W. (1980): Effects of aspirin on salivary and serum phenytoin kinetics in healthy subjects. *Clin. Pharmacol. Ther.*, 27:170–176.
343. Pedersen, A. K. (1978): Dipyridamole and platelet aggregation. *Lancet*, ii:270.
344. Pedersen, A. K. (1979): Specific determination of dipyridamole in serum by high-performance liquid chromatography. *J. Chromatogr.*, 162:98–103.
345. Pederson, A. K., and Jakobsen, P. (1981): Sulfinpyrazone metabolism during long term therapy. *Br. J. Clin. Pharmacol.*, 11:597–603.
346. Pederson, A. K., and Jakobsen, P. (1979): Two new metabolites of sulfinpyrazone in the rabbit. A possible cause of prolonged in vivo effect. *Thromb. Res.*, 6:871–876.
347. Pedersen, N. T. (1978): Occurrence of megakaryocytes in various vessels and their retention in the pulmonary capillaries in man. *Scand. J. Haematol.*, 21:396–402.
348. Peterson, D. A., Gerrad, J. M., Rao, G. H. R., and White, J. G. (1981): Salicylic acid inhibition of the irreversible effect of acetylsalicylic acid on prostaglandin synthetase may be due to competition for the enzyme cationic binding site. *Prostaglandins Med.*, 6:161–164.
349. Perel, J. M., Snell, M. M., Chen, W., and Dayton, P. G. (1964): A study of structure activity relationships in regard to species difference in the phenylbutazone series. *Biochem. Pharmacol.*, 13:1305–1317.
350. The Persantine-Aspirin Reinfarction Study Group. (1980): Persantine and aspirin in coronary heart disease. *Circulation*, 62:449–461.
351. Pfister, R., and Hafliger, F. (1961): Uber derivate und analoge des phenylbutazons. IV. Analoge mit schwefelhaltigen Seitenketten. *Helv. Chim. Acta*, 44:232–237.
352. Pick, R., Chediak, J., and Glick, G. (1979): Aspirin inhibits development of coronary atherosclerosis in cynomolgus monkey (Macaca fascicularis) fed an atherogenic diet. *J. Clin. Invest.*, 63:158–162.
353. Pierson, Jr., R. N., Holt, P. R., Watson, R. M., and Keating, R. P. (1979): Aspirin and gastrointestinal bleeding: chromate[51] blood loss studies. *Am. J. Med.*, 31:259–265.
354. Piper, P. J., and Vane, J. R. (1969): Release of additional factors in anaphylaxis and its antagonism by antiinflammatory drugs. *Nature*, 233:29–35.
355. Piper, P. J., and Vane, J. R. (1971): The release of prostaglandins from the lung and other tissues. *Ann. NY Acad. Sci.*, 180:363–385.
356. Piper, D. W., Greig, M., Coupland, G. A., Hobbin, E., and Shinners, J. (1975): Factors relevant to the prognosis of chronic gastric ulcer. *Gut*, 16:714–718.
357. Poch, G., and Kukovetz, W. R. (1972): Studies on the possible role of cyclic AMP in drug induced coronary vasodilatation. In: *Advances in Cyclic Nucleotide Research, Vol. 1*, edited by P. Greengard and G. A. Robinson, pp. 195–211. Raven Press, New York.
358. Povalski, H. J., Olson, R., Kopia, S.,, and Furness, P. (1970): Comparative effects of sulfinpyrazone and aspirin in the coronary occlusion—reperfusion dog model. In: *Cardiovascular Actions of Sulfinpyrazone—Basic and Clinical Research*, edited by M. McGregor, J. F. Mustard, M. Oliver, and S. Sherry, pp. 153–173. Symposium Specialists Inc., Miami.

359. Preston, F. E., Greaves, M., and Jackson, G. A. (1981): Cumulative inhibitory effect of daily 40 mg aspirin on prostacyclin synthesis. *Lancet*, i:211–222.
360. Preston, F. E., Whipps, S., Jackson, C. A., French, A. J., Wyld, P. J., and Stoddard, C. J. (1981): Inhibition of prostacyclin and platelet thromboxane A₂ after low dose aspirin. *N. Engl. J. Med.*, 304:76–79.
361. Pure, E., and Needleman, P. (1979): The effect of endothelial damage on prostaglandin synthesis by the isolated perfused rabbit mesenteric vasculature. *J. Cardiovas. Pharmacol.*, 3:299–309.
362. Quick, A. J. (1966): Salicylates and bleeding: The aspirin tolerance test. *Am. J. Med. Sci.*, 252:265–269.
363. Rajah, S. M., Crow, M. J., Penny, A. F., Ahmad, R., and Watson, D. A. (1977): The effect of dipyridamole on platelet function: correlation with blood levels in man. *Br. J. Clin. Pharmacol.*, 4:129–133.
364. Rajah, S. M., Penny, A., and Kester, R. (1978): Aspirin and bleeding-time. *Lancet*, ii:1104.
365. Rajah, S. M., Penny, A. F., Crow, M. J., Pepper, M. D., and Watson, D. A. (1979): The interaction of varying doses of dipyridamole and acetyl salicylic acid on the inhibition of platelet functions and their effect on the bleeding time. *Br. J. Clin. Pharmacol.*, 8:483–489.
366. Rampton, D. S., Sladen, G. E., Bhakoo, K. K., Heinzelmann, D. I., and Youlten, L. J. F. (1980): Rectal mucosal prostaglandin E release and electrolyte transport in ulcerative colitis. *Advances in Prostaglandin and Thromboxane Research, Vol. 8*, edited by B. Samuelsson, P. Ramwell, and R. Paoletti, pp. 1621–1626. Raven Press, New York.
367. Rainsford, K. D., and Whitehouse, M. W. (1976): Gastric irritancy of aspirin and its dangers: Anti-inflammatory activity without this side-effect. *J. Pharm. Pharmacol.*, 28:599–601.
368. Rainsford, K. D., and Whitehouse, M. W. (1977): Non-steroidal antiinflammatory drugs: Combined assay for anti-emetic potency and gastric ulcerogeneses in the same animal. *Life Sci.*, 21:371–378.
369. Randall, L. O., and Selitto, J. J. (1957): A method for the measurement of analgesic activity on inflamed tissue. *Arch. Int. Pharmacodyn. Ther.*, 111:409–419.
370. Rees, W. D. W., and Turnberg, L. A. (1980): Reappraisal of the effects of aspirin on the stomach. *Lancet*, ii:410–413.
371. Renaud, S., and Lecompte, F. (1970): Thrombosis prevention by coagulation and platelet aggregation inhibitors in hyperlipemic rats. *Thromb. Diath. Haemorrh. (Stuttg.)*, 24:577–589.
372. Reyers, I., Mussoni, L., Donati, M. B., and de Gaetano, G. (1980): Failure of aspirin at different doses to modify experimental thrombosis in rats. *Thromb. Res.*, 18:669–674.
373. Rich, R. R., and Johnson, J. S. (1973): Salicylate hepatotoxicity in patients with juvenile rheumatoid arthritis. *Athritis Rheum.*, 16:1–9.
374. Rittenhouse, E. A., Hessel, E. A., Ho, C. S., and Merendino, K. A. (1972): Effects of dipyridamole on microaggregate formation in the pump oxygenator. *Ann. Surg.*, 175:1–9.
375. Robert, A. (1980): Prostaglandins and digestive diseases. In: *Advances in Prostaglandin and Thromboxane Research, Vol. 8*, edited by B. Samuelsson, P. Ramwell, and R. Paoletti, pp. 1533–1542. Raven Press, New York.
376. Roberts, A. J., Jacobstein, J. G., Cipriano, P. R., Alonso, D. R., Combes, J. R., and Gay, W. A. (1980): Effectiveness of dipyridamole in reducing the size of experimental myocardial infarction. *Circulation*, 61:228–236.
377. Robertson, R. P., and Chen, M. (1977): A role for prostaglandin E in defective insulin secretion and carbohydrate intolerance in diabetes mellitus. *J. Clin. Invest.*, 60:747–751.
378. Robin, E., Davies, R., and Rees, G. (1959): Salicylate intoxication with special reference to the development of hypokalaemia. *Am. J. Med.*, 26:869–871.
379. Rollins, P. G. (1980): Ultrastructural observations on the pathogenesis of aspirin induced gastric erosions. *Br. J. Exp. Pathol.*, 61:497–504.
380. Rogers, P. H., and Sherry, S. (1976): Current status of antithrombotic therapy in cardiovascular disease. *Prog. Cardiovasc. Dis.*, 19:235–253.
381. Rome, L. H., Lands, W. E. M., Roth, G. J., and Majerus, P. W. (1976): Aspirin as a quantitative acetylating reagent for the fatty acid oxygenase that forms prostaglandins. *Prostaglandins*, 11:23–29.
382. Roos, H., and Pfleger, K. (1972): Kinetics of adenosine uptake by erythrocytes, and the influence of dipyridamole. *Mol. Pharmacol.*, 8:417–425.
383. Rosenberg, J. C., and Sell, T. L. (1975): *In vitro* evaluation of inhibitors of platelet release and aggregation. *Arch. Surg.*, 110:980–983.

384. Rosenblum, W. I., El-Sabban, F., and Ellis, E. F. (1980): Aspirin and indomethacin enhance platelet aggregation in mouse mesenteric arterioles. *Am. J. Physiol.*, 239:H220–H226.
385. Rosenthal, R. K., Bayler, T. B., and Fremont-Smith, K. (1964): Simultaneous salicylate concentrations in synovial fluid and plasma in rheumatoid arthritis. *Arthritis Rheum.*, 7:103–108.
386. Roth, G. J., and Majerus, P. W. (1975): The mechanism of the effect of aspirin on human platelets. I. Acetylation of a particulate fraction protein. *J. Clin. Invest.*, 56:624–632.
387. Roth, G. J., and Siok, C. J. (1978): Acetylation of the NH_2-terminal serine of prostaglandin synthase by aspirin. *J. Biol. Chem.*, 253:3782–3784.
388. Roth, G. J., Stanford, N., and Majerus, P. W. (1978): Acetylation of prostaglandin synthetase by aspirin. *Proc. Natl. Acad. Sci. USA*, 72:3073–3076.
389. Rowland, M., Riegelman, S., Harris, P. A., Sholkoff, S. D., and Eyring, E. J. (1967): Kinetics of acetylsalicylic acid disposition in man. *Nature*, 215:413–414.
390. Rowland, M., Riegelman, S., Harris, P. A., and Sholkoff, S. D. (1972): Absorption kinetics of aspirin in man following oral administration of an aqueous solution. *J. Pharm. Sci.*, 61:379–385.
391. Rowland, M., and Riegelman, S. (1968): Pharmacokinetics of acetyl salicylic acid and salicylic acid after intravenous administration in man. *J. Pharm. Sci.*, 57:1313–1319.
392. Royer, R. J., Gross, A., Netter, P., Favre, G., Mur, J. M., and Zannad, F. (1980): Pharmacokinetics of salicylates in renal failure. *Proc. of First World Congress Clinical Pharmacology (Lond)*, (Abstract 0152).
393. Rozenberg, M. C., and Walker, C. M. (1973): The effect of pyrimidine compounds on the potentiation of adenosine inhibition of aggregation, on adenosine phosphorylation and phosphodiesterase activity of blood platelet. *Br. J. Haematol.*, 24:409–418.
394. Rubio, R., Berne, R. M., and Katori, M. (1969): Release of adenosine in reactive hyperaemia of the dog heart. *Am. J. Physiol.*, 216:56–62.
395. Ruegg, M., Riesterer, L., and Jaques, R. (1970): The euglobulin clot lysis time. A method for evaluating plasma fibrinolytic activity of normal and arthritic rats and the therapeutic values of anti-inflammatory (steroidal and nonsteroidal) agents. *Pharmacology*, 4:242–254.
396. Ruegg, M. (1976): Antithrombolic effects of sulfinpyrazone in animals. Influence of fibrinolysis and sodium arachidonate-induced pulmonary embolism. *Pharmacology*, 14:422–536.
397. Rumble, R. H., Brooks, P. M., and Roberts, M. S. (1980): Metabolism of salicylate during chronic aspirin therapy. *Br. J. Clin. Pharmacol.*, 9:41–45.
398. Russell, P. T., Alan, N., and Clary, P. (1973): Impaired placental conversion of prostaglandin E_1 to A_1 in toxaemia of pregnancy. *Fed. Proc.*, 32:3304A.
399. Salem, H. H., Koutts, J., and Firkin, B. G. (1980): Circulating platelet aggregates in ischaemic heart disease and their correlation to platelet life span. *Thromb. Res.*, 17:707–711.
400. Samter, M., and Beers, R. F. (1967): Concerning the nature of intolerance to aspirin. *J. Allergy*, 40:281–293.
401. Samter, M., and Beers, R. F. (1968): Intolerance to aspirin. Clinical studies and consideration of this pathogenesis. *Am. Intern. Med.*, 68:975–983.
402. Samuelsson, B. (1977): The role of prostaglandin endoperoxides and thromboxanes as bioregulators. In: *Biochemical Aspects of Prostaglandins and Thromboxanes: Proceedings Intra-Science Symposium on New Biochemistry of Prostaglandins and Thromboxanes, Santa Monica, California*, edited by N. Kharsch and J. Fried, pp. 133–154. Academic Press, New York.
403. Samuelsson, B., Hammarström, S., and Borgeat, P. (1979): Pathways of arachidonic acid metabolism. In: *Advances in Inflammation Research*, edited by G. Weissmann et al., pp. 405–412. Raven Press, New York.
404. Schmidt, C. R., Beazell, J. M., Atkinson, A. J., and Ivy, A. C. (1938): The effect of therapeutic agents on the volume and the constituents of bile. *Am. J. Dig. Diseases*, 5:613–617.
405. Schneeweiss, J., and Pook, G. W. (1960): Hyperuricaemia due to pyrazinamide. *Br. Med. J.*, 2:830–832.
406. Schrader, J., Berne, R. M., and Rubio, R. (1972): Uptake and metabolism of adenosine by human erythrocyte ghosts. *Am. J. Physiol.*, 223:159–166.
407. Schreiner, G. E. (1962): The nephrotoxicity of analgesic abuse. *Ann. Intern. Med.*, 57:1047–1052.
408. Schraer, K., and Rosen, P. (1979): The cyclic AMP level in coronary arteries, *Nauyn-Schmeideberg's Arch. Pharmacol.*, 306:101–103.
409. Schrör, K., Link, H. B., Rösen, R., Klaus, W., and Rösen, P. (1980): Prostacyclin-induced vasodilatation interactions with adenosine and energy change in the rat heart in vitro. *Eur. J. Pharmacol.*, 64:341–348.

410. Schrör, K., Smith, E. F., Bickerton, M., Smith, J. B., Nicolaou, K. C., Magolda, R., and Lefer, A. M. (1980): Preservation of the ischaemic myocardium by pinane thromboxane A_2. *Am. J. Physiol.*, 238:H87–H92.

411. Schwartz, D. B., Norman, N. E., and Simons, E. R. (1980): Effect of sulfinpyrazone and its thioether metabolite on platelets and their response to thrombin. *Circulation (Suppl. III)*, 62:274.

412. Seaman, W. E., and Plotz, P. H. (1976): Effect of aspirin on liver tests in patients with RA or SLE and in normal volunteers. *Arthritis Rheum.*, 19:155–160.

413. Settipane, G. (1981): Adverse reactions to aspirin and related drugs. *Arch. Int. Med.*, 141:328–332.

414. Settipane, R. A., Constantine, H. P., and Settipane, G. A. (1980): Aspirin intolerance and recurrent urticaria in normal adults and children. *Allergy*, 35:149–154.

415. Shakali, M., and Tarassoli, M. (1979): Cellular relationship in the rat bone marrow studied by freeze-fracture and lanthanum impregnation thin sectioning electron microscopy. *J. Ultrastructr. Res.*, 69:343–361.

416. Sharma, H. M., Moore, S., Merrick, H. W., and Smith, M. R. (1972): Platelets in early hyperacute allograft rejection in kidneys and their modification by sulfinpyrazone (Anturane) therapy. *Am. J. Pathol.*, 66:445–460.

417. Sharma, H. M. (1975): Drugs, platelets and the prevention of transplant rejection. In: *Platelets, Drugs and Thrombosis*, edited by Hirsch, Cade, Gallus, and Schonbaum, pp. 204–211. Karger, Basel.

418. Sherry, S. (1980): Drug trials in myocardial infarction. Lessons to be learned from the Anturane Reinfarction Trial. *Eur. J. Clin. Pharmacol.*, 17:401–408.

419. Sholkoff, S. D., Erving, E. I., Rowland, M., and Riegelman, S. (1967): Plasma and synovial fluid concentrations of acetylsalicylic acid in patients with rheumatoid arthritis. *Arthritis Rheum.*, 10:348–351.

420. Shuman, M. A., and Levine, S. P. (1978): Thrombin generation and secretion of platelet factor 4 during blood clotting. *J. Clin. Invest.*, 61:1102–1106.

421. Shuman, M. A., Botney, M., and Fenton II, J. W. (1979): Thrombin-induced platelet secretion. *J. Clin. Invest.*, 63:1211–1218.

422. Silver, M. J., Hoch, W., and Kocsis, J. J. (1974): Arachidonic acid causes sudden death in rabbits. *Science*, 183:1085–1087.

423. Silvoso, G. R., Ivey, K. J., Butt, J. H., Lockard, O. O., Holt, S. D., Sisk, C., Baskin, W. N., MacKercher, P. A., and Hewitt, J. (1979): Incidence of gastric lesions in patients with rheumatic disease on chronic aspirin therapy. *Ann. Intern. Med.*, 91:517–520.

424. Simon, B., Kather, H., and Kommerell, B. (1980): Activation of human colonic mucosal adenylate cyclase by prostaglandins. In: *Advances in Prostaglandin and Thromboxane Research, Vol. 8*, edited by B. Samuelsson, P. Ramwell, and R. Paoletti, pp. 1617–1620. Raven Press, New York.

425. Siurla, M., Mustala, F. O., and Jussila, J. (1969): Absorption of acetylsalicylic acid by a normal and an atrophic gastric mucosa. *Scand. J. Gastroenterol.*, 4:269–273.

426. Smith, M. J. H. (1978): Aspirin and prostaglandins, some recent developments. *Agents Actions*, 8:427–429.

427. Smith, M. J. H., and Smith, P. K. (1966): *The Salicylates. A Critical Bibliographic Review.* In: *The Salicylates*, edited by M. J. H. Smith and K. Smith, pp. 86–90. Wiley Interscience Publishers, New York.

428. Smith, M. J. H., and Dawkins, P. D. (1971): Salicylate and enzymes. *J. Pharm. Pharmacol.*, 23:729–744.

429. Smith, W. L., and Lands, W. E. M. (1971): Stimulation and blockade of prostaglandin biosynthesis. *J. Biol. Chem.*, 21:6700–6702.

430. Smith, J. B., and Willis, A. L. (1971): Aspirin selectively inhibits prostaglandin production in human platelets. *Nature (New Biol.)*, 231:235–237.

431. Smith, W. L., and Lands, W. E. M. (1972): Oxygenation of polyunsaturated fatty acids during prostaglandin biosynthesis by sheep vesicular gland. *Biochemistry*, 11:3276–3285.

432. Smith, J. B., Ogletree, M., Lefer, A. M., and Nicolau, K. C. (1978): Antibodies which antagonize the effects of prostacyclin. *Nature*, 274:64–65.

433. Smith, M. J. H., Ford-Hutchinson, A. W., Walker, J. R., and Slack, J. A. (1979): Aspirin salicylate and prostaglandins. *Agents Actions*, 9:483–487.

434. Smith, P. H., Gleason, H. L., Stoll, C. G., and Ogorzalek, S. (1946): Studies on the pharmacology of salicylates. *J. Pharmacol. Exp. Ther.*, 87:237–255.

435. Smythe, H. A., Ogryzlo, M. A., and Murphy, E. A. (1965): The effect of sulfinpyrazone (Anturane) on platelet economy and blood coagulation in man. *Can. Med. Assoc. J.*, 92:818–821.
436. Solomon, L. M., Juhlin, L., and Kirschenbaum, M. B. (1968): Prostaglandin on cutaneous vasculature. *J. Invest. Dermatol.*, 51:280–282, 292.
437. Somolyo, A. V., Vinall, P., and Somolyo, A. P. (1969): Excitation-contraction coupling and electrical events in two types of vascular smooth muscle. *Microvasc. Res.*, 1:354–373.
438. Somova, L. (1973): Inhibition of prostaglandin synthesis in kidneys by aspirin-like drugs. In: *Supplementation to Advances in The Biosciences, Vol. 9*, edited by S. Bergström and S. Bernhard, Int. Conf. Prostaglandins, Vienna, p. 53. Pergamon Press, Braunschweig.
439. Soren, A. (1979): Kinetics of salicylates in blood and joint fluid. *Eur. J. Clin. Pharmacol.*, 16:279–282.
440. Steelman, S. L., Smit Sibinga, C. T., Schulz, P., Van den Heuvel, W. J. H., and Tempero, K. F. (1976): The effect of diflunisal on urinary prostaglandin excretion, bleeding time and platelet aggregation in normal human subjects. In: *Proc. XIII Int. Congress Internal Medicine*, p. 215.
441. Stephen, F. O., and Lawrenson, K. B. (1969): ^{51}Cr excretion in bile. *Lancet*, i:158–159.
442. Stewart, J. H., and Gallery, E. H. (1976): Analgesic abuse and kidney disease. *Aust. N. Z. J. Med.*, 6:498–508.
443. Stevenson, D. D., Arroyare, G. M., Bhat, K. N., and Tan, E. M. (1976): Oral aspirin challenges in asthmatic patients. *Clin. Allergy*, 6:493–499.
444. Stevenson, D. D., Simon, R. A., and Mathison, D. A. (1980): Aspirin sensitive asthma: tolerance to aspirin after positive oral challenges. *J. Allergy Clin. Immunol.*, 66:82–88.
445. St. John, C. J. B., Yeomans, M. D., and de Boer, W. G. R. N. (1973): Chronic gastric ulcer induced by aspirin; an experimental model. *Gastroenterology*, 65:634.
446. Stuart, R. K. (1970): Platelet function studies in human beings receiving 300 mg of aspirin per day. *J. Lab. Clin. Med.*, 75:462–471.
447. Szeczeklik, A., Gryglewski, R. J., and Czerniawska-Mysik, G. (1975): Relationship of inhibition of prostaglandin biosynthesis by analgesics to asthma attacks in aspirin sensitive patients. *Br. Med. J.*, 1:67–71.
448. Szeczeklik, A., Gryglewski, R. J., and Czerniawska-Mysik, G. (1977): Clinical patterns of hypersensitivity to nonsteroidal anti-inflammatory drugs and their pathologenesis. *J. Allergy Clin. Immunol.*, 60:276–284.
449. Szeczeklik, A., Czerniawska-Mysik, G., Serwonska, M., and Kublinski, P. (1980): Inhibition by ketotifen of idiosyncratic reactions to aspirin. *Allergy*, 35:421–424.
450. Szeczeklik, A., Pieton, R., Sieradzki, J., and Nizankowski, R. (1980): The effects of prostacyclin on glycaemia and insulin release in man. *Prostaglandins*, 19:959–968.
451. Takeguchi, C., and Sih, C. J. (1972): A rapid spectrophotometric assay for prostaglandin synthetase: Application to the study of non-steroidal, antiinflammatory agents. *Prostaglandins*, 2:169–184.
452. Talbert, R. L., Ludden, T. M., and West, R. E. (1979): Rapid establishment of therapeutic serum concentrations of salicylates. *J. Clin. Pharmacol.*, 19:108–112.
453. Talbert, R. L., Ludden, T. M., Littlefield, L. C., and Reed, W. E. (1980): Development of a loading regimen for aspirin. *Curr. Ther. Res.*, 27:584–594.
454. Tateson, J. E., Moncada, S., and Vane, J. R. (1977): Effects of prostacyclin (PGX) on cyclic AMP concentrations in human platelets. *Prostaglandins*, 13:389–397.
455. Tavassoli, M. (1980): Megakaryocyte-platelet axis and the process of platelet formation and release. *Blood*, 55:537–545.
456. Trnavska, Z., and Trnavsky, K. (1980): Characterization of salicylate binding to synovial fluid and plasma protein in patients with rheumatoid arthritis. *Eur. J. Clin. Pharmacol.*, 18:403–406.
457. Treacher, D., Warlow, C., and McPherson, K. (1978): Aspirin and bleeding time. *Lancet*, ii:1378.
458. Turpie, A. G. G., Lernesky, M. A., and Larke, R. P. B. (1973): Effect of Newcastle disease virus on human or rabbit platelets. Aggregation and loss of constituents. *J. Lab. Invest.*, 28:575–583.
459. Tweedale, M., and Ogilvie, R. (1973): Antagonism of spironolactone-induced natriuesis by aspirin in man. *N. Engl. J. Med.*, 289:198–200.
460. Tyce, G. M., Fuster, V., and Owen, C. A., Jr. (1979): Dipyridamole levels in plasma of man and other species. *Res. Commun. Chem. Pathol. Pharmacol.*, 26:495–508.
461. Tyler, H. M., Saxton, C. A., and Perry, M. J.: Administration to man of UK-37, 248-01, a selective inhibitor of thromboxane synthetase. *Lancet*, ii:629–632.
462. Vaessen, L. M. B., Bonthuis, F., Hesse, C. J., and Lameijer, L. O. F. (1977): Effect of sulfinpyrazone (Anturane) on degree of vascular lesions and survival of cardiac allograft in rats. *Transplantation Proc.*, 9:993–996.

463. Vane, J. R. (1971): Inhibition of prostaglandin synthesis as a mechanism of action for aspirin-like drugs. *Nature (New Biol.),* 231:232–235.
464. Vane, J. R. (1972): Prostaglandins and the aspirin like drugs. *Hosp. Prac.,* 7:61–71.
465. Vergaftig, B. B. (1978): The inhibition of cyclo-oxygenase of rabbit platelets by aspirin is prevented by salicylic acid and phenanthrolines. *Eur. J. Pharmacol.,* 50:231–241.
466. Vermylen, J., Defreyn, G., Comeras, Lo., Machin, S. J., VanScharen, J., and Verstràete, M. (1981): Thromboxane synthetase inhibition as antithrombotic strategy. *Lancet,* i:1073–1075.
467. Vicic, W. J., Lages, B., and Weiss, H. J. (1980): Release of human platelet factor V activity is induced by both collagen and ADP and is inhibited by aspirin. *Blood,* 56:448–455.
468. Walker, J. L. (1972): The regulatory function of prostaglandins in the release of histamine and SRS-A from passively sensitized human lung tissue. In: *Advances in the Biosciences, Vol. 9,* edited by S. Bergstrom and S. Bernhard, pp. 235–243. Pergamon Press, Braunschweig.
469. Walter, E., Staiger, C., deVries, J., Zimmerman, R., and Weber, T. (1981): Induction of drug metabolizing enzymes by sulfinpyrazone. *Eur. J. Clin. Pharmacol.,* 19:353–358.
470. Weiss, H. J. (1978): Antiplatelet therapy. *N. Engl. J. Med.,* 298:1344–1347.
471. Weiss, H. J., Aledort, L. M., and Kochwa, S. J. (1968): The effect of salicylates on the haemostatic properties of platelets in man. *J. Clin. Invest.,* 47:2169–2180.
472. Weiss, H. J., Turitto, V. T., Vicic, W. J., and Baumgartner, H. R. (1981): Effect of aspirin and dipyridamole on the interaction of human platelets with sub-endothelium: studies using citrated and native blood. *Thromb. Hameostas.,* 45:136–141.
473. Weksler, B., Ley, C. W., and Jaffe, E. A. (1978): Stimulation of endothelial cell prostacyclin production by thrombin, trypsin and the ionophore A23187. *J. Clin. Invest.,* 62:923–930.
474. Weltman, J. K., Szaro, R. P., and Settipane, G. A. (1978): An analysis of the role of IGE in intolerance to aspirin and tartarazine. *Allergy,* 33:273–281.
475. West, J. W., Bellet, S., Manzoli, V. C., and Müller, O. (1962): Effects of persantin (RA 8), a new coronary vasodilator, on coronary blood flow and cardiac dynamics in the dog. *Circ. Res.,* 10:35–44.
476. White, A. M., and Butler, C. D. (1975): The effect of sulfinpyrazone (Anturane®) on immulogically derived thrombocytopenia and on platelet survival. *Thromb. Diath. Haemorrh. (Stuttg.),* 34:553.
477. White, J. G., and Gerrard, J. M. (1979): Interaction of microtubules and microfilaments in platelet contractile physiology. In: *Methods and Achievements in Experimental Pathology,* edited by G. Gabiani, G. Jasmin, and M. Cantin, pp. 1–39. Karger, Basel.
478. Whitehouse, M. W., and Rainsford, M. D. (1980): Esterification of acidic antiinflammatory drugs suppresses their gastrotoxicity without adversely affecting their antiinflammatory activity in rats. *J. Pharm. Pharmacol.,* 32:795–796.
479. Whiting, J., Salata, K., and Bailey, J. M. (1980): Aspirin: An unexpected side effect of prostacyclin synthesis in cultured vascular smooth muscle cells. *Science,* 210:663–665.
480. Whittle, B. J. R., Higgs, G. A., Eakins, K. E., Moncada, S., and Vane, J. R. (1980): Selective inhibition of prostaglandin production in inflammatory exudates and gastric mucosa. *Nature,* 284:271–273.
481. Wiedeman, M. P. (1970): Microscopic observation of small blood vessels in sulfinpyrazone-treated animals. In: *Cardiovascular Action of Sulfinpyrazone: Basic and Clinical Research,* edited by M. McGregor, J. F. Mustard, M. F. Oliver, and S. Sherry, pp. 99–108. Symposium Specialists Inc., Miami.
482. Wilcken, D. E. L., Paoloni, H. J., and Eikens, E. (1971): Evidence for intravenous dipyridamole (Persantin) producing a "coronary steal" effect in ischaemic myocardium. *Aust. N. Z. J. Med.,* 1:8.
483. Williams, S., and Turnberg, L. A. (1979): Studies of the "protective" properties of gastric mucus: evidence for a "mucus bicarbonate" barrier. *Gut,* 20:922–923.
484. Willis, A. L., Davison, R., Ramwell, P. W., Brockelhurst, W. D., and Smith, B. (1972): Release and actions of prostaglandins in inflammation and fever: Inhibition by antiinflammatory and antipyretic drugs. In: *Prostaglandins in Cellular Biology,* edited by P. W. Ramwell, and B. B. Pharris, pp. 227–259. Plenum Press, New York.
485. Winder, C. V. (1959): Aspirin and algesimetry. *Nature,* 184:494–497.
486. Wishinsky, H., Glasser, E. J., and Perkel, S. (1967): Protein interactions of sulfonylurea compounds. *Diabetes (Suppl.),* 2:18–25.
487. Wojnar, R. J., Hearn, T., and Starkweather, S. (1980): Augmentation of allergic histamine release from human leukocytes by nonsteroidal anti-inflammatory–analgesic agents. *J. Allergy Clin. Immunol.,* 66:37–45.

488. Wong, P. Y. D., Bedwani, J. R., and Cuthbert, A. W. (1972): Hormone action and the levels of cyclic AMP and prostaglandins in the toad bladder. *Nature (New Biol.)*, 238:27–31.
489. Woslait, W. (1976): Theoretical analysis of the binding of salicylate by human serum albumin. The relationship between free and bound drug and therapeutic levels. *Eur. J. Clin. Pharmacol.*, 9:285–290.
490. Wright, J. H. (1910): The histogenesis of blood platelets. *J. Morphol.*, 21:263–266.
491. Young, V. P., Giles, A. R., Pater, J., Corbett, W. E. N. (1980): Sex differences in bleeding time and blood loss in normal subjects following aspirin ingestion. *Thromb. Res.*, 20:705:709.
492. Zak, S. B., Tallan, H. H., Quinn, G. P., Fratta, I., and Greengard, P. (1963): The determination and physiological distribution of dipyridamole and its glucuronides in biological material. *J. Pharmacol. Exp. Ther.*, 141:392–398.
493. Zucker, M. B., and Peterson, J. (1970): Effect of acetylsalicylic acid, other nonsteroidal antiinflammatory agents, and dipyridamole on human blood platelets. *J. Lab. Clin. Med.*, 76:66–75.

Prostaglandins and the Cardiovascular System,
edited by John A. Oates. Raven Press,
New York © 1982.

Effect of Prostaglandin-Mediated Platelet-Suppressant Drugs on Acute Cardiovascular Catastrophes

Sol Sherry

*Department of Medicine, Temple University School of Medicine,
Philadelphia, Pennsylvania 19140*

There are two major classifications of thrombi, those that form in areas of slow flow and low pressure, and those that form in the presence of rapid flow and high pressure. Although there may be some overlap in the biochemical and physiological mechanisms producing these entities, it is recognized that a thrombus forming in the veins, slow flow and low pressure, is primarily a coagulation thrombus and consists mostly of red blood cells and fibrin. In contrast, those occurring in the systemic arteries, rapid flow and high pressure, consist of a prominent white head, composed of platelets that have adhered and aggregated at a site of injured or destroyed endothelium, and a variable amount of superimposed fibrin-red-cell coagulum. Since the latter type of thrombus is the one most likely to be affected by platelet-suppressant drugs, the action of such drugs on arterial thromboembolic events will be the focus of this chapter.

Sulfinpyrazone, aspirin, and dipyridamole will be the only drugs under consideration. All three have undergone extensive clinical investigation for their antithrombotic effects in arterial vascular disease, and each of these drugs, despite differences in their pharmacological actions, influences platelet activity through prostaglandin-mediated pathways. Clofibrate, beta-blockers, and other drugs also have demonstrated platelet-inhibitory activity, but they will be excluded from this review because either their mechanism of action is unclear, they have not undergone extensive testing, or the rationale for their use in various trials was unrelated to their platelet effects.

CARDIAC STUDIES

In recent years there has been considerable interest in testing whether agents that affect prostaglandin metabolism and thereby inhibit the ability of platelets to aggregate at sites of vascular injury might decrease the risk of a coronary death. This is because the two major immediate causes of coronary death, sudden cardiac death, presumably due to an acute fatal arrhythmia, and the more classical myocardial infarction, may primarily be due to platelet phenomena. Platelet thrombi readily form on injured coronary vessels that frequently occur in coronary artery disease and also are likely to shed platelet emboli. Such thrombi and emboli could readily produce areas of transient ischemia both by physical obstruction and by the vaso-constrictive properties of the released serotonin and thromboxane A_2. The resulting ischemia could precipitate an arrhythmia sufficient to cause sudden death. In areas of more extensive injury to a coronary artery, such as a sudden crack, fissure, or ulcer in an atheromatous plaque, a plug of platelets can rapidly fill the lesion and serve to initiate a large arterial thrombus sufficient in size to occlude the entire vessel and cause an extensive transmural infarction. There is reason to suspect that agents that inhibit platelet function could significantly influence the incidence of major coronary events.

SECONDARY PREVENTION OF DEATH IN ISCHEMIC HEART DISEASE

To test the hypothesis that treatment with platelet-active drugs could prevent death from acute coronary events or their sequelae, several large-scale secondary intervention trials have been undertaken in patients with chronic ischemic heart disease. The population chosen for study were patients who had experienced one or more acute myocardial infarctions—an almost certain indicator of ischemic heart disease. In addition, this population has the advantage of being at higher risk of mortality from subsequent acute coronary events, thereby providing a better op-portunity for assessing the efficacy of these drugs.

In North America, aspirin, alone, or in combination with dipyridamole, and sulfinpyrazone, has recently been the subject of intensive investigation in large multicenter studies of patients with previous myocardial infarction. The results of three studies were published in 1980. Other controlled, clinical trials have also been conducted, especially with aspirin. Still other clinical studies are being planned or in progress.

Problems Associated with Clinical Studies in Patients Who Have Recovered from Myocardial Infarction

Evaluating a platelet-active drug in the secondary prevention of death among patients who have had a previous myocardial infarction presents many problems other than the details of trial design, operation of the study, and its analysis. These problems are considerable and make an accurate evaluation very difficult. They may be considered from at least three aspects. These are those problems related to the type of study being undertaken, those related to the drugs under investigation, and those related to the analysis of mortality.

Type of Study

Retrospective studies do not, by themselves, meet the requirements for an ade-quately controlled experiment. Data obtained from retrospective studies are of value only in providing a rationale for appropriate prospective trials.

In general, prospective studies can be divided into two types; intent-to-treat trials and clinical efficacy studies. In the former, all patients are randomized into the study on the basis of an intent to treat either with the active drug or an appropriate control, usually a placebo. Once randomized, regardless of whether the patient is subsequently shown not to have met the eligibility criteria, never received any medication, stopped taking it, or withdrew from the trial, the patient is counted in the drug group to which he was assigned. While this approach, which dominates the methodology currently employed by most biometricians, protects against bias, the results are so diluted, by inclusion in the analysis of significant numbers of ineligible patients, drop-ins, and drop-outs, that only a qualitative effect of the true efficacy of the drug can be shown. With current sample sizes, a positive result can be demonstrated only when the drug's effect is very striking. A moderate effect is unlikely to reach statistical significance unless the number of endpoints being measured is very, very large.

However, clinical efficacy studies where only those events among eligible patients being actively treated with adequate amounts of the drug, active agent or control, are analyzed, have the advantage of allowing for a quantitative assessment of the drug's true effect. However, such studies may not effectively control against bias, as do intent-to-treat studies, and the interpretation of the results from such trials is likely to be more suspect.

Drugs

Multiple pharmacological actions in vivo

Each of the drugs under investigation has multiple pharmacological actions, and a positive trial result does not necessarily prove the hypothesis upon which the study was based. Even if an effect were to be related to the action of these drugs on prostaglandin metabolism, the fact that prostaglandins are ubiquitous in their distribution in tissues precludes the conclusion that the result is attributable to the drug's action on platelets. This only can be proven when a direct relationship can be established between the desired pharmacological action under investigation and the clinical results achieved. Unfortunately, in the evaluation of platelet-active drugs, no single test, or combination of tests, has been shown to be specifically related to an effective pharmacological state *in vivo*.

Dose

Considering the lack of a test that truly measures the *in vivo* state of the interaction of platelets with a normal or impaired vessel, the dosage of the drug employed in trials has been empirical and fixed. The former dosage may prove inappropriate and the latter does not allow for individual variation based on an appropriate titration. Cyclo-oxygenase inhibitors may not only affect thromboxane A_2 synthesis but also impair prostacyclin production and the critical or determining factor regulating platelet-vessel wall interaction may be the local thromboxane A_2: prostacyclin ratio.

This knowledge has raised the serious question of whether daily doses of 150 to 300 mg of aspirin might be much more effective than the usually employed doses of 900 mg or more. Similar concern can be expressed about dipyridamole and sulfinpyrazone, since even less is known about their pharmacodynamics *in vivo*.

Sex differences

In several of the clinical trials, evidence has been presented that the therapeutic benefit from platelet-active drugs is restricted to only males. This was first reported in the Canadian Cooperative Study (14) and similar sex differences are suggested in other trials (28; Anturane Reinfarction Trial, personal communication). Experimental evidence supporting such a contention has been obtained in rabbits (52).

Analysis of Mortality

Potential contribution of platelet-active agents to reduction of mortality in myocardial infarction patients

The hypothesis underlying the use of platelet-active drugs is that platelets may play a significant role in the pathogenesis of sudden death and fatal myocardial infarction. Yet most trials have used total deaths, regardless of cause, as the endpoint analyzed. This inclusion of deaths from other causes serves only to dilute any benefit that could be attributed to these agents. Even when cardiac mortality has been the primary endpoint, as in the Anturane Reinfarction Trial (4), deaths from other cardiac causes, from which myocardial infarction patients are also at risk, can impair the analysis of the benefit.

Even more important is the question of the contribution of platelet-mediated phenomena to sudden death and fatal acute myocardial infarction. It is unlikely that these fatalities always occur through a similar pathogenetic mechanism. There may well be multiple causes for the initiation of these lethal events and platelet-mediated phenomena may be an important, but not exclusive, trigger. If so, only a percentage of deaths can be prevented by platelet-active drugs, and if that percentage is a limited one, trials of the size currently being undertaken would be unlikely to demonstrate significant benefit even if the drugs were effective. The argument may be made that the demonstration of moderate benefit should not be the goal of this type of research. However, from the perspective of the magnitude of the public health problem posed, fatal acute coronary events being the single largest cause of death in the Western World and the number of annual deaths from this cause being enormous, even a moderate benefit, would represent an important development.

Further clinical considerations pertinent to the evaluation of mortality: natural history of cardiac mortality following an acute myocardial infarction

Mortality following an acute myocardial infarction is not linear with time, an observation originally stressed by Zumoff et al. (94), nor are the causes of death similar during different time-frames. These considerations also complicate the evaluation of a drug effect in this disorder. In describing mortality following an acute myocardial infarction, three periods with different rates and different primary causes of death can be readily identified.

Natural History of Cardiac Mortality Following an Acute Myocardial Infarction: By Period

In-hospital or recovery period

This is generally recognized as a time of very high mortality. In-hospital mortality is not linear with time but is highest during the 1st day and progressively decreases on a daily basis during the entire period of hospitalization, as is well documented in the literature (7,17,44,57,70,92). Illustrative of this point is the study by Beard et al. (7) of patients admitted to the U.S. Veterans Administration Hospitals who were 50 years of age or over. They observed annualized mortality rates of 438.9% for 0 to 7 days, 248.6% for 8 to 14 days, and 84% for 15 to 28 days.

The mortality during this in-hospital or recovery period (the latter usually refers to the first 30 days) varies considerably among reports since there are differences among the patient groups in length of hospitalization, age, sex, smoking habits, geographical areas, ethnic background, types of therapy, hospital facilities (coronary care units, etc.) and various other aspects. Ibrahim et al. (48) after a careful review of an extensive literature, concluded that mortality from the 1st hr to 30 days following hospitalization for an acute myocardial infarction averages 14.5% (the annual rate would be approximately 174%).

Early Post-Recovery Period

Following the recovery period, the mortality among survivors of a recent myocardial infarction progressively declines over approximately the next six months, and then reaches a steady and much lower level, as illustrated in Fig. 1. This figure, adapted from Cannom et al. (15), shows combined data on 188 patients discharged from the Yale-New Haven Hospital, 148 patients with a transmural infarction and 40 patients with a non-transmural infarction. The break in the survival curve, noted approximately 6 months after discharge, has been well recognized for many years (94) and has received adequate confirmation in the literature (7,8,15,44,70,92). This break serves to separate the entire postrecovery period into two periods; an early and a late postrecovery period based on different mortality rates. The early postrecovery period is a high mortality time during which mortality progressively decreases. The late postrecovery period is characterized by a low and constant mortality which extends for five or more years after the early period.

The differences in mortality between the first 6 months after discharge, early postrecovery period, and subsequent time periods is quite striking. Cannom et al. (15) found an 11.7% mortality during the first six months after discharge and 5.5% during the next six months. Weinblatt et al. (92) observed a cardiac mortality of

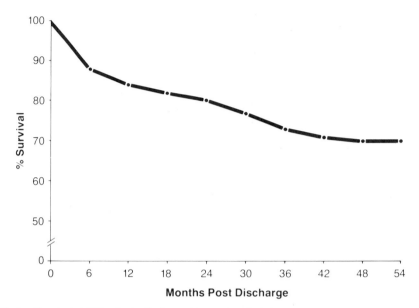

FIG. 1. Survival of 188 patients discharged from a hospital after an acute myocardial infarction. Adapted from Cannom et al. (Ref. 15). [Sherry, S. (1980): *Eur. J. Clin. Pharmacol.*, 17:401–407].

8.5% for the five-month period ending six months after the index infarction. The cardiac mortality for the periods 7 to 30 months and 31 to 54 months after the index infarction was 3.7% and 2.9%, respectively. Helmers et al. (44) described a 17.9% mortality during the first year after hospital discharge. Mortality during the first six months was 11.2% and during the second six months, 7.6%. In another study involving 12 different Swedish hospitals, Helmers and Lundman (43) reported 8.5% cardiac mortality during the first six months after discharge, mortality during the first two months was double that of the last two, and this accounted for 25% of all of the deaths encountered over a four- to five-year follow-up. Beard et al. (7) in their study observed a 28-day to 6-month (5-month period) mortality of 6.4%, and the mortality for the next six months was 4.6%. A Cooperative Study (17) formed a 29- to 90-day mortality of 4.52% (2.26% per month), a 91- to 120-day mortality of 4.56% (1.52% per month), and a 120- to 360-day mortality of 6.05% (0.76% per month). Bigger et al. (8) followed 100 patients discharged from the Presbyterian Hospital in New York City. Of the 19 cardiac deaths that occurred during the one-year observation period, 15 or 79% occurred during the first six months.

Estimates of the mortality during the early postrecovery period have varied widely, undoubtedly because of the many differences among the patient groups. However, a reasonable approximation for an average group would be that 6 to 10% of the survivors of the recovery period will die during the early postrecovery period (an annualized mortality rate of 12 to 20%).

Late Postrecovery Period

This period is characterized by a constant and low mortality extending for several years after the index infarction. The mortality during the late postrecovery period has been estimated at about 3 to 4% per year (70,92).

The data obtained from the placebo group in the Anturane Reinfarction Trial (ART) are also consistent with the previously published data on the natural history of cardiac mortality following an acute myocardial infarction (4). In Fig. 2, which presents the life-table cumulative mortality curve for the placebo group, note the break in the curve which occurs at period 7. Since each period is 28 days, this break falls 6 to 7 months after trial entry. The second break noted at period 18 is probably artifactual since it was produced by a small number of deaths at a time when the number of patients under observation was falling rapidly and subsequent mortality was no different than before.

Fifty-six percent of all the placebo deaths occurred during the first six months and the annualized mortality for the first six months of this trial was 10.3%. This is somewhat lower than the previous estimate, based on the literature, of 12 to 20%. However, in ART, deaths within the first seven days of entry, when mortality is highest, were non-analyzable. Patients with significant cardiomegaly or a classification greater than Killip Class II at trial entry, and consequently at high risk of dying of pump failure, were not eligible. Considering these restrictions the mortality would appear to be within predictable limits. As for the survivors who entered the 7- to 24-month period, the mortality observed in ART, 4.1%, was consistent with observations of others.

Based on the literature, Fig. 3 provides a schematic representation of the cumulative mortality following an acute myocardial infarction from the onset of the infarct and extending over a two-year period. Three periods are identified: the very-high-mortality recovery period of 30 days, the high-mortality early postrecovery period, and the low-mortality late postrecovery period. Note that mortality is progressively changing during the first two periods and constant during the last period.

This description of the natural history of mortality following acute myocardial infarction from a temporal standpoint emphasizes certain aspects essential to the proper design and interpretation of any therapeutic intervention: Unless the time frames of observation are exactly similar in both groups, errors in interpretation may arise. It is most desirable to have all patients enter the study at the same time after the infarct and to have them followed serially during the natural history of the disease. As Bigger et al. (8) have stated, "Because the excess influence on mortality exerted by infarction is almost dissipated by six months, any therapeutic intervention, such as antiarrhythmic prophylaxis or a cardiac surgical procedure, designed to alter favorably the post-hospital course of high risk patients should be applied early after acute myocardial infarction." A proper interpretation of the effect of any therapeutic intervention must take into account the disparate mortalities during each period, and the effect of any intervention should be analyzed separately for each period of different mortality.

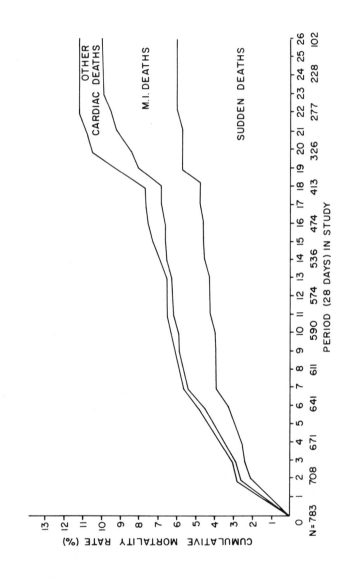

FIG. 2. Cumulative mortality by causes of analyzable death for eligible patients receiving placebo in the Anturane Reinfarction Trial. [Sherry, S. (1980): *Eur. J. Clin. Pharmacol.*, 17:401–407].

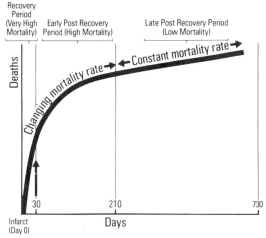

FIG. 3. Schematic representation of cumulative mortality following an acute myocardial infarction. [Sherry, S. (1980): *Eur. J. Clin. Pharmacol.*, 17:401–407].

The Natural History of Cardiac Mortality Following an Acute Myocardial Infarction: By Cause

While it is generally recognized that many different causes exist for cardiac mortality among survivors of myocardial infarction, recurrent myocardial infarction, sudden death, congestive heart failure, it is less well appreciated that the contribution of each of these causes of death varies during different periods, and these periods coincide well with the three distinct mortality periods described above.

Mortality during the Recovery Period

Aggressive monitoring of patients and prompt antiarrhythmic therapy, as practiced in hospitals today, has largely eliminated electrical instability as a prominent cause of in-hospital mortality among infarction patients. Currently, probably 90% of the deaths are mechanical, such as pump failure arising from the infarct itself or one of its direct complications. The observations reported of the in-hospital mortality at the Montreal Cardiological Institute (P. Theroux, *personal communication*) are fairly typical and include shock, 62%; congestive heart failure, 10%; cardiac rupture, 13%; renal failure, 5%; thromboembolism, 4%; sudden death, 2%; and all others, 4%. The most important prognostic indicator for survival during the recovery period appears to be the effect of the infarction itself on the mechanical efficiency of the heart as a pump.

Mortality During the Early Postrecovery Period

By the end of the recovery period, the mechanical aspects are no longer very prominent. They have either improved or are under control, or the patient has succumbed. However, the electrical instability of the heart, which accompanies the infarction, subsides only slowly over the next several months, and it and its lethal counterpart, sudden death, dominate mortality during the early postrecovery period. Bigger et al. (8) reported that 80% of the deaths during the first six months after discharge were sudden deaths, and a similar incidence was reported by Schulze et al. (78) from their study at Johns Hopkins Hospital. Helmers et al. (44) reported that a third of all of the sudden deaths observed in a five-year follow-up of a group of 475 patients occurred within the first six months. Others have commented that the first two- to three-month period following discharge from the hospital is remarkable for its high incidence of sudden death. Since electrical instability is the main factor determining mortality during this period, it is not surprising that the presence of complex ventricular arrhythmias on Holter monitoring has proven to be a useful indicator of prognosis (55,65,78).

Mortality During the Late Postrecovery Period

The cardiac death rate during this period (3 to 4% per year) is similar to that described for chronic ischemic heart disease in general (4,8) and the major causes of mortality are the same, recurrent myocardial infarction, congestive heart failure, sudden death, etc. In contrast to earlier periods, no one cause predominates. The enhanced risk of mortality associated with the acute infarction itself has essentially disappeared at the end of the early postrecovery period, and the patient entering the low-mortality late postrecovery period now has the same probability for survival as any patient with chronic ischemic heart disease and similar risk factors. Therefore, it is not surprising that the most important prognostic factor for patients in the late postrecovery period appears to be the nature and distribution of the underlying coronary vascular disease, as demonstrated by coronary angiography. Mechanical and electrical phenomena continue to play a contributory, but less important, role.

Based on these considerations, two additional points may be made concerning the interpretation of the results of long-term intervention trials of the effects of a drug on mortality following an acute myocardial infarction. Cognizance must be taken of the fact that cardiac mortality varies by cause during different time periods. Drugs used in long-term intervention trials are not likely to influence the various causes of mortality to the same degree and the effect may be expected to be more prominent at one time than another. Proper interpretation of a drug's effect, assuming great care has been taken in properly classifying the deaths by cause, requires an independent evaluation by cause as well as by period. This may be particularly important for sudden death, since the electrical instability of the heart during the early post-recovery period appears to be related to the acute infarct. Since the pathogenesis of a lethal reentry arrhythmia during the early and late postrecovery periods may be different, the drug's effect should be considered independently by period, as well as *in toto*.

Clinical Trials with Aspirin Alone

More studies have been conducted with aspirin than with the other drugs. Interest in the possible role of aspirin in coronary events was first expressed by Craven in the early 1950's when he reported that in 1,465 sedentary, overweight men, aged 45 to 65 years, placed on a daily regimen of 300 mg of aspirin over a 7-year period, no coronary occlusion or insufficiency occurred (20). While Cobb et al. (16) did not speculate on the association of aspirin therapy and the unexpectedly low incidence of myocardial infarction as the cause of death in the autopsy findings of a large series of patients dying with rheumatoid arthritis at the Massachusetts General Hospital, their observations, in retrospect, could be interpreted as providing evidence for Craven's view. However, it is only in the last decade that Craven's remarkable claims have found any support in subsequent studies.

In an epidemiological survey reported in 1974 (10), the Boston Collaborative Drug Surveillance Group found that the percentage of patients who had regularly, usually daily, but of undetermined dosage, taken aspirin during the month before hospitalization was significantly lower in 325 patients hospitalized with acute myocardial infarction than in 3,807 patients hospitalized for other causes (0.09% versus 4.9%). In an update of their retrospective data published two years later (11), the group reported that this negative association between aspirin use and risk of myocardial infarction was maintained with the accumulation of approximately twice the original data. The findings could not be taken as conclusive but they provided important impetus for several subsequent controlled prospective studies.

Another study was an American Cancer Society survey of records of over 1,000,000 men and women maintained during a 5-year period (37). A review of these records showed that the rate of death from coronary heart disease was no lower for those who took aspirin often than for those who took the drug seldom or never. Unfortunately, the use of aspirin and the cause of deaths were loosely defined in the records surveyed.

In an early attempt to study the issue prospectively, no benefit was found for aspirin. In a Finnish double-blind, prospective study conducted for a year in 430 aged people, all more than 70 years of age (mean, 79), no difference was found in morbidity (hospitalization) or mortality between the aspirin-treated (1 g daily) and control (placebo) groups (42). However, later studies have shown somewhat more interesting results.

Medical Research Council Studies

More direct support for aspirin's role in the secondary prevention of mortality from myocardial infarction came with the publication in 1974 of the results of a prospective, randomized, controlled Medical Research Council study conducted in England by Elwood et al. (27). In a double-blind trial, the investigators compared the effects on mortality of daily treatment with 300 g of aspirin for 2 years with those of placebo in 1,239 men who had a confirmed diagnosis of myocardial infarction. The low dosage of aspirin was chosen on the basis that it was well above the level needed to inhibit collagen- or ADP-induced platelet aggregation. In the aspirin-treated group, reductions in total mortality of 12% and 25% over that in the placebo group were found at 6 and 12 months, respectively. These reductions were not statistically significant. However, when the results were analyzed in respect to the interval between myocardial infarction and admission to the study, a stronger difference was found. Approximately half the patients entered the study less than 6 weeks after myocardial infarction. The mortality rate for the aspirin-treated group that entered the study within 6 weeks after myocardial infarction was 7.8% as compared to a 13.5% rate in the placebo group.

The same investigators recently completed another Medical Research Council Study of a similar multicenter, randomized, double-blind design (28). However, for this study, a higher daily dosage of aspirin, 900 mg (300 mg three times daily), was used, for a period of just one year. Women also were included in the study and comprised 15% of the total 1,682 patients in the study. In addition to the total mortality, mortality from ischemic heart disease, rehospitalization resulting from myocardial infarction, ischemic heart disease without myocardial infarction, or other causes were measured. The investigators attempted to measure compliance, on the basis of tests for salicylate made at unannounced home visits, and they estimated it to be at least 72%, and probably much higher. Although the withdrawal rate, primarily due to side effects, was high, it was evenly distributed, 228 patients, or 27%, from each group, and the withdrawals were included in the analysis.

The total mortality rate in patients given aspirin was 12.3%, compared to a rate of 14.8% in those receiving placebo. The 17.3% reduction in mortality attributable to aspirin was not statistically significant. However, these data may have been influenced by the fact that two factors strongly prognostic of death, pulmonary congestion and cardiac enlargement, were more common in the aspirin-treated group. The analysis of specific mortality resulting from ischemic heart disease suggested a greater, statistically significant reduction in the aspirin-treated group, but when this rate was adjusted for slight age differences between the groups, it was no longer significant.

There were only slight differences between the treatment groups in numbers of rehospitalizations for ischemic heart disease without myocardial infarction or for other causes. However, 7.1% of the aspirin-treated group were readmitted for infarction as compared with 10.9% for the placebo group—a 34% reduction that was statistically significant. The total mortality and the nonfatal ischemic heart disease morbidity increased with age in men but not consistently so in women. The combined rate was significantly reduced in the aspirin-treated group by 28% ($p < 0.05$) in all patients. However, in their report of their findings, the investigators note that the data on nonfatal reinfarctions were limited and uncertain.

The investigators found that the results consistently suggested a smaller benefit from aspirin for women than for men. They noted that their data "suggested that the difference between the treatments emerges very early and about three months after infarction little further difference developed." Their findings in this respect could not be considered conclusive.

Comment

The Elwood trials illustrate many of the problems previously discussed. In the first trial, the intent was to admit all patients within the first six weeks after their infarction and follow them for a period of two years. Later, so that the number of patients in the trial could be increased, patients were admitted who had had an infarction at any time during the previous six months. Although there was equal randomization between the patients in terms of their trial entry, each group now contained patients in whom not only the mortality risk had been markedly reduced but also possibly the preventable causes of death. The initial trend based on the early entry group, which was markedly in favor of aspirin, was soon blunted, and the benefit achieved never reached significance. Therefore, the second trial was designed to admit all patients early. However, the original design was not followed, and patients were admitted much earlier during the in-hospital period and as early as three days after infarction, the dose was changed from 0.3 g to 0.9 g daily, and women were included. In this intent-to-treat trial, a large number of dropouts were included in the analysis. As with the first trial, a difference between the treatment groups favoring aspirin appeared to emerge early after the infarction but after three months little further difference developed. It is unfortunate that both trials were not run similarly except for the entry point and that the trial size was not large enough to allow for an independent analysis of the late postrecovery period. These inconclusive studies still leave one with the impression that aspirin may reduce mortality during the early postrecovery period.

Coronary Drug Project Aspirin Study

The Coronary Drug Project Aspirin Study, completed in 1975, evaluated total mortality, cause-specific mortality, nonfatal events, and combinations of fatal and nonfatal events in aspirin-treated and control (placebo) groups (18). The study population was selected from groups who had been receiving dextrothyroxine or estrogen therapy in another coronary drug project study, but had stopped treatment. The 1,529 patients, all male, had had at least one documented myocardial infarction. One-third of them had had serious complications or more than one infarction. Five or more years had elapsed since the last infarction for approximately 75% of the patients, and more than 60% of them were over 55 years of age.

The patients were randomly assigned, on a double-blind basis, to daily treatment with 972 mg of aspirin (324 mg three times per day) or placebo, for a period ranging from 10 to 28 months. Patients were evaluated at 4-month intervals and compliance was monitored. Overall mortality was 5.8% in the aspirin group and 8.3% in the placebo group, a difference of 30%. In regard to cause-specific mortality, the aspirin group had a reduction relative to the placebo group of 27% for coronary death and 19% for sudden cardiovascular deaths, deaths occurring within 60 min after onset of symptoms.

The incidence of definite nonfatal myocardial infarction was only slightly lower in the aspirin group (3.7%) than in the placebo group (4.2%). The largest clinical difference in definite or suspect nonfatal cardiovascular events was for the development of hypertension since entry, which occurred in 12.2% and 9.6% of the aspirin and placebo groups, respectively—an incidence that was 27% higher in the aspirin group. All observed side effects were reported more frequently by the aspirin group than by the placebo group. The largest difference was for stomach pain and twice as many aspirin patients complained of such pains as did placebo patients, 12.5% for aspirin, 6.3% for placebo.

Comment

In this study, 75% or more of the patients had had their myocardial infarction five years or more earlier, and therefore, the placebo group mortality was low, approximately 4% per year. The number of patients in the trial was never enough to provide a statistically significant difference even if mortality in the aspirin group was reduced by 30%. Only one period of mortality was under study, the late postrecovery period. Finally, the study was complicated through the admission into the trial of three cohorts of patients from the Coronary Drug Project (those previously on high-dose estrogen, dextrothyroxine, and low-dose estrogen, with the latter being entered more than a year later than the others). The death rates in the placebo group of each of these cohorts differed, and the effect of aspirin, while positive in two, was negative in the other. While the data suggest that there may be some benefit from treatment with aspirin in patients whose infarct occurred many years earlier, during the late postrecovery period, the evidence supporting this conclusion is far from impressive.

German-Austrian Multicenter Study

In a German-Austrian, multicenter, prospective study, completed in 1977, aspirin was compared with phenprocoumon or placebo for the secondary prevention of myocardial infarction or sudden death (12,13). Of the 946 patients admitted to the study 4 to 6 weeks after their qualifying infarction, 78.5% were male. Patients were randomly placed in one of three treatment groups; aspirin, 1.5 g daily; placebo; or phenprocoumon.

Phenprocoumon, an anticoagulant widely used in Germany and Austria for the prevention of reinfarction, was given at a dosage adjusted individually to maintain prothrombin time values between 15% and 25% or thrombotest values around 10%. The trial was double-blind regarding the placebo or aspirin groups but open about treatment with phenprocoumon. Randomization was within strata, including hospital, age, sex, secondary infarction, cardiac failure, and hyperlipidemia or cholesterolemia.

Over a two-year period, patients received clinical and laboratory evaluations at 2- to 4-week intervals. Compliance was checked in subgroups through urine salicylate determinations. Nonfatal myocardial infarction and sudden death, as well as total and cardiac mortality, were selected as endpoints for the trial, and patients experiencing a nonfatal event were not returned to the study.

A final analysis of the data has not yet been published. However, some results have been reported (12). A total of 61 patients died of verified myocardial infarction or sudden death during the trial, most during the first half year. The highest numbers of coronary deaths occurred in the phenprocoumon group with 26 and the placebo group with 22. Only 13 such deaths occurred in the aspirin group. This reduction reaches a level of statistical significance close to a p value of 0.05. When compared to the placebo, the benefit from aspirin was restricted to the first six months, although, because of the relatively small numbers of deaths during this period, a statistically significant benefit could not be established.

The investigators analyzed risk factors in relation to their results and found that the most relevant risk factors for death were reinfarction as the qualifying event for entry into the study and heart failure within four weeks after the initial infarction. Side effects occurred most frequently in the aspirin group, especially gastrointestinal complaints.

Comment

The trial, while not conclusive because of the relatively small numbers of patients studied (309 placebo, 317 aspirin, and 320 phenprocoumon), is, like the Elwood studies, highly suggestive that aspirin may reduce mortality from acute coronary events during the early postrecovery period but not thereafter. The dose of aspirin, 1.5 g daily, is the largest used in any of the aspirin trials and is at a level likely to interfere with prostacyclin production. However, the beneficial effects claimed, 42% reduction in deaths as compared to placebo group, are as great, if not greater, than those observed in Elwood's study using 0.3 g daily.

Aspirin Myocardial Infarction Study

The largest prospective trial of aspirin for the secondary prevention of death from myocardial infarction has been the Aspirin Myocardial Infarction Study (AMIS) (5). This double-blind, controlled study, sponsored by the National Heart, Lung, and Blood Institute and conducted at 30 clinical centers in the United States, was designed to test whether the regular administration of aspirin to patients who had experienced at least one documented myocardial infarction would result in a significant reduction in total mortality over a three-year period. Secondary objectives, such as cause-specific mortality and nonfatal cardiovascular events, were also evaluated.

Over a 13-month period, 4,524 patients with a previous, documented myocardial infarction were enrolled in the study. Of these, 4,021 (89%) were men. The patients were between the ages of 30 to 69 years, with a mean age of 54.8 years. Patients were randomly assigned to treatment with aspirin or placebo in a double-blind fashion. Based on the experience of the Coronary Drug Project Aspirin Study (18), a total daily dosage of 1.0 g (0.5 g twice daily) of aspirin was selected.

The time of entrance into the study after the qualifying myocardial infarction ranged anywhere from eight weeks to as long as five years, with a mean of 25 months. Results were further compromised by the fact that, by an accident in the randomization process, seven baseline characteristics were distributed unevenly enough between the two groups to make the discrepancies statistically significant.

These risk factors included previous heart failure, angina pectoris, cardiomegaly, and histories of using digitalis, nitroglycerin, propranolol, or other drugs. For all seven, the inferred risk fell more heavily on the aspirin group. During the minimum three-year follow-up period, the initial baseline characteristics were reviewed at four-month intervals. Various biochemical measurements also were recorded during the course of the study. Compliance was checked and estimated to be very good.

Fatal events were analyzed with the Cox statistical procedure based on a proportional hazard model. For nonfatal events, such as recurrent myocardial infarction, angina pectoris, stroke, intermittent cerebral ischemic attacks, and cardiovascular surgery, a 2×2 table analysis was employed. All patients were included in the analysis. In terms of the study's endpoint, total mortality, no significant benefit from aspirin was found. The total mortality rate after 38 months of follow-up was 10.8% in the aspirin group and 9.7% in the placebo group. The cardiovascular-morbidity tallies favored the aspirin-treated group. The percentage of nonfatal myocardial infarction was 6.3% in the aspirin group versus 8.1% in the placebo group. Only unimpressive differences were found between men's and women's responses to aspirin, although the women had a lower overall mortality rate.

In reference to side effects, symptoms suggestive of peptic ulcer, gastritis, or erosion of the gastric mucosa, bloody stools, and symptomatic gout occurred in 23.7% of those taking aspirin and 14.9% of those receiving placebo. Three times as many patients receiving aspirin as those receiving placebo complained of gastrointestinal problems, including heartburn, stomach pain, nausea, vomiting, and constipation. On the basis of their findings, the investigator stated that "aspirin is not recommended for routine use in patients who have survived an MI."

Comment

This study, involving a very large number of patients followed for a three-year period, was designed to be the *definitive* study on aspirin. Unfortunately, it was based on the findings of the Coronary Drug Project Aspirin study and did not take into account the findings of the first Elwood study, nor the natural history of mortality following an acute myocardial infarction. It was primarily a study of a dose of 1 g of aspirin given daily during the late postrecovery period. The findings are not dissimilar from those reported in the two Elwood trials or the German-Austrian multicenter study for this particular period. It is sad that the trial was not designed as a study of the effect of aspirin on the natural history of mortality following an acute infarction, with all patients entering during a rather narrow window shortly after survival from an acute infarction. The trial offers no useful data for the period during which others claim that aspirin may have a beneficial effect.

Single-Dose Study

Another study, sponsored by the Medical Research Council in England, investigated the effects upon mortality of a *single* dose of aspirin, 300 mg, given to patients who had experienced acute symptoms suggestive of myocardial infarction. They measured mortality within three days. In an analysis of 1,705 such patients (29), no benefit was found within 28 days.

Other Studies in Progress or Unpublished

An open, randomized study of the effects of aspirin, 1.5 g daily, compared to those of oral anticoagulants on reinfarction and cardiac death in patients with myocardial infarction has been conducted in 15 hospitals in France under the Institut National de la Santé et de la Recherche Médicale (INSERM). Details of the study have not yet been published. An enrollment of 1500 patients to be followed for 2 years is planned (88).

No other studies known to us are presently in progress for the investigation of treatment with aspirin alone for the *secondary* prevention of death in patients with ischemic heart disease, as indicated by prior myocardial infarction. However, two studies have been started to study the effects of aspirin on myocardial infarction and death in patients with unstable angina pectoris. One double-blind, randomized study, being conducted in 10 Veterans Administration hospitals in the United States, compares the effects of low doses of aspirin, 324 mg, and of placebo given daily for 12 weeks (89). The patients are men who have been admitted to a coronary care unit for new or worsening angina and have evidence of coronary artery disease but not acute myocardial infarction.

The other double-blind, randomized study, sponsored by the Medical Research Council of Canada and designed to cover a two-year period will measure the effects of aspirin (1.3 g daily) and sulfinpyrazone (800 mg daily), singly and in combination, compared to a placebo in 700 patients admitted to a coronary care unit with unstable angina pectoris. The study, scheduled for completion in 1984, will have acute myocardial infarction and death as its endpoints (M. Gent, *personal communication*).

A large study of aspirin in the primary prevention of death and cardiovascular events, stroke and heart attack, is being conducted in 4,200 healthy subjects (all physicians) in England (89). Patients have been randomly allocated to a control (untreated) group or treatment with aspirin, 500 mg daily.

General Comment on Studies with Aspirin Alone

The results of the various prospective studies with aspirin alone in reducing cardiac mortality following an acute myocardial infarction remain inconclusive. In those trials where aspirin was tested soon after an infarction, there appears to be a beneficial effect in reducing the high mortality during the early postrecovery period. In general, the findings are reminiscent of those more clearly established with sulfinpyrazone in the Anturane Reinfarction Trial. When beneficial results have been claimed, they have been observed with doses of aspirin varying from 0.3 to 1.5 g daily. This suggests that the dosage of aspirin may not be as critical *in vivo* as postulated on the basis of *in vitro* studies.

Clinical Trials with Dipyridamole and Aspirin

The rationale for combined treatment with dipyridamole and aspirin is based on a possible synergistic effect, since aspirin inhibits production of the platelet-aggregating substance, thromboxane A_2, while dipyridamole enhances the action of prostacyclin, an inhibitor of platelet aggregation (61), which is inhibited by aspirin. The recent Persantine®-Aspirin Reinfarction Study (PARIS) compared the effects of combined treatment with dipyridamole (Persantine®) and aspirin with those of aspirin alone or placebo on mortality and morbidity in patients with previous myocardial infarction (71).

In the double-blind trial conducted at 20 clinical centers in the United States and England, 2,026 patients, aged 30 to 74 years, of whom 1,759 (87%) were men, were randomly given one of the following treatments three times daily: dipyridamole, 75 mg, and aspirin 324 mg; aspirin, 324 mg, and one placebo tablet; two placebo tablets. There were 810 patients allocated to each of the two active treatment groups, and 406 to the placebo group. Patients were started in the trial anytime from 8 weeks to as long as 5 years after a myocardial infarction documented by EKG changes and enzyme elevations. The primary endpoints evaluated were total mortality, coronary mortality, and coronary incidence defined as coronary death or definite but nonfatal myocardial infarction.

Follow-up visits were scheduled one month after entry into the study and at 4-month intervals thereafter, for an average follow-up period of 44 months. Compliance was monitored at these visits by tablet count and urine testing for drugs and was found to be similar in the three groups. Of the total 2,026 patients, 1,666 completed the trial. Another 224 patients were reported deceased. The remaining 136 patients withdrew from the study; of these one was known to have died, 128 were known to be alive, and the fate of seven was unknown at the time the results were reported.

Total mortality was 16% and 18% lower in the dipyridamole/aspirin and aspirin groups than in the placebo group. Three-quarters of the deaths were coronary in nature. There were 24% and 21% fewer coronary deaths in the dipyridamole/aspirin and aspirin groups, than in the placebo group. Coronary *incidence* was reduced by 25% and 24% in these groups. The aspirin group had the highest incidence of sudden coronary death, with 5.6% of the group's patients dying within one hr after the onset of symptoms. The aspirin group showed the lowest incidence of non-sudden coronary death—2.5%, compared to 5.7% and 4.0% in the placebo and dipyridamole/aspirin groups.

None of the differences were statistically significant at a Z value greater than 2.6, the critical value chosen for the study. However, significant differences in coronary *incidence* between the dipyridamole/aspirin and placebo groups were found after 4, 8, 12, 16, 20, and 24 months of treatment. Patients enrolled within 6 months after myocardial infarction had fewer deaths in the active treatment groups, a reduction of 44% in the combination group and 51% in the aspirin group. However, the number of patients enlisted so soon after myocardial infarction was limited to

179 in the dipyridamole/aspirin group, 173 in the aspirin group, and 95 in the placebo group.

Both active treatment groups showed a reduction in incidence of definite nonfatal MI, angina pectoris requiring hospitalization, and stroke. Both showed a higher incidence of acute coronary insufficiency than the placebo group. The largest difference occurred for congestive heart failure; both active treatment groups showed a lower incidence than the placebo group, but neither difference was statistically significant.

Several additional analyses were conducted to assess the occurrence of angina during the trial. Between-group differences were small, with no detectable effect, adverse or beneficial, in either active treatment group. The expected aspirin-related side effects appeared in both active treatment groups. These reactions included stomach pain, heartburn, nausea, gastrointestinal irritation, and gastrointestinal bleeding. The combination group also showed a significant increase in headache incidence.

Because of the marked reductions in total and coronary deaths in patients entering the PARIS trial within 6 months after infarction and treated with aspirin and dipyridamole, another large-scale study is being undertaken by the same investigators in patients enrolled within four months after myocardial infarction. This study will compare the combination treatment with placebo only.

Comment

While this study did not show a statistically significant benefit from treatment with aspirin alone or in combination with dipyridamole, in contrast to the results of AMIS, it does suggest an appreciable reduction in fatal coronary events and in combined fatal and nonfatal coronary episodes (coronary incidence). Furthermore, this beneficial effect could more readily be demonstrated among those patients who entered the trial within six months of their qualifying myocardial infarction, during a period of increased mortality risk (early postrecovery period). In this respect, the findings in the aspirin group of PARIS are reminiscent of the observations previously reported in the Elwood studies (27,28) and the German-Austrian multicenter trial (12,13).

Whether the addition of dipyridamole to aspirin in the dosages employed provided any additional benefit over that claimed for aspirin alone was not determined by this trial. While some of the clinical endpoints appeared to favor the combination therapy, others favored aspirin alone.

While PARIS and AMIS had an essentially common protocol and were undertaken at the same time, their results appear to be dissimilar and have been interpreted differently. Perhaps this discrepancy is due to a major difference in the size of the placebo group relative to the test group. In PARIS there were only 400 placebo patients, compared to 800 patients in each of the active drug compartments. In essence, PARIS was designed to take advantage of the large placebo compartment of 2,257 patients in AMIS, on the assumption that the PARIS and AMIS placebo results would be similar, and for this reason, only a small placebo compartment would be necessary. However, as seen in Table 1, this supposition proved to be incorrect.

In effect, the benefits ascribed to aspirin and the combination therapy in PARIS may be related to a spuriously high mortality observed in the small placebo compartment of PARIS rather than to the positive effect of the active drugs being tested. If the mortality rates in the aspirin and dipyridamole/aspirin compartments of PARIS are compared to that of the large placebo compartment of AMIS, which involved patients of a similar type studied at the same time, no difference is apparent.

The small placebo compartment in PARIS also creates problems in interpretation of the differences in results for those patients who entered the trial within six months of their qualifying infarction and those who entered later. Since approximately 20% entered less than 6 months after infarction, the benefit claimed is based on a study of only 95 placebo patients and 173 and 179 aspirin and dipyridamole/aspirin patients, and is related more to the soft endpoints, coronary events requiring hospitalization, than to the hard endpoint, mortality. A new study is underway, that may provide an answer to the questions raised by the first PARIS study.

Clinical Trials with Sulfinpyrazone

Sulfinpyrazone, a uricosuric agent used since the 1950's for the treatment of gout, was first reported to have platelet-regulating action in 1965 (79). In the ensuing decade, its effects were studied in the prevention of arteriovenous shunt thrombosis (49), recurrent venous thrombosis (80), and thromboembolism in patients with prosthetic cardiac valves (82). In 1975, in a double-blind, placebo-controlled study of 291 elderly male patients, sulfinpyrazone was reported to significantly reduce mortality from vascular causes in a subgroup of 166 atherosclerotic patients (9).

Anturane Reinfarction Trial

In 1975 a large-scale, double-blind study of the effects of sulfinpyrazone on cardiac mortality in patients with a recent myocardial infarction was undertaken (3,4). The study, conducted over a 3-year period at 26 clinical centers in the United States and Canada, and designated the Anturane Reinfarction Trial, compared sulfinpyrazone, 800 mg daily (200 mg four times per day), with placebo for an average period of 16 months. Patients were enrolled in the study 25 to 35 days after the occurrence of a documented myocardial infarction.

TABLE 1. *Cumulative annual mortality (%) by drug group in AMIS and PARIS*

	Placebo	Aspirin	Dipyridamole/Aspirin
AMIS	8.8	9.6	
PARIS	11.4	9.0	9.4

In contrast to previous, intent-to-treat trials, the Anturane Reinfarction trial was designed as a clinical efficacy study. This was considered possible without creating bias for the following reasons: (a) sulfinpyrazone could not be differentiated from the placebo by either patient or physician on the basis of taste, color, or appearance; (b) sulfinpyrazone would produce no unique symptoms or signs that would allow it to be identified either by the patient or physician; (c) all laboratory determinations were carried out in a central laboratory and, in addition, uric acid determinations were blanked out from any laboratory assays conducted on trial patients at the respective participating institutions; (d) all criteria were set forth clearly in the protocol and operations manual before the trial was initiated; (e) the accuracy of the data collected was reviewed both during the trial and retrospectively by several audits carried out at different levels by independent groups with expertise in the conduct of such audits, and (f) all decisions were made on a blind basis without knowledge of drug assignment, and were reviewed at three independent levels.

It was deemed feasible to establish beforehand that the primary analysis would be of cardiac deaths only among eligible patients with analyzable events, according to clearly defined criteria for eligibility and analyzability established before the inception of the trial. Prior to the start of the trial, specific criteria were established for the classifications of death as "sudden death," "myocardial infarction," or "other cardiac" deaths. Sudden death was an unobserved death or one that occurred within 60 min of the onset of symptoms. Myocardial infarction had to be documented at autopsy, or by clinical evidence of pain, EKG findings, and by elevation of a serum enzyme, serum glutamic oxaloacetic transaminase, lactic dehydrogenase, or creatinine phosphokinase, to twice the normal level. The other cardiac category included congestive heart failure, arrhythmia, or cardiogenic shock.

All deaths in eligible patients were further classified as analyzable or nonanalyzable. A death was considered nonanalyzable if it occurred within seven days after the initiation or termination of therapy, in a patient who did not comply with instructions, of if it could be attributed directly to surgery without association with a nonfatal event occurring during treatment. Analyzable deaths formed a basis for the primary analysis of the efficacy of sulfinpyrazone.

Of the original 1,629 patients in the study, 1,143 (73%) completed the protocol and were included in the primary analysis. Of the remainder, 415 withdrew prematurely for various medical and nonmedical reasons, and 71 were excluded from analysis by the study's policy committee because they were judged, on a blind basis, not to meet the protocol criteria.

Follow-up visits were scheduled at 4, 8, 10, 14, 16, 20, and 22 months after entry into the study. Eighty-seven percent of the patients consistently took at least 80% of their medication, as measured by tablet counts at these visits. Serum uric acid levels were also measured as an indication of compliance with sulfinpyrazone therapy.

Side effects were recorded at each visit according to frequency, severity, and duration. Thromboembolic events were reported in 36 patients (5%) receiving placebo and only 19 patients (2%) of those receiving sulfinpyrazone. Gastrointestinal problems were reported by 214 patients taking sulfinpyrazone and 185 placebo-treated patients. Side effects were reported by 84% of the placebo-treated patients and 81% of those receiving sulfinpyrazone. Fifty-eight patients withdrew from the trial because of these events, but they were equally distributed between the groups.

All 106 analyzable deaths reported in the study were cardiovascular in nature, 105 were cardiac, the primary endpoint, and one was cerebrovascular. After 24 months the observed reduction in cardiac mortality from sulfinpyrazone treatment was approximately 32% ($p = 0.058$). Over half of the deaths were sudden cardiac deaths and the reduction in this category was mainly responsible for the overall reduction. There were 37 sudden deaths in the placebo group versus 22 in the sulfinpyrazone-treated group, a reduction of 43% ($p = 0.041$). This advantage occurred during the first 6 months of treatment when the rate of analyzable sudden deaths was 7% in the placebo group versus 1.8% in the sulfinpyrazone-treated group, a highly significant reduction of 74% ($p = 0.003$). After this time the rates of sudden death were comparable for the two groups, 2.0% with placebo versus 2.3% with sulfinpyrazone treatment.

The reduction in sudden deaths, when nonanalyzable sudden deaths were included, was 68% at six months for the sulfinpyrazone-treated group. By this time, the majority of sudden deaths had already occurred. For the entire 24-month observation period, the reduction rate was 41%. Sulfinpyrazone had no effect upon analyzable deaths from myocardial infarction. There were 18 deaths in the placebo group and 17 in the sulfinpyrazone group after 24 months.

In reporting these findings, the investigators noted that the first six months after myocardial infarction are a period of high risk, particularly from sudden death, directly related to the previous myocardial infarction. It is during this period, early postrecovery period, that sulfinpyrazone exerts its effect. They also noted that while the study was undertaken because of sulfinpyrazone's known effects upon platelet function, the fact that it was effective in reducing sudden cardiac deaths, but not deaths from myocardial infarction, suggests that another, yet unknown, mechanism of action exists.

Anturane Reinfarction Italian Study

A trial, similar in design to the Anturane Reinfarction Trial, and designated "The Anturane Reinfarction Italian Study" (ARIS), is just reaching completion. This study differed from the larger American counterpart in several respects (74). The daily dosage of sulfinpyrazone, 800 mg, was given in two doses of 400 mg per day instead of four 200 mg doses. Patients also were enrolled in the study a week or two earlier after their qualifying infarction—10 to 20 days. In addition to fatal reinfarction and sudden cardiac death, nonfatal myocardial infarction serves as an endpoint for the study. Finally, platelet function tests were performed during the course of the study to see if a correlation exists between therapeutic effects and effects on platelet function.

The study was designed for a population of 650 patients of both sexes, to be followed for a period of at least one year. A preliminary report described details of 400 patients enrolled at the time and preliminary findings of the platelet function studies (19). Final results have yet to be published. As mentioned previously, a large Canadian study comparing the effects of sulfinpyrazone and aspirin, singly and in combination, in patients with unstable angina is currently in progress.

General Comment on Studies with Sulfinpyrazone

A great deal of publicity has been given to sulfinpyrazone. The Anturane Reinfarction Trial is the only study that has claimed a major benefit for the agent in reducing cardiac mortality following an acute myocardial infarction, and this through a striking reduction in sudden death during the first six-months, high-risk early postrecovery period, following discharge of the patient from the hospital. This claim was possible because of the unique features of the trial design, as a clinical efficacy study. By avoiding the various dilution factors inherent in intent-to-treat trials, this study allowed for a quantitative assessment of the drug's actual effect in compliant patients. In addition, because of the early and narrow entry window, 25–35 days after the qualifying infarction, the trial studied the effect of this drug on the natural history of mortality among recent survivors of an infarct by both period and cause.

Considering the negative results of the Aspirin Myocardial Infarction Study (AMIS) and the inconclusive results of the Persantine®-Aspirin Reinfarction Study (PARIS), it is not surprising that the trial has come under considerable criticism. The U.S. Food and Drug Administration has raised serious questions as to the classification of certain of the deaths, sudden, myocardial infarction, other cardiac, within each treatment group. A review of the deaths by an independent panel of cardiologists recently convened for this purpose should clarify this issue.

While the emphasis on the reduction of sudden death alone may or may not require modification, the overall reduction in cardiac mortality during the early postrecovery period is not dissimilar to the beneficial effects ascribed to aspirin during this period in both the Elwood studies (27,28), and the German-Austrian multicenter trial (12,13). This also was true of those patients receiving the combination of aspirin and dipyridamole in the Persantine®-Aspirin Reinfarction Study who were entered within the first six months of their qualifying infarction.

The claim that sulfinpyrazone reduces the incidence of sudden death and not fatal myocardial infarction has stimulated research on possible other actions of this drug that could account for this finding. Since most sudden deaths are due to the appearance of a lethal ventricular arrhythmia, the effect of this drug on experimentally-induced ventricular arrhythmias arising from an ischemic myocardium in animals has been under study and a number of interesting observations have been made (51,64,75). Since an observation of a similar action by aspirin was reported (63), an effect of these agents on prostaglandin pathways other than platelets may be involved in any possible beneficial therapeutic effect.

The striking results of the Anturane Reinfarction Trial require confirmation. Great interest can be attached to the results of the Italian study. Unfortunately, the size of this trial, approximately 650 patients, is probably too small to yield statistically significant differences even if the differences observed are similar to those described in the Anturane Reinfarction Trial. The importance of this study probably will relate more to whether the various period and cause mortality rates are or are not influenced in a similar fashion to that described in the North American study.

PREVENTION OF THROMBOEMBOLISM ASSOCIATED WITH PROSTHETIC HEART VALVES AND RHEUMATIC HEART DISEASE

Although innovations in the technique and materials used in cardiovascular prostheses have improved the general prognosis of patients receiving artificial heart valves and arterial grafts, these prostheses still tend to be thrombogenic. Shortened platelet survival time is observed in the majority of patients receiving prosthetic heart valves, and this high platelet consumption correlates significantly with the frequency of thrombosis and thromboembolism.

Conventional anticoagulant therapy (e.g., warfarin) is essential and frequently anticoagulant prophylaxis is continued for life. However, these drugs do not alter platelet survival time (39,91). Sulfinpyrazone, dipyrimadole, and aspirin have been tested for their antithrombotic effect in patients with prosthetic heart valves. Simultaneous laboratory testing of platelet reactivity in these patients has demonstrated that platelet survival time does correlate with thromboembolic risk and that normalization of platelet turnover reduces the risk of thromboembolism (81,85,91).

Studies with Sulfinpyrazone

In one of the earliest studies of platelet inhibitors in patients with cardiac prostheses, 800 mg/day of sulfinpyrazone, was found to increase platelet survival time in seven of nine patients with prosthetic mitral valves. During the 16-week postoperative follow-up, however, no decrease in platelet adhesiveness or aggregation was noted (90). In a later study (91) involving 55 patients with mitral or aortic valve replacements, 22 with identified shortened platelet survival time were treated with sulfinpyrazone, 800 mg/day, in conjunction with warfarin. Platelet survival time became normal in 11 patients and increased in another seven. This study was important, for it demonstrated that the thrombogenic potential may not only be related to preoperative platelet abnormalities in a given patient but also to the particular valve used. Patients with mitral valve disease were more prone to thromboembolism than those with aortic valve disease.

In a further refinement of this suggestion of the thrombogenic potential of certain grafts, Steele et al. (82) found that a directly sewn aortic homograft was superior to stented valves. The patients at highest risk remained those with a history of thromboembolism. These patients invariably had shortened platelet survival and were immediately considered for platelet suppressant therapy. Six such patients received sulfinpyrazone (800 gm/day) and two received dipyridamole (100 mg/day) plus aspirin (1200 mg/day). Warfarin was maintained concomitantly throughout treatment with the platelet inhibitors. A platelet survival test was performed before and three months after treatment. Dipyridamole and aspirin prolonged platelet survival in one patient and sulfinpyrazone significantly prolonged platelet survival in five patients, from 2.5 ± 0.18 to 3.4 ± 0.14 days ($p < 0.001$). During the subsequent 18 months, none of the eight patients developed thromboembolism.

Steele and coworkers later confirmed that platelet survival time provides a reliable measure of thromboembolic risk (84–86). In one of their studies of 126 patients with aortic or mitral valve replacement, they found that thromboembolism tends not to occur in patients with normal postoperative platelet survival time. When 94 patients at risk with shortened platelet survival time were placed on sulfinpyrazone therapy, 800 mg per day, for up to one year, usually in conjunction with warfarin, eleven developed thromboembolism, five following mitral valve replacement and six after aortic valve replacement. Among the remaining patients treated with sulfinpyrazone, platelet survival time increased significantly. When the results were analyzed by type of valve, it was found that platelet survival times were shorter in patients with mitral valve replacements. The Björk-Shiley aortic valve was associated with significantly longer platelet survival times than several Starr-Edwards models.

Studies with Dipyridamole and Aspirin

Aspirin and dipyridamole have been studied individually and in combination in several double-blind studies in patients with prosthetic heart valves. In a double-blind study by Sullivan et al. (87), dipyridamole (400 mg/day) was compared to placebo in 163 patients with prosthetic valve replacements. Warfarin was employed concomitantly in all patients. After one year survival rates in both groups were comparable, but the incidence of embolism was significantly lower in the dipyridamole-treated group.

There have been two double-blind studies in which the possible additive effect of 1 g of aspirin per day with anticoagulants was compared to that of anticoagulants alone (22,24). The patients had received aortic ball valves. During the observation period of 1 to 2 years, the aspirin-anticoagulant combination provided significantly better protection. In one study, the incidence of emboli occurred at a rate of 1.76 episodes/100 patients per year with the combination versus 9.32 episodes/100 patients per year with anticoagulants alone. Dale (22) also tested the effect of aspirin alone by gradually withdrawing anticoagulants from 77 patients. However, embolic events increased considerably within 5 months and anticoagulant therapy had to be reinstated.

Hetzer et al. (45) studied the incidence of thromboembolic complications in groups of patients receiving either warfarin or aspirin, 600 mg/day, or no anticoagulation medication at all. The patients had received mitral valve replacement with the Hancock xenograft. The authors concluded that aspirin was useful as long-term postoperative therapy in combination with warfarin, particularly in patients with a history of systemic emboli or atrial clots.

Dale et al. (23) conducted a small pilot study in which five patients were given three 3-week sequences of the following antithrombotic regimens: (a) dipyridamole:

150 mg/day, 75 mg/day, 150 mg/day; (b) aspirin, 1 g twice daily; and (c) dipyrid-amole, 150 mg/day; dipyridamole, 75 mg/day, and aspirin, 0.5 g/day; aspirin, 0.5 g/day. Starr-Edwards aortic ball valve prostheses had been placed one to four years previously and digitoxin and warfarin had been maintained throughout that period. Prior to treatment, mean platelet half-life was 3.52 days. Dipyridamole alone, aspirin alone, or the combination of dipyridamole and aspirin did not increase platelet survival time significantly. With aspirin and with the combination, collagen-induced platelet aggregation was markedly reduced ($p < 0.001$) and bleeding time was prolonged.

Like Dale, Moggio et al. (60) singled out patients given cloth-covered Starr-Edwards mitral or aortic valves. Of 183 patients, 58 received no anticoagulation, 48 received warfarin, 70 received aspirin, 10 g twice daily, and seven received dipyridamole, 100 mg four times daily. The incidence of emboli in the dipyridamole group was 10 per 100 patients per year as compared to 1.2 for warfarin, 2.6 for aspirin, and 4.0 for those without anticoagulation therapy. The authors favored either warfarin or the warfarin-aspirin combination, as both demonstrated compa-rable prophylaxis against thromboembolism.

Sands et al. (77) agreed that adequate anticoagulant therapy is a most important factor in the postoperative prognosis of patients receiving cardiovascular prostheses. They reported excellent postoperative responses in two patients who received 100 mg of dipyridamole, 600 mg of aspirin, and warfarin daily following implantation of Björk-Shiley aortic valves. When warfarin was electively withdrawn after five months, severe thrombus formation developed around the valve, leading to irre-versible complications in both cases.

Acute thrombotic obstruction with Björk-Shiley mitral or aortic valves was also reported in 8 of 159 patients who had received these prostheses (62). Of six patients with occluded mitral prostheses, one survived, as did the two patients with occluded aortic valves. The onset of symptoms, occurring 10 to 53 months after placement, was sudden, as described by Sands et al. (77), and progressed rapidly. At the time of onset, seven of the eight patients were on a regimen of aspirin (900 to 1200 mg/day) plus dipyridamole (100 to 400 mg/day). Coumarin derivatives had been discontinued because of hemorrhaging. The authors recommended that when an-ticoagulants cannot be maintained, patients be observed very closely and that im-mediate surgical intervention is indicated whenever prosthetic clicks disappear or when there is echocardiographic or fluoroscopic evidence of impaired disc function.

General Comment

In the presence, but not in the absence, of anticoagulation, sulfinpyrazone, as-pirin, and the combination of dipyridamole and aspirin appear to be effective in reducing the incidence of thromboembolic complications associated with prosthetic heart valves (the effectiveness for dipyridamole alone, i.e., without aspirin, remains unclear). However, it should be recognized that combined therapy increases the bleeding risk associated with anticoagulant therapy due to: (a) enhancement of the anticoagulant activity of the coumarins by aspirin or sulfinpyrazone, since the latter compete for the coumarin binding sites on plasma proteins; and (b) inhibition of platelet function and coagulation is a more severe hemostatic defect than either alone. Consequently, combined therapy requires more careful monitoring and adjustment of coumarin dosage as well as increasing the risk of bleeding episodes. This becomes an important factor in the selection of patients for combined therapy.

While the studies of Steele and Weily appear to relate the action of these platelet-active drugs to their effects in improving platelet survival, the positive clinical response attributed to aspirin, which does not influence platelet survival, casts doubt on the validity of this hypothesis.

PREVENTION OF OCCLUSION OF AN AORTOCORONARY BYPASS

The effect of platelet-active drugs in patients with an aortocoronary bypass has been studied within only the last several years. As with prosthetic heart valves, there appears to be a definite relationship between shortened platelet survival time and saphenous vein graft occlusion (83).

A study in dogs using dipyridamole combined with aspirin suggested that platelet-active drugs may be useful in reducing platelet deposition following a saphenous vein bypass graft (34). However, McEnany and coworkers (56) found that warfarin was superior to both placebo and aspirin in maintaining graft patency 6 to 40 months after aortocoronary bypass.

In a controlled randomized study by Pantely et al. (68), three groups of patients who underwent aortocoronary bypass graft surgery received one of the following three regimens: dipyridamole (75 mg) and aspirin (325 mg) three times daily; warfarin therapy; or no medication at all. Treatment began on the third postoperative day and continued for six months. At the end of that period, no significant difference was found between groups as to vein-graft patency or various hemodynamic, angiographic, or clinical findings. Similar results were reported by Phillips et al. (72), except that they found that patients who had received the dipyridamole-aspirin combination experienced fewer embolic episodes than control patients.

It has been suggested (36) that the dipyridamole-aspirin combination would have proven more effective in the Pantely study had it been initiated earlier after surgery before mechanisms of platelet activation and release could proceed. It was also suggested that the dose of aspirin in the Pantely study was too high (53,69).

The only study to date using sulfinpyrazone in this regard was conducted by Baur and his associates (6). Sulfinpyrazone (800 mg/day) was compared to placebo in 255 patients. The drug was started 24 hr after surgery. The incidence of early graft closure was 3.8% in the sulfinpyrazone group versus 9.1% in the placebo group ($p < 0.025$). Sulfinpyrazone was particularly effective in reducing the early closure rate in grafts with a flow of more than 30 ml/min.

Comment

The evaluation of platelet-active drugs in preventing the late closure of coronary bypass remains an area of active investigation but, at present, no firm conclusion can be drawn. As with the thromboembolic complications associated with prosthetic valves, it may be difficult to show an effect of these agents in the absence of anticoagulation. Both platelets and fibrin appear to play an important role in these situations and a combined form of therapy may be necessary to achieve maximal benefit.

CEREBROVASCULAR DISEASE STUDIES

Secondary Prevention of Transient Ischemic Attacks (TIAs), Stroke, and Death in Patients with TIAs

Cerebral transient ischemic attacks (TIAs) are known to be frequent precursors of stroke and death (25), and thromboembolism is thought to play a major role in their pathogenesis (35). An early double-blind study (1) of the effect of dipyridamole in 169 patients with cerebral ischemia, however, showed no benefit from treatment with the drug. The first evidence for an effect by platelet-active drugs came in 1971 and 1972 in the form of case reports (40,66) of two patients and one patient, respectively, with amaurosis fugax. Aspirin was found to reduce, or, in the latter case, abolish attacks of transient blindness in these patients. When dipyridamole was given to one of these patients, it had no effect.

In 1972, Evans (30) published findings of a 12-week, double-blind crossover comparison of sulfinpyrazone (200 mg four times daily) and placebo in 20 patients with amaurosis fugax. He found that treatment with sulfinpyrazone significantly reduced the number of subsequent TIAs. In 1973, Dyken et al. (26) reported on their retrospective study of patients with TIAs, in which they found that 15 patients treated with aspirin had a marked reduction in subsequent TIAs compared to nine patients who did not receive aspirin.

Another double-blind study comparing sulfinpyrazone and placebo, conducted by Blakely and Gent (9) included 99 elderly institutionalized men who had a stroke. A significant reduction in death from vascular causes was found in the men in the sulfinpyrazone-treated group. Steele et al. (84) reported a marked reduction in subsequent TIAs in 19 TIA patients treated with sulfinpyrazone when compared with six untreated patients over an average 27-month period. Similarly, in a prospective, double-blind trial conducted in Heidelberg (76), aspirin (1500 mg/day) caused a significant reduction in TIAs and cerebral infarcts in 31 patients with carotid TIAs, when compared to placebo over a 24-month period.

The Canadian Cooperative Study: Aspirin and Sulfinpyrazone

The Canadian Cooperative Study Group (14) assessed the relative efficacy of aspirin and sulfinpyrazone, singly and in combination, in the reduction of recurrent transient ischemic attacks, stroke or death. In their trial, conducted at 24 clinical centers in Canada, 585 patients with threatened stroke, defined as at least one cerebral or retinal ischemic attack within the preceding three months, were studied for an average of 26 months. Patients were stratified for each clinical center on the basis of the presumed site of ischemia and the presence or absence of a residual deficit, prior to random assignment on a double-blind basis, to one of four treatment groups. In approximately 65% of the patients, the symptoms of the ischemic attack were referable to the carotid circulation, in 25% to the vertebrobasilar, and in 10% to both. More than half of the patients for each site were free of residua.

The four regimens, each four times daily, were: sulfinpyrazone, 200 mg, plus a placebo; aspirin, 325 mg, plus a placebo; sulfinpyrazone, 200 mg, plus aspirin, 325 mg; and two placebos. Because sulfinpyrazone was believed to require 1 week to produce a biologically significant effect, any events occurring in the first week of therapy with any of the four regimens were excluded from the analysis of the results. Since the reason for withdrawal of any patient from the trial might be a deterioration in their neurological status, patients who withdrew were followed for 6 months and any events occurring were charged against the corresponding study regimen. Any bias caused by their inclusion would be against showing a benefit from treatment. The endpoints were TIA and stroke or death. The latter were grouped together on the basis that those who died could not proceed to stroke.

Follow-up visits were scheduled 1 and 3 months after entry into the study, and every 3 months thereafter. Pill counts were made, and at the final follow-up visit compliance was estimated to be 92%. The average follow-up period was 26 months. Aspirin produced a risk reduction of 19% for all events—continuing TIAs, stroke or death. For the clinically more important events of stroke or death, aspirin produced an observed risk reduction of 31%, with a 48% reduction occurring in men. The greatest response, a reduction of 62%, was found in the 331 aspirin-treated men who entered the study without a previous myocardial infarction. There was no significant reduction for women.

Of the total population included in the study, 114 patients suffered stroke or death, or both. There were 23 additional events of stroke or death which were ruled ineligible because they occurred within the first 7 days of treatment or more than 6 months after withdrawal from the study. If these 23 events were included in the main analysis, the statistical significance of the observed aspirin effect would increase.

No statistically significant reductions in TIAs or stroke or death occurred in the sulfinpyrazone-treated group as compared to the placebo group, nor in the group treated with a combination of aspirin and sulfinpyrazone as compared to aspirin alone. However, the fewest events, strokes or deaths, occurred in the group receiving combined treatment. No statistically significant differences were found to be associated with the different sites of ischemia, the presence or absence of residua, single and multiple attacks, amaurosis fugax, age, smoking, obesity, hypercholesterolemia, and hypertension.

Among the various side effects reported during the 3-month follow-up visits, pain in the upper abdomen and heartburn were more common among patients allocated to aspirin-containing regimens. A total of 41% of the patients starting the study withdrew from treatment. Of these, 24% were due to side effects, and 72% of those withdrawing because of side effects were receiving aspirin.

AITIA Study: Aspirin

The Aspirin in Transient Ischemic Attacks (AITIA) study compared the effects of aspirin with those of placebo upon reduction or prevention of TIAs, cerebral infarction, and stroke-related mortality in patients with carotid TIAs (32,33). The study, conducted at ten clinical centers in the United States, included only patients who had experienced TIAs of the hemispheric type or attacks of monocular blindness (amaurosis fugax). Upon entry into the study, a clinical decision regarding surgical intervention was made for each patient. The patient was then assigned to either a medical or surgical group. Within each group patients were randomly allocated in a double-blind fashion to treatment with aspirin, 1300 mg daily (650 mg twice a day) or placebo. The medical group consisted of 178 eligible patients, and the surgical group 125. The absolute endpoints were total mortality and cause-specific mortality, from stroke and cardiovascular causes, and both cerebral and retinal infarction.

The number of carotid TIAs occurring within the 3 months prior to randomization was compared with the number reported in the first six months of follow-up. Based on this comparison, and in combination with the absolute endpoints, the patient's response was classified as either favorable or unfavorable. Those patients who did not complete the full six months of observation were labelled as "less than six months follow-up."

Follow-up visits were scheduled monthly for the first 6 months and at 3-month intervals thereafter. Compliance was checked by pill counts and urine salicylate testing.

The results of the 178 medically treated patients were reported as follows (32): an analysis for the first 6 months of follow-up showed that within the placebo group, 34 of 77 cases (44.2%) were classified as unfavorable because of continuing TIAs, whereas only 15 of 78 cases (19.2%) were classified as unfavorable in the aspirin group. This difference was considered statistically significant. When analysis was extended from 6 to 12 months, 48 out of the 178 patients (24 in each of the treatment groups) could not be classified as favorable or unfavorable because of a lack of follow-up. Due to the large number of such cases (27%), further analysis of the TIA results was confined to six months.

The analysis of absolute endpoints showed no significant difference for the aspirin and placebo treatments. It was when patients having as many TIAs in the first six months of follow-up as they had had in the three months prior to randomization were included with those having an absolute endpoint in the first six months that aspirin emerged as the superior treatment.

Within the subgroup of patients diagnosed as having stenotic lesions of the carotid artery, significantly fewer (29.3%) absolute endpoints were reached in the aspirin-treated group. When the occurrence of carotid TIAs in six months of follow-up was also considered in this subgroup, the differential was even more pronounced in favor of aspirin. Various side effects reported by the medically treated patients included upset stomach, weakness, dizziness, and urticaria, but none was of sufficient magnitude to cause withdrawal from the study.

Results for the 125 patients who had carotid TIAs and one or more accessible carotid lesions and underwent reconstructive surgery of the carotid artery were reported separately (33). Most of these patients (60 to 70%) were randomized to either aspirin or placebo treatments within one week of surgery. Results and analyses for the surgical patients were generally consistent with findings reported for the medical group. Life-table analysis of absolute endpoints for 24 months follow-up did not reveal a statistically significant difference between the aspirin and placebo treatments. When deaths which were not stroke-related were eliminated from the life-table analysis, a significant difference was observed in favor of aspirin. Because of the small number of patients and the short period of follow-up, it was not possible to conclude that aspirin has an effect in preventing cerebral infarction.

Eight patients from the placebo group suffered brain infarcts as absolute endpoints within 24 months. Among aspirin-treated patients, there was one cerebral infarct, one retinal infarct, and six cardiovascular deaths. This cardiovascular mortality was claimed to be related to the much higher percentage of patients with cardiovascular risk factors remaining in the aspirin group, 12 months after randomization. The absolute level of cases having an unfavorable outcome in the surgical treatment group was about half of those reported for the medically treated patients.

Comment

There is little question that TIAs represent an excellent model for testing platelet-active drugs. Thromboembolic phenomena have long been implicated as playing a prominent role in most cases of TIA and stroke. Anticoagulation has been shown to be a useful secondary intervention in selected situations (54,59), and the importance of platelets in the pathogenesis of these morbid events is as important (if not more important) than fibrin formation. This is in contrast to acute coronary events where the significance of thromboembolic phenomena precipitating sudden death or myocardial infarction is much less clear, the effects of anticoagulation are still controversial, and where the role of platelets remains to be clarified.

From early observations and the more recent large double-blind controlled trials, reasonable evidence has been provided that aspirin at a dosage of 1300 mg daily has a therapeutic effect in males suffering from transient ischemic episodes. It reduces the incidence of subsequent ischemic episodes and also appears to lessen the occurrence of strokes and stroke-related mortality. The lack of benefit from this medication in females is quite surprising (14; W. S. Fields, *personal communication*). The biological or pharmacological basis for the difference is unclear at present.

As for the other platelet-active drugs, dipyridamole given alone appears to have no effect. Whether it will act synergistically with aspirin, as it does in improving platelet survival (38), could be clarified by contemplated studies.

The sulfinpyrazone data are conflicting. The observations of Evans (30), of Steele (84), and of Blakely and Gent (9) that a significant reduction in thromboembolic phenomena primarily due to decreased incidence of TIAs and strokes was found in the sulfinpyrazone group all suggest a positive effect for this agent. Sulfinpyrazone had no demonstrable effect when used alone in the Canadian Cooperative

Study although there is a suggestion of some benefit, in terms of hard endpoints, when sulfinpyrazone was combined with aspirin. No further studies with sulfinpyrazone are contemplated at present and the issue of its effectiveness, or lack thereof, remains unresolved.

PERIPHERAL VASCULAR DISEASE STUDIES

Prevention of Thrombotic Occlusion of Arteriovenous Shunts

Thrombi found in synthetic shunts are indistinguishable from those found in natural vessels (47). In the animal model, dipyridamole, aspirin, and sulfinpyrazone have all been shown to inhibit thrombus formation in these shunts (21,31,67). In their study of sulfinpyrazone, Woods and coworkers (93) found that when the drug is administered to dialysis patients, fibrin deposition within the dialyzers is significantly reduced. At the same time arterial platelet counts and fibrinogen levels during dialysis increase indicating that sulfinpyrazone reduces coagulation triggered by the interaction of platelets with the foreign surface within the dialyzer. The drug may also decrease dialysis-induced occult intravascular coagulation in the body.

Clinically, thrombotic episodes in patients with arteriovenous shunts occur with less frequency than those associated with coronary prostheses or bypasses. Nevertheless, they constitute a major complication in patients with severe renal disease requiring chronic hemodialysis. In preliminary work with platelet-active drugs in hemodialysis patients, sulfinpyrazone was found to be more effective than either aspirin or dipyridamole in preventing arteriovenous shunt thrombosis (46,73).

In the case of aspirin, however, dosage may be a critical factor. Low doses effectively reduce the activity of platelet cyclooxygenase, but high doses block the production of prostacyclin, a potent antithrombotic agent (41). To demonstrate that low doses of aspirin are adequate for preventing shunt thrombosis, Harter conducted a randomized double-blind trial with 44 chronic hemodialysis patients with arteriovenous shunts. They received either 160 mg of aspirin per day or placebo for an average of five months. The incidence of thrombosis was 0.46 thrombi per patient-month in the placebo group versus 0.16 in the aspirin group ($p < 0.005$). At this low dose, aspirin was not only effective in reducing shunt thrombosis, but also less toxic. Harter observed no gastrointestinal hemorrhage or bleeding.

By contrast, a high incidence of gastrointestinal complications was reported by Albert and Schmidt (2), who administered 500 mg of aspirin three times daily to patients with chronic renal failure. With this dosage, aspirin did provide protection against thrombosis comparable to that provided by sulfinpyrazone (600 mg/day), but the latter was preferred because it was better tolerated.

In a randomized double-blind study, Kaegi and coworkers (49) compared sulfinpyrazone, 600 mg/day, to placebo in 52 patients with straight arteriovenous shunts. After six months of observation, thrombi developed in 12 sulfinpyrazone and 24 placebo patients. This corresponded to 0.18 thrombi per patient-month and 0.76 thrombi per patient-month, respectively ($p < 0.001$). The frequency of shunt revisions was also lower with sulfinpyrazone.

Kaegi subsequently crossed over these two treatment groups and observed them for an additional six months. The results achieved with sulfinpyrazone in the first half of the study were confirmed (50). The therapeutic effect was observed within one week and was more apparent in men than in women.

The antithrombotic effect of sulfinpyrazone in patients with arteriovenous shunts was again corroborated in an independent double-blind study conducted by Michie and Wombolt (58). They compared sulfinpyrazone (600 mg/day) to placebo in 16 patients with end-stage renal disease. After a three-month period, thrombus formation in the shunt had occurred in three placebo patients but in only one sulfinpyrazone patient. Once again, men seemed better protected than women. Sulfinpyrazone was well tolerated and extensive laboratory analyses revealed that sulfinpyrazone exerts its antithrombotic effect without altering prothrombin time or partial thromboplastin time.

Comment

External arteriovenous shunts in patients undergoing chronic hemodialysis have served as an excellent model for evaluating the antithrombotic effects of platelet-active drugs in man. Consistent with the findings in experimental animals, both aspirin and sulfinpyrazone have proven effective in humans in preventing thrombosis in this type of shunt, and they have yielded comparable results. Also, on the basis of current and admittedly limited observations, both low and high doses of aspirin appear to be approximately equal in their effectiveness. However, it should be noted that in models involving a prosthetic surface, (external arteriovenous shunts and prosthetic heart valves) the surface is not protected by local prostacyclin production. Therefore, the observations made in these models with agents that suppress prostaglandin synthesis may not be applicable to their effects on endothelialized surfaces.

CONCLUDING COMMENTS AND FUTURE PROSPECTS

The investigation of drugs affecting prostaglandins as antithrombotic agents, particularly for preventing acute arterial vascular catastrophes, has opened a new and exciting chapter in medical therapeutics. While a clear picture of their usefulness in various selected clinical situations still remains to be defined, it is evident that benefits can be ascribed to their use. In some situations, as described in this chapter, their value appears to be established, while in others much further work is required to determine whether there is an effect and, if so, to what extent.

The agents so far investigated not only vary in their effect on various prostaglandins but also have additional pharmacological actions that may influence the final clinical result. Consequently, we need to know much more about the differing effects of these drugs and what may be expected from each of these agents either singly or in combination. Particularly relevant to the investigation of these agents is the need to establish optimal dosages, to improve on trial design, and to clarify whether there are sex differences in responsiveness.

We still do not know whether dipyridamole by itself has any antithrombotic effect *in vivo* or whether, when used in combination with aspirin, the clinical effect is greater than that with aspirin alone. One could also speculate that the combination of dipyridamole with sulfinpyrazone, from a theoretical standpoint, may well be superior to that of dipyridamole with aspirin. Considering that arterial thrombosis involves both the interaction of platelets with the vessel wall and the coagulation of blood with fibrin formation, it is likely that maximal benefits will not be achieved until platelet-active drugs are tested in combination with anticoagulants.

The explosion of knowledge concerning both platelet and endothelial cell function and the mediators of their regulation will undoubtedly lead to the development and testing of many new drugs in the future. One can only hope that the scientific basis for their evaluation will be more firmly established than the empiricism that appears to dominate our current approach.

If the platelet-vessel wall interaction proves to be the key or initiating step in the pathogenesis of arteriosclerosis, then the research which has begun in this field may ultimately lead to primary preventive measures rather than the secondary interventions that appear to be the goal of most of our current endeavors for the major catastrophic vascular accidents.

ACKNOWLEDGMENTS

We thank Lucinda M. Pitcairn, Sue Wehner, and Stephen Lee for their help in the preparation of this manuscript, and Patricia Leppin for her efforts in typing.

REFERENCES

1. Acheson, J., Danta, G., and Hutchinson, E. C. (1969): Controlled trial of dipyridamole in cerebral vascular disease. *Br. Med. J.*, 1:614–615.
2. Albert, F. W., and Schmidt, U. (1979): Sulfinpyrazone or acetylsalicylic acid to prevent post-operative thrombus formation in arteriovenous fistulas of haemodialysis patients. *Thromb. Haemost.*, 42:63.
3. The Anturane Reinfarction Trial Research Group (1978): Sulfinpyrazone in the prevention of cardiac death after myocardial infarction. *N. Engl. J. Med.*, 298:289–295.
4. The Anturane Reinfarction Trial Research Group (1980): Sulfinpyrazone in the prevention of sudden death after myocardial infarction. *N. Engl. J. Med.*, 302:250–256.
5. Aspirin Myocardial Infarction Study Research Group (1980): A randomized controlled trial of aspirin in persons recovered from myocardial infarction. *JAMA*, 243:661–669.
6. Baur, H. R., Van Tassel, R. A., and Gobel, F. L. (1979): Effect of sulfinpyrazone on early graft closure rate after myocardial revascularization. *Circulation, [Part II]* 60:105.
7. Beard, O. W., Hipp, H. R., Robins, M., Taylor, J. S., Ebert, R. V., and Beran, L. C. (1960): Initial myocardial infarction among 503 veterans. Five-year survival. *Am. J. Med.*, 28:871–883.
8. Bigger, J. T., Jr., Heller, C. A., Wenger, T. L., and Weld, F. M. (1978): Risk stratification after acute myocardial infarction. *Am. J. Cardiol.*, 42:202–210.
9. Blakely, J. A., and Gent, M. (1975): Platelets, drugs, and longevity in a geriatric population. In: *Platelets, Drugs, and Thrombosis*, edited by J. Hirsh, J. F. Cade, A. S. Gallus, and E. Schonbaum, pp. 284–291. S. Karger, Basel.
10. Boston Collaborative Drug Surveillance Group (1974): Regular aspirin intake and acute myocardial infarction. *Br. Med. J.*, 1:440–443.
11. Boston Collaborative Drug Surveillance Program (1976): Regular aspirin use and myocardial infarction. *Br. Med. J.*, 2:1057.
12. Breddin, K., Uberla, K., and Walter, E. (1977): German-Austrian multicenter two year prospective study on the prevention of secondary myocardial infarction by ASA in comparison to phenprocoumon and placebo. Sixth International Congress on Thrombosis and Haemostasis. *Thromb. Haemost.*, 38:168.

13. Breddin, K., Loew, D., Lechner, K., Uberla, K., and Walter, E. (1979): Secondary prevention of myocardial infarction: comparison of acetylsalicylic acid, phenprocoumon and placebo. *Thromb. Haemost.*, 40:225–236.
14. The Canadian Cooperative Study Group (1978): A randomized trial of aspirin and sulfinpyrazone in threatened stroke. *N. Engl. J. Med.*, 299:53–59.
15. Cannom, D. S., Levy, W., and Cohen, L. S. (1976): The short- and long-term prognosis of patients with transmural and non-transmural myocardial infarction. *Am. J. Med.*, 61:452–458.
16. Cobb, S., Anderson, F., and Bauer, W. (1953): Length of life and cause of death in rheumatoid arthritis. *N. Engl. J. Med.*, 249:553–556.
17. Cooperative Study (1966): Death rate among 795 patients in their first year after myocardial infarction. *JAMA*, 197:184–186.
18. The Coronary Drug Project Research Group (1976): Aspirin in coronary heart disease. *J. Chron. Dis.*, 29:625–642.
19. Cortellaro, M., Fassio, G., Boschetti, C., Basagni, M., and Polli, E. E. (1979): Controlled *ex-vivo* effect of sulfinpyrazone on platelet function of myocardial infarction patients. *Haematologia*, 64:173–189.
20. Craven, L. L. (1953): Experiences with aspirin (acetylsalicylic acid) in the nonspecific prophylaxis of coronary thrombosis. *Miss. Valley Med. J.*, 75:38–44.
21. Cucuianu, M. P., Nishizawa, E. E., and Mustard, J. F. (1971): Effect of pyrimido-pyrimidine compounds on platelet function. *J. Lab. Clin. Med.*, 77:958–974.
22. Dale, J. (1975): Prevention of arterial thromboembolism with acetylsalicylic acid in patients with prosthetic heart valves. Sixth International Congress on Thrombosis and Haemostasis. *Thromb. Haemost.*, 38:66.
23. Dale, J., Myhre, E., and Rootwelt, K. (1975): Effects of dipyridamole and acetylsalicylic acid on platelet functions in patients with aortic ball-valve prostheses. *Am. Heart J.*, 89:613–618.
24. Dale, J. (1977): Prevention of arterial thromboembolism with acetylsalicylic acid. A controlled clinical study in patients with aortic ball valves. *Am. Heart J.*, 94:101–111.
25. Didisheim, P., and Fuster, V. (1978): Actions and clinical status of platelet-suppressive agents. *Semin. Hematol.*, 15:55–72.
26. Dyken, M. L., Kolar, O. J., and Jones, F. H. (1973): Differences in the occurrence of carotid transient ischemic attacks associated with antiplatelet aggregation therapy. *Stroke*, 4:732–736.
27. Elwood, P. C., Cochrane, A. L., Burr, M. L., Sweetnam, P. M., Williams, G., Welsby, E., Hughes, S. J., and Renton, R. (1974): A randomized controlled trial of acetylsalicylic acid in the secondary prevention of mortality from myocardial infarction. *Br. Med. J.*, 1:436–440.
28. Elwood, P. C., and Sweetnam, P. M. (1979): Aspirin and secondary mortality after myocardial infarction. *Lancet*, 2:1313–1315.
29. Elwood, P. C., and Williams, W. O. (1979): A randomized controlled trial of aspirin in the prevention of early mortality in myocardial infarction. *J.R. Coll. Gen. Pract.*, 29:413–416.
30. Evans, G. (1972): Effect of drugs that suppress platelet surface interaction on incidence of amaurosis fugax and transient cerebral ischemia. *Surg. Forum*, 23:239–241.
31. Evans, G., Packham, M. A., Nishizawa, E. E., Mustard, J. F., and Murphy, E. A. (1968): The effect of acetylsalicylic acid on platelet function. *J. Exp. Med.*, 128:877–894.
32. Fields, W. S., Lemak, N. A., Frankowski, R. F., and Hardy, R. J. (1977): Controlled trial of aspirin in cerebral ischemia. *Stroke*, 8:301–316.
33. Fields, W. S., Lemak, N. A., Frankowski, R. F., and Hardy, R. J. (1978): Controlled trial of aspirin in cerebral ischaemia. Part II: Surgical group. *Stroke*, 9:309–319.
34. Fuster, V., Dewanjee, M. K., Kaye, M. P., Josa, M., Metke, M. P., and Chesebro, J. H. (1979): Noninvasive radioisotopic technique for detection of platelet deposition in coronary artery bypass grafts in dogs and its reduction with platelet inhibitors. *Circulation*, 60:1508–1512.
35. Genton, E., Barnett, H. J. M., Fields, W. S., Gent, M., and Hoak, J. C. (1977): XIV. Cerebral ischemia: the role of thrombosis and of antithrombotic therapy. *Stroke*, 8:150–175.
36. Goldberg, I. D., and Stemerman, M. B. (1980): Antiplatelet and anticoagulant therapy after coronary bypass (Letter). *N. Engl. J. Med.*, 302:865.
37. Hammond, E. C., and Garfinkel, L. (1975): Aspirin and coronary heart disease: findings of a prospective study. *Br. Med. J.*, 2:269–271.
38. Harker, L. A., and Slichter, S. J. (1970): Studies of platelet and fibrinogen kinetics in patients with prosthetic heart valves. *N. Engl. J. Med.*, 283:1302–1305.
39. Harker, L. A., Slichter, S. J., and Sauvage, L. R. (1977): Platelet consumption by arterial prostheses: The effects of endothelialization and pharmacologic inhibition of platelet function. *Ann. Surg.*, 186:594–601.

40. Harrison, M. J. G., Marshall, J., Meadows, J. C., and Ross Russell, R. W. (1971): Effect of aspirin in amaurosis fugax. *Lancet*, 2:743–744.
41. Harter, H. R., Burch, J. W., Majerus, P. W., Stanford, N., Delmez, J. A., Anderson, C. B., and Weerts, C. A. (1979): Prevention of thrombosis in patients on hemodialysis by low-dose aspirin. *N. Engl. J. Med.*, 301:577–579.
42. Heikinheimo, R., and Järvinen, K. (1971): Acetylsalicylic acid and arteriosclerotic-thromboembolic diseases in the aged. *J. Am. Geriatr. Soc.*, 19:403–405.
43. Helmers, C., and Lundman, T. (1978): Sudden coronary death after acute myocardial infarction. *Adv. Cardiol.*, 25:176–182.
44. Helmers, C., Lundman, T., Massing, R., and Wester, P. O. (1976): Mortality pattern among initial survivors of acute myocardial infarction using a life-table technique. *Acta Med. Scand.*, 200:469–473.
45. Hetzer, R., Hill, J. D., Kerth, W. J., Ansbro, J., Adappa, M. G., Rodvien, R., Kamm, B., and Gerbode, F. (1978): Thromboembolic complications after mitral valve replacement with Hancock xenograft. *J. Thorac. Cardiovasc. Surg.*, 75:651–658.
46. Hirsh, J. (1978): Platelet inhibitors in the treatment of thrombosis. *Clin. Invest. Med.*, 1:191–206.
47. Hovig, T., Jorgensen, L., Rowsell, H. C., and Mustard, J. F. (1970): The structure of thrombus-like deposits formed in extracorporeal shunts. *Am. J. Pathol.*, 59:75–100.
48. Ibrahim, M. A., Sackett, D. L., and Winkelstein, W., Jr. (1969): Acute myocardial infarction: magnitude of the problem. In: *Thrombosis*, edited by S. Sherry, K. M. Brinkhous, E. Genton, and J. M. Stengle, pp. 106–116. National Academy of Science, Washington, D.C.
49. Kaegi, A., Pineo, G. F., Shimizu, A., Trivedi, H., Hirsh, J., and Gent, M. (1974): Arteriovenous shunt thrombosis. *N. Engl. J. Med.*, 290:304–306.
50. Kaegi, A., Pineo, G. F., Shimizu, A., Trivedi, H., Hirsh, J., and Gent, M. (1975): The role of sulfinpyrazone in the prevention of arterio-venous shunt thrombosis. *Circulation*, 52:497–499.
51. Kelliher, G. J., Dix, R. K., Jurkiewicz, N., and Lawrence, T. L. (1980): Effects of sulfinpyrazone on arrhythmia and death following coronary occlusion in cats. In: *Cardiovascular Actions of Sulfinpyrazone: Basic and Clinical Research*, edited by M. McGregor, J. F. Mustard, M. Oliver, and S. Sherry, pp. 193–209. Symposia Specialists, Miami.
52. Kelton, J. E., Hirsh, J., Carter, C. J., and Buchanan, M. R. (1978): Sex differences in the antithrombotic effects of aspirin. *Blood*, 52:1073–1076.
53. Klotz, L. (1980): Letter to the Editor. *N. Engl. J. Med.*, 302:866.
54. Link, H., Lebram, G., Johansson, I., and Rodberg, C. (1979): Prognosis in patients with infarction and TIA in carotid territory during and after anticoagulant therapy. *Stroke*, 10:529–532.
55. Luria, M. H., Knoke, J. D., Margolis, R. M., Hendriks, F. H., and Kuplic, J. B. (1976): Acute myocardial infarction: Prognosis after recovery. *Ann. Int. Med.*, 85:561–565.
56. McEnany, M., DeSanctis, R. W., Hawthorne, J. W., Mundth, E. D., Wintraub, R. M., Austen, W. G., and Salzman, E. W. (1976): Effect of antithrombotic therapy on aorto-coronary vein graft patency rates. *Circulation*, 54:124.
57. Madsen, E. B., Svendsen, T. L., Rasmussen, S., and Pedersen, A. (1978): Prognostic factors in acute myocardial infarction occurring within the first five days of ECG-monitoring. *Dan. Med. Bull.*, 25:155–159.
58. Michie, D. D., and Wombolt, D. G. (1977): Use of sulfinpyrazone to prevent thrombus formation in arteriovenous fistulas and bovine grafts of patients on chronic hemodialysis. *Curr. Ther. Res.*, 22:196–204.
59. Millikan, C. H., and McDowell, F. H. (1978): Treatment of transient ischemic attacks. *Stroke*, 9:299–308.
60. Moggio, R. A., Hammond, G. L., Stansel, H. C., and Glenn, W. W. L. (1978): Incidence of emboli with cloth-covered Starr-Edwards valve without anticoagulation and with varying forms of anticoagulation. *J. Thorac. Cardiovasc. Surg.*, 75:296–299.
61. Moncada, S., and Korbut, R. (1978): Dipyridamole and other phosphodiesterase inhibitors act as antithrombotic agents by potentiating endogenous prostacyclin. *Lancet*, 1:1286–1289.
62. Moreno-Cabral, R. J., McNamara, J. J., Mamiya, R. T., Brainard, S. C., and Chung, G. K. T. (1978): Acute thrombotic obstruction with Bjork-Shiley valves. Diagnostic and surgical considerations. *J. Thorac. Cardiovasc. Surg.*, 75:321–330.
63. Moschos, C., Haider, B., DeLaCruz, C., Jr., Lyons, M. M., and Regan, T. J. (1978): Antiarrhythmic effects of aspirin during nonthrombotic coronary occlusion. *Circulation*, 57:681–684.

64. Moschos, C. B., Escobinas, A. J., and Jorgensen, D. B. (1980): Effects of sulfinpyrazone on ischemic myocardium. In: *Cardiovascular Actions of Sulfinpyrazone: Basic and Clinical Research*, edited by M. McGregor, J. F. Mustard, M. Oliver, and S. Sherry, pp. 175–191. Symposia Specialists, Miami.
65. Moss, A. J., DeCamilla, J., and Davis, H. (1977): Potential for mortality reduction in the early posthospital period. *Am. J. Cardiol.*, 39:816–820.
66. Mundall, J., Quintero, P., von Kaulla, K. N., Harmon, R., and Austin, J. (1972): Transient monocular blindness and increased platelet aggregability treated with aspirin: A case report. *Neurology*, 22:280–285.
67. Mustard, J. F., Rowsell, H. C., Smythe, H. A., Senyi, A., and Murphy, E. A. (1967): The effect of sulfinpyrazone on platelet economy and thrombus formation in rabbits. *Blood*, 29:859–866.
68. Pantely, G. A., Goodnight, S. H., Rahimtoola, S. H., Harlan, B. J., DeMots, H., Calvin, L., and Rösch, J. (1979): Failure of antiplatelet and anticoagulant therapy to improve patency of grafts after coronary-artery bypass. *N. Engl. J. Med.*, 301:962–966.
69. Pantely, G. A., Goodnight, S. H., and Rahimtoola, S. H. (1980): (Letter) *N. Engl. J. Med.*, 302:866.
70. Pell, S., and D'Alonzo, C. A. (1964): Immediate mortality and five-year survival of employed men with a first myocardial infarction. *N. Engl. J. Med.*, 270:916–922.
71. The Persantine®-Aspirin Reinfarction Study Research Group (1980): Persantine® and aspirin in coronary heart disease. *Circulation*, 62:449–461.
72. Phillips, S. J., Kongtahworn, C., Zeff, R. H., and Beshany, S. E. (1980): (Letter) *N. Engl. J. Med.*, 302:866.
73. Pineo, G. F., Kaegi, A., Hirsh, J., and Gent, M. (1975): Platelets, drugs and thrombosis of arteriovenous shunts. *Platelets, Drugs, and Thrombosis*, edited by J. Hirsh, J. F. Cade, A. S. Gallus, and E. Schonbaum, pp. 276–283. S. Karger, Basel.
74. Polli, E. E., and Cortellaro, M. (1978): Anturane Reinfarction Italian Study Research Group (Letter). *N. Engl. J. Med.*, 298:1258–1259.
75. Povalski, H. J., Olson, R., Kopia, S., and Furness, P. (1980): Comparative effects of sulfinpyrazone and aspirin in the coronary occlusion-reperfusion dog model. In: *Cardiovascular Actions of Sulfinpyrazone: Basic and Clinical Research*, edited by M. McGregory, J. F. Mustard, M. Oliver, and S. Sherry, pp. 153–171. Symposia Specialists, Miami.
76. Reuther, R., and Dorndorf, W. (1978): Aspirin in patients with cerebral ischemia and normal angiograms or non-surgical lesions. Results of a double-blind trial. In: *Acetylsalicylic Acid in Cerebral Ischemia and Coronary Heart Disease*, edited by K. Breddin, W. Dorndorf, D. Loew, and R. Marx, pp. 97–106. F. K. Schautlauer Verlag, Stuttgart.
77. Sands, M. J., Leach, C. N., Lachman, A. S., and Levine, H. (1978): Thrombosis of the Bjork-Shiley aortic valve prosthesis. Recognition and management. *JAMA*, 240:1411–1413.
78. Schulze, R. A., Jr., Strauss, H. W., and Pitt, B. (1977): Sudden death in the year following myocardial infarction. Relation to ventricular premature contractions in the late hospital phase and left ventricular ejection fraction. *Am. J. Med.*, 62:192–199.
79. Smythe, H. A., Ogryzlo, M. A., Murphy, E. A., and Mustard, J. F. (1965): The effect of sulfinpyrazone (Anturan) on platelet economy and blood coagulation in man. *Can. Med. Assoc. J.*, 92:818–821.
80. Steele, P. P., Weily, H. S., and Genton, E. (1973): Platelet survival and adhesiveness in recurrent venous thrombosis. *N. Engl. J. Med.*, 288:1148–1152.
81. Steele, P. P., Weily, H. S., Davies, H., and Genton, E. (1974): Platelet survival in patients with rheumatic heart disease. *N. Engl. J. Med.*, 290:537–539.
82. Steele, P., Weily, H., Davies, H., Pappas, G., and Genton, E. (1975): Platelet survival time following aortic valve replacement. *Circulation*, 51:358–362.
83. Steele, P., Battock, D., Pappas, G., and Genton, E. (1976): Correlation of platelet survival time with occlusion of saphenous vein aorto-coronary bypass grafts. *Circulation*, 53:685–687.
84. Steele, P., Carroll, J., Overfield, D., and Genton, E. (1977): Effect of sulfinpyrazone on platelet survival time in patients with transient cerebral ischemic attacks. *Stroke*, 8:396–398.
85. Steele, P., Weily, H., Rainwater, J., and Vogel, R. (1979): Platelet survival time and thromboembolism in patients with mitral valve prolapse. *Circulation*, 60:43–45.
86. Steele, P., Rainwater, J., and Vogel, R. (1979): Platelet suppressant therapy in patients with prosthetic cardiac valves. Relationship of clinical effectiveness to alteration of platelet survival time. *Circulation*, 60:910–913.

87. Sullivan, J. M., Harken, D. E., and Gorlin, R. (1971): Pharmacologic control of thromboembolic complications of cardiac-valve replacement. *N. Engl. J. Med.*, 284:1391–1394.
88. Verstraete, M. (1978): Registry of prospective clinical trials. Third report. *Thromb. Haemost.*, 39:759–767.
89. Verstraete, M. (1980): Registry of prospective clinical trials. Fourth report. *Thromb. Haemost.*, 43:176–181.
90. Weily, H. S., and Genton, E. (1970): Altered platelet function in patients with prosthetic mitral valves. Effects of sulfinpyrazone therapy. *Circulation*, 42:967–972.
91. Weily, H. S., Steele, P. P., Davies, H., Pappas, G., and Genton, E. (1974): Platelet survival in patients with substitute heart valves. *N. Engl. J. Med.*, 290:534–537.
92. Weinblatt, E., Shapiro, S., Frank, C. W., and Sager, R. V. (1968): Prognosis of men after first myocardial infarction: Mortality and first recurrence in relation to selected parameters. *Am. J. Public Health*, 58:1329–1347.
93. Woods, H. F., Ash, G., and Weston, M. J. (1978): Sulfinpyrazone reduces fibrin deposition of dialyzer membranes. *Clin. Sci. Mol. Med.*, 55:19P–20P.
94. Zumoff, B., Hart, H., and Hellman, H. (1966): Considerations of mortality in certain chronic diseases. *Ann. Int. Med.*, 63:595–601.

Prostaglandins and the Cardiovascular System,
edited by John A. Oates. Raven Press,
New York © 1982.

Metabolic Fate of Thromboxane A_2 and Prostacyclin

L. Jackson Roberts II, Alan R. Brash, and John A. Oates

Departments of Medicine and Pharmacology, Vanderbilt University Medical Center, Nashville, Tennessee 37232

Information regarding the metabolic fate of prostaglandins and thromboxanes contributes importantly to our understanding of the biological activity of these compounds *in vivo* and is of value in attempting to quantitatively assess their endogenous production. For example, the efficient metabolic conversion of greater than 95% of PGE_2 and $PGF_{2\alpha}$ entering the pulmonary circulation to 15-keto-13,14-dihydro metabolites by the lung represents the primary mechanism by which PGE_2 and $PGF_{2\alpha}$ are biologically inactivated and is the primary determinant of the extent to which the biological actions of these two prostaglandins are limited to their local site of production as opposed to exerting systemic effects (1,2,15,23,28). Therefore, except under grossly abnormal pathologic conditions, circulating levels of unmetabolized prostaglandins are extremely low (60). Because of the low levels of the parent prostaglandins that normally circulate and because substantial artifacts can be introduced as a result of the formation of prostaglandins and thromboxanes by cellular elements of blood during blood collection and plasma isolation, it has been established that quantification of metabolites of prostaglandins and thromboxanes represents a more reliable means to assess endogenous production of these compounds than does quantification of the parent compounds (60,61).

The metabolic fate of PGE_2 and $PGF_{2\alpha}$ has been studied in detail in both experimental animals and man (10,22–29,66,67,72). More recently, the metabolic fate of thromboxanes, prostacyclin, and 6-keto-$PGF_{1\alpha}$ has been investigated (39,52–58, 69–71). We will attempt to outline the current knowledge regarding the metabolism of these compounds. The majority of our discussion will pertain to the metabolic fate of thromboxanes and prostacyclin in man, although selected studies involving experimental animals will be discussed where potentially important information has been obtained that awaits analogous studies in man or human tissues. We have chosen to discuss the metabolic fate of the thromboxanes and prostacyclin together both because of similarities in the biochemical aspects of the metabolism of these compounds and because of the presumed important quantitative relationship in the production of these compounds as a determinant of platelet activation *in vivo*.

211

BIOLOGICAL INACTIVATION OF TxA_2 AND PGI_2

TxA_2 and PGI_2 are both chemically unstable (12,30). Therefore, in addition to enzymatic metabolic transformation, spontaneous chemical degradation of TxA_2 and PGI_2 to biologically inactive products also may be a contributing factor that determines the duration of the biological activity of these compounds formed endogenously. The relative importance of enzymatic and nonenzymatic mechanisms of biological inactivation of these two compounds *in vivo*, however, is not entirely clear.

INACTIVATION OF PGI_2

PGI_2 has been shown to be a better substrate for the 15-hydroxy-prostaglandin dehydrogenase than 6-oxo-$PGF_{1\alpha}$ (47). Although the lung effectively inactivates PGE_2 and $PGF_{2\alpha}$ entering the pulmonary circulation by metabolic transformation to their respective 15-keto-13,14-dihydro metabolites, the majority of PGI_2 entering the pulmonary circulation has been found to escape inactivation by the lung (4,19,59,75,81). As lung homogenates have been shown to readily metabolize PGI_2, this has been interpreted as indicative of a limited capacity of the lung to extract PGI_2 from the pulmonary circulation (31). It is noteworthy that identical findings were made for PGA_2 in the late 1960s (33,46). At least under normal circumstances, therefore, compared to other prostaglandins, the lung may be a much less important site of biological inactivation of PGI_2. Whether pathological conditions involving the lung and its circulation may alter the ability of the lung to extract and inactivate PGI_2 remains to be investigated.

Although the lung is apparently not a major site of metabolic inactivation of PGI_2, both the liver and kidney have been shown to readily metabolize PGI_2 by pathways involving the 15-hydroxy-prostaglandin dehydrogenase and β-oxidation (78,79,82). In addition, 15-hydroxy-prostaglandin dehydrogenase activity has been found in arteries and veins that are capable of metabolizing PGI_2 (83). The quantitative importance of metabolic inactivation of PGI_2 *in vivo* by vasculature remains to be defined.

Because intravenous infusion of PGI_2 has been found to result in increased urinary excretion of 6-oxo-$PGF_{1\alpha}$ (70), this indicates that at least to some extent, the duration of the biological activity of PGI_2 *in vivo* is limited by its direct renal excretion or by spontaneous nonenzymatic degradation to 6-oxo-$PGF_{1\alpha}$.

The recent finding that both PGI_2 and 6-oxo-$PGF_{1\alpha}$ can be converted metabolically to 6-oxo-PGE_1, which has been shown to be chemically stable and to have a spectrum biological activity similar to PGI_2, has added complexities to our understanding of the major determinants of inactivation of prostacyclin-like biological activity *in vivo* (5,9,20,42,48,76–78,80). Conflicting data, however, have been presented concerning the relative potencies of the antiplatelet effect of PGI_2 and 6-keto-PGE_1. Although Wong et al. (80) have reported that the antiaggregatory effects of these compounds on platelets are of similar potency, more recently, Miller et al. (48) have shown that 6-keto-PGE_1 is a substantially less potent antiaggregatory agent than PGI_2. Although all excreted metabolites have not been identified, previous studies investigating the metabolic fate of PGI$_2$ of the rat, monkey, and man have failed to identify metabolites with a PGE ring structure (58,69,70). These studies employed [16,17,18,19-³H]PGI$_2$ or [11-³H]PGI$_2$ as the tracer, so that any compounds that had undergone dehydrogenation of the alcohol group of C-9 would have retained the tritium label. This suggests that conversion of PGI$_2$ to 6-oxo-PGE$_1$ *in vivo* may not occur to any major extent. Nevertheless, the presence of a stable inhibitor of platelet aggregation in the plasma of patients with Bartter's syndrome (51,65) is a finding that provokes interest in the possibility that 6-keto-PGE$_1$ might have pathophysiologic importance. Definitive answers to these questions, however, can only be obtained when a means to accurately quantify the levels and production of 6-oxo-PGE$_1$ *in vivo* in man have been developed.

INACTIVATION OF TxA$_2$

Analogous to PGI$_2$, the determinants of the duration of biological action of endogenously formed TxA$_2$ also appear complex (Fig. 1). Because of the extreme lability of TxA$_2$ in aqueous medium at pH 7.4, nonenzymatic degradation of TxA$_2$ to TxB$_2$, which is essentially devoid of biological activity, is probably a major mechanism that limits the duration of the biological action of TxA$_2$. Evidence also has been presented to suggest that TxA$_2$ formed in plasma becomes covalently bound to serum albumin (44). Such covalent binding to serum albumin would render TxA$_2$ biologically inactive and may represent an additional mechanism of biological inactivation of TxA$_2$ formed endogenously. Other studies, however, have shown

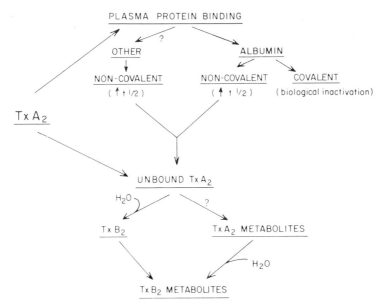

FIG. 1. Biological fate and determinants of the duration of biological action of endogenously formed TxA$_2$.

that the half-life of TxA$_2$ formed in plasma is actually longer than TxA$_2$ formed in aqueous buffer, and that this stabilization of TxA$_2$ is apparently a consequence of noncovalent binding to serum albumin (18,41). In addition, Smith, et al. (64) have found that the prolongation of biological activity of TxA$_2$ formed in plasma persists longer than the biological activity of TxA$_2$ formed in aqueous buffer. However, in this latter study, it was found that prolongation of the biological activity of TxA$_2$ did not occur when albumin was added to aqueous buffer or when plasma was replaced with Cohn fractions I, II, III, IV-1, IV-4, IV-6, V, or VI. The effect seen with plasma, however, also was found using serum. These findings suggest that serum proteins other than albumin are capable in some way of prolonging the biological activity of TxA$_2$.

In interpreting *in vitro* studies on binding to plasma proteins, consideration must be given to the equilibrium achieved at the capillary level between TxA$_2$ in plasma and in the extravascular compartment. Thus, clearance of TxA$_2$ by covalent binding to albumin is a function of the volume of distribution of TxA$_2$ relative to the volume of the plasma compartment, as well as the relative rates at which covalent binding to albumin, hydrolysis, and any direct metabolism of TxA$_2$ occur in the intra- and extravascular compartments.

In summary, therefore, it appears that plasma proteins can affect the biochemical fate of TxA$_2$ in complex ways including biological inactivation by covalent binding to serum albumin, stabilization of formed TxA$_2$ by noncovalent binding to serum albumin, and prolongation of the biological activity of TxA$_2$ by serum proteins possibly other than albumin. Potentially important questions remain to be explored regarding possible effects of clinical disease and drugs on the biochemical and biological fate of endogenously formed TxA$_2$ as a result of alterations in plasma proteins and protein binding of TxA$_2$ (18).

Studies involving Tx metabolism in sensitized guinea pig lung have suggested the possibility that TxA$_2$ also may be biologically inactivated directly by enzymatic metabolic transformation. Sensitized guinea pig lung challenged with antigen releases substantial quantities of 15-keto-13,14-dihydro-TxB$_2$ (3,13). Because studies of the metabolic fate of TxB$_2$ in the nonhuman primate and man have failed to identify any 15-keto-13,14-dihydro metabolites that had retained the original TxB$_2$ ring suggests that TxB$_2$ itself is not, under normal circumstances, a good substrate for the 15-hydroxy-prostaglandin dehydrogenase (39,53–56). We also have confirmed this *in vitro* by the incubation of TxB$_2$ with the 100,000 $\times$ g supernatant of guinea pig liver with added NAD$^+$ *(unpublished observations)*. In these studies, PGE$_2$ was efficiently converted by the 100,000 $\times$ g liver supernatant to 15-keto-13,14-dihydro-PGE$_2$. TxB$_2$, however, was converted predominantly to 11-dehydro-TxB$_2$ with lesser quantities of 15-keto-13,14-dihydro-11-dehydro-TxB$_2$. We were unable to detect any conversion of TxB$_2$ to 15-keto-13,14-dihydro-TxB$_2$ in this *in vitro* system. Further studies with sensitized guinea pig lungs have shown that the proportion of 15-keto-13,14-dihydro-TxB$_2$ compared to TxB$_2$ released in the effluent of challenged lungs increased with successive antigen challenges. In addition, the 100,000 $\times$ g supernatant of sensitized guinea pig lung was found to convert TxB$_2$

itself, in part, to 15-keto-13,14-dihydro-TxB$_2$ (7,8). Thus, although these studies have raised the question that TxA$_2$ may be metabolized directly by the 15-hydroxy-prostaglandin dehydrogenase, the evidence is certainly not conclusive. They do quite definitively illustrate, however, an interesting immunologic-dependent modulation of thromboxane metabolism by the guinea pig lung. Although the mechanisms responsible for this immunologic modulation of thromboxane metabolism are not known, changes in the metabolism of prostaglandins have been demonstrated previously to occur in association with the administration of anti-inflammatory steroids (35) and in certain pathophysiologic and altered physiologic states such as hyperthyroidism, (36) pregnancy, (6,68) gastric ulceration and diabetes (34), and primary pulmonary hypertension (38).

In summary, although enzymatic metabolic transformation in the lung is the primary mechanism by which prostaglandins E$_2$ and F$_{2\alpha}$ are biologically inactivated, the processes leading to biological inactivation of PGI$_2$ and TxA$_2$ *in vivo* are more complex and incompletely understood. In addition to enzymatic metabolic transformation, additional factors include nonenzymatic degradation of both PGI$_2$ and TxA$_2$ to biologically inactive products, enzymatic conversion of PGI$_2$ and 6-oxo-PGF$_{1\alpha}$ to the stable biologically active product 6-oxo-PGE$_1$, extraction of PGI$_2$ from the pulmonary circulation, the influence of plasma protein binding on the pharmacologic half-life and biochemical fate of TxA$_2$, and factors such as immunologic activation that may modulate metabolism.

METABOLIC FATE OF TxB$_2$ IN MAN

Due to the potent adverse biological actions of TxA$_2$, the metabolic fate of TxA$_2$ itself cannot be studied in man. However, the metabolic fate of TxB$_2$ in man has been investigated. As previously mentioned, it is possible that TxA$_2$ may undergo some metabolic transformation directly prior to spontaneous degradation to TxB$_2$, in which case the profile of metabolic products derived from endogenous Tx biosynthesis may differ to some extent from what appears following intravenous infusion of TxB$_2$. However, because TxA$_2$ at least in part degrades to TxB$_2$ prior to metabolic transformation, it was expected that the identification of products of TxB$_2$ metabolism would provide the biochemical information necessary for eventual quantification of endogenous Tx biosynthesis. As discussed later, measurement of the excretion of the major urinary metabolite of TxB$_2$ has in fact proven to be a sensitive index to Tx production *in vivo*.

In the single study investigating the metabolism of TxB$_2$ in man (54,56), 1.25 mg tritium-labeled TxB$_2$ was infused intravenously at a maximum rate of 67.4 ng/kg/min. Total infusion time was 6.5 hr, and 74% of the infused radioactivity was recovered in urine collected for 13 hr from the beginning of the infusion. The urine was extracted by Amberlite XAD-2, purified by silicic acid chromatography, Lipidex-1000 liquid gel chromatography, and both straight and reversed phase high pressure liquid chromatography. Elucidation of the structure of isolated metabolites was accomplished by gas chromatography-mass spectrometry. Twenty urinary metabolites were identified. The structures of these identified metabolites and proposed pathways of metabolic transformation of TxB$_2$ are illustrated in Fig. 2.

The metabolism of TxB$_2$ may be viewed as three distinct pathways based on the fate of the original TxB$_2$ ring. A minor pathway, comprised of two identified metabolites and only 1% of the total recovered radioactivity, yielded acyclic compounds with an alcohol group attached at both C-11 and C-12. A major pathway that yielded only two metabolites but comprised approximately 23% of the total recovered radioactivity consisted of compounds that had been metabolically transformed only by β-oxidation and retained the original TxB$_2$ ring structure. The remaining major pathway yielded sixteen identified metabolites and comprised approximately 29% of the total recovered radioactivity. These metabolites had all undergone dehydrogenation of the original hemiacetal alcohol group at C-11.

The major urinary metabolite that singly accounted for approximately 23% of total recovered radioactivity was the product of a single step of β-oxidation and was identified as 9α,11,15(S)-trihydroxy-2,3-dinor-thromba-5Z,13E-dienoic acid (62) (2,3-dinor-TxB$_2$). The second most abundant metabolite comprised approximately 8% of the total recovered radioactivity and was the initial product formed by dehydrogenation of the C-11 alcohol group of TxB$_2$ and was identified as 9α,15(S)-dihydroxy-11-oxothromba-5Z,13E-dienoic acid (11-dehydro-TxB$_2$).

In summary, metabolism of TxB$_2$ in man yields essentially products which have only undergone β-oxidation and retain the original TxB$_2$ ring structure and a series of compounds which have initially undergone dehydrogenation of the hemiacetal alcohol group followed by metabolic transformation by processes of β and ω-oxidation, dehydrogenation of the C-15 alcohol group, and reduction of the Δ^5 and Δ^{13} double bonds.

METABOLIC FATE OF PROSTACYCLIN

In a qualitative sense, the urinary metabolites of PGI$_2$ and 6-keto-PGF$_{1α}$ have undergone reactions which are typical of the metabolism of the prostaglandins. These compounds are formed by β and ω-oxidation, dehydrogenation of the C-15 alcohol group, reduction of the Δ^{13} double bond, and combinations of these reactions. The mixture of urinary metabolites of PGI$_2$ identified by Sun and Taylor (70) in the monkey is shown in Figure 3. A similar spectrum of compounds was identified in the rat (69,70).

The main features of the metabolic conversion of PGI$_2$ can be summarized as follows:

1. All known metabolites of PGI$_2$ are structural analogs of 6-keto-PGF$_{1α}$.
2. Most urinary metabolites have undergone one step of β-oxidation and thus have the 2,3-dinor structure in the upper side chain. A major urinary metabolite of PGI$_2$ in the rat (52,69), monkey (70), and man (57) is 2,3-dinor-6-keto-PGF$_{1α}$.

Tetranor derivatives of 6-keto-PGF$_{1α}$ have not been detected. However, a pentanor derivative of PGF$_{1α}$ has been identified in the bile of rats given an intravenous bolus

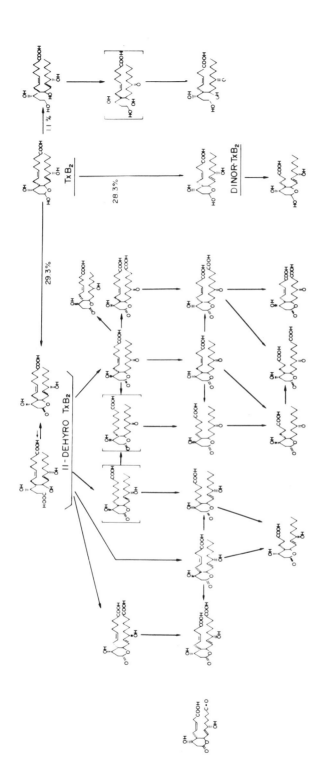

FIG. 2. Identified metabolites and proposed pathways of metabolic transformation of TxB$_2$ in man. Compounds in brackets have not been identified but are proposed intermediates in the formation of identified metabolites.

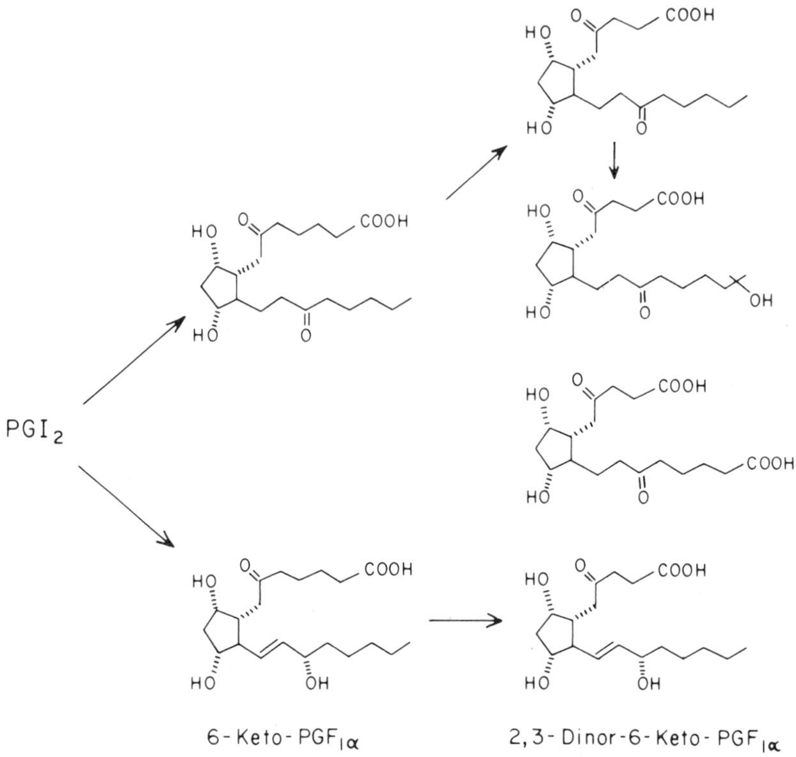

6 - Keto - PGF₁α   2, 3 - Dinor - 6 - Keto - PGF₁α

FIG. 3.   Identified metabolites of PGI₂ in the monkey (70).

of PGI₂ (73) and in the effluent of isolated perfused preparations of rabbit kidney (79) and rabbit liver (78); it also was reported as a urinary metabolite of PGI₂ in the rat (73). Pentanor PGF₁α is thought to be formed by two steps of β-oxidation of 6-keto-PGF₁α followed by oxidative decarboxylation of the α-keto acid.

3. A substantial fraction of metabolites are converted to the 15-keto-13,14-dihydro derivative. In this context, it is worth recalling that every known PGE and PGF urinary metabolite in monkey and in man has been converted through the 15-keto-13,14-dihydro pathway (22,24,25,28,66). This is certainly not the case with PGI₂. In this regard, the metabolic fate of PGI₂ more closely parallels that of the thromboxanes. It is probably because PGI₂ largely escapes metabolism in the lungs that there is more opportunity for direct renal excretion of the compound or of its hydrolysis product, 6-keto-PGF₁α. Also, 6-keto-PGF₁α is a comparatively poor substrate for the 15-hydroxy prostaglandin dehydrogenase (47) which will bias against the formation of the 15-keto-13,14-dihydro derivative.

4. It has been shown that the spectrum of PGI₂ metabolism is not completely relfected by the metabolite profile in urine. The liver is an important organ in PGI₂ inactivation (14,19,58,73,74) and biliary excretion of PGI₂ metabolites

in some species may be quantitatively more important than renal excretion (69). We also know that selected metabolites may be excreted preferentially in bile.

The studies of Sun and Taylor (73) using the conscious rat with cannulated bile duct were the first to elucidate pathways of hepatic metabolism of PGI$_2$. The main findings were that within 3 hr of an intravenous dose of [^{3}H]PGI$_2$, an average of 37% of the radioactivity was recovered in the bile. The major components of the metabolite mixture in the bile were 2,3-dinor-6-keto-PGF$_{1\alpha}$ and the glucuronide conjugate of 6,15-diketo-13,14-dihydro-2,3-dinor-PGF$_{1\alpha}$. The latter compound was not detected in urine. Studies by Wong et al. (78) on the metabolism of PGI$_2$ in the perfused rabbit liver were compatible with the results obtained *in vivo* in the rat. The venous effluent of the perfused liver contained 6-keto-PGF$_{1\alpha}$, β-oxidation and ω-oxidation products of 6-keto-PGF$_{1\alpha}$, and a partially characterized substance thought to be 6-keto-PGE$_1$. However, there were no 15-keto-13,14-dihydro derivatives detected. It appears that the pathway that contributes most to the loss of PGI$_2$ bioactivity in the liver is β-oxidation.

In conclusion, we should reemphasize that all known metabolites of PGI$_2$ are analogs of the hydrolysis product 6-keto-PGF$_{1\alpha}$. Although PGI$_2$ conceivably could react with nucleophiles other than water, this does not appear to happen to any significant extent *in vivo*. As previously mentioned, there is evidence that TxA$_2$ can, to some extent, become covalently bound to serum albumin (44). However, because infusion of small quantities of [3H]PGI$_2$ accounts for appearance of most of the radioactivity in urine and bile in the form of metabolites related to 6-keto-PGF$_{1\alpha}$, it seems unlikely that covalent protein binding is a principal metabolic fate of endogeneously synthesized prostacyclin.

QUANTITATIVE ASPECTS OF THROMBOXANE AND PROSTACYCLIN PRODUCTION IN MAN

Knowledge of the metabolic fate of TxB$_2$ and PGI$_2$ obtained from the above studies provided the basis for the development of quantitative assays of metabolites of Tx and PGI$_2$ as a means to assess endogenous production of these compounds in man. In this regard, we have developed stable isotope dilution mass spectrometric assays for the major urinary metabolite of TxB$_2$, 2,3-dinor-TxB$_2$, and the major urinary metabolite of prostacyclin, 2,3-dinor-6-oxo-PGF$_{1\alpha}$.

The levels of excretion of 2,3-dinor-TxB$_2$ in six normal subjects has been determined to be 206 ± 58 pg/mg creatinine (43). Preliminary studies suggest that the source of 2,3-dinor-TxB$_2$ in normal man derives almost exclusively from platelet Tx production. Substantially elevated excretion of 2,3-dinor-TxB$_2$ has been found to occur in patients with a variety of clinical disorders felt to be associated with abnormal platelet consumption including thrombocytosis, myocardial infarction, variant angina, and peripheral vascular disease (43). In a dose-ranging study of aspirin given to five normal volunteers, we have found that 20 mg/day aspirin decreased the urinary excretion of 2,3-dinor-TxB$_2$ to 33 ± 16% of control level *(unpublished observations).* In contrast, much higher doses of aspirin (2.6 g/day) have been found to result in only 44.6 to 69.9% inhibition of endogenous production of PGE$_2$, which is not derived primarily from the platelet cyclooxygenase (63). In addition, intravenous infusion of prostacyclin in a patient with thrombotic thrombocytopenic purpura was found to reduce the excretion of 2,3-dinor-TxB$_2$ to essentially undetectable levels (17). Thus, it appears that quantification of the urinary excretion of 2,3-dinor-TxB$_2$ will provide a useful and sensitive index of platelet activation occurring *in vivo.* Although it appears that the majority of urinary 2,3-dinor-TxB$_2$ derives from platelet thromboxane production under normal circumstances, there is undoubtedly a component of urinary 2,3-dinor-TxB$_2$ that results from thromboxane biosynthesis from extra-platelet sources—for instance, the lung. Thus, it is not unreasonable to suspect that 2,3-dinor-TxB$_2$ excretion also may be found to be increased in association with pathophysiological processes other than abnormal platelet consumption—for example, pulmonary disease.

QUANTIFICATION OF PGI$_2$ METABOLITE LEVELS IN MAN

The urinary excretion of 2,3-dinor-6-keto-PGF$_{1\alpha}$ in young healthy males is approximately 500 ng/day and approximately one-half of this amount of 13,14-dihydro-6,15-diketo-2,3-dinor-PGF$_{1\alpha}$ is excreted daily (49). This level of metabolite excretion is at least one order of magnitude lower than that of the major urinary metabolites of the E and F prostaglandins. However, it would appear that the proportion of PGI$_2$ production accounted for by 2,3-dinor-6-keto-PGF$_{1\alpha}$ is of a similar order of magnitude to the proportions of PGE and PGF production accounted for by their respective major metabolites (24,28,57). The implication is that there is an extremely low level of endogenous PGI$_2$ synthesis. One finding that would invalidate this conclusion would be if the proportion of endogenous PGI$_2$ metabolized to the dinor metabolites was substantially different from the proportion found in metabolism studies. Comparatively high doses of PGI$_2$ are often used in metabolism studies, and this could result in the appearance of a different metabolite profile in urine. Hensby et al. (32) found that the level of 6-keto-PGF$_{1\alpha}$ measured in plasma was not linearly related to the rate of infusion of exogenous PGI$_2$. A possible explanation for this result could have been the existence of dose-dependent changes in PGI$_2$ metabolism. We have attempted, therefore, to determine the endogenous rate of secretion of prostacyclin by measurement of its fractional elimination as the dinor urinary metabolites during very low level infusion rates of PGI$_2$.

Healthy male volunteers received infusions of prostacyclin in amounts of 0.1, 0.4 and 2.0 ng/kg/min over a 6-hr period. This range of infusion rates was chosen to include some doses that were near the apparent endogenous rate of PGI$_2$ production. No changes in blood pressure and heart rate were seen during these infusions. It was found that the excretion of 2,3-dinor-6-keto-PGF$_{1\alpha}$ was linearly related to the infusion rate and that urinary excretion of this metabolite accounted for 7% of the infused PGI$_2$. From the fraction of prostacyclin eliminated as this metabolite, it was calculated that the maximal secretion of prostacyclin into the circulation was less than 0.1 ng/kg/min. This estimate is lower than the infusion rate considered to be necessary for achieving a pharmacologic effect on platelets. Infusion rates of 2 ng/kg/min are required to achieve the threshold for inhibition of platelet aggregation *(ex vivo)* in man (16).

It was concluded, therefore, that PGI$_2$ is not a circulating antiplatelet hormone under normal circumstances in man.

A major question that remains unanswered is: What are appropriate and effective doses of antiplatelet agents that exert their effect primarily via inhibition of platelet cyclooxygenase (11)? Ideally, these drugs should be administered in doses that effectively inhibit platelet cyclooxygenase synthesis of proaggregatory Tx without substantially reducing endothelial cyclooxygenase production of antiaggregatory PGI$_2$. Although some *in vitro* studies suggest that platelet and endothelial cyclo-oxygenase may have different susceptibilities to inhibition by drugs such as aspirin and sulfinpyrazone (21,37,40,45) and high doses of aspirin may have been shown to reverse the prolongation of bleeding time observed at lower doses (50), it remains to be established definitively whether it is possible to achieve differential inhibition of platelet and endothelial cyclooxygenase in man to any great extent *in vivo* with drugs such as aspirin and sulfinpyrazone, and precisely at what doses of these drugs is a differential effect quantitatively maximal.

Having now developed the means to accurately quantify endogenous production of Tx and PGI$_2$ by measurement of the urinary excretion of 2,3-dinor-TxB$_2$ and 2,3-dinor-6-oxo-PGF$_{1\alpha}$, respectively, it should now be possible to conduct the appropriate pharmacological studies evaluating the comparative effects of varying doses of these drugs on endogenous Tx and PGI$_2$ production. Such information once obtained will undoubtedly prove valuable both in interpreting results of previous studies evaluating the effects of anti-platelet agents and in the rational design of future clinical trials of antiplatelet therapy of human disease.

ACKNOWLEDGMENT

Supported by Grant GM 15431 from the National Institutes of Health.

REFERENCES

1. Ånggard, E., and Samuelsson, B. (1964): Prostaglandins and related factors. *J. Biol. Chem.*, 239:4097–4102.
2. Ånggard, E., Larsson, C., and Samuelsson, B. (1971): The distribution of 15-hydroxy prostaglandin dehydrogenase and prostaglandin- Δ^{13}-reductase in tissues of the swine. *Acta Physiol. Scand.*, 81:396–404.
3. Anhut, A., Peskar, B. A., and Bernauer, W. (1978): Release of 15-keto-13,14-dihydro-thromboxane B$_2$ and prostaglandin D$_2$ during anaphylaxis as measured by radioimmunoassay. *Nauyn-Schmiedeberg's Arch. Pharmacol.*, 305:247–252.
4. Armstrong, J. M., Lattimer, N., Moncada, S., and Vane, J. R. (1978): Comparison of the vasodepressor effects of prostacyclin and 6-oxo-prostaglandin F$_{1\alpha}$ with those of prostaglandin E$_2$ in rat and rabbits. *Br. J. Pharmacol.*, 62:125–129.
5. Axen, U. F., Lincoln, F. H., Thompston, J. L., Honohan, T., and Nishizawa, E. E. (1978): Chemistry of prostaglandins and prostacyclins. In: *Prostaglandins in Cardiovascular and Renal Function*, edited by A. Scriabine, A. M. Lefer, and F. A. Kuehl, Jr., pp. 3–8. Spectrum Publications, New York.

6. Bedwani, J. R., and Morley, P. B. (1975): Enhanced inactivation of prostaglandin E$_2$ by the rabbit lung during pregnancy and progesterone treatment. *Br. J. Pharmacol.*, 53:547–554.
7. Boot, J. R., Cockerill, A. F., Dawson, W., Mallen, D. N. B., and Osborne, D. J. (1978): Modification of prostaglandin and thromboxane release by immunological sensitization and successive immunological challenges from guinea pig lung. *Int. Arch. Allergy Appl. Immunol.*, 57:159–164.
8. Boot, J. R., Dawson, W., and Osborne, D. J. (1976): The biological significance of prostaglandin-like substances released from immunologically challenged guinea-pig lungs. *Br. J. Pharm. Pharmacol.*, 58:471 P.
9. Borda, E. S., Lazzari, M. A., Gimeno, M. F., and Gimeno, A. L. (1980): Human platelet-rich plasma and human serum protects from inactivation the antiaggregatory capacity of prostacyclin-like material (PGI$_2$) produced by the rat stomach fundus. *Prostaglandins*, 19:889–905.
10. Brash, A. R., and Baillie, T. A. (1978): A comparison to t-butyldimethylsilyl and trimethylsilyl ether derivatives for the characterization of urinary metabolites of prostaglandin F$_{2\alpha}$ by gas chromatography mass spectrometry. *Biomed. Mass Spectrometry*, 5:346–356.
11. Burch, J. W., Stanford, N., and Majerus, P. W. (1978): Inhibition of platelet prostaglandin synthesis by oral aspirin. *J. Clin. Invest.*, 61:314–319.
12. Cho, M. J., and Allen, M. A. (1978): Chemical stability of prostacyclin (PGI$_2$) in aqueous solutions. *Prostaglandins*, 15:943–954.
13. Dawson, W., Boot, J. R., Cockerill, A. F., Mallen, D. N. B., and Osborne, D. J. (1976): Release of novel prostaglandins and thromboxanes after immunological challenge of guinea pig lung. *Nature*, 262:699–702.
14. Dusting, G. C., Moncada, S., and Vane, J. R. (1978): Recirculation of prostacyclin (PGI$_2$) in the dog. *Br. J. Pharmacol.*, 64:315–320.
15. Ferreira, S. H., and Vane, J. R. (1967): Prostaglandins: Their disappearance from and release into the circulation. *Nature*, 216:868–873.
16. FitzGerald, G. A., Friedman, L. A., Migamori, I., O'Grady, J., and Lewis, P. J. (1979): A double-blind placebo controlled cross-over study of prostacyclin in man. *Life Sci.*, 25:665–672.
17. FitzGerald, G. A., Maas, R. L., Brash, A. R., Stein, R., Oates, J. A., and Roberts, L. J., II. (1981): Intravenous prostacyclin in thrombotic thrombocytopenic purpura. *Ann. Int. Med.*, 95:319–321.
18. Folco, G., Granström, E., and Kindahl, J. (1977): Albumin stabilizes thromboxane A$_2$. *FEBS Lett.*, 82:321–324.
19. Gerkens, J. F., Friesinger, G. C., Branch, R. A., Shand, D. G., and Gerber, J. C. (1978): A comparison of the pulmonary, renal and hepatic extractions of PGI$_2$—a potential circulating hormone. *Life Sci.*, 22:1837–1842.
20. Gimeno, M. F., Sterin-Borda, L., Borda, E. S., Lazzari, M. A., and Gimeno, A. L. (1980): Human plasma transforms prostacyclin (PGI$_2$) into a platelet antiaggregatory substance which contracts isolated bovine coronary arteries. *Prostaglandins*, 19:907–916.
21. Gordon, J. L., and Pearson, J. D. (1978): Effects of sulphinopyrazone and aspirin on prostaglandin I$_2$ (prostacyclin) synthesis by endothelial cells. *Br. J. Pharmacol.*, 64:481–483.
22. Granström, E. (1972): On the metabolism of prostaglandin F$_{2\alpha}$ in female subjects. Structure of two C$_{14}$ metabolites. *Eur. J. Biochem.*, 25:581–589.
23. Granström, E. (1972): On the metabolism of prostaglandin F$_{2\alpha}$ in female subjects. Structures of two metabolites in blood. *Eur. J. Biochem.*, 27:462–469.
24. Granström, E., and Samuelsson, B. (1971): On the metabolism of prostaglandin F$_{2\alpha}$ in female subjects. *J. Biol. Chem.*, 246:5254–5263.
25. Granström, E., and Samuelsson, B. (1971): On the metabolism of prostaglandin F$_{2\alpha}$ in female subjects. II. Structures of six metabolites. *J. Biol. Chem.*, 246:7470–7485.
26. Green, K. (1971): Metabolism of prostaglandin E$_2$ in the rat. *Biochemistry*, 10:1072–1080.
27. Green, K. (1971): The metabolism of prostaglandin F$_{2\alpha}$ in the rat. *Biochem. Biophys. Acta*, 231:419–444.
28. Hamberg, M., and Samuelsson, B. (1972): On the metabolism of prostaglandins E$_1$ and E$_2$ in man. *J. Biol. Chem.*, 246:6713–6721.
29. Hamberg, M., and Samuelsson, B. (1972): On the metabolism of prostaglandins E$_1$ and E$_2$ in the guinea pig. *J. Biol. Chem.*, 247:3495–3502.
30. Hamberg, M., Svensson, J., and Samuelsson, B. (1975): Thromboxanes: A new group of biologically active compounds derived from prostaglandin endoperoxides. *Proc. Natl. Acad. Sci. USA*, 72:2994–2998.

31. Hawkins, H. J., Smith, J. B., Nicolaou, K. C., and Eling, T. E. (1978): Studies of the mechanisms involved in the fate of prostacyclin (PGI$_2$) and 6-keto-PGF$_{1\alpha}$ in the pulmonary circulation. *Prostaglandins*, 16:871–884.

32. Hensby, C. N., FitzGerald, G. A., Friedman, L. A., Lewis, P. J., and Dollery, C. T. (1979): Measurement of 6-oxo-PGF$_{1\alpha}$ in human plasma using gas chromatography-mass spectrometry. *Prostaglandins*, 18:731–736.

33. Horton, E., and Jones, R. L. (1969): Prostaglandins A$_1$, A$_2$ and 19-hydroxy A$_1$: Their actions on smooth muscle and their inactivation on passage through the pulmonary and hepatic portal vascular beds. *Br. J. Pharmacol.*, 37:705–722.

34. Hoult, J. R. S., and Moore, P. K. (1980): Adaptive changes in activity of prostaglandin synthesizing and metabolizing enzymes are coupled. *Br. J. Pharmacol.*, 69:272P–273P.

35. Hoult, J. R. S., and Moore, P. K. (1980): *In vivo* administration of antiinflammatory steroids alters activities of enzymes which synthesize and metabolize prostaglandins. *Br. J. Pharmacol.*, 69:271P–272P.

36. Hoult, J. R. S., and Moore, P. K. (1978): Thyroxine-induced hyperthyroid state in rats suppresses renal prostaglandin metabolism. *Br. J. Pharmacol.*, 62:416P.

37. Jaffe, E., and Weksler, B. B. (1979): Recovery of endothelial cell prostacyclin production after inhibition by low doses of aspirin. *J. Clin. Invest.*, 63:532–535.

38. Jose, P., Niederhauser, U., Piper, P. J., Robinson, C., and Smith, A. P. (1976): Degradation of prostaglandin F$_{2\alpha}$ in the human pulmonary circulation. *Thorax*, 31:713–719.

39. Kindahl, H. (1977): Metabolism of thromboxane B$_2$ in the cynomolgus monkey. *Prostaglandins*, 13:619–629.

40. Korbut, R., and Moncada, S. (1978): Prostacyclin (PGI$_2$) and thromboxane A$_2$ interaction *in vivo*. regulation by aspirin and relationship with antithrombotic therapy. *Thromb. Res.*, 13:489–500.

41. Lagarde, M., Velardo, B., Blanc, M., and Dechavanne, M. (1980): Fatty acids bound to serum albumin decrease the half-life of thromboxane A$_2$. *Prostaglandins*, 20:275–283.

42. Lee, W. H., McGiff, J. C., Householder, R. W., Sun, F. F., and Wong, P. Y.-K. (1979): Inhibition of platelet aggregation by 6-keto-prostaglandin E$_1$ (6-KPGE$_1$) a metabolite of 6-keto-prostaglandin F$_{1\alpha}$ (6-KPGF$_{1\alpha}$) *Fed. Proc. Am. Soc. Exp. Biol.*, 38:419.

43. Maas, R. L., Roberts, L. J., II, Taber, D. F., and Oates, J. A. (1980): Urinary dinor-thromboxane B$_2$: Levels in normal males and in cardiovascular disease. *Clin. Res.*, 28:319A.

44. Maclouf, J., Kindahl, H., Granström, E., and Samuelsson, B. (1980): Thromboxane A$_2$ and prostaglandin H$_2$ form covalently linked derivatives with human serum albumin. In: *Advances in Prostaglandin and Thromboxane Research, Vol. 6*, edited by B. Samuelsson, P. W. Ramwell, and R. Paoletti, pp. 283–286. Raven Press, New York.

45. Masotti, G., Galanti, G., Poggesi, Abbaye, R., and Neri Sermeri, G. G. (1979): Differential inhibition of prostacyclin production and platelet aggregation by aspirin. *Lancet*, i:1213–1216.

46. McGiff, J. C., Terragno, N. A., Strand, J. C., Lee, J. B., Lonigro, A. J., and Ng, K. K. F. (1969): Selective passage of prostaglandins across the lung. *Nature*, 223:742–745.

47. McGuire, J. C., and Sun, F. F. (1978): Metabolism of prostacyclin. I. Oxidation by rhesus monkey lung 15-hydroxy prostaglandin dehydrogenase. *Arch. Biochem. Biophys.*, 189:92–98.

48. Miller, O. V., Aiken, J. W., Shebuski, R. J., and Gorman, R. R. (1980): 6-keto-prostaglandin E$_1$ is not equipotent to prostacyclin (PGI$_2$) as an antiaggregatory agent. *Prostaglandins*, 20:391–400.

49. Oates, J. A., Falardeau, P., FitzGerald, G. A., Branch, R. A., and Brash, A. R. (1981): Quantitation of urinary prostacyclin metabolites in man: Estimates of the rate of secretion of prostacyclin into the general circulation: In: *Clinical Pharmacology of Prostacyclin*, edited by P. J. Lewis and J. O'Grady, pp. 21–24. Raven Press, New York.

50. O'Grady, J., and Moncada, S. (1978): Aspirin: A paradoxical effect on bleeding time. *Lancet*, ii:780.

51. O'Regan, S., Rivard, G. E., Mongeau, J.-G., and Robitaille, P. O. (1979): A circulating inhibitor of platelet aggregation in Bartter's syndrome. *Pediatrics*, 64:939–941.

52. Pace-Asciak, C. R., Carrara, M. C., and Domazet, Z. (1977): Identification of the major urinary metabolites of 6-ketoprostaglandin F$_{1\alpha}$ (6K-PGF$_{1\alpha}$) in the rat. *Biochem. Biophys. Res. Commun.*, 78:115–121.

53. Roberts, L. J., II, Sweetman, B. J., Morgan, J. L., Payne, N. A., and Oates, J. A. (1977): Identification of the major urinary metabolite of thromboxane B$_2$ in the monkey. *Prostaglandins*, 13:631–647.

54. Roberts, L. J., II, Sweetman, B. J., and Oates, J. A. (1981): Metabolism of thromboxane B$_2$ in man. Identification of twenty urinary metabolites. *J. Biol. Chem.*, 256:8384–8393.

55. Roberts, L. J., II, Sweetman, B. J., and Oates, J. A. (1978): Metabolism of thromboxane B$_2$ in the monkey. *J. Biol. Chem.*, 253:5305–5318.
56. Roberts, L. J., II, Sweetman, B. J., Payne, N. A., and Oates, J. A. (1977): Metabolism of thromboxane B$_2$ in man. Identification of the major urinary metabolite. *J. Biol. Chem.*, 252:7415–7417.
57. Rosenkranz, B., Fischer, C., Reimann, I., Weimer, K. E., Beck, G., and Frölich, J. C. (1980): Identification of the major metabolite of prostacyclin and 6-keto-prostaglandin F$_{1\alpha}$ in man. *Biochem. Biophys. Acta*, 619:207–213.
58. Rosenkranz, B., Fischer, C., Weimer, K. E., and Frölich, J. C., (1980): Metabolism of prostacyclin and 6-keto-prostaglandin F$_{1\alpha}$ in man. *J. Biol. Chem.*, 255:10194–10198.
59. Salmon, J. A., Mulhane, K. M., Dusting, C. J., Moncada, S., and Vane, J. R. (1979): Elimination of prostacyclin (PGI$_2$) and 6-oxo-PGF$_{1\alpha}$ in anesthetized dogs. *J. Pharm. Pharmacol.*, 31:529–532.
60. Samuelsson, B. (1973): Quantitative aspects on prostaglandin synthesis in man. *Adv. Biosci.*, 9:7–14.
61. Samuelsson, G., and Green, J. (1974): Endogenous levels of 15-keto-dihydro-prostaglandins in human plasma. *Biochem. Med.*, 11:298–303.
62. Samuelsson, B., Hamberg, M., Roberts, L. J., II, Oates, J. A., and Nelson, N. A. (1978): Nomenclature for thromboxanes. *Prostaglandins*, 16:857–860.
63. Seyberth, H. W., Sweetman, B. J., Frölich, J. C., and Oates, J. A. (1976): Quantification of the major urinary metabolite of the E prostaglandins by mass spectrometry: Evaluation of the method's application to clinical studies. *Prostaglandins*, 11:381–397.
64. Smith, J. B., Ingerman, C., and Silver, M. J. (1976): Persistence of thromboxane A$_2$-like material and platelet release-inducing activity in plasma. *J. Clin. Invest.*, 58:1119–1122.
65. Stoff, J. S., Stemerman, M., Steer, M., Salzman, E., and Brown, R. S. (1980): A defect in platelet aggregation in Bartter's syndrome. *Am. J. Med.*, 68:171–180.
66. Sun, F. F. (1974): Metabolism of prostaglandin F$_{2\alpha}$ in rhesus monkeys. *Biochem. Biophys. Acta*, 369:95–110.
67. Sun, F. F. (1974): Metabolism of prostaglandin F$_{2\alpha}$ in the rat. *Biochem. Biophys. Acta*, 348:249, 262.
68. Sun, F. F., and Armour, S. B. (1974): Prostaglandin 15-hydroxy dehydrogenase and f13-reductase levels in the lungs of maternal fetal and neonatal rabbits. *Prostaglandins*, 7:327–338.
69. Sun, F. F., and Taylor, B. M. (1978): Metabolism of prostacyclin in rat. *Biochemistry*, 17:4096–4101.
70. Sun, F. F., Taylor, B. M., McGuire, G. C., Wong, P. Y-K, Malik, K. V., and McGiff, J. C. (1979): Metabolic disposition of prostacyclin. In: *Prostacyclin*, edited by J. R. Vane and L. Bergstrom, pp. 119–131. Raven Press, New York.
71. Sun, F. F., Taylor, B. M., Sutter, D. M., and Weeks, J. R. (1979): Metabolism of prostacyclin. III. Urinary metabolite profile of 6-keto-PGF$_{1\alpha}$ in rat. *Prostaglandins*, 17:753–759.
72. Svanborg, K., and Bygdeman, M. (1972): Metabolism of prostaglandin F$_{2\alpha}$ in the rabbit. *Eur. J. Biochem.*, 28:127–135.
73. Taylor, B. M., and Sun, F. F. (1980): Tissue distribution and biliary excretion of prostacyclin metabolites in the rat. *J. Pharmacol. Exp. Ther.*, 214:24–30.
74. Van Dam, J., Fitzpatrick, T. M., Stinger, R. B., Penkos, J. C., Ramwell, P. W., and Kot, P. A. (1979): Hepatectomy selectivity increases the duration of prostacyclin-induced systemic hypotension in the rat. *Clin. Res.*, 27:569A.
75. Waldman, H. M., Alter, I., Kot, P. A., Rose, J. C., and Ramwell, P. W. (1978): Effect of lung transit on systemic depressor responses to archidonic acid and prostacyclin in dogs. *J. Pharmacol. Exp. Ther.*, 204:289–293.
76. Wong, P. Y-K, Lee, W. H., Chao, P. H-W, Reiss, R. F., and McGiff, J. C. (1980): Metabolism of prostacyclin by 9-hydroxydehydrogenase in human platelets. *J. Biol. Chem.*, 255:9021–9024.
77. Wong, P. Y-K, Lee, W. H., and McGiff, J. C. (1979): Metabolism of prostacyclin (PGI$_2$) by the 9-hydroxytprostaglandin dehydrogenase (9-OHPGDH) in human platelets. *Circulation (Suppl. II)*, 59 and 60:II–269.
78. Wong, P. Y-K, Malik, K. V., Desiderio, D. M., McGiff, J. C., and Sun, F. F. (1980): Hepatic metabolism of prostacyclin (PGI$_2$) in the rabbit: Formation of a potent novel inhibitor of platelet aggregation. *Biochem. Biophys. Res. Commun.*, 93:486–494.
79. Wong, P. Y-K, McGiff, J. C., Dagen, L., Malik, K. V., and Sun, F. F. (1979): Metabolism of prostacyclin in the rabbit kidney. *J. Biol. Chem.*, 254:12–14.

80. Wong, P. Y-K, McGiff, J. C., Sun, F. F., and Lee, W. H. (1979): 6-Keto-prostaglandin E₁ inhibits aggregation of human platelets. *Eur. J. Pharmacol.*, 60:245–248.
81. Wong, P. Y-K, McGiff, J. C., Sun, F. F., and Malik, K. V. (1978): Pulmonary metabolism of prostacyclin (PGI₂) in the rabbit. *Biochem. Biophys. Res. Commun.*, 83:731–738.
82. Wong, P. Y-K, Sun, F. F., Malik, K. V., Cagen, L., and McGiff, J. C. (1979): Metabolism of prostacyclin in the isolated kidney and lung of the rabbit. In *Prostacyclin*, edited by J. R. Vane and L. Bergstrom, pp. 133–145. Raven Press, New York.
83. Wong, P. Y-K, Sun, F. F., and McGiff, J. C. (1978): Metabolism of prostacyclin in blood vessels. *J. Biol. Chem.*, 253:5555–5557.

Prostaglandins and the Cardiovascular System,
edited by John A. Oates. Raven Press,
New York © 1982.

Prostaglandins and the Regulation of Renal Circulation and Function

*John G. Gerber, **Robert J. Anderson, **Robert W. Schrier,
and *Alan S. Nies

*Department of Medicine and *Divisions of Clinical Pharmacology and **Renal Diseases,
University of Colorado Health Sciences Center, Denver, Colorado 80262*

The role of prostaglandins in the control of renal circulation and function is one of the most extensively studied fields in renal physiology. However, the literature is filled with reports that contradict each other. In this review we will try to take an objective view of the literature, present evidence from all sides, and reconcile some of the differences that researchers have reported in studying the role of prostaglandins in renal function and hemodynamics.

Prostaglandin Production by the Kidney

The kidney is a heterogenous organ consisting of numerous cell types with specialized functions. Since protaglandins are local hormones usually affecting the function of the cells where they are produced, measuring the production of prostaglandins by homogenates of whole organs carries very little specificity in determining which prostaglandin is important for any given effect.

It has been known for some time that the renal medulla and papilla have a much greater capacity to produce prostaglandins than the renal cortex (106). However, the capacity to metabolize prostaglandins resides mainly with the renal cortex (106). It was hypothesized that the medullary prostaglandins might affect renal cortical function via the tubular transit of these prostaglandins from the medulla to the cortex (64,114). This hypothesis was questionable because the renal cortex is very active in metabolizing the prostaglandins, and it was unlikely that the medulary prostaglandins could reach their site of action in the cortex before being metabolized. Also, if protaglandins are involved in the fine tuning of the renal vascular resistance, the tubular route would seem too circuitous for the prostaglandins to have instantaneous effects on renal blood flow.

Evidence against transport of prostaglandins from the medulla to the cortex in tubular fluids came from experiments performed in dogs with non-filtering kidneys. In these animals intrarenal infusion of arachidonic acid produced a marked decrease in renal vascular resistance (4) that was blocked by a non-steroidal anti-inflammatory drug (71). Since the non-filtering kidney had no tubular fluid flow from the medulla to the cortex, the vasodilator protaglandins had to be synthesized from arachidonic acid in the renal cortex in order to affect renal blood flow. Numerous researchers have been able to demonstrate that the renal cortex has the ability to synthesize protaglandins, although at rates lower than the medulla and papilla (105,129,175). Terragno et al. (163) have demonstrated that the renal cortex contains an inhibitor of prostaglandin synthesis which may account for the low rate of protaglandin production (8). The fetal renal cortex, which does not contain this inhibitor, demonstrates a high capacity to synthesize prostaglandin. However, whether this inhibitor is produced *in vivo* in sites that could affect prostaglandin biosynthesis in the renal vasculature is unlikely.

Once it had been established that both the cortex and the medulla have prostaglandin biosynthetic capacity, the question still remained as to which cells were actually producing these prostaglandins. Smith and Bell (149), using immunohistochemical techniques in the renal cortices of various animal species, have been able to determine that the cyclo-oxygenase is located in the endothelial cells lining the arterioles and the cortical collecting tubules (9). Cyclo-oxygenase was present in the glomeruli of rabbits, cows and sheep but not in rats. However, since Hassid et al. (84) have shown that isolated rat glomeruli produce significant quantities of prostaglandins (10), while histochemically identified cyclo-oxygenase was not detected in the rat glomeruli, histochemical localization of cyclo-oxygenase may not always correlate with prostaglandin production. Even the availability of the cyclo-oxygenase in a particular cell type does not guarantee prostaglandin production *in vivo* because the rate-limiting step in the generation of prostaglandins is the liberation of arachidonic acid from membrane phospholipids. In addition to containing cyclo-oxygenase, the cell must have the capacity to respond to a stimulus that activates a phospholipase to release arachidonic acid.

The components of the renal cortex that have been shown to have the capacity to produce prostaglandins are dissected afferent arterioles from pig kidneys and isolated glomeruli from rats (84,163). The afferent arterioles produce prostacyclin (PGI_2) almost exclusively, while the isolated glomeruli produce all the known primary prostaglandins with $PGF_{2\alpha}$ predominating. The cellular components responsible for the glomerular prostaglandin synthesis are not known.

Isolated interstitial cells from both rats and rabbits have been shown to synthesize PGE_2 (40,185) in the renal medulla that increases in response to hormonal and osmotic stimuli. Collecting ducts also have prostaglandin biosynthetic capacity (25). In addition, the loop of Henle may have prostaglandin biosynthetic capacity because cyclo-oxygenase inhibitors seem to affect salt excretion in that part of the nephron (45). Since so many components of the mammalian kidney have the capacity to synthesize prostaglandins, it is quite likely that prostaglandin synthesis is compartmentalized to the point that the cell that produces the prostaglandin is the only one it affects.

How can one assess the prostaglandin production by the kidney in both man and experimental animals? In man the only non-invasive assessment of renal prostaglandin production is the measurement of the urinary prostaglandin excretion rate.

It has been reported that all of the primary prostaglandins are found in the human urine (83), but which part of the renal excretory system is responsible for this prostaglandin production is not known. In males, the contribution of seminal prostaglandins to the urinary prostaglandins can be considerable so most of the experimental studies that require measurements of urinary prostaglandin synthesis are performed in females. Urinary PGE_2 and $PGD_{2\alpha}$ in dogs, and probably in man, are of renal origin (64). However, the origins of the urinary 6-keto $PGF_{1\alpha}$ and thromboxane B_2 have not been rigorously examined and it is possible that these prostaglandins in the urine are of extrarenal origin. Perhaps the most judicious use of urinary prostaglandin measurement may be to evaluate the extent of cyclo-oxygenase inhibition by non-steroidal anti-inflammatory drugs. However, even in that situation the urinary prostaglandins may be representative only of prostaglandins of renal medullary origin and none of cortical origin.

In addition to the problems with the interpretation of the urinary prostaglandin values, variations in baseline measurements from one laboratory to another may be due to the use of different analytical techniques for urinary prostaglandins. The three most common techniques are gas chromatography—mass spectroscopy (GC-MS), radioimmunoassay, and radioreceptor assay. Of the three, the radioreceptor assay has consistently produced urinary PGE_2 values that are too high (49). The radioimmunoassay in most laboratories compares favorably with GC-MS (32,182), but interventions that increase urine flow rates sometimes give spuriously high prostaglandin values. Consistent, reproducible results are given by GC-MS but the procedure is painstakingly laborious.

Although there are problems with the interpretation of the urinary measurements of protaglandins, there are even more problems with the measurement and interpretation of the renal venous plasma concentration of prostaglandins. The measurement of PGE_2, $PGF_{2\alpha}$ and thromboxane B_2 in plasma is fraught with errors related to platelet prostaglandin production during blood collection. Accurate measurement of the circulating metabolite of PGE_2, 15-keto 13, 14 dihydro PGE_2, is difficult because of the instability of this prostaglandin in aqueous media (79). In addition to the technical problems, the renal venous plasma concentration of prostaglandins is not any more specific than urinary prostaglandins in determining the site of prostaglandin production in the kidney.

The true plasma concentration of all the primary prostaglandins is probably in the very low picogram per milliliter range making accurate determinations very difficult. In studying renal prostaglandin production in man and experimental animals, one must interpret urinary and renal venous prostaglandins levels conservatively. The most accurate we can be is to say that the prostaglandin system was activated or inactivated somewhere in the kidney.

THE EFFECT OF PROSTAGLANDINS ON RENAL HEMODYNAMICS

The evidence is consistent with the hypothesis that the renal prostaglandins can modulate the renal hemodynamic response to stress and mediate the vasodilation produced by some drugs. In order to demonstrate such a physiologic role for prostaglandins in controlling renal hemodynamics, several lines of evidence need to be examined. First, the kidney must be shown to be capable of generating prostaglandins which have an appropriate pharmacologic action (vasodilation). Second, the precursor of the prostaglandins must produce the expected effect that can be blocked by cyclo-oxygenase inhibitors. Third, renal prostaglandin synthesis must be increased in those circumstances where prostaglandins are thought to play a physiologic role. Fourth, inhibition of prostaglandin synthesis must produce an altered response to stress or drug infusion, producing enhanced vasoconstriction or lack of vasodilation.

Effects of Exogenous Prostaglandins and Arachidonic Acid

The evidence that the renal cortex is capable of generating all of the known primary prostaglandins has already been reviewed, and renal infusion studies have been reported for all of them. In dogs, intrarenal infusion of PGI_2, PGE_2, and PGD_2 causes renal vasodilation and a redistribution of renal blood flow towards the inner cortex (30,63,76). The significance of this redistribution of the renal blood flow is not known, but this pattern of vasodilation is not unique to the prostaglandin vasodilators (116). In contrast to findings in the dog, PGE_2 has been shown to be a renal vasoconstrictor in the rat (74). The rat seems to be the unusual species in this regard because PGE_2 is a renal vasodilator in all other mammals studied. PGI_2 vasodilates the rat renal vasculature similar to its effects in other species. Prostaglandin $F_{2\alpha}$ is devoid of activity in the dog renal circulation (30). The lability of thromboxane A_2 has deterred exploration of its effects *in vivo*, but the cyclic endoperoxide analogue, which mimics many of the properties of thromboxane A_2 *in vitro*, is a potent renal vasoconstrictor (72).

Intrarenal infusion of the precursor of the dienoic prostaglandins, arachidonic acid, produces renal vasodilation in the dog and a redistribution of intrarenal blood flow towards the inner cortical glomeruli (30). Cyclo-oxygenase inhibitors totally inactivate arachidonic acid indicating that a prostaglandin product rather than arachidonic acid itself is responsible for the vasodilation. Of the three prostaglandin vasodilators, PGI_2 is the most likely to play a role in modulating renal hemodynamics because isolated renal afferent arterioles generate PGI_2 almost exclusively (163). It is unlikely that a vasoconstrictor substance such as thromboxane A_2 has any significant role in control of the renal circulation under most circumstances because arachidonic acid produces renal vasodilation, and prostaglandin synthesis inhibition produces either no effect or vasoconstriction.

Effects of Blocking Prostaglandin Synthesis

The most useful technique to assess the effects of endogenously produced prostaglandins has been to block cyclo-oxygenase with non-steroidal anti-inflammatory drugs and measure the hemodynamic changes. In unanesthetized dogs, Swain et al. (158) found that indomethacin administration did not alter renal vascular resistance, but meclofenamic acid significantly reduced renal blood flow. There is no good explanation for the different responses to these two drugs. Terragno et al. (164) reported that indomethacin does not alter renal blood flow in conscious dogs.

In conscious rabbits, Beilin and Bhattacharya (12) demonstrated that both indomethacin and meclofenamic acid reduce renal blood flow. In contrast, Bill (22), utilizing microspheres to study regional blood flows in rabbits, could not demonstrate that a dose of 20 mg/kg of indomethacin altered renal blood flow.

An important contribution to our understanding of the effect of prostaglandin synthesis inhibitors on renal hemodynamics in normal conscious animals has been recently reported by Blasingham and co-workers (24). They studied the renal hemodynamic effect of sodium meclofenamate on conscious dogs maintained on normal salt and low-salt diets. Prostaglandin inhibition had no effect on renal blood flow in animals ingesting a normal salt diet, but caused significant renal vasoconstriction in salt-depleted animals. The normal response to sodium depletion is an increase in plasma renin activity and an activation of the sympathetic nervous system. Angiotensin II, norepinephrine, and renal nerve stimulation have all been shown to release vasodilator prostaglandins from the kidney. These vasodilator prostaglandins normally oppose the vasoconstriction and diminish the observed hemodynamic effects of the vasoconstrictor stimuli (2,67,121). However, when the synthesis of prostaglandins is blocked, then the full effect of the vasoconstrictors can occur.

Detailed micropuncture studies of the effects of angiotensin II in the rat support the concept that inhibition of prostaglandin synthesis augments the effects of angiotensin II on glomerular filtration rate and renal plasma flow. Baylis and Brenner (11a) used volume-expanded Munich-Wistar rats to investigate the dynamics of glomerular filtration during an infusion of angiotensin II. They found that angiotensin II in animals with an intact prostaglandin system, produced a decrease in glomerular plasma flow rate and glomerular ultrafiltration coefficient but that single nephron, (or whole kidney) glomerular filtration rate (GFR), was not affected because of an increase in transglomerular hydraulic pressure difference. However, when infused into animals pretreated with indomethacin or meclofenamate, angiotensin II produced a more profound decrease in glomerular capillary plasma flow rate due to a greater increase in arteriolar resistance, and this hemodynamic change resulted in a fall in single nephron and total kidney GFR. Prostaglandin synthesis inhibition did not change the angiotensin II-induced decrease in the glomerular ultrafiltration coefficient. From these studies it appears that the influence of endogenous prostaglandins on the renal effects of angiotensin II is to buffer against excessive vasoconstriction. The GFR may be secondarily influenced by the hemodynamic effects but not by a direct effect of endogenous prostaglandins on the glomerular ultrafiltration coefficient.

Studies in man generally indicate that endogenous prostaglandins modulate vasoconstrictor influences. Inhibition of prostaglandin synthesis in volunteers with a normal sodium intake produced either no change in renal function (16,23) or a slight change in GFR (-4.47%) (36). However, when volunteers were studied during low sodium intake and in the supine position, a greater reduction in GFR was produced by indomethacin (− 9%) (36), and when the low sodium intake was coupled with upright posture to further increase the plasma renin activity, indomethacin reduced the GFR by 12% (124). These findings suggest that the renal effects of inhibiting prostaglandin synthesis in normal man are dependent upon sodium balance and perhaps on the level of the plasma renin activity. Although some investigators have attempted to separate the effects of prostaglandin synthesis inhibition on the GFR from the effects on renal plasma flow (36,119a), studies in animals clearly indicate that the effects on GFR are linked to, and probably result from, the hemodynamic changes. Methods for measuring renal plasma flow in man, based on clearance techniques are sufficiently variable to suggest that small changes may not be discerned.

In order to correctly interpret the results of studies on the effect of prostaglandin inhibition on renal hemodynamics, one must know the activity of both the sympathetic nervous system, and the renin angiotensin system. When the activity of these vasoconstrictor systems is high, as in states of sodium depletion, there is the greatest influence of the prostaglandin system to modulate the vasoconstriction. Under these circumstances, inhibition of prostaglandin synthesis results in renal vasoconstriction and a reduction in GFR. On the other hand, when the vasoconstrictor activity is low, as is usually the case in salt-repleted normal animals, the vasodilator prostaglandin system is not active and inhibition of prostaglandin synthesis produces little or no hemodynamic effects.

Specific Pathologic Conditions in which Prostaglandins Contribute to the Maintenance of Renal Blood Flow

The general concept of vasodilator prostaglandins modulating vasoconstrictor influences on the renal circulation during salt restriction in normals also holds true for pathologic conditions. If the activity of the renin-angiotensin and/or sympathetic nervous system is high, vasodilator prostaglandins appear to be important in modulating renal hemodynamics. Terragno et al. (164) reported that pentobarbital anesthesia together with laparotomy stimulated renal prostaglandin production in a way that indicated inhibition of prostaglandin synthesis was associated with renal vasoconstriction. Pentobarbital or chloralose anesthesia alone, however, was not sufficient to stimulate renal prostaglandin synthesis. Presumably the additional stress of the surgical procedure with its attendant fluid loss was responsible for activation of the renin-angiotensin and/or the sympathetic nervous systems.

During hypotensive hemorrhage in dogs, Henrich et al. (86) reported that renal prostaglandins play a very key role in opposing the renal vasoconstriction secondary to the activation of the renin-angiotensin system and the renal sympathetics. In control animals a 30% hypotensive hemorrhage was associated with only a slight decline in renal blood flow and GFR. However, in dogs pretreated with indomethacin, the decline in renal blood flow and GFR was several fold higher, showing that vasodilatory prostaglandins protect the kidney from excessive vasoconstriction during hypotensive hemorrhage. Since renal denervation together with an angiotensin II receptor antagonist also prevented the renal vasoconstriction during hypotensive hemorrhage in indomethacin-treated dogs, the authors concluded that both angiotensin II and norepinephrine mediated the renal vasoconstriction and vasodilatory prostaglandins cushioned these responses. Data et al. (33) found that prostaglandin inhibitors, indomethacin and aspirin, effectively blocked the decrease in renal vascular resistance during hypotensive hemorrhage in dogs, and also prevented the redistribution of renal blood flow from the outer to inner cortex.

There are several pathologic conditions in man where prostaglandins are important in maintaining renal function. In patients with Bartter's syndrome there is excessive production of renal prostaglandins, and administration of indomethacin leads to a 20% reduction in the glomerular filtration rate (11). Hypokalemia is another situation where renal prostaglandins are overproduced and may contribute to renal hemodynamics. It is not clear whether the increased renal prostaglandin production in patients with Bartter's syndrome is secondary to hypokalemia.

Radfar et al. (136) found that patients with hypokalemia secondary to psychogenic vomiting had an elevated urinary PGE_2 excretion rate, high plasma renin activity, and resistance to the vascular effects of angiotensin II. Galvez et al. (68) reported similar findings in experimental hypokalemia in dogs, and indomethacin corrected both the elevated plasma renin activity, and the angiotensin resistance, suggesting that enhanced prostaglandin synthesis was responsible for these defects. Düsing et al. (43) could not demonstrate an increase in urinary prostaglandin excretion or plasma renin activity after induction of mild hypokalemia in normal female volunteers, although the pressor effect of infused angiotensin II was diminished. It is possible that the potassium deficit must be fairly severe before urinary PGE_2 increases, and urinary PGE_2 excretion does not necessarily reflect the synthesis of prostaglandins in sites that regulate renin secretion or vascular responsiveness to angiotensin II.

Congestive heart failure with prerenal azotemia is associated with an elevated excretion of immunoreactive PGE in the urine. Patients with heart failure also are known to have increases in plasma renin activity and activation of the sympathetic nervous system. In one patient with heart failure, indomethacin produced acute oliguric renal failure, probably because of inhibition of prostaglandin synthesis (173).

The administration of indomethacin or ibuprofen to patients with alcoholic cirrhosis has been associated with a marked decrease of renal plasma flow, and glomerular filtration rate (28,183). The degree of impairment of renal function produced by the non-steroidal anti-inflammatory drug in these patients was better correlated with indices of a renal salt-retaining state, a low urinary sodium excretion rate and high plasma renin activity, than with parameters of hepatic function. In conjunction with these effects of inhibiting prostaglandin synthesis, cirrhotic patients have been found to have an increased urinary PGE excretion rate (183). These studies lend some support to the intriguing hypothesis that the hepatorenal syndrome may be secondary to a relative deficiency in renal prostaglandin production.

Patients with chronic renal diseases of several etiologies may have further deterioration or renal function when given prostaglandin synthesis inhibitors. When investigated many of these patients have been found to have increased urinary PGE excretion. The administration of indomethacin (36) or aspirin (15) to patients with chronic renal disease resulted in a reduction of GFR and renal plasma flow. Patients with lupus erythematosus and probable lupus nephritis have a dramatic decrease in renal blood flow and glomerular filtration rate when treated with aspirin (98). Patients with nephrotic syndrome who were on sodium restricted diets and presumably had a reduced effective plasma volume, had a marked reduction in GFR and renal plasma flow when given indomethacin (8a). These findings suggest that prostaglandins are important in maintaining renal blood flow and glomerular filtration in patients with chronic renal disease.

The effect of prostaglandin inhibitors on the course of acute renal failure is variable in animal studies. In rabbits, indomethacin potentiated acute glycerol-induced renal failure but not mercuric chloride-induced renal failure (167). In rats, however, indomethacin had no effect on either glycerol- or mercuric chloride-induced renal failure (125,167). The effects of prostaglandin inhibition on the course of acute tubular necrosis in man is unknown.

In summary, in pathologic conditions associated with elevations of plasma renin activity and/or activation of the sympathetic nervous system, the renal prostaglandin system seems to be necessary to preserve renal blood flow. There is a suggestion that prostaglandins also are important for maintenance of renal blood flow in some patients with preexisting renal disease. In these cases, inhibition of prostaglandin synthesis with non-steroidal anti-inflammatory drugs will result in a decrease in renal blood flow and a decrease in GFR.

Prostaglandins as Mediators of Drug-Induced Vasodilation

Renal prostaglandins are thought to be important in mediating some of the physiologic effects of bradykinin and furosemide. The interrelationship between the renal kallikrein and the renal prostaglandin system is complex and incompletely understood. Numerous stimuli will activate both systems simultaneously. Bradykinin in cultured interstitial cells, as well as in intact kidneys, is a potent activator of phospholipase A_2 that releases arachidonic acid from tissue phospholipids (92,185). Most likely any stimulus that activates the renal kallikrein-kinin system will activate the prostaglandin system through the generation of bradykinin. Nasjletti et al. (120), utilizing mineralocorticoid administration in rats to stimulate both the renal kallikrein-kinin and prostaglandin systems, were able to demonstrate that the enhanced urinary prostaglandin excretion was the consequence of the activation of the renal kallikrein-kinin system by the steroids and not a co-stimulation of these two systems. Changes in intrarenal kallikrein activity can modulate renal prostaglandin production. However, whether prostaglandin production in vascular sites is affected by activation of the renal kallikrein-kinin system is not known. Since renal kallikrein is located largely in the brush border of the tubules, it seems an unlikely candidate to affect prostaglandin synthesis at non-tubular sites.

Since bradykinin is such a potent stimulator of prostagandin release, some researchers have proposed that the renal vasodilatory effect of bradykinin may be prostaglandin mediated (162). However, neither Lonigro et al. (113), nor Blasingham and Nasjletti (23), were able to alter the renal vascular effect of bradykinin with the use of prostaglandin synthetase inhibitors. This suggests that prostaglandins do not participate in bradykinin's vascular effects. In contrast, the natriuresis associated with intrarenal bradykinin infusion was blunted with the use of prostaglandin synthesis inhibitors. The activation of the renal kallikrein-kinin system can stimulate renal prostaglandin synthesis, and these prostaglandins can modulate the renal tubular sodium handling associated with enhanced kinin generation.

The interrelationship between furosemide administration and renal prostaglandin synthesis also is incompletely understood. It has been known for some time that both the renal vasodilation and renin release following administration of furosemide to animals and man, are totally blocked by cyclo-oxygenase inhibitors (135, 176). The mechanism of the interaction between furosemide and the prostaglandin system is a controversial subject. Furosemide in high concentrations *in vitro* will inhibit both the 15-hydroxydehydrogenase and 9-keto reductase to retard the metabolism of prostaglandin E_2 (156,159). However, *in vivo* this inhibition of prostaglandin metabolism has not been demonstrated (73). Furosemide administration *in vivo* is associated with an increase in urinary excretion of all the prostaglandins suggesting that furosemide interacts with the prostaglandin system by activating renal phospholipases releasing arachidonic acid rather than inhibiting the catabolism of PGE_2 (32). We have reported that furosemide-induced renal vasodilation in dogs is associated with the release of arachidonic acid from the kidney, and that this release is dependent on an intrarenal mechanism rather than a direct effect of furosemide on the vasculature (75).

Prostaglandins as Mediators of Renal Autoregulation

Renal prostaglandins have been reported by Herbaczynska-Cedro and Vane (87), to participate in the autoregulation of renal blood flow in the *in situ* pump-perfused dog kidney. Numerous well designed studies in the isolated canine kidney, the pump-perfused kidney *in situ*, or *in vivo*, have not confirmed the necessity of intact prostaglandin synthesis for the autoregulation of renal blood flow (6,35,96). Although renal blood flow does decrease in anesthetized dogs after the administration of prostaglandin synthesis inhibitors, autoregulation is not affected.

Prostaglandins as Mediators of Tubuloglomerular Feedback

Tubuloglomerular feedback is the process whereby a decrease in the rate of sodium chloride delivery to the distal tubule results in a decrease in the single nephron glomerular filtration rate via afferent arteriolar constriction (28). Experiments with cyclo-oxygenase inhibitors have implied that prostaglandins play a permissive role in the full expression of the tubuloglomerular feedback (96). The exact site where prostaglandins might participate in the tubuloglomerular feedback is not known. Cyclo-oxygenase inhibitors have been shown to blunt the tubulo-glomerular feedback in rats on a normal or high-salt diet, but not on a low-salt diet (142). Since the activity of the tubuloglomerular is very much dependent on the salt balance of the animal (141), the possiblity that cyclo-oxygenase inhibitors cause salt retention, which in itself will blunt the tubuloglomerular feedback, has to be considered as an explanation for these findings.

Thromboxane as a Mediator of Renal Vasoconstriction

Studies with isolated perfused kidneys from rabbits with chronic ureteral obstruction, glycerol-induced renal failure, and renal venous obstruction, have shown an increase in the amount of prostaglandins and thromboxane A_2 released into the renal venous effluent (13,119,184). Microsomes from these kidneys also produce thromboxane in increased amounts. The physiological significance of these findings is not known. The possibility that thromboxane A_2 may have vascular effects is suggested by *in vitro* experiments where bradykinin infusions into the renal artery produced constriction in the isolated, perfused kidney from a rabbit with one of the models of renal disease mentioned. Constriction produced by bradykinin was not a consistent finding but when it occurred, it could be inhibited by non-steroidal anti-inflammatory drugs. These investigators have not reported *in vivo* experiments. However, experiments *in vivo* with a similar model in the rat have been reported by Yarger et al. (179). These investigators found that imidazole but not indomethacin was effective in improving the blood flow and function of the kidney that had a 24-hr ureteral obstruction. Imidazole, *in vitro*, will inhibit thromboxane synthesis. Although it was suggested that imidazole produced its beneficial effects in the rat by inhibiting thromboxane synthesis, no data has proven that, in fact, imidazole decreased thromboxane synthesis in the *in vivo* model. Since indomethacin does not improve renal function in the rat model, the assumption must be that the predominant prostaglandin produced is not thromboxane and that imidazole may be producing its effects by another mechanism.

PROSTAGLANDINS AND WATER METABOLISM

The identification of cyclo-oxygenase in the interstital cells of the renal medulla and papilla and in the collecting ducts, has lent support to the hypothesis that prostaglandins may be involved in the regulation of renal water excretion (7). This hypothesis was devised to explain *in vitro* findings that some prostaglandins antagonize the hydrosomotic effects of antidiuretic hormone (ADH). Studies, *in vivo*, have generally supported this hypothesis.

Prostaglandins in the Control of Thirst and ADH-Release

Normal homeostasis requires fluid intake to replace water loss. The brain is responsible for the regulation of thirst and the release of ADH, while the kidney is responsible for the control of water loss. Although ADH is required for maximal renal water conservation, the renal response to ADH is dependent on the tonicity of the interstitial fluid in the renal medulla and the rate of flow and tonicity of collecting tubular fluid. Present evidence indicates that prostaglandins may be involved in ADH-release, thirst, and the renal response to ADH.

Prostaglandin E_2 has been shown to stimulate ADH-release *in vitro* from both an isolated pituitary preparation (66), and from an organ culture of the guinea pig neurohypophysial complex (93). In the latter studies, indomethacin suppressed the ability of hypertonicity or angiotensin II to release ADH but did not influence basal ADH-release.

Intracarotid infusion of PGE_2 *in vivo*, into rats, produced an increase in urine osmolality without changes in arterial pressure suggesting that ADH-release may be a direct effect of PGE_2 (169). Other *in vivo* studies of the effects of PGE_1 or PGE_2 in goats, rats or dogs, suggested release of ADH. However, the hemodynamic effects produced by the prostaglandins in these studies obviated any interpretation of a direct effect of the prostaglandins on ADH-release (8,21,75,88,108,178). Indomethacin was shown to reduce urinary ADH excretion in normal volunteers (78). These findings do not necessarily imply a direct role for prostaglandins in ADH-release since it has been shown that indomethacin enhances the renal response to ADH that would lead to a feedback decrease in ADH secretion. It is premature to make the definitive statement that prostaglandins mediate ADH-release *in vivo*. Investigations of the role of prostaglandins in the regulation of thirst have produced contradictory results (8,21,122) and additional data will be required before conclusions can be drawn.

Prostaglandins in the Intrarenal Regulation of Water Excretion

In Vitro Studies

Abundant evidence has accumulated that PGE_1 and PGE_2 will antagonize the effects of ADH to stimulate water transport *in vitro* both in the toad bladder and in the isolated perfused rabbit renal collecting duct (80,112,132,133). Cyclo-oxygenase inhibitors have enhanced the *in vitro* response to ADH implying a role for endogenous prostaglandins to modulate the effects of ADH (3,133).

The mechanism whereby PGE inhibits the action of ADH is not entirely clear. ADH stimulates adenylate cyclase in the toad bladder, kidney slice, and isolated collecting tubules, whereas PGE and arachidonic acid antagonize this effect of ADH (94,112). Since PGE_1 does not antagonize the effects of cyclic AMP (cAMP) in the toad bladder (59,112,132,177), prostaglandins seem to act proximal to the formation of cAMP. However, in some studies, cyclo-oxygenase inhibitors also increase the effects of cAMP to produce enhanced water transport suggesting the possibility of a site of PG action beyond cAMP formation (3,58).

Studies by Lum et al. (115) showed that ADH produced a greater increase in renal medullary cAMP content in indomethacin-treated rats than in control rats, supporting the concept that endogenous prostaglandins interfere with ADH-induced cAMP formation. The possibility that phosphodiesterase inhibition produced by indomethacin was responsible for the effect was disproved by showing normal medullary phosphodiesterase activity in the kidneys of indomethacin-treated animals.

The interpretation of all these studies on cAMP formation is complicated by the observation that PGE ($> 10^{-6}$M) can increase adenylate cyclase of renal tissue independent of an effect of ADH (59,131,47). Many of the cyclo-oxygenase inhibitors also inhibit other enzymes which can affect the response observed (60). Finally, there are many ADH-sensitive cell types within the kidney including cells in the glomeruli, vasculature, interstitial cells and tubules. This cellular heterogenicity limits the interpretation that can be made from the results of an analysis of whole tissue. Studies using more specific prostaglandin inhibitors and homogenous cell populations are necessary to clarify the issue.

In Vivo Studies

The interpretation of data generated *in vivo* is even more difficult than interpretation of the *in vitro* studies because renal prostaglandins can affect renal hemodynamics and solute excretion that by themselves can alter renal water handling. These interactions between the various effects of renal prostaglandins will be discussed in the final section of this chapter.

Infusion of PGE_1 or PGE_2 into the renal artery of dogs suggested an anti-ADH action because of an increase in free-water clearance (81,95,118). However, dissociating this effect from the effect of PGE on renal blood flow and solute excretion is difficult. Similar increase in free-water excretion produced by PGE_1 were observed in animals without circulating ADH, suggesting that PGE may enhance water excretion by increasing fluid delivery out of the proximal tubule (21). Such an effect on the proximal tubule, does not exclude an additional direct effect on the distal nephron or an effect on the action of ADH.

A more direct assessment of the role of endogenous prostaglandins in the control of water excretion *in vivo* was made by Anderson et al. (5) in anesthetized, hypophysectomized dogs undergoing a water diuresis. In these dogs indomethacin or meclofenamate potentiated the action of exogenous vasopressin without altering hemodynamics or solute excretion. A similar enhancement of the effects of ADH by non-steroidal anti-inflammatory drugs has been demonstrated in conscious animals and in man (20,53,104,147). These results are consistent with the hypothesis that endogenous prostaglandins modulate the effects of ADH on the water permeability of the collecting duct. However, the possibility that non-steroidal anti-inflammatory drugs increase medullary toxicity, thereby increasing the osmotic gradient for water movement, (165) has not been entirely ruled out.

Prostaglandins and Water Excretion in Disease

Hypokalemia can produce polyuria and a renal concentrating defect, the etiology of which is not clear (19,77,89,137). Some investigators have suggested that potassium depletion results in a decrease in medullary interstitial tonicity (48), but evidence *in vivo* and *in vitro* indicates that hypokalemia may also produce a defect in the cellular action of ADH (57,117). The cellular defect could be because of structural abnormalities in the collecting duct or because of a biochemical change in the collecting duct produced by the hypokalemic state (97,151). Evidence links potassium concentration and prostaglandin synthesis (41,43,185,187). Increasing potassium concentration inhibits PGE_2 synthesis by rabbit renomedullary interstitial cells and rabbit and human renal papillary slices. It is possible that hypokalemia may stimulate prostaglandin synthesis. In man and experimental animals, potassium depletion has been reported to increase urinary PGE excretion in some studies (43,55,185), but not in others (18,90). Similar contradictory results are reported in studies of the effects of non-steroidal anti-inflammatory drugs on the concentrating defect of hypokalemia (42,77,152). More work is needed in this area to resolve the conflicting data.

Angiotensin II will increase renal prostaglandin synthesis, that may then affect renal water excretion. In recent experiments, Galvez et al. (69) clamped one renal artery and observed a contralateral increase in urine volume, urinary PGE excretion, and free-water clearance independent of changes in renal or systemic hemodynamics, glomerular filtration or solute excretion. Saralasin, a competitive inhibitor of Angiotensin II, inhibited this effect as did indomethacin, suggesting the involvement of both a prostaglandin and angiotensin II. The effect was not due to inhibition of ADH-release, since it was also observed in hypophysectomized animals receiving a constant infusion of ADH. These results indicate that the increase in angiotensin II generation induced by renal artery stenosis, produced an increase in prostaglandin production by the contralateral kidney. The prostaglandin then antagonized the effects of ADH resulting in increased free-water excretion by the contralateral kidney.

Pyelonephritis results in a defect in renal concentrating ability that is independent of histologic changes and is rapidly reversible when the infection is controlled. In rats with pyelonephritis, indomethacin or meclofenamate improved the renal concentrating ability (110). The mechanism of this improvement is unknown, but measurements indicate that the beneficial effect of indomethacin is independent of changes in papillary blood flow. No measurements of glomerular filtration, medullary tonicity, or protaglandins were made.

Reports have suggested the involvement of prostaglandins in several other types of nephrogenic diabetes insipidus. It has been suggested that the polyuria that occurs in some patients on lithium therapy is due to increased prostaglandin synthesis (37,61,138,139,171). Indomethacin given to the patients with lithium-induced polyuria, diminished the excretion of PGE, decreased urine flow rate, and increased urinary osmolality without altering the glomerular filtration rate or solute excretion (171). These preliminary observations suggest that prostaglandins antagonize the renal effect of ADH and contribute to the lithium-induced polyuria.

The polyuria of hypercalcemia also has been suggested to involve the prostaglandin system. The initial step in prostaglandin synthesis is the release of arachidonic acid from phospholipids by a calcium-dependent phospholipase. Calcium ionophores augment, and calcium uptake inhibitors suppress, prostaglandin formation in renal slices (101,181). One can speculate that hypercalcemia may produce nephrogenic diabetes insipidus via a prostaglandin mechanism. In a preliminary report, Serros and Kirschenbaum (143) produced hypercalcemia in rats with 1,25 dihydroxyvitamin D_3, that resulted in increases in urine volume and prostaglandin excretion, and indomethacin reversed the process.

Continuous ADH administration leads to escape from its hydroosmotic effects (133). A role for prostaglandins was suggested by the observation that ADH stimulates PG synthesis from cultured renomedullary interstitial cells, kidney slices, and toad urinary bladder in some (185,186), but not all (22a,62) studies. Urinary PGE excretion has also been found to increase following ADH administration to rats with diabetes insipidus (172,38). Gross and Anderson (82) found that the early escape from ADH in the rat was associated with an increase in urinary PGE_2 excretion, and indomethacin not only prevented the increase in PGE_2 excretion, but also prevented the early escape. However, escape from ADH ultimately occurred, although at a lower plasma sodium concentration. These observations implicate prostaglandin involvement in only the early escape from the water-retaining effect of ADH.

In summary, a role for prostaglandin in the maintenance of water balance has been established. Prostaglandin E_1 and PGE_2 antagonize the effects of ADH. Although the mechanism of this effect is still not entirely understood, there is substantial evidence that prostaglandins decrease the cellular cAMP response to ADH. However, effects of prostaglandin on hemodynamics, solute excretion, and medullary tonicity also can be important determinants of ADH responsiveness. The beneficial effects of inhibition of prostaglandin synthesis in a variety of polyuric states may be related not only to enhanced responsiveness to ADH, but also to ADH independent influences on renal concentrating ability, such as an increased medullary tonicity.

EFFECT OF PROSTAGLANDINS ON SODIUM METABOLISM

Despite extensive study, the precise influence of renal prostaglandins on renal sodium handling remains unclear. Since the kidney is the major organ regulating sodium balance, and since sodium balance is the major determinant of extracellular fluid volume, the role of prostaglandins in renal sodium transport is an important subject. Four types of studies have been carried out to investigate this issue: (1) *in vitro* studies utilizing a variety of animal membranes; (2) studies utilizing infusions of pharmacologic doses of prostaglandins into the renal or systemic circulation; (3) balance studies that examine the effects of altering sodium balance on renal prostaglandin biosynthesis; and (4) determinations of the effect of prostaglandin inhibition, usually with non-steroid anti-inflammatory agents, on sodium balance. Conflicting evidence for a natriuretic role for prostaglandins can be found in most of these areas.

In Vitro Studies

Data from *in vitro* studies support conclusions that PGE can enhance, inhibit, or have no effect on sodium transport. When PGE_1 was applied to the serosal surface of the toad bladder, significant increases in short circuit current and active sodium transport resulted (112). Similar findings have been demonstrated using frog skin (9,51). Since the mechanisms of sodium transport in these membranes are thought to be similar to transport in renal collecting duct, and distal tubular epithelium, it is possible that prostaglandins could decrease renal sodium excretion by enhancing tubular sodium reabsorption. This antinatriuretic effect might be obscured *in vivo* by prostaglandin induced renal vasodilation that would decrease proximal tubular sodium reabsorption.

Utilizing several *in vitro* preparations, Dunn and Howe (39) were unable to find an effect of prostaglandins A, E, and F on electrolyte transport in rabbit cortical and medullary tubular suspensions, in renal cortical slices from rat and guinea pig, in rabbit renal medullary slices, or in human erythrocytes. Consistent with these findings, Fine and Trizna (56) demonstrated that PGE_2 applied to either the peritubular or luminal surface of isolated medullary collecting tubules, or medullary thick ascending limbs of Henle, had no effect on sodium transport.

In direct contrast, Stokes and Kokko (155) found that PGE_2 applied to the peritubular surface of isolated collecting tubules from DOCA-treated rabbits resulted in an inhibition of the negative transepithelial potential in cortical and outer medullary collecting tubules. It also produced a decrease of net luminal sodium transport by inhibition of sodium efflux without affecting sodium backflux. The effects of PGE_2 on the collecting tubules were dose-dependent, rapid, and generally reversible. Stokes (154) noted that PGE_2 inhibits chloride reabsorption in the medullary thick ascending limb of Henle but not in the cortical thick asending limb. Iino and Imai (91) using both normal and DOCA-loaded rabbits also observed that PGE_1, PGE_2, and $PGF_{2\alpha}$ could inhibit sodium efflux when these lipids were applied to the peritubular surface of isolated cortical and medullary collecting tubules. Conflicting data on the effects of prostaglandin on collecting tubule and ascending limb of Henle sodium transport cannot be resolved with the available information.

In Vivo Studies

Infusion of Prostaglandins and Arachidonic Acid

When infused either intravenously or into the renal artery, prostaglandins of the E and A series cause a concomitant increase in renal blood flow and an increase in renal sodium excretion in anesthetized dogs (81,95,118) and conscious man (29,103,107). On the basis of clearance studies that demonstrate an increase in free-water clearance associated with the natriuresis of prostaglandin infusion, it appears that intrarenal prostaglandin infusions decrease sodium reabsorption in the proximal tubule. A natriuretic response following intrarenal prostacyclin and cyclic endoperoxides also has been observed (76,126). It is important to note that all of these studies utilized pharmacologic doses of prostaglandins, and that the intrarenal infusion of these substances may not mimic their intrarenal site of biosynthesis and action. Furthermore, the natriuresis of prostaglandin infusion appears to be similar to that obtained with the intrarenal infusion of other renal vasodilators (118), suggesting a non-specific hemodynamic effect. Shea and coworkers (144) found that intrarenal prostaglandin administered during intrarenal vasodilation with acetylcholine resulted in a further increase in natriuresis without additional vasodilation. This suggests a direct *in vivo* effect of prostaglandin to inhibit tubular sodium reabsorption.

The most convincing evidence that endogenous prostaglandins may be natriuretic has been the demonstration of Tannenbaum et al. (160) that the intrarenal infusion of arachidonic acid to anesthetized dogs results in ipsilateral increases in sodium excretion and prostaglandin-like substances in renal venous effluent. Furthermore, enhanced renal sodium excretion could be demonstrated with doses of arachidonate (< 3 μg/kg/min) that did not alter glomerular filtration rate or renal blood flow. This natriuresis could be stopped by the administration of an inhibitor of prostaglandin synthesis.

In *in vivo* micropuncture studies, Strandhoy et al. (157) investigated whether alterations in intrarenal physical forces associated with increased renal blood flow could be detected following renal arterial infusions of PGE. They noted both an increase in peritubular capillary hydrostatic pressure, and a decrease in peritubular oncotic pressure. However, only PGE_1 decreased fractional and absolute sodium reabsorption by the proximal tubule. No changes in proximal sodium reabsorption were seen with PGE_2 infusions despite quantitatively similar alterations in hydrostatic and oncotic pressure. Fülgraff and Meiforth (65) reported similar results and also noted that PGE_2 had no effect on sodium transport in the loop of Henle but did result in decreased fractional sodium reabsorption along the distal nephron. Infusion studies indicate that prostaglandins can increase renal sodium excretion. The mechanism, site and physiologic significance of these observations in health and disease remain to be determined.

Effects of Alterations in Sodium Balance on Renal Prostaglandin Biosynthesis

Saline loading has been reported to diminish urinary PGE excretion in rabbits and rats (111,140,146,166,174). In contrast, Lifschitz et al. (111) found no relationship between sodium intake, and urinary PGE_2 excretion in the rabbit. Experiments with cyclo-oxygenase inhibitors suggest that salt restriction does activate vascular prostaglandin synthesis (24). Some studies have shown saline infusions increases PGE in renal venous blood in humans and dogs (134,146,161). These conflicting results may be due to limitations in the prostaglandin assays employed, the variability in the experimental conditions utilized, awake versus anesthetized, acute versus chronic, various magnitudes of sodium loading, and species differences. There also is the possibility that urinary PGE excretion may not always reflect intrarenal prostaglandin synthesis when there are major changes in urine flow. At present it is difficult to reconcile these results into a coherent hypothesis regarding prostaglandins and renal sodium excretion.

Effects of Prostaglandin Inhibition on Sodium Balance and Diuretic Action

In the majority of published studies, inhibition of prostaglandin synthesis has resulted in decreases in urinary sodium excretion in rats, dogs, and man (4,10, 27,36,46,52,54,85). Donker et al. (36) studied the effects of conventional therapeutic doses of indomethacin, 150 mg/day, in humans with normal or reduced renal function. A decrease in sodium excretion was clearly apparent after one day. Sodium and water retention also occurred with the acute administration of indomethacin to conscious rats during mild saline volume expansion (44,85). Altsheler et al. (4) studied conscious dogs during sodium loading both before and after administration of either indomethacin orally or meclofenamate intravenously. In dogs given a sodium load, administration of either inhibitor of prostaglandin synthesis led to a decrease in sodium excretion over a 5-hr period. There were no significant changes in glomerular filtration rate, renal plasma flow, or filtration fraction during any of the experimental periods.

Fewer studies suggest that, under certain circumstances, inhibition of prostaglandin synthesis may have either no effect or may enhance renal sodium excretion. Berl et al. (20) and Altsheler et al. (4) studying rats and dogs, respectively, showed no effect on sodium excretion when these animals were given prostaglandin synthesis inhibitors during water diuresis. Zambraski and Dunn (180) found no effect of indomethacin and meclofenamate to alter sodium excretion in conscious dogs. Chronic treatment of rabbits with either indomethacin or meclofenamate did not alter renal sodium excretion at different levels of sodium intake (111). Kirschenbaum and Stein (99) administered two structurally dissimilar inhibitors of prostaglandin biosynthesis to conscious dogs during water diuresis and noted significant increases in sodium excretion without changes in potassium excretion, urine volume, glomerular filtration rate, or renal plasma flow. Since potassium excretion and urine volume were unaltered, the authors suggested that the natriuretic effect of these agents occurred somewhere in the distal nephron. Using an isolated blood-perfused dog kidney, Vanherweghem et al. (168) demonstrated that indomethacin decreased the fractional reabsorption of sodium while the GFR and renal plasma flow were constant. Oliw et al. (128) acutely expanded the extracellular fluid volume of rabbits with Ringer's solution with and without prior administration of two different inhibitors of prostaglandin synthesis. They demonstrated that the prostaglandin-inhibited animals had a significantly greater natriuresis than those not given an inhibitor. These observations suggest that inhibition of prostaglandin synthesis does not always result in an antinatriuretic response and sometimes promotes sodium excretion.

Epstein and colleagues (49,50) have proposed that the underlying volume status is an important determinant of renal response to prostaglandin synthesis inhibition. Renal sodium handling was assessed systematically in subjects during different states of sodium balance. The natriuretic response to central volume expansion induced by head-out water immersion was assessed in the sodium-replete state with and without indomethacin pretreatment. Six of the subjects were restudied in an identical manner following dietary sodium restriction to 10 mEq/day. During the sodium-replete studies, the natriuresis of immersion following indomethacin administration did not differ from that observed during immersion without indomethacin. The natriuresis of immersion was markedly attenuated by indomethacin pretreatment during the sodium-depleted state. The demonstration that prostaglandin synthetase inhibition blunted sodium excretion in the sodium-depleted state only is consistent with the formulation that renal prostaglandins are critical modulators of renal function during conditions or disease states of volume contraction.

Several studies have evaluated the role of prostaglandins in diuretic action. The potent loop diuretic, furosemide, results in an increase in urinary prostaglandin excretion in humans (32,1). Administration of a non-steroidal anti-inflammatory agent has been demonstrated to blunt the natriuresis of furosemide in anesthetized animals and in normotensive man (14,17,102,127,130,135). The mechanism(s) whereby prostaglandin inhibition antagonizes the natriuretic effect of furosemide is questionable. The greatest effect of prostaglandin inhibition, causing renal sodium retention and antagonizing the effect of diuretic agents, is seen in states of diminished glomerular filtration rate and/or renal perfusion. In this situation, prostaglandin inhibition often results in further deterioration in the glomerular filtration rate and renal blood flow that can lead to sodium retention so that a direct effect of prostaglandins on sodium transport cannot be assessed. Furosemide also increases renal blood flow by a prostaglandin-related mechanism, and it is possible that such vascular effects could mediate some of the natriuretic effect of furosemide by increasing sodium delivery to the loop of Henle. Finally, furosemide is an organic acid requiring either glomerular filtration or tubular secretion to gain access to the luminal surface of the renal tubule where it exerts its action. The non-steroidal anti-inflammatory agents utilized as prostaglandin inhibitors are also organic acids secreted by the proximal tubule (34). Inhibition of furosemide tubular secretion could be another pathway of diuretic antagonism. However, Brater has found that the antagonistic effect of indomethacin on furosemide natriuresis occurs independent of an affect on the urinary excretion of furosemide (148).

Although prostaglandins can be shown to have pharmacologic effects that alter sodium transport in some *in vitro* systems, whether endogenously produced prostaglandins produce important direct effects on renal tubular sodium handling *in vivo* is far from certain. In experimentally-induced water diuresis where urinary solute concentration is very low, some investigators have found that the non-steroidal anti-inflammatory drugs produce natriuresis. In most circumstances the literature supports the conclusion that the non-steroidal anti-inflammatory drugs produce sodium retention *in vivo* that, at least in part, is related to inhibition of prostaglandin synthesis.

INTERACTIONS BETWEEN RENAL HEMODYNAMICS, SODIUM EXCRETION AND FREE WATER CLEARANCE

In order to integrate the information presented in this chapter, one must know the potential interrelations that exist between renal hemodynamics, salt excretion, and free-water clearance. Because of these interrelationships, statements about direct effects of prostaglandin *in vivo* on renal tubular sodium handling or water reabsorption must be made with caution.

The vasodilator prostaglandins increase renal blood flow and shift the intrarenal distribution of blood flow toward the inner cortical nephrons. These hemodynamic effects alter the physical factors such as hydrostatic and osmotic pressure differentials between the tubular fluid and peritubular interstitial fluid, resulting in a decreased proximal reabsorption of sodium and an increased delivery of fluid and solute out of the proximal tubules. Vasodilation per se can enhance sodium delivery to the distal nephron and may account for much of the natriuresis observed. However, when pharmacologic doses of prostaglandins are infused into a renal vasculature that is already maximally dilated with acetylcholine, an additional natriuresis occurs, suggesting effects on sodium balance unrelated to vasodilation (144).

The increase in distal delivery of fluid and solute produced by prostaglandins also can result in an augmented free-water clearance because of an increase in the amount of solute available for reabsorption in the diluting segments of the nephron. Even in the absence of ADH, prostaglandins can increase free-water clearance (153). However, the fact that PGE_1 can increase free-water clearance more than acetylcholine, in spite of comparable effects on solute excretion in saline expanded dogs, suggests additional effects on the water permeability of the collecting duct (118).

In addition to affecting sodium delivery to the distal nephron, the vasodilation produced by prostaglandins can affect free-water clearance by influencing local environmental factors that provide the osmotic driving force for water movement across the collecting tubule. An increase in inner cortical, medullary, and papillary blood flow produced by prostaglandins can wash out solutes from the medulla and reduce interstitial hypertonicity thereby reducing water reabsorption, increasing free-water clearance, and producing ADH hyporesponsiveness (145). However, the renal prostaglandins do not appear to mediate the effect of ADH to redistribute the renal blood flow toward the inner cortical nephrons (170). In addition to hemodynamic effects, any direct effect of prostaglandins reducing sodium reabsorption from the tubular fluid into the medullary interstitial fluid also would result in a reduction of the osmotic gradient for water movement which could increase free-water clearance.

In contrast to the effects of vasodilator prostaglandins, the non-steroidal anti-inflammatory drugs can decrease renal blood flow under conditions of stress in which prostaglandin synthesis is enhanced and vasoconstrictor hormones are present in increased amounts. Indomethacin has been shown to reduce renal blood flow to the inner cortex, plasma flow to the papilla, and red cell velocity in medullary vasa rectae (31,100,109,150). These hemodynamic effects may not only increase proximal tubular sodium and water reabsorption, resulting in an anti-natriuresis and decreased solute available for free-water generation by the nephron, but also can decrease solute washout from the medullary interstitial fluid and enhance the osmotic gradient for water reabsorption. Indomethacin will increase medullary interstitial solute concentration in rats (70,165). If endogenous prostaglandins directly inhibit sodium reabsorption by the nephron, then the non-steroidal anti-inflammatory drugs can increase sodium reabsorption on this basis that may contribute to medullary interstitial hypertonicity and enhance the maximum urinary concentration produced by ADH.

CONCLUSIONS

Renal prostaglandins are important in maintaining the renal blood flow and glomerular filtration rate in conditions where vasoconstrictor hormones are increased and in diseases where renal function is impaired. Inhibition of prostaglandin synthesis produces profound effects on renal hemodynamics and function, resulting in sodium and water retention. Under normal unstressed conditions, the renal prostaglandins do not appear to be of critical importance in controlling renal blood flow. However, the prostaglandins are involved in determining the magnitude of response to ADH and may be important in some conditions where urinary concentrating ability is impaired. Finally, although the direct effect of renal prostaglandins on sodium metabolism is controversial, the usual effect of inhibition of prostaglandin synthesis is to produce sodium retention.

ACKNOWLEDGMENTS

This work was supported by a research grant from NIH HL 21308. Dr. Gerber is an Established Investigator of the American Heart Association and Dr. Anderson has an RCDA from NIH, HL 00316.

REFERENCES

1. Abe, K., Yasujima, M., Chiba, S., Irokawa, N., Ito, T., and Yoshinaga, K. (1977): Effect of furosemide on urinary excretion of prostaglandin E in normal volunteers and patients with essential hypertension. *Prostaglandins*, 14:513-521.
2. Aiken, J. W., and Vane, J. R. (1973): Intrarenal prostaglandin release attenuates the renal vasoconstrictor activity of angiotensin. *J. Pharmacol. Exp. Ther.*, 184:678-687.
3. Albert, W. C., and Handler, J. S. (1974): Effect of PGE_1, indomethacin, and polyphloretin phosphate on toad bladder response to ADH. *Am. J. Physiol.*, 226:1382–1386.
4. Altsheler, P., Klahr, S., Rosenbaum, R., and Slatopolsky, E. (1978): Effects of inhibitors of prostaglandin synthesis on renal sodium excretion in normal dogs and dogs with decreased renal mass. *Am. J. Physiol.*, 235:F338–F344.
5. Anderson, R. J., Berl, T., McDonald, K. M., and Schrier, R. W. (1975): Evidence for an *in vivo* antagonism between vasopressin and prostaglandin in the mammalian kidney. *J. Clin. Invest.*, 56:420–426.
6. Anderson, R. J., Taher, M. S., Cronin, R. E., McDonald, K. M., and Schrier, R. W. (1975): Effect of β-adrenergic blockade and inhibitors of angiotensin II and prostaglandins on renal autoregulation. *Am. J. Physiol.*, 229:731–736.

7. Anderson, R. J., Berl, T., McDonald, K. M., and Schrier, R. W. (1976): Prostaglandins: Effects on blood pressure, renal blood flow, sodium and water excretion (editorial review). *Kidney Int.*, 10:205–215.

8. Anderson, B., and Leksell, L. G. (1975): Effects on fluid balance of intraventricular infusions of prostaglandin E_1. *Acta Physiol. Scand.*, 93:286–288.

8a. Arisz, L., Donker, A. J. M., Brentjins, J. R. H., and van der Hem, G. K. (1976): The effect of indomethacin on proteinuria and kidney function in the nephrotic syndrome. *Acta Med. Scand.*, 199:121–125.

9. Barry, E., and Hall, W. J. (1969): Stimulation of sodium movement across frog skin by prostaglandin E_1. *J. Physiol. (Lond.)*, 200:83–84.

10. Bartha, J. (1977): Effect of indomethacin on renal function in anesthetized dogs. *Int. Urol. Nephrol.*, 9:81–90.

11. Bartter, F. C., Gill, J. R., Frölich, J. C., Bowden, R. E., Hollifield, J. W., Radfar, N., Keiser, H. R., Oates, J. A., Seyberth, H., and Taylor, A. A. (1976): Prostaglandins are overproduced by the kidneys and mediate hyperreninemia in Bartter's syndrome. *Trans. Assoc. Am. Physicians*, 89:77–91.

11a. Baylis, C., and Brenner, B. M. (1978): Modulators by prostaglandin synthesis inhibitors of the action of exogenous angiotensin II on glomerular ultrafiltration in the rat. *Circ. Res.*, 43:889–898.

12. Beilin, L. J., and Bhattacharya, J. (1976): The effects of prostaglandin synthesis inhibitors on renal blood flow distribution within the kidney. *J. Physiol.*, 256:9P–10P.

13. Benabe, J. E., Klahr, S., Hoffman, M. D., and Morrison, A. R. (1980): Production of thromboxane A_2 by the kidney in glycerol-induced acute renal failure. *Prostaglandins*, 19:333–347.

14. Berg, K. J., and Bergan, A. (1976): Effects of different doses of acetylsalicylic acid on renal function in the dog. *Scand. J. Clin. Lab. Invest.*, 36:779–786.

15. Berg, K. J. (1977): Acute effects of acetylsalicylic acid on renal function in normal man. *Eur. J. Clin. Pharm.*, 11:111–116.

16. Berg, K. J. (1977): Acute effects of acetylsalicylic acid on renal function in normal man. *Eur. J. Clin. Pharm.*, 11:117–123.

17. Berg, K. J., and Loew, D. (1977): Inhibition of furosemide-induced natriuresis by acetylsalicylic acid in dogs. *Scand. J. Clin. Lab. Invest.*, 37:125–131.

18. Berl, T., Aisenbrey, G. A., and Linas, S. L. (1980): Renal concentrating defect in the hypokalemic rat is prostaglandin independent. *Am. J. Physiol.*, 238:F37–F41.

19. Berl, T., Linas, S. L., Aisenbrey, G. A., and Anderson, R. J. (1977): On the mechanism of polyuria in potassium depletion: The role of polydipsia. *J. Clin. Invest*, 60:620–625.

20. Berl, T., Raz, A., Wald, H., Horowitz, J., and Czaczkes, W. (1977): Prostaglandin synthesis inhibition and the action of vasopressin: Studies in man and rat. *Am. J. Physiol.*, 232:F529–F537.

21. Berl, T., and Schrier, R. W. (1973): Mechanism of effect of prostaglandin E_1 on renal water excretion. *J. Clin. Invest.*, 52:463–471.

22. Bill, A. (1979): Effects of indomethacin on regional blood flow in conscious rabbits—A microsphere study. *Acta Physiol. Scand.*, 105:437–442.

22a. Bisordi, J. E., Schlondorff, D., and Hays, R. M. (1980): Interaction of vasopressin and prostaglandins in the toad urinary bladder. *J. Clin. Invest.*, 66:1200–1210.

23. Blasingham, M. C., and Nasjletti, A. (1979): Contributions of renal prostaglandins to the natriuretic action of bradykinin in the dog. *Am. J. Physiol.*, 237:F182–F187.

24. Blasingham, M. C., Shade, R. E., Share, L., and Nasjletti, A. (1980): The effect of meclofenamate on renal blood flow in the unanesthetized dog: Relation to renal prostaglandins and sodium balance. *J. Pharmacol. Exp. Ther.*, 214:1–4.

25. Bohman, S. O. (1977): Demonstration of prostaglandin synthesis in collecting duct cells and other cell types of the rabbit renal medulla. *Prostaglandins*, 14:729–741.

26. Boyer, T. D., Zia, P., and Reynolds, T. B. (1979): Effect of indomethacin and prostaglandin A_1 on renal function and plasma renin activity in alcoholic liver disease. *Gastroenterology*, 77:215–222.

27. Brater, D. C. (1979): Effect of indomethacin on salt and water homeostasis. *Clin. Pharmacol. Ther.*, 25:322–330.

28. Briggs, J. P., and Wright, F. S. (1979): Feedback control of glomerular filtration rate: Site of effector mechanism. *Am. J. Physiol.*, 236:F40–F47.

29. Carr, A. A. (1970): Hemodynamic and renal effects of a prostaglandin, PGA_1, in subjects with essential hypertension. *Am. J. Med. Sci.*, 259:21–26.

30. Chang, L. C. T., Splawinski, J. A., Oates, J. A., and Nies, A. S. (1975): Enhanced renal prostaglandin production in the dog. II. Effects on intrarenal hemodynamics. *Circ. Res.*, 36:204–207.
31. Chuang, E. L., Reineck, H. J., Osgood, R. W., Kunau, R. T., Jr., and Stein, J. H. (1978): Studies on the mechanism of reduced urinary osmolality after exposure of the renal papilla. *J. Clin. Invest.*, 61:633–639.
32. Ciabattoni, G., Pugliese, F., Cinotti, G. A., Stirati, G., Ronci, R., Castrucci, G., Pierucci, A., and Patrono, C. (1979): Characterization of furosemide-induced activation of the renal prostaglandin system. *Europ. J. Pharmacol.*, 60:181–187.
33. Data, J. L., Chang, L. C. T., and Nies, A. S. (1976): Alteration of canine renal vascular response to hemorrhage by inhibitors of prostaglandin synthesis. *Am. J. Physiol.*, 230:940–945.
34. Data, J. L., Rane, A., Gerber, J., Wilkerson, G. R., Nies, A. S., and Branch, R. A. (1978): The influence of indomethacin on the pharmacokinetics, diuretic response, and hemodynamics of furosemide in the dog. *J. Pharmacol. Exp. Ther.*, 206:431–438.
35. Dighe, K. K., Hall, J. C., Smith, G. W., and Ungar, A. (1977): Renal blood flow autoregulation and renal venous prostaglandins in the pump-perfused canine kidney. *Br. J. Pharmacol.*, 59:571–575.
36. Donker, A. J. M., Ansz, L., Brentjens, J. R. H., vander Hem, G. K., and Hollemans, H. J. G. (1976): The effect of indomethacin on kidney function and plasma renin activity in man. *Nephron*, 17:288–296.
37. Donker, A. J., Prins, E., Meijer, S., Sluiter, W. J., van Berkestign, W. B. M., and Dols, L. C. W. (1979): A renal function study in 30 patients on long-term lithium therapy. *Clin. Nephrol.*, 12:254–262.
38. Dunn, M. J., Greely, H. P., Valtin, H., Kinter, L. B., and Beeuwkes, R. III. (1978): Renal excretion of prostaglandins E_2 and $F_{2\alpha}$ in diabetes insipidus rats. *Am. J. Physiol.*, 235:E624–E627.
39. Dunn, M. J., and Howe, D. (1977): Prostaglandins lack a direct inhibitory action on electrolyte and water transport in the kidney and the erythrocyte. *Prostaglandins*, 13:417–429.
40. Dunn, M. J., Staley, R. S., and Harrison, M. (1976): Characterization of prostaglandin production in tissue culture of rat renal medullary cells. *Prostaglandins*, 12:37–49.
41. Düsing, R., Attallah, A. A., Prezyna, A. P., and Lee, J. B. (1978): Renal biosynthesis of prostaglandin E_2 and $F_{2\alpha}$: Dependence on extracellular potassium. *J. Lab. Clin. Med.*, 92:669–677.
42. Düsing, R., Gill, J. R., Jr., and Bartter, F. C. (1978): The role of prostaglandins in the renal response to desoxycorticosterone (DOCA) in the dog. *Kidney Int.*, 14:693.
43. Düsing, R., Gill, J. R., Bartter, F. C., and Güllner, H. G. (1980): The effect of potassium depletion on urinary prostaglandins in normal man. In: *Advances in Prostaglandin and Thromboxane Research*, Vol. 7, edited by B. Samuelsson, P. W. Ramwell, and R. Paoletti, pp. 1189–1192. Raven Press, New York.
44. Düsing, R., Melder, B., and Kramer, J. J. (1976): Prostaglandins and renal function in acute extracellular volume expansion. *Prostaglandins*, 12:3–10.
45. Düsing, R., Nicolas, V., Glanzer, K., Kipnowski, J., and Kramer, J. H. (1980): Evidence that prostaglandins participate in the regulation of NaCl absorption in the ascending limb of Henle *in vivo*. In: *Proceedings from International Symposium on Prostaglandins and the Kidney*, Abstract No. 1, Stuttgart, Germany.
46. Düsing, R., Opitz, W. D., and Kramer, H. J. (1977): The role of prostaglandins in the natriuresis of acutely salt-loaded rats. *Nephron*, 18:212–219.
47. Eakins, K. E. (1971): Prostaglandin antagonism by polymeric phosphates of phloretin and related compounds. *Ann. N.Y. Acad. Sci.*, 180:386–395.
48. Eigler, J. O., Salassa, R. M., Bahn, R. C., and Owen, C. A., Jr. (1962): Renal distribution of sodium in potassium-depleted and vitamin D-intoxicated rats. *Am. J. Physiol.*, 202:1115–1120.
49. Epstein, M., Lifschitz, M. D., Hoffman, D. S., and Stein, J. H. (1979): Relationship between renal prostaglandin E and renal sodium handling during water immersion in normal man. *Circ. Res.*, 45:71–80.
50. Epstein, M., and Lifschitz, M. D. (1980): Volume status as a determinant of the influence of renal PGE on renal function. *Nephron*, 25:157–159.
51. Fassina, G., Carpenedo, F., and Santi, R. (1969): Effect of prostaglandin E_1 on isolated short-circuited frog skin. *Life Sci.*, 8:181–187.
52. Feigen, L. P., Klainer, E., Chapnick, B. M., and Kadowitz, P. J. (1976): The effect of indomethacin on renal function in pentabarbital-anesthetized dogs. *J. Pharmacol. Exp. Ther.*, 198:457–463.

53. Fejes-Toth, G., Magyra, A., and Walter, J. (1977): Renal response to vasopressin after inhibition of prostaglandin synthesis. *Am. J. Physiol.*, 232:F416–F423.
54. Feldman, D., Loose, D. S., and Tan, S. Y. (1978): Nonsteroidal anti-inflammatory drugs cause sodium and water retention in the rat. *Am. J. Physiol.*, 234:F490–F496.
55. Ferris, T. F. (1978): Prostaglandins, potassium and Bartter's syndrome. *J. Lab. Clin. Med.*, 92:663–668.
56. Fine, L. G., and Trizna, W. (1977): Influence of prostaglandins on sodium transport of isolated medullary nephron segments. *Am. J. Physiol.*, 232:F383–390.
57. Finn, A. L., Handler, J. S., and Orloff, J. (1966): Relation between toad bladder potassium content and permeability response to vasopressin. *Am. J. Physiol.*, 210:1279–1284.
58. Flores, A. G. A., and Sharp, G. W. G. (1972): Endogenous prostaglandins and osmotic water flow in the toad bladder. *Am. J. Physiol.*, 233:1392–1397.
59. Flores, J., Witkum, P. A., Beckman, B., and Sharp, G. W. G. (1975): Stimulation of osmotic water flow in toad bladder by prostaglandin E_1. *J. Clin. Invest.*, 56:256–262.
60. Flower, R. J.: Drugs which inhibit prostaglandin biosynthesis. *Pharmacol. Rev.*, 36:33–67.
61. Forrest, J. N., Jr., Cohen, A. D., Torretti, J., Himmelhoch, J. M., and Epstein, F. H. (1974): On the mechanism of lithium-induced diabetes insipidus in man and the rat. *J. Clin Invest.*, 53:1115–1123.
62. Forrest, J. N., Jr., and Goodman, D. B. P. (1980): Prostaglandin E_2 mediates the effect of pH on ADH-stimulated water flow but ADH does not stimulate prostaglandin E_2 production in the toad urinary bladder. *Clin. Res.*, 28:445A.
63. Friesinger, G. C., Oelz, O., Sweetman, B. J., Nies, A. S., and Data, J. L. (1978): Prostaglandin D_2, another renal prostaglandin. *Prostaglandins*, 15:969–981.
64. Frölich, J. C., Wilson, T. W., Sweetman, B. J., Smigel, M., Nies, A. S., Carr, K., Watson, J. T., and Oates, J. A. (1975): Urinary prostaglandins. Indentification and origin. *J. Clin. Invest.*, 55:763–770.
65. Fülgraff, G., and Meiforth, A. (1971): Effects of prostaglandin E_2 on excretion and reabsorption of sodium and fluid in rat kidneys (micropuncture studies). *Pfluegers Arch.*, 330:243–256.
66. Gagnon, D. J., Cousineau, D., and Boucher, P. J. (1973): Release of vasopressin by angiotensin II and prostaglandin E_2 from the rat neurohypophysis *in vitro*. *Life Sci. (Part I)*, 12:487.
67. Gagnon, D. J., Gauthier, R., and Regoli, D. (1974): Release of prostaglandins from the rabbit perfused kidney: Effects of vasoconstrictors. *Br. J. Pharmacol.*, 50:553–558.
68. Galvez, O. G., Bay, W. H., Roberts, B. W., and Ferris, T. F. (1977): The hemodynamic effects of potassium deficiency in the dog. *Circ. Res. (Suppl. I)*, 40:11–16.
69. Galvez, O. G., Roberts, B. W., Mishkind, M. H., Bay, W. H., and Ferris, T. F. (1977): Studies of the mechanism of contralateral polyuria after renal artery stenosis. *J. Clin. Invest.*, 59:609–615.
70. Ganguli, M., Tobian, L., Azar, S., and O'Donnell, M. (1977): Evidence that prostaglandin synthesis inhibitors increase the concentration of sodium and chloride in rat renal medulla. *Circ. Res. (Suppl I)*, 49:I35–I139.
71. Gerber, J. G., Data, J. L., and Nies, A. S. (1978): Enhanced renal prostaglandin production in the dog. The effect of sodium arachidonate in non-filtering kidney. *Circ. Res.*, 42:43–45.
72. Gerber, J. G., Ellis, E., Hollifield, J., and Nies, A. S. (1979): Effect of prostaglandin endoperoxide analogue on canine renal function, hemodynamics and renin release. *Euro. J. Pharmacol.*, 53:239–246.
73. Gerber, J. G., Hubbard, W. C., Branch, R. A., and Nies, A. S. (1978): The lack of an effect of furosemide on uterine prostaglandin metabolism *in vivo*. *Prostaglandins*, 15:663–670.
74. Gerber, J. G., and Nies, A. S. (1979): The hemodynamic effects of prostaglandins in the rat. Evidence for important species variation in renovascular responses. *Circ. Res.*, 44:406–410.
75. Gerber, J. G., and Nies, A. S. (1980): Furosemide induced renal vasodilation: The role of the release of arachidonic acid. In: *Advances in Prostaglandin and Thromboxane Research*, Vol. 7, edited by B. Samuelsson, P. W. Ramwell, and R. Paoletti, pp. 1079–1082. Raven Press, New York.
76. Gerber, J. G., Nies, A. S., Friesinger, G. C., Gerkens, J. F., Branch, R. A., and Oates, J. A. (1978): The effects of PGI_2 on canine renal function and hemodynamics. *Prostaglandins*, 16:519–528.
77. Giebisch, G., and Lozano, R. (1959): The effects of adrenal steroids and potassium depletion on the elaboration of an osmotically concentrated urine. *J. Clin. Invest.*, 38:843–853.

78. Glasson, P., Gaillard, R., Riondel, A., and Vallotton, M. B. (1979): Role of renal prostaglandins and relationship to renin, aldosterone, and antidiuretic hormone during salt depletion in man. *J. Clin. Endocrinol. Metab.*, 49:176–181.
79. Granstrom, E., and Kindahl, H. (1980): Radioimmunologic determination of 15-keto-13,14-di-hydro-PGE_2: A method for its stable degradation product, 11-deoxy-15-keto-13,14-dihydro-11β, 16-cyclo-PGE_2. In: *Advances in Prostaglandin and Thromboxane Research*, Vol. 6, edited by B. Samuelsson, P. W. Ramwell, and R. Paoletti, pp. 181–182. Raven Press, New York.
80. Grantham, J. J., and Orloff, J. (1968): Effect of prostaglandin E_1 on the permeability response of the isolated collecting tubule to vasopressin, adenosine 3′,5′-monophosphate and theoglylline. *J. Clin. Invest.*, 47:1154–1161.
81. Gross, J. B., and Bartter, F. C. (1973): Effects of prostaglandins E_1, A_1 and $F_{2\alpha}$ on renal handling of salt and water. *Am. J. Physiol.*, 225:218–224.
82. Gross, P. A., and Anderson, R. J. (1980): Mechanisms of escape from antidiuretic hormone. *Clin. Res.*, 28:446A.
83. Gülner, H.-G., Smith, J. B., and Bartter, F. C. (1980): The principal metabolites of arachidonic acid are overproduced in Bartter's syndrome. In: *Advances in Prostaglandin and Thromboxane Research*, Vol. 7, edited by B. Samuelsson, P. W. Ramwell, and R. Paoletti, pp. 1185–1187. Raven Press, New York.
84. Hassid, A., Konieczkowski, M., and Dunn, M. J. (1979): Prostaglandin synthesis in isolated rat kidney glomeruli. *Proc. Natl. Acad. Sci. USA*, 76:1155–1159.
85. Haylor, J., and Lote, C. J. (1978): Renal excretion of solutes and water in conscious rats after inhibition of prostaglandin synthetase by indomethacin. *J. Physiol.*, 281:46–47.
86. Henrich, W. L., Berl, T., McDonald, K. M., Anderson, R. J., and Schrier, R. W. (1978); Angiotensin II, renal nerves, and prostaglandins in renal hemodynamics during hemorrhage. *Am. J. Physiol.*, 235:F46–F51.
87. Herbaczynska-Cedro, K., and Vane, J. R. (1973): Contribution of intrarenal generation of prostaglandin to autoregulation of renal blood flow in the dog. *Circ. Res.*, 33:428–436.
88. Hoffman, W. E., and Schmid, P. G. (1979): Cardiovascular and antidiuretic effects of central prostaglandin E_2. *J. Physiol. (Lond.)*, 288:159–169.
89. Hollander, W., Jr., Winters, R. W., Williams, T. F., Bradley, J., Oliver, J., and West, L. G. (1957): Defect in the renal tubular reabsorption of water associated with potassium depletion in rats. *Am. J. Physiol.*, 189:557–563.
90. Hood, V. L., and Dunn, M. J. (1978): Urinary excretion of PGE_2 and $PGF_{2\alpha}$ in potassium-deficient rats. *Prostaglandins*, 15:273–283.
91. Iino, Y., and Imai, M. (1978): Effects of prostaglandins on Na transport in isolated collecting tubules. *Pfluegers Arch.*, 373:125–132.
92. Isakson, P. C., Raz, A., Denny, S. E., Wyche, A., and Needleman, P. (1977): Hormonal stimulation of arachidonic acid release from isolated perfused organs. Relationship to prostaglandin synthesis. *Prostaglandins*, 14:853–872.
93. Ishikawa, S., Saito, T., and Yoshida, S. (1981): The effect of prostaglandins on the release of arginine vasopressin from the Guinea pig hypothalamo-neurohypophyseal complex in organ culture. *Endocrinology*, 108:193–198.
94. Jackson, B. A., Edwards, R. M., and Dousa, T. P. (1980): Vasopressin-prostaglandin interactions in isolated tubules from rat outer medulla. *J. Lab. Clin. Med.*, 96:119–128.
95. Johnston, H. H., Herzog, J. P., and Lauler, D. P. (1968): Effect of prostaglandin E_1 on renal hemodynamics, sodium and water excretion. *Am. J. Physiol.*, 213:939–946.
96. Kaloyanides, G. J., Ahrens, R. E., Shepherd, J. A., and DiBona, G. F. (1976): Inhibition of prostaglandin E_2 secretion. Failure to abolish autoregulation in the isolated dog kidney. *Circ. Res.*, 38:67–73, 1976.
97. Kim, J. R., Schrier, R. W., and Berl, T. (1979): Effect of hypokalemia on renal medullary cyclic AMP (cAMP) generation, metabolism and action. *Clin. Res.*, 27:420A.
98. Kimberly, R. P., Gill, J. R., Bowden, R. E., Keiser, H. R., and Plotz, P. H. (1978): Elevated urinary prostaglandins and the effects of aspirin on renal function in lupus erythematosus. *Ann. Int. Med.*, 89:336–341.
99. Kirschenbaum, M. A., and Stein, J. H. (1976): The effect of inhibition of prostaglandin synthesis on urinary sodium excretion in the conscious dog. *J. Clin. Invest.*, 57:517–521.
100. Kirschenbaum, M. A., White, N., Stein, J. H., and Ferris, T. F. (1974): Redistribution of renal cortical blood flow during inhibition of prostaglandin synthesis. *Am. J. Physiol.*, 227:801–805.

101. Knapp, H. R., Oelz, O., Roberts, L. J., Sweetman, B. J., Oates, J. A., and Reed, P. W. (1977): Ionophores stimulate prostaglandin and thromboxane biosynthesis. *Proc. Natl. Acad. Sci. USA*, 74:4251–4255.

102. Kover, G., and Tost, H. (1977): The effect of indomethacin on kidney function: Indomethacin and furosemide antagonism. *Pfluegers Arch.*, 372:215–220.

103. Krakoff, L. R., DeGuia, D., Vlachakis, N., Sticker, J., and Goldstein, M. (1973): Effect of sodium balance on arterial blood pressure and renal responses to prostaglandin A in man. *Circ. Res.*, 33:539–546.

104. Kramer, H. J. (1978): Effects of inhibition of prostaglandin synthesis on renal electrolyte excretion and concentrating ability in healthy man. *Prostaglandins Med.*, 1:341–349.

105. Larrson, C., and Änggård, E. (1976): Mass spectrometric determination of prostaglandin E_2, $F_{2\alpha}$ and A_2 in the cortex and medulla of the rabbit kidney. *J. Pharm. Pharmacol.*, 28:326–328, 1976.

106. Larrson, C., and Änggård, E. (1976): Regional differences in the formation and metabolism of prostaglandins in the rabbit kidney. *Eur. J. Pharmacol.*, 21:30–36.

107. Lee, J. B., McGiff, J. C., Kannegiessir, H., Aykent, Y. Y., Mudd, J. G., and Frawley, T. F. (1971): Antihypertensive renal effects of prostaglandin A_1 in patients with essential hypertension. *Ann. Intern. Med.*, 74:703–710.

108. Leksell, L. G. (1976): Influence of prostaglandin E_1 on cerebral mechanisms involved in the control of fluid balance. *Acta Physiol. Scand.*, 98:85–93.

109. Lemley, K. V., Robertson, C. R., and Jamison, R. L. (1980): Effect of prostaglandin inhibition on erythrocyte velocities in vasa recta of water-loaded rats. *Clin. Res.*, 28:63A.

110. Levison, S. P., and Levison, M. E. (1976): Effect of indomethacin and sodium meclofenamate on the renal concentrating defect in experimental enterococcal pyelonephritis in rats. *J. Lab. Clin. Med.*, 88:958–964.

111. Lifschitz, M. D., Patak, R. V., Fadem, S. Z., and Stein, J. H. (1978): Urinary prostaglandin E excretion: Effect of chronic alterations in sodium intake and inhibition of prostaglandin synthesis in the rabbit. *Prostaglandins*, 16:607–619.

112. Lipson, L. C., and Sharp, G. W. (1971): Effect of prostaglandin E_1 on sodium transport and osmotic water flow in the toad bladder. *Amer. J. Physiol.*, 220:1046–1052.

113. Lonigro, A. J., Hagemann, M. H., Stephenson, A. H., and Fry, C. L. (1978): Inhibition of prostaglandin synthesis by indomethacin augments the renal vasodilator response to bradykinin in the anesthetized dog. *Circ. Res.*, 43:447–455.

114. Lonigro, A. J., Itskovitz, H. D., Crowshaw, K., and McGiff, J. C. (1973): Dependency of renal blood flow on prostaglandin synthesis in the dog. *Circ. Res.*, 32:712–717.

115. Lum, G. M., Aisenbrey, G. A., Dunn, M. J., Berl, T., Schrier, R. W., and McDonald, K. M. (1977): *In vivo* effect of indomethacin to potentiate the renal medullary cyclic AMP response to vasopressin. *J. Clin. Invest.*, 59:8–13.

116. McNay, J. L., and Abe, Y. (1970): Redistribution of cortical blood flow during renal vasodilation in dogs. *Circ. Res.*, 27:1023–1032.

117. Mannitius, A., Levitin, H., Beck, D., and Epstein, F. H. (1960): On the mechanism of impairment of renal concentrating ability in potassium depletion. *J. Clin. Invest.*, 39:684–692.

118. Martinez-Maldonado, M., Tsparas, M. N., Eknoyan, G., and Suki, W. N. (1972): Renal actions of prostaglandins: Comparison with acetylcholine and volume expansion. *Am. J. Physiol.*, 222:1147–1152.

119. Morrison, A. R., Nishikawa, K., and Needleman, P. (1978): Thromboxane biosynthesis in the ureter obstructed isolated perfused kidney of the rabbit. *J. Pharmacol. Exp. Ther.*, 205:1–8.

119a. Muther, R. S., Potter, D. M., and Bennett, W. M. (1981): Aspirin-induced depression of glomerular filtration rate in normal humans: Role of sodium balance. *Ann. Int. Med.*, 94:317–321.

120. Nasjletti, A., McGiff, J. C., and Colina-Chourio, J. (1978): Interrelations of the renal kallikrein-kinin system and renal prostaglandins in the conscious rat. Influence of mineralocorticoids. *Circ. Res.*, 43:799–807.

121. Needleman, P., Marshall, G. R., and Johnson, E. M. (1974): Determinants and modification of adrenergic and vascular resistance in the kidney. *Am. J. Physiol.*, 227:665–669.

122. Nicholaides, S., and Fitzsimmons, J. T. (1975): La dependance de la prise d'eau induite par l'angiotensine II envers la fenction vasomotrice cerebrale locale chez le rat. *C.R. Acad. Sci. [D] (Paris)*, 201:1417–1420.

123. Nielson, I. L., Rasmussen, S., and Hilden, T. (1980): Acetylsalicylic acid and renal function. *Br. Med. J.*, 1:610.

124. Oates, J. A., Frölich, J. C., and Nies, A. S. (1978): Prostaglandins and the kidney. In: *Renal Function*, edited by G. H. Giebisch, and E. F. Purcell, pp. 299–308. Josiah Macy, Jr., Foundation.
125. Oken, D. E. (1976): Local mechanisms in the pathogenesis of acute renal failure. *Kidney Int.*, 10:S94–99.
126. Oliver, J. A., Sciacca, R. R., and Cannon, R. J. (1979): Renal vascular and excretory responses to prostaglandin endoperoxides in the dog. *Am. J. Physiol.*, 236:H427–H433.
127. Oliw, E., Kover, G., Larsson, C., and Änggård, E. (1976): Reduction by indomethacin of furosemide effects in the rabbit. *Eur. J. Pharm.*, 38:95–100.
128. Oliw, E., Kover, G., Larsson, C., and Änggård, E. (1978): Indomethacin and diclofenac sodium increase sodium and water excretion after extracellular volume expansion in the rabbit. *Eur. J. Pharmacol.*, 49:381–388.
129. Oliw, E., Lundén I., Sjöquist, B., and Änggård, E. (1978): Determination of 6-keto-prostaglandin $F_{1\alpha}$ in rabbit kidney and urine and its relation to sodium balance. *Acta Physiol. Scand.*, 105:359–366.
130. Olsen, U. B. (1975): Indomethacin inhibition of bumetanide diuresis in dogs. *Acta Pharmacol. Toxicol.*, 37:65–78.
131. Omachi, R. S., Robbie, D. E., Handler, J. S., and Orloff, J. (1974): Effect of ADH and other agents on cyclic AMP accumulation in toad bladder epithelium. *Am. J. Physiol.*, 226:1152–1157.
132. Orloff, J., Handler, J. S., and Bergstrom, S. (1965): Effect of prostaglandin (PGE$_1$) on the permeability response of toad bladder to vasopressin, theophylline and adenosine 3',5'-monophosphate. *Nature*, 205:397–398.
133. Ozer, A., and Sharp, G. W. G. (1972): Effects of prostaglandins and their inhibitors on osmotic water flow in the toad bladder. *Am. J. Physiol.*, 222:674–680.
134. Papanicolaou, N., Safar, M., Hornych, A., Fontaliran, F., Weiss, Y., Bariety, J., and Milliez, P. (1975): The release of renal prostaglandins during saline infusion in normal and hypertensive subjects. *Clin. Sci. Mol. Med.*, 49:459–463.
135. Patak, R. V., Mookerjee, B. K., Bentzel, C. J., Hysert, P. E., Babej, M., and Lee, J. B. (1975): Antagonism of furosemide by indomethacin in normal and hypertensive man. *Prostaglandins*, 10:649–661.
136. Radfar, N., Gill, J. R., Bartter, F. C., Bravo, E., Taylor, A. A., and Bowden, R. E. (1978): Hypokalemia in Bartter's syndrome and other disorders produces resistance to vasopressors via prostaglandin overproduction. *Proc. Soc. Exp. Biol. Med.* 158:502–507.
137. Relman, A. S., and Schwartz, W. B. (1956): The nephropathy of potassium depletion: A clinical and pathological entity. *N. Engl. J. Med.*, 255:195–203.
138. Robin, E. Z., Garston, R. G., Weir, R. V., and Posen, G. A. (1979): Persistent nephrogenic diabetes insipidus associated with long-term lithium carbonate treatment. *Can. Med. Assoc. J.* 121:194–198.
139. Rutecki, G. W., Nally, J. F., Bay, W. H., and Ferris, T. F. (1977): The acute effects of lithium (Li) on renal function. *Kidney Int.*, 12:571.
140. Scherer, B., Schnermann, J., Sofroniev, M., and Weber, P. (1977): Prostaglandin analysis in urine of humans and rats by different radioimmunoassays: Effect on PG excretion by PG-synthetase inhibitors, laparotomy and furosemide. *Prostaglandins*, 15:255–266.
141. Schnermann, J., Hermle, M., Schmidmeier, E., and Dahlheim, H. (1975): Impaired potency for feedback regulation of glomerular filtration rate in DOCA excaped rats. *Pfluegers Arch.*, 358:325–338.
142. Schnermann, J., and Weber, P. C. (1980): A role of renal cortical prostaglandins in the control of glomerular filtration rate in rat kidneys. In: *Advances in Prostaglandin and Thromboxane Research*, Vol. 7, edited by B. Samuelsson, P. W. Ramwell, and R. Paoletti, pp. 1047–1052. Raven Press, New York.
143. Serros, E. R., Lowe, A., and Kirschenbaum, M. A. (1979): Prostaglandin-dependent polyria in conscious hypercalcemic rats. *Clin. Res.*, 27:430A.
144. Shea, P. T., Eisner, G. M., and Slotkoff, M. (1978): Evidence for a direct tubular effect of prostaglandin E$_2$ induced natriuresis. *Clin. Res.*, 26:43A.
145. Shimizu, Kurosawa, T., Maeda, T., and Yoshitoshi, Y. (1969): Free water excretion and washout of renal medullary urea by prostaglandin E$_1$. *Jpn. Heart. J.*, 10:437–455.
146. Shimizu, K., Yamamoto, M., and Yoshitoshi, Y. (1973): Effects of saline infusion on prostaglandin-like materials in renal venous blood and medulla of canine kidney. *Jpn. Heart J.*, 14:140–145.

147. Silverstein, M. E., Feldman, R. C., Henderson, L. W., and Engelman, K. (1974): Effects of indomethacin (INDO) on human renal clearance of sodium (Na) and H$_2$O. *Clin. Res.*, 22:721A.
148. Smith, D. E., Brater, D. C., Lin, E. T., and Benet, L. Z. (1979): Attenuation of furosemide's diuretic effect by indomethacin: Pharmaco-kinetic evaluation. *J. Pharmacokinet. Biopharm.*, 7:265–274.
149. Smith, W. L., and Bell, T. G. (1978): Immunohistochemical localization of the prostaglandin-forming cyclooxygenase in renal cortex. *Am. J. Physiol.*, 235:F451–F457.
150. Solez, K., Fox, J. A., Miller, M., and Heptinstall, R. H. (1974): Effects of indomethacin on renal inner medullary plasma flow. *Prostaglandins*, 7:91–97.
151. Stetson, D. L., Wade, J. B., and Giebisch, G. (1980): Morphologic alterations in the rat medullary collecting duct following potassium depletion. *Kidney Int.*, 16:45–56.
152. Stoff, J. S., Rosa, R. M., and Epstein, F. H. (1979): The concentrating defect of acute potassium depletion in man is independent of renal prostaglandins. *Kidney Int.*, 16:874.
153. Stoff, J. S., Silva, P., Rosa, R., and Epstein, F. H. (1978): Effect of indomethacin on water excretion in diabetes insipidus; possible action of prostaglandins independent of antidiuretic hormone. *Clin. Res.*, 26:477A.
154. Stokes, J. B. (1979): Effect of prostaglandin E$_2$ on chloride transport across the rabbit thick ascending limb of Henle. *J. Clin. Invest.*, 64:495–502.
155. Stokes, J. B., and Kokko, J. P. (1977): Inhibition of sodium transport by prostaglandin E$_2$ across the isolated, perfused rabbit collecting tubule. *J. Clin. Invest.*, 59:1099–1104.
156. Stone, K. J., and Hart, M. (1976): Inhibition of renal PGE$_2$-9-keto reductase by diuretics. *Prostaglandins*, 12:197–207.
157. Strandhoy, J. W., Ott, C. E., Schneider, E. G., Willis, L. R., Beck, N. P., Davis, B. B., and Knox, F. G. (1974): Effects of prostaglandins E$_1$ and E$_2$ on renal sodium reabsorption and Starling forces. *Am. J. Physiol.*, 226:1015–1021.
158. Swain, J. A., Heyndricks, G. R., Boettcher, D. H., and Vatner, S. F. (1975): Prostaglandin control of renal circulation in the unanesthetized dog and baboon. *Am. J. Physiol.*, 229:826–830.
159. Tai, H. H., and Hollander, C. S. (1976): Kinetic evidence of a distinct regulatory site on 15-OH prostaglandin dehydrogenase. In: *Advances in Prostaglandin and Thromboxane Research*, Vol. 1, edited by B. Samuelsson and R. Paoletti, pp. 171–175. Raven Press, New York.
160. Tannenbaum, J., Splawinski, J. A., Oates, J. A., and Nies, A. S. (1975): Enhanced renal prostaglandin production in the dog: I. Effect on renal function. *Circ. Res.*, 36:197–203.
161. Terashima, R., Anderson, F. L., and Jubitz, W. (1976): Prostaglandin E release in the dog: Effect of sodium. *Am. J. Physiol.*, 231:1429–1432.
162. Terrango, N. A., Lonigro, A. J., Malik, K. U., and McGiff, J. C. (1972): The relationship of the renal vasodilator action of bradykinin to the release of a prostaglandin E-like substance. *Experientia*, 28:437–439.
163. Terragno, N. A., McGiff, J. C., and Terragno, D. A. (1979): Synthesis of prostaglandins by vascular and non-vascular renal tissues and the presence of an endogenous prostaglandin synthesis inhibitor in the cortex. Proc. 7th Int'l. Congr. Pharmacol. In: *Advances in Pharmacology and Therapy*, edited by B. B. Vargaftig, pp. 39–46. Pergamon Press, New York.
164. Terragno, N. A., Terragno, D. A., and McGiff, J. C. (1977): Contribution of prostaglandins to the renal circulation in conscious, anesthetized, and laparotomized dogs. *Circ. Res.*, 40:590–595.
165. Tobian, L., O'Donnell, M., and Ganguli, M. (1971): Relationship of prostaglandins and sodium in renal papilla in kyoto hypertensive rats and during high sodium diets. *Trans. Am. Assoc. Physicians*, 84:281–288.
166. Tobian, L., O'Donnell, M., and Smith, P. (1974): Intrarenal prostaglandin levels during normal and high sodium intake. *Circ. Res.*, 34,35 *(Suppl.)*:83–89.
167. Torres, V. E., Strong, C. G., Romero, J. C., and Wilson, D. M. (1975): Indomethacin enhancement of glycerol-induced acute renal failure in rabbits. *Kidney Int.*, 7:170–178.
168. Vanherweghem, J. L., Ducobu, J., and D'Hollander, A. (1975): Effects of indomethacin on renal hemodynamics and on water and sodium excretion by the isolated dog kidney. *Pflugers Arch.*, 357:243–252.
169. Vilhardt, J. and Hedqvist, P. (1970): A possible role of prostaglandin E$_2$ in the regulation of vasopressin secretion in rats. *Life Sci. (Part I)*, 9:825.
170. Walker, L. A., Gerber, J. G., Frölich, J. C., and Nies, A. S. (1978): Redistribution of intrarenal blood flow following ADH administration: Lack of inhibition by blockade of prostaglandin cyclooxygenase. *Prostaglandins Med.*, 1:295–303.

171. Walker, R. M., Stoff, J. S., Brown, R. S., and Epstein, F. H. (1980): The relation of renal prostaglandins to urinary dilution in lithium induced nephrogenic diabetes insipidus and normal subjects. *Clin. Res.*, 28:463A.
172. Walker, L. A., Whorton, A. R., Smigel, M., France, R., and Frölich, J. C. (1978): Antidiuretic hormone increases renal prostaglandin synthesis *in vivo*. *Am. J. Physiol.*, 235:F180–F185.
173. Walshe, J. J., and Venuto, R. C. (1979): Acute oliguric renal failure induced by indomethacin: Possible mechanism. *Am. Int. Med.*, 91:47–49.
174. Weber, P. C., Larson, C., and Scherer, B. (1977): Prostaglandin E_2 9-ketoreductase as a mediator of salt intake-related prostaglandin-renin interaction. *Nature*, 266:65–66.
175. Whorton, A. R., Smigel, M., Oates, J. A., and Frölich, J. C. (1978): Regional differences in prostaglandin formation by the kidney. *Biochim. Biophys. Acta*, 529:176–180.
176. Williamson, H. E., Bourland, W. A., and Marchand, G. R. (1975): Inhibition of furosemide increase in renal blood flow by indomethacin. *Proc. Soc. Exp. Biol. Med.*, 148:164–166.
177. Wong, P. Y. D., Bedwani, J. R., and Cuthbert, A. W. (1972): Hormone action and the levels of cyclic AMP and prostaglandins in the toad bladder. *Nature*, 238:27–31.
178. Yamamoto, M., Share, L., and Shade, R. E. (1976): Vasopressin release during ventriculocisternal perfusion with prostaglandin E_2 in the dog. *J. Endocrinol.*, 71:325–331.
179. Yarger, W. E., Schocken, D. D., and Harris, R. H. (1980): Obstructive nephropathy in the rat. Possible role for the renin-angiotensin system, prostaglandins, and thromboxanes in post-obstructive renal function. *J. Clin. Invest*, 65:400–412.
180. Zambraski, E. J., and Dunn, M. J. (1979): Renal prostaglandin E_2 secretion and excretion in conscious dogs. *Am. J. Physiol.*, 236:F552–558.
181. Zenser, J. V., and Davis, B. B. (1978): Effects of calcium on prostaglandin E_2 synthesis by rat medullary slices. *Am. J. Physiol.*, 235:F213–218.
182. Zia, P., Zipser, R., Speckart, P., and Horton, R. (1978): The measurement of urinary prostaglandin E in normal subjects and in high renin states. *J. Lab. Clin. Med.*, 92:415–422.
183. Zipser, R. D., Hoefs, J. C., Speckart, P. F., Zia, P. K., and Horton, R. (1979): Prostaglandins: Modulators of renal function and pressor resistance in chronic liver disease *J. Clin. Endocrinol. Metab.*, 48:895–900.
184. Zipser, R., Myers, S., and Needleman, P. (1980): Exaggerated prostaglandin and thromboxane synthesis in the renal vein constricted rabbit. *Circ. Res.*, 47:231–237.
185. Zusman, R. M., and Keiser, H. R. (1977): Prostaglandin E_2 biosynthesis by rabbit renomedullary interstitial cells in tissue culture. *J. Biol. Chem.*, 252:2069–2071.
186. Zusman, R. M., Keiser, H. R., and Handler, J. S. (1977): Vasopressin-stimulated prostaglandin E biosynthesis in the toad urinary bladder. *J. Clin. Invest.*, 60:1339–1347.
187. Zusman, R. M., and Keiser, H. R., (1980): Regulation of prostaglandin E_2 synthesis by angiotensin II, potassium, osmolality, and dexamethasone. *Kidney Int.* 17:277–283.

Prostaglandins and the Cardiovascular System,
edited by John A. Oates. Raven Press,
New York © 1982.

Participation of Prostaglandins in the Control of Renin Release

Edwin K. Jackson, Robert A. Branch, and John A. Oates

Departments of Medicine and Pharmacology, Vanderbilt University Medical Center, Nashville, Tennessee 37232

The renin–angiotensin system is an important determinant of arterial blood pressure and sodium homeostasis. Consequently, an elucidation of the factors controlling the release of renin is essential to a thorough understanding of cardiovascular physiology and pharmacology. During the past several years, considerable evidence has emerged linking prostaglandins to the control of renin release. The purpose of the present discussion is to review critically the data relating prostaglandins to renin release, pinpoint areas requiring additional research and clarification, offer possible models of renin release control, and apply, whenever possible, the significance of these data to clinical medicine. In an effort to provide more than a mere recitation of available data, we have chosen to emphasize new developments and controversial issues rather than dwell on well resolved facts.

PHYSIOLOGICAL MECHANISMS CONTROLLING RENIN RELEASE

There is now an enormous body of literature that relates to the basic physiological mechanisms controlling renin release. An understanding of these mechanisms is prerequisite for a discussion of the participation of prostaglandins in renin secretion. Consequently, the physiological control of renin secretion will be reviewed briefly in this discussion; however, for a more detailed account of this subject, the reader is referred to the excellent review by Keeton and Campbell (68). The three most important physiological mechanisms controlling renin release are: 1) the intrarenal baroreceptor, 2) the macula densa, and 3) the intrarenal beta-adrenoreceptors.

Intrarenal Baroreceptor

A reduction in renal perfusion pressure, either as a consequence of systemic hypotension or renal artery stenosis, is a potent stimulant for renin release. Moreover, renin release induced by renal artery hypotension occurs despite the absence of glomerular filtration, renal sympathetic innervation, and circulating adrenal catecholamines (5). That component of renin release following renal artery hypotension in the absence of glomerular filtration and catecholaminergic influences has been termed baroreceptor-mediated renin release. The exact anatomical structure of the intrarenal baroreceptor that is activated during renal artery hypotension is unknown. The intrarenal baroreceptor is thought to reside in the wall of the afferent arteriole because papaverine, which dilates renal afferent arterioles, blocks baroreceptor-mediated renin release (138). However, the use of papaverine as a pharmacological tool does not incontrovertibly localize the baroreceptor mechanism. Also somewhat enigmatic is the exact stimulus that activates the intrarenal baroreceptor. The current consensus is that the stimulus to the intrarenal baroreceptor is a decrease in either afferent arteriolar stretch (123,124), wall tension (27,126), circumferential stress (38), or volume strain (39) secondary to a decrease in afferent arteriolar transluminal pressure. Since both the stimulus that activates the intrarenal baroreceptor and the exact anatomical structure that responds to the stimulus remain controversial, it is perhaps more appropriate to conceptualize the definition of baroreceptor-mediated renin release as that component of renin release that occurs during renal artery hypotension, independent of the macula densa and beta-adrenoreceptors.

Macula Densa

The macula densa is a group of cells at the junction between the thick region of the ascending limb of the loop of Henle and the distal tubule. These cells make intimate contact with the granular juxtaglomerular cells of the afferent arteriole and are presumed to influence the release of renin. Historically, stimulation of macula densa-induced renin release was considered to be triggered by a reduction in distal tubular sodium load. However, recent studies indicate that the chloride ion, rather than the sodium ion, regulates macula densa-mediated renin release (69,72,73). This conclusion was suggested by the observations that intrarenal infusions of both sodium chloride and lysine chloride inhibit renin release in sodium depleted dogs, while sodium sulfate is without effect (13). Further, it was found that the suppression of renin release by NaCl in sodium depleted dogs is blocked by furosemide (13). Since furosemide inhibits the chloride pump in the ascending limb of the loop of Henle (70), these studies indicate that macula densa-mediated renin secretion is an inverse function of chloride flux into the macula densa. Accordingly, during sodium chloride depletion, distal tubular chloride concentrations would decrease, which in turn would reduce chloride flux into the macula densa and, consequently, increase renin release. The converse would occur during sodium repletion.

Intrarenal Beta-Adrenoreceptor

Electrical stimulation of the renal nerves in both the intact kidney (79,125) and in the papaverine-treated, nonfiltering kidney (65) stimulates a release of renin that can be blocked by prior propranolol administration. Furthermore, beta agonists stimulate renin release in the isolated kidney (127), in renal cortical slices (86), and in renal cortical cells (64). These observations strongly support a direct independent capability of the beta-adrenoreceptor to influence renin release. In addition, it also appears that the adrenergic nervous system can modulate the sensitivity of the renin release mechanisms to baroreceptor or macula densa-mediated stimuli (121).

Integration of Renin Release Control

In the intact kidney, the three mechanisms discussed above usually integrate their activity such that in many situations, the renin release response to a given stimulus involves all three physiological mechanisms. In order to delineate the independent ability of each mechanism to influence renin release, it is necessary to ablate two of the mechanisms and then study the isolated remaining mechanism. As previously mentioned, intrarenal papaverine blocks baroreceptor-mediated renin release (138). Macula densa-mediated renin release can be ablated by rendering the kidney non-filtering, thus preventing alterations in NaCl flux to the macula densa. This maneuver is easily accomplished by combining 2 hr of renal artery occlusion with several days of ureteral ligation (6). Ablation of beta-adrenoreceptor-mediated renin release can be obtained by coupling renal denervation with beta-adrenoreceptor antagonism. Witty et al. (138) have illustrated the usefulness of these techniques in their studies that elucidated the mechanisms of renin release in hypotensive hemorrhage. In these studies, renin secretion was increased by hypotensive hemorrhage in nonfiltering, papaverine-treated kidneys, in papaverine-treated, denervated kidneys, and in denervated, nonfiltering kidneys. It was only in the denervated, nonfiltering papaverine-treated kidney that the renin release response to hypotensive hemorrhage was blocked. These data indicated that all three physiological mechanisms contribute to the increase in renin release during hypotensive hemorrhage.

EVIDENCE LINKING PROSTAGLANDINS AND RENIN RELEASE

Inhibition of Renin Release by Prostaglandin Cyclooxygenase Inhibitors

Studies with prostaglandin cyclooxygenase inhibitors have contributed in a major way to our current understanding of the involvement of prostaglandins in renin release. A reduction in basal plasma renin activity occurs following cyclooxygenase inhibition in the rabbit (75,98,131), rat (16,18,77), and man (31,40,93,102). In addition, cyclooxygenase inhibition attenuates renin secretion induced by furosemide (2,93,102,120), sodium depletion (31,41,110,144), endotoxemia (59), captopril (1), prazosin (100), saralasin (18), hydralazine (16), adrenalectomy (85), chlorisondamine (16), low potassium (76), insulin (19), and orthostasis (102).

Although studies with cyclooxygenase inhibitors are consistent with the hypothesis that prostaglandins are involved in renin release, they are by no means conclusive. In each study it is assumed that the effect of cyclooxygenase inhibitors on renin release is due to the inhibition of prostaglandin biosynthesis rather than to some other pharmacological action of the drug. Renin release suppression following cyclooxygenase inhibition also could be the result of either an indirect effect due to sodium retention or an action of prostaglandin synthesis inhibitors on a prostaglandin-independent mechanism. The sodium retaining property of a cyclooxygenase inhibitor such as indomethacin is well known (40). Since sodium retention reduces renin release, it is important to exclude changes in sodium balance as a possible explanation for the reduction in renin release following cyclooxygenase inhibition. Accordingly, the effects of indomethacin on renin release have been examined in situations where sodium retention does not occur, i.e., dietary sodium deprivation. These studies have revealed that cyclooxygenase inhibitors reduce renin secretion in humans (31,41,110) or animals (144) in steady-state balance on low sodium diets independent of sodium retention.

The major criticism of studies using cyclooxygenase inhibitors is that these drugs may inhibit some enzyme or other basic components of the renin release mechanism independent of cyclooxygenase inhibition. Indeed, the prototype of the cyclooxygenase inhibitors and the drug most often used in renin release studies, indomethacin, inhibits a variety of enzymes other than cyclooxygenase (37). Since the synthesis of cAMP may be involved in the renin release mechanism and since cAMP acts via protein kinases, the report that submicromolar concentrations of indomethacin can inhibit protein kinase (66) is particularly disturbing. The usual approach in addressing this pitfall is to investigate the effect of more than one cyclooxygenase inhibitor in an individual setting. The underlying assumption of this approach is that chemically dissimilar moieties will have the inhibition of cyclooxygenase as their only common activity. Reassuringly, cyclooxygenase inhibitors besides indomethacin have been shown to inhibit renin release (16,18,85,87). This approach, however, has the obvious fallacy that if two drugs are similar enough to inhibit one system in common, they could certainly act similarly at other sites as well. An alternative approach is that if the drug acts at a prostaglandin-independent site, then the drug should shift the renin release dose–response curves of exogenous prostaglandins to the right. Conversely, if the site of action of the drug is the cyclooxygenase enzyme, infusions of exogenous prostaglandins will bypass the enzyme and the renin release dose–response curves will not be altered. To our knowledge, a systematic study examining the effects of cyclooxygenase inhibitors at various doses on prostaglandin-induced renin release has not been reported. However, prostaglandin infusions certainly stimulate renin release in indomethacin-pretreated kidneys (42,44), and 10^{-4}M indomethacin does not block renin release induced by 10^{-5}M prostaglandin endoperoxide analogue in rat cortical slices (116).

Stimulation of Renin Release by Arachidonic Acid

One of the strong arguments for the involvement of prostaglandins in renin secretion is the observation that the precursor of the dienoic prostaglandins, arachidonic acid, is a potent stimulant to renin release. Larsson et al. (75) noted that in the anesthetized rabbit, an intrarenal infusion of arachidonic acid increased renal venous plasma renin activity twofold. Similar results have been reported in the anesthetized rat (129,131), anesthetized dog (10,108), and conscious dog (45). Data et al. (25) and Seymour and Zehr (108) have examined the effects of intrarenal arachidonic acid infusions on renin secretion in nonfiltering, denervated as well as nonfiltering, denervated, papaverine-treated dogs. In both studies, arachidonic acid significantly enhanced renin release despite functional isolationof the juxtaglomerular cells from the macula densa and beta-adrenoreceptors and, in the latter study, from the intrarenal baroreceptor as well. Thus, arachidonic acid enhanced renin release by exerting a direct effect on the juxtaglomerular cells. A direct effect of arachidonic acid on the renin release mechanism in juxtaglomerular cells also is supported by the observations that arachidonic acid induces renin release in rabbit (130,131,133,134), rat (116), and mouse (78) renal cortical slices. Prior administration of indomethacin blocks the renin release response to arachidonic acid, both *in vivo* (10,108) and *in vitro* (78,116,130,131,134). These observations suggest that exogenous administration of arachidonic acid is able to bypass the initiating stimulus to the prostaglandin cascade, utilize available cyclooxygenase, and form a product that can trigger renin release. Along these lines, it is of interest that infusions of the precursors of the monoenoic and trienoic prostaglandin series to denervated, nonfiltering canine kidneys fail to induce renin release (45), suggesting that a dienoic prostaglandin is responsible for renin release *in vivo*.

Stimulation of Renin Release by Prostaglandins

Obviously, any model of renin release that proposes that prostaglandin biosynthesis plays a pivotal role in renin release control requires that one or more of the prostaglandins synthesized by renal tissue stimulates renin secretion by a direct effect on the juxtaglomerular cells. Studies in the rabbit renal cortex have revealed that of the arachidonic acid metabolites, only PGI_2, PGE_2, PGD_2, and $PGF_{2\alpha}$ are synthesized by this tissue to any significant degree (135). Similar findings have been reported for human renal cortex except that no PGD_2 biosynthesis was observed and a small amount of thromboxane A_2 production occurred (56). Whereas the published effects of $PGF_{2\alpha}$ and PGD_2 on renin release have been variable (Tables 1 and 2), PGI_2 and PGE_2 are renin secretagogues. The actions of PGI_2 and PGE_2 on renin release appear to be mediated via direct stimulation of the juxtaglomerular cells. This conclusion is supported by the observations that 1) these prostanoids

TABLE 1. *Effect of prostanoids on renin release in renal cortical slices*

Author (ref.)	Species	Prostanoid						
		PGI_2	PGE_2	$PGF_{2\alpha}$	PGD_2	PGG_2	EPA[+]	AA[±]
Weber et al. (130)	Rabbit		NE	↓	—	↑	↑ c	↑
Whorton et al. (133)	Rabbit	↑	↑ a	↑ a	NE	—	—	↑
Suzuki et al. (116)	Rat	↑	↑ b	↑	↑ b	—	↑	↑
Lin et al. (78)	Mouse	↑	↑ a	↑	NE	—	↑	↑

+, Stable endoperoxide analogs, ±, arachidonic acid; *a*, less potent than PGI_2; *b*, maximal effect less than PGI_2; *c*, blocked by indomethacin; NE, no effect; ↑, indicates stimulation; ↓, indicates inhibition.

TABLE 2. *Effect of prostanoids on renin release when infused into the renal artery of dogs*

Author (ref.)	Prostanoid				
	PGI_2	PGE_2	$PGF_{2\alpha}$	PGD_2	EPA
Gerber et al. (42)	↑	↑	—	NE	—
Yun et al. (143)	—	↑	NE	—	—
Seymour et al. (106)	↑	—	—	↑	—
Gerber et al. (43)	—	—	—	—	↑ [a]

[a], Blocked by indomethacin; NE, indicates no effect; ↑, indicates stimulation; ↓, indicates inhibition.

release renin when infused intrarenally into beta-adrenoreceptor blocked, nonfiltering kidneys (44), 2) the renin releasing action of PGI_2 and PGE_2 is unrelated to renal vasodilation (42,44,92) and 3) both PGI_2 and PGE_2 release renin in cortical slices (Table 1). It can be concluded firmly then that the kidney is capable of biosynthesizing PGI_2 and PGE_2 and that these prostaglandins are capable of releasing renin via direct action on the juxtaglomerular cells.

The direct actions of the unstable prostaglandin endoperoxides (PGG_2 and PGH_2) on renin secretion require further clarification. PGG_2 does increase renin release *in vitro* (130); however, since PGG_2 is converted rapidly to other prostanoids, it is not possible to conclude that endoperoxides directly stimulate renin secretion. Stable analogs of endoperoxides (EPA) release renin both *in vitro* (78,116,130) and *in vivo* (43). However, in two studies, the effects of EPA on renin release were blocked by inhibition of prostaglandin biosynthesis (43,130). These data suggest that EPA releases renin via activation of prostaglandin biosynthesis rather than by direct effect on juxtaglomerular cells. In contrast, Suzuki et al. (116) recently reported that in rat renal cortical slices, EPA stimulated renin release equally in the presence and absence of indomethacin. Like the prostglandin endoperoxides, the direct action of TxA_2 on renin secretion remains to be elucidated. The current availability of highly potent thromboxane synthetase inhibitors should facilitate assessment of the participation of TxA_2 in renin release control.

Relationship Between Arachidonic Acid Release, Prostaglandin Biosynthesis, and Renin Release

A fourth type of evidence implicating prostaglandins in the control of renin release is the apparent association between renin release, arachidonic acid release, and renal prostaglandin biosynthesis. Relevant to this discussion is the study by Weber et al. (132) who observed that intravenous furosemide increased plasma renin activity, plasma arachidonic acid levels, and urinary $PGF_{2\alpha}$ excretion rates in man. Furthermore, indomethacin pretreatment abolished the rise in plasma renin activity and prostaglandin synthesis following furosemide, indicating the dependency of furosemide-stimulated renin release on prostaglandin synthesis. Other studies also have indicated a dramatic increase in either urinary PGE_2 excretion (14,90) or renal venous PGE_2 concentrations (136,137) following furosemide administration. Sodium depletion, another potent stimulant of renin release, also enhances renal PGE_2 biosynthesis as assessed by either urinary PGE_2 excretion (26,74,112) or renal venous PGE_2 concentrations (89). For example, Kramer and Dusing (74) reported that the urinary excretion rate of PGE_2 tripled after 2 days of low salt diet in human subjects, an effect which was readily reversed by the renin release suppressing maneuver of a high salt diet. Finally, Satoh and Zimmerman (103) found that renal artery constriction increased both renal renin secretion and renal PGE_2 production in anesthetized dogs. Thus, there is supporting evidence that physiological and pharmacological stimuli that result in increases and decreases in renin release also show concomitant changes in activation of renal PGE_2 biosynthesis.

However, the interpretation of those studies as evidence linking prostaglandins to renin release is limited by several considerations: 1) The changes in urinary PGE_2 excretion following furosemide might be secondary to increases in urine flow, since increases in urine flow per se also enhance urinary PGE_2 excretion (36,67). 2) The increase in both urinary PGE_2 excretion and renal venous PGE_2 levels following either furosemide, low salt diet, or renal artery constriction might be the result of, rather than the cause of, elevated angiotensin II levels. Indeed, the increase in renal venous PGE_2 levels following renal artery constriction is most likely secondary to elevated angiotensin II levels produced by the renal artery occlusion (103). 3) The studies mentioned above measured renal PGE_2 biosynthesis; however, the best evidence indicates that if prostanoids participate in renin release it is PGI_2 rather than PGE_2 that is involved.

Since it cannot be said that the biosynthesis of one prostanoid necessarily reflects the production of another prostanoid, relationships between renin release and PGE_2 production are not strong evidence linking PGI_2 to renin release mechanisms. In view of the latter statement, before resuming the discussion of the relationship between renin release and renal prostanoid production, it seems appropriate at this point to digress into a brief consideration of why it is suspected that PGI_2 rather than PGE_2 is involved in renin release mechanisms.

Before any particular prostanoid can be considered a possible mediator or modulator of renin release several criteria must be fulfilled:

1. The prostanoid must be synthesized by the kidney.
2. The prostanoid must be a potent stimulus for renin secretion.
3. A correlation should exist between the release of renin and the secretion of the prostanoid following activation of renin release by an appropriate stimulus.
4. Selective synthesis inhibition of the prostanoid should abolish or reduce the renin release induced by an appropriate stimulus.

As noted earlier, arachidonic acid is metabolized to PGI_2, PGE_2, $PGF_{2\alpha}$, PGD_2, and TxA_2 by the renal cortex (56,135) and, of these metabolites, only PGI_2 and PGE_2 have been shown to consistently stimulate renin release from the juxtaglomerular cells (Tables 1 and 2). In addition, renin secretion has been associated with both increases in PGI_2 biosynthesis (60) and PGE_2 biosynthesis (74,89). Thus, three of the four criteria have been fulfilled by both PGI_2 and PGE_2.

It is relevant to note, however, that PGI_2 is several times more potent than PGE_2 as a renin secretagogue (78,133). Furthermore, studies with the selective PGI_2 synthesis inhibitor, U-51605, in rabbit renal cortical slices demonstrate that the release of renin by arachidonic acid is inhibited by this compound at doses which block the conversion of arachidonic acid to 6-keto-$PGF_{1\alpha}$ while enhancing the conversion to PGE_2 (133). Thus, *in vitro* the stimulant effect of arachidonic acid on renin secretion is dependent upon PGI_2 biosynthesis, but independent of PGE_2 biosynthesis. It is critical to note that the rate-limiting step in prostaglandin bio-synthesis is the release of arachidonic acid from phospholipids (83). It is precisely at this point that any stimulus to renin release that involves activation of the pros-taglandin system must act. It follows then that application of arachidonic acid to tissues *in vitro* to a certain extent mimics the activation of the prostaglandin system by any stimulus *in vivo*. Therefore, if the *in vitro* findings with U-51605 and arachidonic acid parallel the *in vivo* situation, stimuli to renin release that involve the prostaglandin system most likely do so through PGI_2 rather than through PGE_2. However, since U-51605 also inhibits thromboxane synthetase, the participation of TxA_2 in renin release cannot be ruled out at this time.

Given the probability that it is PGI_2 rather than PGE_2 that participates in renin release, a relationship between renal PGI_2 biosynthesis and renin secretion would be important supporting evidence in favor of a link between the renal prostaglandin system and renin release. Recently, Jackson et al. (60) examined the relationship between PGI_2 biosynthesis and renin release following renal artery stenosis in conscious dogs. In these experiments, arteriovenous differences in 6-keto-$PGF_{1\alpha}$ and plasma renin activity were measured before and 10 min into a one-third reduction in renal blood flow. Interestingly, renal artery stenosis was accompanied by a marked increase in both 6-keto-$PGF_{1\alpha}$ secretion rates and renin secretion rates, indicating a close association between renin release and PGI_2 biosynthesis.

Recently, a possible metabolite of PGI_2, 6-keto-PGE_1, has been described (139). This compound possesses vasodilator (62,96) and platelet aggregation-inhibiting activity (139,140) similar to that of PGI_2 but is more stable than PGI_2 under phys-iological conditions of temperature and pH. Since 6-keto-PGE_1 has pharmacological actions similar both quantitatively and qualitatively to PGI_2, the possibility exists that 6-keto-PGE_1 is also a potent renin secretagogue and therefore might mediate a portion of the renin-releasing action of PGI_2 *in vivo*. Studies in our laboratory have revealed that, when infused intrarenally into nonfiltering beta-adrenoreceptor-blocked kidneys, 6-keto-PGE_1 was approximately 5 times more potent than PGI_2 as a renin secretagogue in the canine kidney (62). Since these studies were conducted in animals without functional intrarenal beta-adrenoreceptors or macula densas, the observed increases in renin secretion induced by 6-keto-PGE_1 were most likely mediated by a direct activation on the renal juxtaglomerular cells. Similarly, McGiff et al. (80) demonstrated that 6-keto-PGE_1 released renin from rabbit renal cortical slices with a potency greater than PGI_2, and Schwertschlag et al. (104) found that

6-keto-PGE₁ was equipotent with PGI₂ in releasing renin from the isolated perfused rat and rabbit kidney. Additionally, Spokas et al. (111) demonstrated the existence of 9-hydroxyprostaglandin dehydrogenase, the enzyme that catalyzes the conversion of PGI₂ to 6-keto-PGE₁, in the rabbit kidney. Interestingly, this enzyme had the same renal zonal distribution as renin, i.e., highest in the cortex and lowest in the renal papilla. Although a potent stimulant of renin release, it still remains to be determined whether 6-keto-PGE₁ is of any physiological importance in the control of renin release.

Summary of the Role of Prostaglandins in Renin Release

In summary, four types of evidence have been presented that link prostaglandin biosynthesis to the contol of renin release: 1) inhibition of prostaglandin biosynthesis prevents renin release; 2) the prostaglandin precursor, arachidonic acid, stimulates renin release by a mechanism dependent on prostaglandin biosynthesis; 3) PGI₂ and PGE₂ are biosynthesized by the kidney and are renin secretagogues; 4) several maneuvers that stimulate renin secretion also activate prostaglandin biosynthesis. It must be admitted that no single experimental approach has provided proof that prostaglandins are involved in renin release *in vivo*. However, the available evidence is convincingly consistent with the hypothesis that prostaglandins mediate or modulate renin release.

The simplest model consistent with the data is that a stimulus releases arachidonic acid and, as a consequence of increased precursor availability, increases prostaglandin biosynthesis (Fig. 1). The newly synthesized prostaglandins then stimulate renin release. The rate-limiting step in this sequence would be the release of ar-

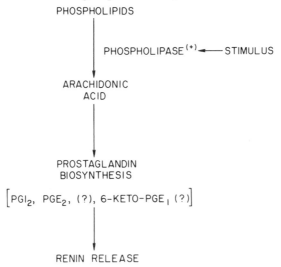

FIG. 1. Possible model of the participation of prostaglandins in the control of renin release.

achidonic acid from phospholipid storage pools. At present, little is known about the coupling between the stimulus and the precursor release. Most likely, the initial stimulus activates a phospholipase, thus resulting in increased arachidonic acid availability. As mentioned previously, current evidence suggests that PGI_2, either directly or through its metabolite 6-keto-PGE_1, is the metabolite of arachidonic acid that mediates renin release; however, the participation of PGE_2 and TxA_2 have not been excluded.

One possible objection to the hypothesis that prostaglandins participate in renin release is that angiotensin II stimulates prostaglandin biosynthesis in a number of tissues including the kidney (7–9,15,33,49,50,54,82,84,109,119). If prostaglandins activate renin release and angiotensin II activates renal prostaglandin biosynthesis, the inter-relationships would exist for a positive feedback cycle between the renin–angiotensin system and the prostaglandin system. Since in normal individuals renin release remains highly controlled, such a positive feedback cycle obviously does not exist. One possible explanation for this apparent dilemma can be found in the extraordinarily selective manner in which angiotensin II activates prostaglandin biosynthesis. In organs other than the kidney such as the mesentery artery (33) and the heart (82), angiotensin II primarily stimulates the biosynthesis of PGI_2. In contrast, in the kidney angiotensin II markedly enhances PGE_2 production while only slightly increasing renal PGI_2 biosynthesis (82). As already discussed, PGI_2 is more potent than PGE_2 as a renin secretagogue. Therefore, the PGE_2 released by angiotensin II intrarenally would not be expected to markedly affect renin secretion. Thus, it may be more than just a quirk of evolution that angiotensin II activates primarily PGI_2 production in nonrenal tissue while increasing primarily PGE_2 biosynthesis in the kidney. An additional consideration is the likely compartmentalization of prostaglandin release and action within the kidney.

PHYSIOLOGICAL MECHANISMS OF RENIN RELEASE WHICH REQUIRE PROSTAGLANDIN BIOSYNTHESIS

As stated previously, *in vivo* renin release is controlled by three mechanisms: 1) an intrarenal baroreceptor, 2) the macula densa, and 3) intrarenal beta-adreno-receptors. Since it is possible to functionally isolate each mechansim by ablating the other two, it is possible to investigate the role of the prostaglandin system in each of these afferent limbs of a reflex arc that results in renin release.

Prostaglandins and the Intrarenal Baroreceptor

The role of prostaglandins in baroreceptor-mediated renin release can be optimally investigated in denervated, beta-adrenoreceptor blocked, nonfiltering dog kidneys. In this preparation, stimulation of the baroreceptor by suprarenal aortic constriction results in a rise in renal venous renin activity in the control situation, but little change in indomethacin pretreated animals (25). This strongly implicates the prostaglandin system in baroreceptor-mediated renin release.

Prostaglandins and the Macula Densa

The optimal mode for investigating the macula densa is the denervated, beta-adrenoreceptor blocked, papaverine-treated, filtering kidney. In this situation, Olson et al. (91) found that a reduction of perfusion pressure with a suprarenal aortic clamp reduced the rate of NaCl delivery to the macula densa and stimulated renin release. Further, the rise in renin release following aortic clamping was abolished by both indomethacin and meclofenamate pretreatment. This observation suggests that the prostaglandin system is an integral component of macula densa-mediated renin release.

Other studies also have indicated the dependency of baroreceptor-mediated and macula densa-mediated renin release on prostaglandin biosynthesis. Berl et al. (4) have examined the effects of indomethacin on renin release induced by renal artery hypotension and have found that indomethacin blocks renin secretion induced by suprarenal aortic constriction in filtering kidneys. Since the renin release in this model was most likely mediated by the baroreceptor and macula densa, these data support the conclusion that both baroreceptor- and macula densa-mediated renin release are prostaglandin-dependent. Further evidence for this conclusion is provided by the study of Henrich et al. (57). These investigators found that in beta-adrenoreceptor blocked dogs, either indomethacin or control of renal artery perfusion pressure abolished the release of renin induced by hypotensive hemorrhage. Again, the most likely mechanisms mediating renin secretion in this model were the baroreceptor and macula densa. Although these latter studies did not use experimental models in which a single renin release mechanism was isolated, these studies do indicate that renin release induced by a combination of macula densa and baroreceptor stimuli requires prostaglandin biosynthesis.

Prostaglandins and the Beta-Adrenoreceptor

The optimal model for investigating the dependence of beta-adrenoreceptor-mediated renin release on prostaglandin biosynthesis would be the papaverine-treated, nonfiltering kidney. However, the majority of experiments have been performed in the intact kidney and have yielded conflicting results. Evidence in favor of prostaglandin involvement in beta-adrenoreceptor-mediated renin release has been obtained by Campbell et al. (16) who demonstrated in the rat that indomethacin inhibited the release of renin induced by suprarenal aortic infusions of the beta-adrenoreceptor agonist, isoproterenol. Similar results were found if, instead of isoproterenol, the $beta_1$-selective adrenoreceptor agonists, H133/22, was given intraperitoneally. The doses of these beta-adrenoreceptor agonist were chosen so that no change in hemodynamics was observed and, since beta-agonists have little effect on the renal vasculature or sodium transport, it was unlikely that alterations in stimuli to the baroreceptor or macula densa occurred. Additionally, indomethacin and meclofenamate inhibited the renin release induced by reflex activation of the sympathetic nervous system by hydralazine in the rat (16) and rabbit (17).

Similarly, Suzuki et al. (115) also reported inhibition by indomethacin of both isoproterenol-induced renin release and the renin release induced by reflex activation of the sympathetic nervous system in the rat. However, Seymour et al. (105) were unable to inhibit the release of renin induced by suprarenal aortic infusions of isoproterenol in the rat. Further evidence in support of a role for prostaglandins in beta-adrenoreceptor-stimulated renin release has been provided by Feuerstein and Feuerstein (35). These investigators found that the renin release induced by an intrarenal infusion of isoproterenol in the cat was abolished by both indomethacin and propranolol. Interestingly, Suzuki et al. (114) recently reported that indomethacin blocked the renin release induced by isoproterenol but not by dibutyryl cAMP in rat renal cortical slices. However, Beierwaltes et al. (3) were unable to inhibit isoproterenol-induced renin release with indomethacin in isolated rat glomeruli. Thames et al. (122) found that renin release could be induced in the dog by low frequency (0.5 Hz) electric stimulation of the renal nerves without altering renal blood flow or sodium excretion. In this model, both indomethacin and beta-adrenoreceptor blockade prevented the rise in renin release following low frequency renal nerve stimulation.

In contrast, indomethacin failed to block renin release induced by intravenous isoproterenol in sodium-deplete humans (41). Further, in contrast to the studies in the rat and cat, isoproterenol-induced renin release in the dog clearly is not blocked by indomethacin (4,105,107). In addition, renin release induced by reflex activation of the sympathetic nervous system in the dog by hypotensive hemorrhage is not inhibited by indomethacin (57). Finally, Jackson et al. (61) found that the release of renin evoked by renal nerve stimulation in the phentolamine-treated dog was abolished by beta-adrenoreceptor blockade, yet was unaltered by indomethacin. Similarly, Kopp et al. (71) reported that beta-adrenoreceptor blockade, but not indomethacin or diclofenac sodium, inhibited the renin response to low level renal nerve stimulation in the dog.

At present, it appears that prostaglandins might participate in renin release induced by beta-adrenoreceptor activation in the rat and cat, but most probably do not in the dog or human. Obviously, a final verdict regarding the role of prostaglandins in beta-adrenoreceptor-mediated renin release must await further clarifying studies. In the meantime, the above discussion should serve to enlighten the reader as to the complexities inherent in the interpretation of studies on renin release control.

PROSTAGLANDIN-MEDIATED RENIN RELEASE IN DISEASE STATES

Renin-Dependent Hypertension

If prostaglandin biosynthesis is central to the control of renin release, it follows that the prostaglandin system may be involved in the pathophysiology of high renin disease states. One situation in which renin release is considered to contribute to the disease process is that of renin-dependent hypertension. If the prostaglandin system is involved in the excessive renin secretion of renin-dependent hypertension, pharmacological manipulation of the prostaglandin system may provide new insights into mechanisms of hypertension, and eventually offer new therapeutic approaches to reduce excessive renin secretion and hence, blood pressure levels.

One approach to evaluate the role of prostaglandins in renin-dependent hypertension would be to inhibit the synthesis of prostaglandins in models of renin-dependent hypertension. If the hyperreninemia is prostaglandin-mediated, inhibition of prostaglandin synthesis should reduce both plasma renin activity and blood pressure. Surprisingly, there is a paucity of data on the effects of indomethacin in patients with hypertension. This lack of information probably reflects a variability in response in preliminary studies that has deterred rather than encouraged investigators to elucidate whether differences in the etiology of the disease process is the basis for the variation. For example, in our study of a small group of hypertensive patients, indomethacin had no significant effect on blood pressure in the whole group; however, one patient with clearly defined bilateral renal artery stenosis had a statistically significant fall in blood pressure and plasma renin activity with administration of indomethacin which returned to control level on withdrawal of indomethacin (41). It was also reported that indomethacin lowered blood pressure and plasma renin activity in two siblings with renin-dependent hypertension, hyperaldosteronism, and hypokalemia (29). In addition, chronic meclofenamate administration has been found to prevent the development of hypertension in rats following renal artery clipping (81).

Recently, DeForrest et al. (28) have examined the effects of indomethacin and meclofenamate on renal hemodynamics in conscious sodium depleted dogs. In these animals, blood pressure was supported in part by elevated levels of plasma renin activity. It is noteworthy that in this study, both indomethacin and meclofenamate produced a significant fall in mean arterial blood pressure that was highly correlated with the decrease in plasma renin activity following cyclooxygenase inhibition. Dietz et al. (30) also reported that indomethacin treatment decreased blood pressure in the high renin phase of 1-clip, 1-kidney Goldblatt hypertension in dogs. Another example of a hypotensive response to indomethacin was reported by Boyer et al. (12). These investigators found that indomethacin significantly lowered mean arterial blood pressure and plasma renin activity in subjects with elevated plasma renin activity secondary to alcoholic liver cirrhosis.

Another model that supports the role of prostaglandins in high-renin hypertension is the rat model in which the aorta is ligated between the renal arteries. This maneuver results in an ischemic left kidney and induces a severe hypertension associated with high plasma renin activities. The high level of renin activity is considered to contribute in a major way to the development of hypertension because the removal or inactivation of the renin–angiotensin system by nephrectomy (21,34,117), antiangiotensin II antibodies (21), angiotensin antagonists (34,117,118), or converting-enzyme inhibitors (117) abolishes the hypertension. Studies in our laboratory (63) have revealed that indomethacin treatment lowers both mean arterial blood pressure and plasma renin activity in aortic ligated rats. Further, there was a significant correlation between the decrease in mean arterial blood pressure and the percentage decrease in plasma renin activity. Given the renin-dependent nature of this model, these data strongly suggest that indomethacin lowers blood pressure in aortic ligated rats by inhibiting prostaglandin-mediated renin release.

If the hypothesis is true that excessive renal prostaglandin production can result in renin-dpendent hypertension, then chronic infusions of renin-releasing prostaglandins into the renal artery of an experimental animal should mimic renovascular hypertension. Support for this hypothesis recently has been reported by Hockel and Cowley (58) who demonstrated that chronic intrarenal PGE_2 infusions produced both elevated plasma renin activity and hypertension in dogs. Further, the rise in blood pressure during intrarenal PGE_2 infusions had an almost perfect linear relationship with the rise in plasma renin activity. Similar results were reported with chronic intravenous PGE_1 infusions (97).

In contrast to the reduction in arterial pressure by prostaglandin synthesis inhibitors in high-renin hypertension, the inhibition of prostaglandin synthesis in other clinical and experimental situations has been reported to have no effect on (141,142,145) or to exacerbate hypertension (20,22,23,94,95,99,113). Romero and Strong (99,113) have unequivocally demonstrated that chronic indomethacin treatment increased the blood pressure of one-kidney Goldblatt rabbits and induced malignant hypertension in those two-kidney Goldblatt rabbits in which the renal artery constriction was associated with a decrease in renal blood flow. In addition, chronic indomethacin treatment has been reported to increase the blood pressure of normotensive rabbits (24). These apparent discrepancies can be resolved by considering the overall pharmacology of drugs that inhibit renal prostaglandin synthesis. Prostaglandin synthesis inhibitors both prevent the synthesis of vasodilatory and natriuretic prostaglandins as well as inhibiting the release of renin. The former effect is potentially hypertensive, whereas the latter effect is potentially antihypertensive. The net effect, then, of prostaglandin synthesis inhibition on blood pressure would depend upon which is more prominent, prostaglandin-mediated vasodilation and natriuresis, or prostaglandin-mediated renin release. This would depend upon the experimental or clinical situation under investigation.

The disparity of effects of prostaglandin synthesis inhibition on blood pressure serves to emphasize the multiple actions of prostaglandins on the regulation of blood pressure. Clearly, the common biosynthetic origins of the prostaglandins do not connote similar functions. Rather, function is linked to the structure of the prostanoid formed and the microenvironment into which it is released.

Bartter's Syndrome

Bartter's syndrome is a rare renal disease characterized by juxtaglomerular hyperplasia, hyperreninemia, hyperaldosteronism, normotension, hyporesponsiveness to the vasoconstrictor effects of angiotensin II, polyuria, increased urinary excretion of PGE_2, and inappropriately elevated excretion of chloride and potassium (46). It appears to be due to a genetic abnormality, and published family studies are consistent with an autosomal recessive trait. The expression of this trait can occur at any age, but usually presents in young people. In childhood, it is often associated with impaired growth. Recently, considerable interest has been aroused by this syndrome as it illustrates a complex interrelating sequence of hormonal changes. The fundamental basis for this syndrome is still uncertain. However, Gill and Bartter (47) have proposed that the primary defect is in chloride reabsorption in the ascending limb of the loop of Henle. This hypothesis was suggested by the observation that fractional chloride reabsorption in the distal tubule is reduced in patients with Bartter's syndrome, leading to a failure to achieve normal free water clearance, as compared to patients with psychogenic vomiting and equivalent degrees of hypokalemia. The physiological consequences of impaired chloride reabsorption at this site can be predicted from existing knowledge of renal physiology.

First, impaired chloride reabsorption would stimulate prostaglandin-mediated renin release by the macula densa. The enhanced renin secretion would elevate circulating angiotensin II levels and, consequently, an increase in aldosterone release from the adrenal cortex would be expected. This oversecretion of aldosterone would then contribute to distal tubule potassium loss.

Second, decreased chloride reabsorption in the ascending limb of Henle's loop would increase NaCl delivery to the distal tubule and, consequently, enhance potassium excretion by a nonmineralocorticoid mechanism. The increase in potassium excretion might be a result of either enhanced sodium–potassium countertransport and/or due to enhanced tubular flow rate. Decreased potassium reabsorption in the loop of Henle secondary to reduced chloride reabsorption also may contribute to the nonmineralocorticoid component of potassium excretion.

Although PGE_2 excretion is elevated in many patients with Bartter's syndrome (11,47,48,51–53,55,146), it also is increased in patients with hypokalemia due to psychogenic vomiting (47) and may be elevated by the potassium supplements administered to these patients (146). Accordingly, the probability that increased urinary excretion of this prostaglandin is an epiphenomenon in Bartter's syndrome must be considered. There is no evidence that urinary excretion of PGE_2 is a specific reflection of the production of the arachidonic acid metabolite that regulates renin release.

Elucidation of decreased chloride reabsorption in the ascending limb of the loop of Henle provides an explanation for a number of abnormalities in Bartter's syndrome. This defect in chloride reabsorption would appear to be the primary pathogenetic mechanism, with increased prostaglandin biosynthesis at the renin regulatory site occurring as a secondary phenomenon. This view is consistent with the findings that inhibition of prostaglandin biosynthesis reverses the hyperreninemia, increased angiotensin II production, and hyperaldosteronism (11,32,55,88,128,146), yet only partially and variably reduces potassium wasting (11,32,48,55,88,101,128,146).

Because cyclooxygenase inhibitors do reduce plasma renin, angiotensin, and aldosterone levels, the mineralocorticoid component of the hypokalemia is reduced. However, the nonmineralocorticoid component of hypokalemia, maximal free water clearance, and growth rate in children are not affected. Thus, whereas cyclooxygenase inhibitors do provide palliative treatment in contributing towards reducing potassium requirements, patients can be managed with large potassium supplements. In most instances, the prognosis is dependent on adequate potassium supplementation. Unfortunately, some patients develop a progressive glomerulonephritis.

REFERENCES

1. Abe, K., Itoh, T., Satoh, M., Haruyama, T., Imai, Y., Goto, T., Satoh, K., Otsuka, Y., and Yoshinaga, K. (1980): Indomethacin (IND) inhibits an enhanced renin release following the captopril, SQ 14225, administration. *Life Sci.*, 26:561–565.
2. Bailie, M. D., Crosslan, K., and Hook, J. B. (1976): Natriuretic effect of furosemide after inhibition of prostaglandin synthetase. *J. Pharmacol. Exp. Ther.*, 199:469–476.
3. Beierwaltes, W. H., Schryver, S., Olson, P. S., and Romero, J. C. (1980): Interaction of the prostaglandin and renin-angiotensin systems in isolated rat glomeruli. *Am. J. Physiol.*, 239:F602–F608.
4. Berl, T., Henrich, W. L., Erickson, A. L., and Schrier, R. W. (1979): Prostaglandins in the beta-adrenergic and baroreceptor-mediated secretion of renin. *Am. J. Physiol.*, 236:F472–F477.
5. Blaine, E. H., Davis, J. O., and Prewitt, R. L. (1971): Evidence for a renal vascular receptor in control of renin secretion. *Am. J. Physiol.*, 220:1593–1597.
6. Blaine, E. H., Davis, J. O., and Witty, R. T. (1970): Renin release after hemorrhage and after suprarenal aortic constriction in dogs without sodium delivery to the macula densa. *Circ. Res.*, 27:1081–1089.
7. Blumberg, A. L., Denny, S. E., Marshall, G. R., and Needleman, P. (1977): Blood vessel-hormone interactions: angiotensin, bradykinin, and prostaglandins. *Am. J. Physiol.*, 232:H305–H310.
8. Blumberg, A., Denny, S., Nishikawa, K., Pure, E., Marshall, G. R., and Needleman, P. (1976): Angiotensin III—induced prostaglandin (PG) release. *Prostaglandins*, 11:195–197.
9. Blumberg, A. L., Nishikawa, K., Denny, S. E., Marshall, G. R., and Needleman, P. (1977): Angiotensin (AI, AII, AIII) receptor characterization. *Circ. Res.*, 41:154–158.
10. Bolger, P. M., Eisner, G. M., Ramwell, P. W., and Slotkoff, L. M. (1976): Effect of prostaglandin synthesis on renal function and renin in the dog. *Nature*, 259:244–245.
11. Bowden, R. E., Gill, Jr., J. R., Radfar, N., Taylor, A. A., and Keiser, H. R. (1978): Prostaglandin synthetase inhibitors in Bartter's syndrome. *JAMA*, 239:117–121.
12. Boyer, T. D., Zia, P., and Reynolds, T. B. (1979): Effect of indomethacin and prostaglandin A_1 on renal function and plasma renin activity in alcoholic liver disease. *Gastroenterology*, 77:215–222.
13. Branch, R. A., Gerber, J. G., and Gerkens, J. (1982): The role of chlorine in macula densa regulation of renin release in the dog. *(Submitted.)*
14. Brater, D. C., Beck, J. M., Adams, B. V., and Campbell, W. B. (1980): Effects of indomethacin on furosemide-stimulated urinary PGE_2 excretion in man. *Eur. J. Pharmacol.*, 65:213–219.
15. Brown, C. A., Zusman, R. M., and Haber, E. (1980): Identification of an angiotensin receptor in rabbit renomedullary interstitial cells in tissue culture. *Circ. Res.*, 46:802–807.
16. Campbell, W. B., Graham, R. M., and Jackson, E. K. (1979): Role of renal prostaglandins in sympathetically mediated renin release in the rat. *J. Clin. Invest.*, 64:448–456.
17. Campbell, W. B., Graham, R. M., Jackson, E. K., Loisel, D. P., and Pettinger, W. A. (1980): Effect of indomethacin on hydralazine-induced renin and catecholamine release in the conscious rabbit. *Br. J. Pharmacol.*, 71:529–531.
18. Campbell, W. B., Jackson, E. K., and Graham, R. M. (1979): Saralasin-induced renin release: Its blockade by prostaglandin synthesis inhibitors in the conscious rat. *Hypertension*, 1:637–642.
19. Campbell, W. B., and Zimmer, J. A. (1980): Insulin-induced renin release: blockade by indomethacin in the rat. *Clin. Sci.*, 58:415–418.
20. Cangiano, J. L., Rodriguez-Sargent, C., and Martinez-Maldonado, M. (1978): Modification of experimental renal hypertension in the rat by indomethacin and hydralazine. *J. Lab. Clin. Med.*, 92:516–520.
21. Carretero, O. A., Kuk, P., Piwonska, S., Houle, J. A., and Marin-Grez, M. (1971): Role of the renin-angiotensin system in the pathogenesis of severe hypertension in rats. *Circ. Research*, 29:654–663.
22. Chrysant, S. G. (1979): Effects of high salt intake and meclofenamate on arterial pressure and renal function in the spontaneously hypertensive rat. *Clin. Sci.*, 57:251s–253s.

23. Chrysant, S. G., Mandal, A. K., and Nordquist, J. A. (1980): Renal functional and organic changes induced by salt and prostaglandin inhibition in spontaneously hypertensive rats. *Nephron*, 25:151–155.

24. Colina-Chourio, J., McGiff, J. C., and Nasjletti, A. (1979): Effect of indomethacin on blood pressure in the normotensive unanaesthetized rabbit: possible relation to prostaglandin synthesis inhibition. *Clin. Sci.*, 57:359–365.

25. Data, J. L., Gerber, J. G., Crump, W. J., Frolich, J. C., Hollifield, J. W., and Nies, A. S. (1978): The prostaglandin system: a role in canine baroreceptor control of renin release. *Circ. Res.*, 42:454–458.

26. Davila, D., Davila, T., Oliw, E., and Anggard, E. (1978): The influence of dietary sodium on urinary prostaglandin excretion. *Acta Physiol. Scand*, 103:100–106.

27. Davis, J. O., and Freeman, R. H. (1976) Mechanisms regulating renin release. *Physiol. Rev.*, 56:1–56.

28. DeForrest, J. M., Davis, J. O., Freeman, R. H., Seymour, A. A., Rowe, B. P., Williams, G. M., and Davis, T. P. (1980): Effects of indomethacin and meclofenamate on renin release and renal hemodynamic function during chronic sodium depletion in conscious dogs. *Circ. Res.*, 47:99–107.

29. deJong, P. E., Donker, A. J. M., van der Wall, E., Erkelens, D. W., van der Hem, G. K., and Doorenbos, H. (1980): Effect of indomethacin in two siblings with a renin-dependent hypertension, hyperaldosteronism and hypokalemia. *Nephron*, 25:47–52.

30. Dietz, J. R., Davis, J. O., DeForrest, J. M., Freeman, R. H., Echtenkamp, S. F., and Seymour, A. A. (1981): Effects of indomethacin in dogs with acute and chronic renovascular hypertension. *Am. J. Physiol.*, 240:H533–H538.

31. Donker, A. J. M., Arisz, L., Brentjens, J. R. H., van der Hem, G. K., and Hollemans, H. J. G. (1976): The effect of indomethacin on kidney function and plasma renin activity in man. *Nephron*, 17:288–296.

32. Donker, A. J. M., deJong, P. E., Statius van Eps, L. W., Brentjens, J. R. H., Bakker, K., and Doorenbos, H. (1977): Indomethacin in Bartter's syndrome. *Nephron*, 19:200–213.

33. Dusting, G. J., Mullins, E. M., and Nolan, R. D. (1981): Prostacyclin release accompanying angiotensin conversion in rat mesenteric vasculature. *Eur. J. Pharmacol.*, 70:129–137.

34. Fernandes, M., Fiorentini, R., Onesti, G., Bellini, G., Gould, A. B., Hessan, H., Kim, K. E., and Swartz, C. (1978): Effect of administration of Sar[1]Ala[8] angiotensin II during the development and maintenance of renal hypertension in the rat. *Clin. Sci. Mol. Med.*, 54:633–637.

35. Feuerstein, G., and Feuerstein, N. (1980): The effect of indomethacin on isoprenaline-induced renin secretion in the cat. *Eur. J. Pharmacol.*, 61:85–88.

36. Fichman, M., Zia, P., and Zipser, R. (1980): Contribution of urine volume to the elevated urinary prostaglandin E in Bartter's syndrome and central and nephrogenic diabetes insipidus. *Adv. Prostaglandin Thrombox. Res.*, 7:1193–1196.

37. Flower, R. J. (1974): Drugs which inhibit prostaglandin biosynthesis. *Pharmacol. Rev.*, 26:33–67.

38. Fray, John C. S. (1976): Stretch receptor model for renin release with evidence from perfused rat kidney. *Am. J. Physiol.*, 231:936–944.

39. Fray, John C. S. (1980): Stimulus secretion coupling of renin. *Circ. Res.*, 47:485–492.

40. Frolich, J. C., Hollifield, J. W., Dormois, J. C., Frolich, B. L., Seyberth, H., Michelakis, A. M., and Oates, J. A. (1976): Suppression of plasma renin activity by indomethacin in man. *Circ. Res.*, 39:447–452.

41. Frolich, J. C., Hollifield, J. W., Michelakis, A. M., Vesper, B. S., Wilson, J. P., Shand, D. G., Seyberth, H. J., Frolich, W. H., and Oates, J. A. (1979): Reduction of plasma renin activity by inhibition of the fatty acid cyclooxygenase in human subjects. *Circ. Res.*, 44:781–787.

42. Gerber, J. G., Branch, R. A., Nies, A. S., Gerkens, J. F., Shand, D. G., Hollifield, J., and Oates, J. A. (1978): Prostaglandins and renin release: assessment of renin secretion following infusion of PGI_2, E_2 and D_2 into the renal artery of anesthetized dogs. *Prostaglandins*, 15:81–88.

43. Gerber, J. G., Ellis, E., Hollifield, J., and Nies, A. S. (1979): Effect of prostaglandin endoperoxide analogue on canine renal function, hemodynamics and renin release. *Eur. J. Pharmacol.*, 53:236–246.

44. Gerber, J. G., Keller, R. T., and Nies, A. S. (1979): Prostaglandins and renin release. *Circ. Res.*, 44:796–799.

45. Gerkens, J. F., Williams, A., and Branch, R. A. (1981): Effect of precursors of the 1,2, and 3 series prostaglandins on renin release and renal blood flow in the dog. *Prostaglandins*, 22:513–520.

46. Gill, J. R. (1980): Bartter's syndrome. *Ann. Rev. Med.*, 31:405–419.
47. Gill, J. R., and Bartter, F. C. (1978): Evidence for a prostaglandin-independent defect in chloride reabsorption in the loop of Henle as a proximal cause of Bartter's syndrome. *Am. J. Med.*, 65:766–772.
48. Gill, J. R., Frolich, J. C., Bowden, R. E., Taylor, A. A., Keiser, H. R., Seyberth, H. W., Oates, J. A., and Bartter, F. C. (1976): Bartter's syndrome: a disorder characterized by high urinary prostaglandins and a dependence of hyperreninemia on prostaglandin synthesis. *Am. J. Med.*, 61:43–51.
49. Grodzinska, L., and Gryglewski, R. J. (1980): Angtiotensin-induced release of prostacyclin from perfused organs. *Pharmacol. Res. Comm.*, 12:339–347.
50. Gryglewski, R. J., Korbut, R., and Splawinski, J. (1979): Angiotensin and bradykinin are the releasers of prostacyclin. *Abstract, Fourth International Prostaglandin Conference*, Washington, D.C., May 27–31, p. 44.
51. Gullner, H., Cerletti, C., Bartter, F. C., Smith, J. B., and Gill, J. R. (1979): Prostacyclin overproduction in Bartter's syndrome. *The Lancet*, 767–768.
52. Gullner, H., Smith, J. B., and Bartter, F. C. (1980): The principal metabolites of arachidonic acid are overproduced in Bartter's syndrome. *Adv. Prostaglandin Thrombox. Res.*, 7:1185–1187.
53. Gullner, H. G., Smith, J. B., Cerlett, C., Gill, Jr., J. R., and Bartter, F. C. (1980): Correction of increased prostacyclin synthesis in Bartter's syndrome by indomethacin treatment. *Prostaglandins Med.*, 4:65–72.
54. Gunther, S., and Cannon, P. J. (1980): Modulation of angiotensin II coronary vasoconstriction by cardiac prostaglandin synthesis. *Am. J. Physiol.*, 238:H895–H901.
55. Halushka, P. V., Wohltmann, H., Privitera, P. J., Hurwitz, G., and Margolius, H. S. (1977): Bartter's syndrome: Urinary prostaglandin E-like material and kallikrein; indomethacin effects. *Ann. Int. Med.*, 87:281–286.
56. Hassid, A., and Dunn, M. J. (1980): Microsomal prostaglandin biosynthesis of human kidneys. *J. Biol. Chem.*, 255:2472–2475.
57. Henrich, W. L., Schrier, R. W., and Berl, T. (1979): Mechanisms of renin secretion during hemorrhage in the dog. *J. Clin. Invest.*, 64:1–7.
58. Hockel, G. M., and Cowley, A. W. Jr. (1979): Prostaglandin E_2 induced hypertension in conscious dogs. *Am. J. Physiol.*, 237:H449–H454.
59. Isakson, P. C., Shofer, F., McKnight, R. C., Feldhaus, R. A., Raz, A., and Needleman, P. (1977): Prostaglandins and the renin-angiotensin system in canine endotoxemia. *J. Pharmacol. Exp. Ther.*, 200:614–622.
60. Jackson, E. K., Gerkens, J. F., and Branch, R. A. (1982): Acute renal artery constriction increases renal PGI_2 biosynthesis and renin release in the conscious dog. *J. Pharmacol. Exp. Ther. (in press)*.
61. Jackson, E. K., Herzer, W. A., Zimmerman, J. B., Oates, J. A., Branch, R. A., and Gerkens, J. F. (1982): Effects of indomethacin on beta-adrenoreceptor stimulated renin release in the dog. *J. Pharmacol. Exp. Ther. (in press)*.
62. Jackson, E. K., Herzer, W. A., Zimmerman, J. B., Branch, R. A., Oates, J. A., and Gerkens, J. F. (1981): 6-keto-prostaglandin E_1 is more potent than prostaglandin I_2 as a renal vasodilator and renin secretagogue. *J. Pharmacol. Exp. Ther.*, 216:24–27.
63. Jackson, E. K., Oates, J. A., and Branch, R. A. (1981): Indomethacin decreases arterial blood pressure and plasma renin activity in rats with aortic ligation. *Circ. Res.*, 49:180–185.
64. Johns, E. J., Richards, H. K., and Singer, B. (1975): Effects of adrenaline, noradrenaline, isoprenaline and salbutamol on the production and release of renin by isolated renal cortical cells of the cat. *Br. J. Pharmacol.*, 53:67–73.
65. Johnson, J. A., Davis, J. O., and Witty, R. T. (1971): Effects of catecholamines and renal nerve stimulation on renin release in the nonfiltering kidney. *Circ. Res.*, 29:646–653.
66. Kantor, H. S., and Hampton, M. (1978): Indomethacin in submicromolar concentrations inhibits cyclic AMP-dependent protein kinase. *Nature*, 276:841–842.
67. Kaye, Z., Zipser, R., Hahn, J., Zia, P., and Horton, R. (1980): Is urinary flow rate a major regulator of prostaglandin E excretion in man? *Prostaglandins Med.*, 4:303–309.
68. Keeton, T. K., and Campbell, W. B. (1980): The pharmacologic alteration of renin release. *Pharmacol. Rev.*, 32:81–227.
69. Kirchner, K. A., Kotchen, T. A., Galla, J. H., and Luke, R. G. (1978): Importance of chloride for acute inhibition of renin by sodium chloride. *Am. J. Physiol.*, 235:F444–F450.
70. Kokko, J. P. (1974): Membrane characteristics governing salt and water transport in the loop of Henle. *Fed. Proc.*, 33:25–30.

71. Kopp, U., Aurell, M., Sjolander, M., and Ablad, B. (1981): The role of prostaglandins in the alpha- and beta-adrenoreceptor mediated renin release response to graded renal nerve stimulation. *Pflügers Arch. Eur. J. Physiol.*, 391:1–8.
72. Kotchen, T. A., Galla, J. H., and Luke, R. G. (1976): Failure of $NaHCO_3$ and $KHCO_3$ to inhibit renin in the rat. *Am. J. Physiol.*, 231:1050–1056.
73. Kotchen, T. A., Galla, J. H., and Luke, R. G. (1978): Contribution of chloride to the inhibition of plasma renin by sodium chloride in the rat. *Kidney Int.*, 13:201–207.
74. Kramer, H. J., and Dusing, R. (1979): Renal prostaglandin—metabolism and salt and water balance in healthy man. *Kidney Int.*, 16:825.
75. Larsson, C., Weber, P., and Anggard, E. (1974): Arachidonic acid increases and indomethacin decreases plasma renin activity in the rabbit. *Eur. J. Pharmacol.*, 28:391–394.
76. Lazar, J. D., and Whorton, A. R. (1980): Prostaglandin mediation of potassium effects on renin release. *Life Sci.*, 27:1327–1333.
77. Leyssac, P. P., Christensen, P., Hill, R., and Skinner, S. L. (1975): Indomethacin blockade of renal PGE-synthesis: Effect on total renal and tubular function and plasma renin concentration in hydropenic rats and on their response to isotonic saline. *Acta. Physiol. Scand.*, 94:484–496.
78. Lin, C.-S., Iwao, H., Puttkammer, S., and Michelakis, A. M. (1981): Prostaglandins and renin release in vitro. *Am. J. Physiol.*, 240:E609–E614.
79. Loeffler, J. R., Stockigt, J. R., and Ganong, W. F. (1972): Effect of alpha- and beta-adrenergic blocking agents on the increase in renin secretion produced by stimulation of the renal nerves. *Neuroendocrinology*, 10:129–138.
80. McGiff, J. C., Spokas, E. G., and Wong, P. Y-K. (1982): Stimulation of renin release by 6-oxo-prostaglandin E_1 and prostacyclin. *Br. J. Pharmacol.*, 75:137–144.
81. McQueen, D., and Bell, K. (1976): The effects of prostaglandin E_1 and sodium meclofenamate on blood pressure in renal hypertensive rats. *Eur. J. Pharmacol.*, 37:223–235.
82. Needleman, P., Bronson, S. D., Wyche, A., and Sivakoff, M. (1978): Cardiac and renal prostaglandin I_2: Biosynthesis and biological effects in isolated perfused rabbit tissues. *J. Clin. Invest.*, 61:839–849.
83. Needleman, P., and Kaley, G. (1978): Cardiac and coronary prostaglandin synthesis and function. *New Engl. J. Med.*, 1122–1128.
84. Needleman, P., Marshall, G. R., and Sobel, B. E. (1975): Hormone interactions in the isolated rabbit heart: Synthesis and coronary vasomotor effects of prostaglandins, angiotensin, and bradykinin. *Circ. Res.*, 37:802–808.
85. Meyer, D. K., and Benzing, A. (1979): Studies on the inhibitory effect of indomethacin and meclofenamate on the adrenalectomy-induced increase in plasma renin concentration. *Naunyn-Schmiedeberg's Arch. Pharmacol.*, 309:25–27.
86. Michelakis, A. M., Caudle, J., and Liddle, G. W. (1969): In vitro stimulation of renin production by epinephrine, norepinephrine, and cyclic AMP. *Proc. Soc. Exp. Biol. Med.*, 130:748–753.
87. Montanaro, D., Punzi, L., Piccoli, A., Pellizzaro, E., Baggio, B., and Todesco, S. (1980): Effects of diclofenac on renin-angiotensin-aldosterone system in normotensive subjects: Comparison with indomethacin. *Curr. Ther. Res.*, 28:253–258.
88. Norby, L., Flamenbaum, W., Lentz, R., and Ramwell, P. (1976): Prostaglandins and aspirin therapy in Bartter's syndrome. *Lancet*, 2:604–606.
89. Oliver, J. A., Pinto, J., Sciacca, R. R., and Cannon, P. J. (1980): Increased renal secretion of norepinephrine and prostaglandin E_2 during sodium depletion in the dog. *J. Clin. Invest.*, 66:748–756.
90. Oliw, E., and Anggard, E. (1979): Different effects of furosemide on urinary excretion of prostaglandins E_2 and $F_{2\alpha}$ in rabbits. *Acta. Physiol. Scand.*, 105:367–373.
91. Olson, R. D., Skoglund, M. L., Nies, A. S., and Gerber, J. G. (1980): Prostaglandins mediate the macula densa stimulated renin release. *Adv. Prostaglandin Thrombox. Res.*, 7:1135–1137.
92. Osborn, J. L., Noordewier, B., Hook, J. B., and Bailie, M. D. (1978): Mechanism of prostaglandin E_2 stimulation of renin secretion. *Proc. Soc. Exp. Biol. Med.*, 159:249–252.
93. Patak, R. V., Mookerjee, B. K., Bentzel, C. J., Hysert, P. E., Babej, M., and Lee, J. B. (1975): Antagonism of the effects of furosemide by indomethacin in normal and hypertensive man. *Prostaglandins*, 10:649–659.
94. Pugsley, D. J., Beilin, L. J., and Peto, R. (1975): Renal prostaglandin synthesis in the Goldblatt hypertensive rat. *Circ. Res.*, 36,37:I81–188.
95. Pugsley, D., Beilin, L. J., and Peto, R. (1975): Renal prostaglandin synthesis in experimental renal-clip hypertension in the rat. *Clin. Sci. Mol. Med.*, 48:303s–306s.

96. Quilley, C. P., Wong, P. Y. K., and McGiff, J. C. (1979): Hypotensive and renovascular actions of 6-keto-prostaglandin E₁, a metabolite of prostacyclin. *Eur. J. Pharmacol.*, 57:273–276.

97. Rocchini, A., and Behrendt, D. (1981): Prostaglandin E₁ induced hypertension, diuresis, naturesis, and polydipsia in conscious dogs. *Circulation*, 64:IV-223.

98. Romero, J. C., Dunlap, C. L., and Strong, C. G. (1976): The effect of indomethacin and other anti-inflammatory drugs on the renin-angiotensin system. *J. Clin. Invest.*, 58:282–288.

99. Romero, J. C., and Strong, C. G. (1977): The effect of indomethacin blockade of prostaglandin synthesis on blood pressure of normal rabbits and rabbits with renovascular hypertension. *Circ. Res.*, 40:35–41.

100. Rubin, P., and Blaschke, T. (1979): Prazosin stimulates renin release and indomethacin reverses this effect. *Clin. Res.*, 27:74A.

101. Rudin, A., Aurell, M., Hansson, L., and Westberg, G. (1979): Effect of Sar¹-ala⁸-angiotensin II on blood pressure and renin in Bartter's syndrome before and after treatment with prostaglandin synthetase inhibitors. *Scand. J. Clin. Lab. Invest.*, 39:543–550.

102. Rumpf, K. W., Frenzel, S., Lowitz, H. D., and Scheler, F. (1975): The effect of indomethacin on plasma renin activity in man under normal conditions and after stimulation of the renin angiotensin system. *Prostaglandins*, 10:641–648.

103. Satoh, S., and Zimmerman, B. G. (1975): Influence of the renin-angiotensin system on the effect of prostaglandin synthesis inhibitors in the renal vasculature. *Circ. Res., (Suppl. I)* 36 and 37:I-89–I-96.

104. Schwertschlag, U., Stahl, T., and Hackenthal, E. (1982): A comparison of the effects of prostacyclin and 6-keto-prostaglandin E₁ on renin release in the isolated rat and rabbit kidney. *Prostaglandins*, 23:129–138.

105. Seymour, A. A., Davis, J. O., Echtenkamp, S. F., Dietz, J. R., and Freeman, R. H. (1981): Adrenergically induced renin release in conscious indomethacin-treated dogs and rats. *Am. J. Physiol.*, 240:F515–F521.

106. Seymour, A. A., Davis, J. O., Freeman, R. H., DeForrest, J. M., Rowe, B. P., and Williams, G. M. (1979): Renin release from filtering and nonfiltering kidneys stimulated by PGI₂ and PGD₂. *Am. J. Physiol.*, 237:F285–F290.

107. Seymour, A. A., Davis, J. O., Freeman, R. H., Echtenkamp, S. E., and Dietz, J. R. (1980): Renin release stimulated via beta-adrenergic receptors independent of renal prostaglandins. *Fed. Proc.*, 39:826.

108. Seymour, A. A., and Zehr, J. E. (1979): Influence of renal prostaglandin synthesis on renin control mechanisms in the dog. *Circ. Res.*, 45:13–25.

109. Shebuski, R. J., and Aiken, J. W. (1979): Angiotensin II induced renal prostacyclin release suppresses platelet aggregation in the anesthetized dog. *Abstract of the Fourth Internation Prostaglandin Conference, Washington, D.C.*, p. 106, May, 1979.

110. Speckart, P., Zia, P., Zipser, R., and Horton, R. (1977): The effect of sodium restriction and prostaglandin inhibition on the renin-angiotensin system in man. *J. Clin. Endocrinol. Metabol.*, 44:832–837.

111. Spokas, E. G., Wong, P. Y-K., and McGiff, J. C. (1981): Prostaglandin mechanisms and renin release. *Fed. Proc.*, 40:548.

112. Stah, R. A. K., Attallah, A. A., Bloch, D. L., and Lee, J. B. (1979): Stimulation of rabbit renal PGE₂ biosynthesis by dietary sodium restriction. *Am. J. Physiol.*, 237:F344–F349.

113. Strong, C. G., and Romero, J. C. (1976): Effects of indomethacin in rabbit renovascular hypertension. *Clin. Sci. Mol. Med.*, 51:249s–251s.

114. Suzuki, S., Franco-Saenz, R., and Mulrow, P. J. (1980): The role of renal prostaglandins in the renin response to isoproterenol in the rat in vitro. *Clin. Res.*, 128:722A.

115. Suzuki, S., Franco-Saenz, R., Tan, S. Y., and Mulrow, P. J. (1981): Effects of indomethacin on plasma renin activity in the conscious rat. *Am. J. Physiol.*, 240:E286–E289.

116. Suzuki, S., Franco-Saenz, R., Tan, S. Y., and Mulrow, P. J. (1981): Direct action of prostaglandins on renin release from rat renal cortical slices. *Proc. Soc. Exp. Biol. Med.*, 166:484–488.

117. Sweet, C. S., and Columbo, J. M. (1979): Cardiovascular properties of antihypertensive drugs in a model of severe renal hypertension. *J. Pharmacol. Meth.*, 2:223–239.

118. Sweet, C. S., Columbo, J. M., and Gaul, S. L. (1976): Central antihypertensive effects of inhibitors of the renin-angiotensin system in rats. *Am. J. Physiol.*, 231:1794–1799.

119. Swies, J., Radomski, M., and Gryglewski, R. J. (1979): Angiotensin-induced release of prostacyclin (PGI₂) into circulation of anaesthetized cats. *Pharmacol. Res. Comm.*, 11:649–655.

120. Tan, S. Y., and Mulrow, P. J. (1977): Inhibition of the renin-aldosterone response to furosemide by indomethacin. *J. Clin. Endocrinol. Metab.*, 45:174–176.
121. Thames, M. D., and DiBona, G. F. (1979): Renal nerves modulate the secretion of renin mediated by nonneural mechanisms. *Circ. Res.*, 44:645–652.
122. Thames, M. D., Osborn, J. L., and DiBona, G. F. (1980): Renin release mediated solely by renal nerves: Inhibition by blockade of prostaglandin synthesis. *Circulation Abstr.*, 62:III–222.
123. Tobian, L. (1960): Interrelationship of electrolytes, juxtaglomerular cells, and hypertension. *Physiol. Rev.*, 40:280–312.
124. Tobian, L. (1962): Relationship of juxtaglomerular apparatus to renin and angiotensin. *Circulation*, 25:189–192.
125. Vander, A. J. (1965): Effect of catecholamines and the renal nerves on renin secretion in anesthetized dogs. *Am. J. Physiol.*, 209:659–662.
126. Vander, A. J. (1967): Control of renin release. *Physiol. Rev.*, 47:359–382.
127. Vandongen, R., and Greenwood, D. M. (1975): The stimulation of renin secretion by non-vasoconstrictor infusions of adrenaline and noradrenaline in the isolated rat kidney. *Clin. Sci. Mol. Med.*, 49:609–612.
128. Vierhapper, H., and Waldhausl, W. (1980): Effect of indomethacin upon the renin-angiotensin system in patients with Bartter's syndrome. *Eur. J. Clin. Invest.*, 10:119–124.
129. Weber, P., Holzgreve, H., Stephan, R., and Herbst, R. (1975): Plasma renin activity and renal sodium and water excretion following infusion of arachidonic acid in rats. *Eur. J. Pharmacol.*, 34:299–304.
130. Weber, P. C., Larsson, C., Ånggard, E., Hamberg, M., Corey, E. J., Nicolaou, K. C., and Samuelsson, B. (1976): Stimulation of renin release from rabbit renal cortex by arachidonic acid and prostaglandin endoperoxides. *Circ. Res.*, 39:868–874.
131. Weber, P. C., Larsson, C., Hamberg, M., Anggard, E., Corey, E. J., and Samuelsson, B. (1976): Effects of stimulation and inhibition of the renal prostaglandin synthetase system on renin release in vivo and in vitro. *Clin. Sci. Mol. Med.*, 51:271s–274s.
132. Weber, P. C., Scherer, B., and Larsson, C. (1977): Increase of free arachidonic acid by furosemide in man as the cause of prostaglandin and renin release. *Eur. J. Pharmacol.*, 41:329–332.
133. Whorton, A. R., Lazar, J. D., Smigel, M. D., and Oates, J. A. (1980): Prostaglandin-mediated renin release from renal cortical slices. *Adv. Prostaglandin Thrombox. Res.*, 7:1123–1129.
134. Whorton, A. R., Misono, K., Hollifield, J., and Frolich, J. C. (1977): Prostaglandins and renin release: Stimulation of renin release from rabbit renal cortical slices by PGI_2. *Prostaglandins*, 14:1095–1104.
135. Whorton, A. R., Smigel, M., Oates, J. A., and Frolich, J. C. (1978): Regional differences in prostacyclin formation by the kidney. *Biochim. Biophys. Acta*, 529:176–180.
136. Williamson, H. E., Bourland, W. A., Marchand, G. R., Farley, D. B., and VanOrden, D. E. (1975): Furosemide induced release of prostaglandin E to increase renal blood flow. *Proc. Soc. Exp. Biol. Med.*, 150:104–106.
137. Williamson, H. E., Marchand, G. R., Bourland, W. A., Farley, D. B., and VanOrden, D. E. (1976): Ethacrynic acid induced release of prostaglandin E to increase renal blood flow. *Prostaglandins*, 11:519–522.
138. Witty, R. T., Davis, J. O., Johnson, J. A., and Prewitt, R. L. (1971): Effects of papaverine and hemorrhage on renin secretion in the nonfiltering kidney. *Am. J. Physiol.*, 221:1666–1671.
139. Wong, P. Y-K., Malik, K. U., Desiderio, D. M., McGiff, J. C., and Sun, F. F. (1980): Hepatic metabolism of prostacyclin in the rabbit: Formation of a potent novel inhibitor of platelet aggregation. *Biochem. Biophys. Res. Comm.*, 93:486–494.
140. Wong, P. Y-K., McGiff, J. C., Sun, F. F., and Lee, W. H. (1979): 6-Keto-prostaglandin E_1 inhibits the aggregation of human platelets. *Eur. J. Pharmacol.*, 60:245–248.
141. Ylitalo, P., Pitkajarvi, T., Metsa-Ketela, T., and Vapaatalo, H. (1976): The effect of inhibition of prostaglandin synthesis on plasma renin activity and blood pressure in essential hypertension. *Prostaglandins Med.*, 1:479–488.
142. Yun, J., Kelly, G., and Bartter, F. C. (1979): Effect of indomethacin on renal function and plasma renin activity in dogs with chronic renovascular hypertension. *Nephron*, 24:278–282.
143. Yun, J. C. H., Kelly, G. D., Bartter, F. C., and Smith, G. W. II. (1978): Role of prostaglandins in the control of renin secretion in the dog. *Life Sci.*, 23:945–952.
144. Yun, J., Kelly, G., Bartter, F. C., and Smith, H. Jr. (1977): Role of prostaglandins in the control of renin secretion in the dog. *Circ. Res.*, 40:459–464.

145. Zimmerman, B. G. (1978): Effect of meclofenamate on renal vascular resistance in early goldblatt hypertension in conscious and anesthetized dogs. *Prostaglandins*, 15:1027–1033.
146. Zipser, R. D., Rude, R. K., Zia, P. K., and Fichman, M. P. (1979): Regulation of urinary prostaglandins in Bartter's syndrome. *Am. J. Med.*, 67:263–267.

Prostaglandins and the Cardiovascular System,
edited by John A. Oates. Raven Press,
New York © 1982.

Prostaglandins and the Ductus Arteriosus

William F. Friedman, *Morton P. Printz, *Randal A. Skidgel, Leland N. Benson, and Mirka Zednikova

*Department of Pediatrics, University of California, Los Angeles, School of Medicine,
Los Angeles, California, and *Division of Pharmacology, Department of Medicine,
University of California, San Diego, School of Medicine, La Jolla, California*

Until recently it was assumed that the ductus arteriosus was a passively open channel during fetal life, and that it constricted postnatally by undefined molecular mechanisms in response to the abrupt rise in arterial PO_2 that accompanies the first breath of life. Recent studies strongly support the concept that control of ductus arteriosus patency and closure is mediated through prostaglandins (14,27,28,36, 60,61,64,65). The identity of the active prostaglandin or prostaglandins, their site(s) of origin, the relationship of the contractile response of the ductus to oxygen tension and to other vasoactive substances, as well as to hemodynamic changes in the pulmonary and systemic circulations remain under investigation.

The ductus arteriosus is an unique structure, since its patency after birth may result in cardiac decompensation (26,32), or it may provide the only life sustaining conduit to preserve systemic (37,38) or pulmonary blood flow (49,50) in the presence of associated cardiac malformations.

Most studies of the vasomotor activity of the ductus arteriosus employed isolated strips or rings of the vessel, often exposed transiently or throughout *in vitro* life to conditions of PO_2, light and temperature which have little or no relation to *in utero* conditions and would have altered the vessel's pharmacological responsiveness (8–11,14,16–21). This report will focus on *in situ* studies performed in the chronically instrumented, undisturbed, fetal lamb. In collaboration with Doctors Stanley Kirkpatrick and Edward Hoskins, techniques were developed in our laboratories that allowed, for the first time, direct observations of ductal caliber *in situ*. These investigations were designed to evaluate the effects of prostaglandins and inhibitors of endogenous prostaglandin synthesis on the hemodynamics and dimensions of the ductus arteriosus, as well as the interaction between these stimuli, other vasoactive agents and the autonomic nervous system.

Data will also be presented examining the question of whether the ductus arteriosus is unique among blood vessels in its ability to synthesize prostaglandins, and of additional investigations into other possible sites for the synthesis and release of prostaglandins which could affect the ductus arteriosus *in utero* and postnatally. An obvious site is the lung, since, in the adult it is a major site for the synthesis and degradation of prostaglandins, and the lung is involved intimately with the changes that take place in the fetal cardiocirculatory patterns at birth. Thus, we will also examine prostaglandin biosynthetic and catabolic pathways in the developing fetal lamb lung.

IN SITU STUDIES

Surgical and technical modifications of sonocardiometry methods reported previously from our laboratory (24,25,40) have been utilized to study the intact fetal lamb ductus. One hundred and sixty-six experiments were performed on 42 time-dated pregnant ewes of mixed western breeds operated upon at gestational ages of 90 to 124 days (term = 148 days). The lambs were instrumented chronically with patent ductus arteriosus sonomicrometer dimension crystals and with pressures determined in the main pulmonary artery and the ascending and descending aorta. Direct serial measurements of the caliber of the ductus arteriosus were recorded, as well as pressures on all sides of the channel. Drugs were infused through a catheter implanted chronically in the superior vena cava so as not to disrupt the monitoring of periductal pressures, or occasionally, through a catheter implanted in the left atrium to see if delivery of a drug principally to the vasovasorum of the ductus arteriosus, rather than the lumen, would influence a response. Fetuses were allowed a one to seven day recovery period prior to pharmacologic intervention.

Experiments were designed to study the direct action of vasoactive agents (Table 1) on the ductus arteriosus, as well as the influence of the prior administration of these agents on the responses to indomethacin or other prostaglandin synthetase inhibitors, and, finally the actions of these agents on the ductus arteriosus already constricted by indomethacin.

Prostaglandin Synthetase Inhibitors

Indomethacin

The effects of inhibiting endogenous prostaglandin synthesis with indomethacin on the contractile behavior *in utero* of the fetal ductus arteriosus were studied in doses ranging from 0.001 to 1.00 mg/kg. Constriction of the fetal channel began at doses as low as 0.01 mg/kg. The plateau of the dose response curve occurred at dosage levels of approximately 0.2 mg/kg. (Fig. 1). Over the gestational age range studied, no age-related differences were observed of the response of the ductus arteriosus to indomethacin. The values for ductal constriction in fetuses of 96 days gestational age were the same as those for the older animals and conformed to the dose response curve.

The time course of response to indomethacin was not evaluated completely, nor were pharmacokinetic studies undertaken. We did note, however, that the time from infusion to maximum constriction averaged 44 min, with an initial increase in pulmonary arterial pressure and heart rate within the first three min after infusion.

TABLE 1. *Pharmacologic agents investigated*

N	Pharmacologic agents	Dose	Effect on Ductus
	Prostaglandin synthetase inhibitors		
61	Indomethacin	0.001–1.0 mg/kg	Constricts
18	Imidazole	2.0–4.0 mg/kg/min	Dilates
	Prostaglandins		
63	PGE_1	0.1–1.0 µg/kg/min	Dilates
2	PGE_2	0.1–1.0 µg/kg/min	Dilates
2	$PGF_{2\alpha}$	0.1–1.0 µg/kg/min	N.E.
2	PGH_2	2.0 µg/kg/min	Dilates
25	PGI_2	1.0–100.0 µg/kg/min	N.E.
		2.5–120.0 µg/kg	N.E.
		510.0–850.0 µg/kg	Dilates
3	PGG_2 ether analogue	0.25–25.0 µg/kg/min	N.E.
	Autonomic nervous system mediators and blockers		
3	Acetylcholine	0.01–1.0 µg/kg/min	N.E.
3	Atropine	0.2 mg/kg	N.E.
2	Norepinephrine	0.1–1.0 µg/kg/min	N.E.
2	Propranolol	1.0 mg/kg	N.E.
5	Phentolamine	0.1 mg/kg	N.E.
2	Methoxamine	50.0 µg/kg/min	N.E.
	Reno-vascular and tryptaminergic agents		
3	Angiotensin I	50.0–100.0 µg/kg/min	N.E.
3	Angiotensin II	50.0–100.0 µg/kg/min	N.E.
4	Angiotensin I converting enzyme blocker (SQ-20881)	10.0–250.0 µg/kg/min 250.0 µg/kg	N.E. N.E.
3	Serotonin	100.0–300.0 µg/kg/min	N.E.
3	Methysergide	20.0–100.0 µg/kg/min	N.E.
	Agents affecting cyclic nucleotides		
2	Aminophylline	14.0,28.0 µg/kg/min	N.E.
2	Adenosine	2.0 mg/kg/min	N.E.
4	Dibutyryl cyclic-AMP	0.4–4.0 mg/kg/min	N.E.

Constricts: Constricts ductus arteriosus; Dilates: Dilates ductus, but only when ductus has been previously constricted with indomethacin; N.E.: No effect on ductus; N: Number.

Indomethacin induced constriction of the ductus arteriosus was always reversed completely and within three to ten min by infusion of PGE_1 (0.1 µg/kg/min) (Fig. 2).

The direct determinations of ductus arteriosus dimensions and the estimated wall thickness (1 mm) of the ductus arteriosus, based on 30 post-sacrificed specimens, were used to calculate the change in the internal cross sectional area of the ductus arteriosus (Fig. 1). In calculating the change in ductus cross sectional area in order to construct the dose/response relation between ductus constriction and indomethacin dose, we assumed that ductal constriction was not accompanied by substantial changes in the length of the vessel. To test this assumption, and in order to ascertain if the ductus arteriosus piezo electric dimension cyrstals were placed at a site allowing detection of maximum constriction, five chronically instrumented fetal

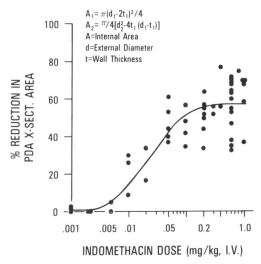

FIG. 1.   The dose effect relationship is shown of inhibiting endogenous prostaglandin synthesis with indomethacin on contraction of the ductus arteriosus in the chronically instrumented, undisturbed fetal lamb *in utero* between 95 and 147 days gestational age. Each point represents a separate experiment on an individual fetus.

lambs underwent selective injections of contrast material, Hypaque M 75%, 1 cc/kg and normal saline 1 cc/kg, into the fetal main pulmonary artery with cineangiographic monitoring (Fig. 3).

These fetal angiographic studies indicated that the ductus arteriosus shortened 3% to 10% during indomethacin constriction. Most importantly, the angiographic studies illustrated that the point of maximum constriction of the ductus arteriosus was not at the mid point of the vascular channel where the piezo electric cystals were monitoring dimension changes, but at the aortic end of the ductus arteriosus (Fig. 3). Thus, it should be recognized that an underestimation exists in our presentation of the magnitude of ductal constriction in response to indomethacin. This underestimation would be less with mild constriction, i.e., at low doses of indomethacin, and greatest with substantial constriction, i.e., at high dose levels of the drug. The vasoconstrictor responses of the ductus arteriosus to indomethacin were accompanied by striking reductions in circulating PGE_2 and significant, but less marked reductions in circulating $PGF_{2\alpha}$ levels measured by radioimmunoassay (Fig. 4).

Imidazole

The effects of imidazole, a thromboxane synthase inhibitor (48), were studied in 18 experiments at the doses indicated in Table 1. The rationale was to assess inhibition of thromboxane synthase activity, although other direct actions of imidazole on the circulation would not be excluded. Imidazole appeared to have no direct effect on ductus arteriosus caliber or pulmonary arterial or aortic blood

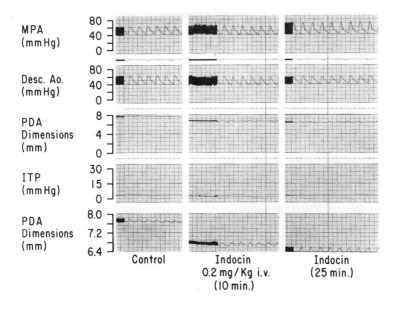

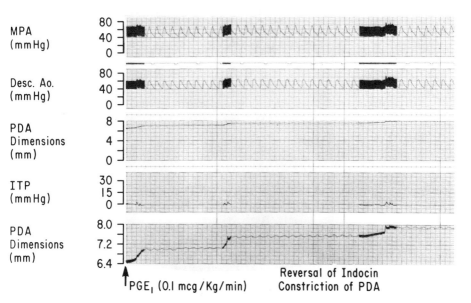

FIG. 2. Top: Representative experiment in which indomethacin (0.2 mg/kg) produced profound constriction of the fetal ductus arteriosus 124 days gestation, 4 days post-op. The constriction is best appreciated in the magnified scale of the lower tracing. Patent ductus arteriosus (PDA) dimensions are measured directly with sonomicrometer crystals and pressures are reported simultaneously from the fetal main pulmonary artery (MPA) and descending aorta (DESC, AO). A rise in MPA pressure was associated with ductal constriction, with little change in aortic pressure. ITP = intratracheal pressure. **Lower:** Recordings occurred 18 hr after the experiment shown in top 125 days gestation, 5 days post-op. The infusion of PGE$_1$ (0.1 mg/kg, i.v.) restored ductus dimensions to normal; little change was observed in MPA pressure during ductus dilatation and aortic pressure rose slightly.

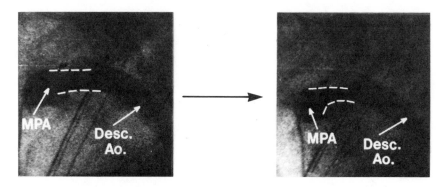

FIG. 3. Fetal lamb angiographic studies (122 days gestation, 11 days post-op) showing the constrictor response to indomethacin. The ductus arteriosus is enclosed by the dashed lines. The sonomicrometer crystals at the level of the mid ductus underestimate the magnitude of constriction which is maximum at the aortic end of the ductus. **Left:** control; **right:** indomethacin (0.2 mg/kg, i.v.). %Δ PDA X-section area: −31% mid-ductus, −71% maximum. MPA, main pulmonary artery, DESC. A., descending aorta.

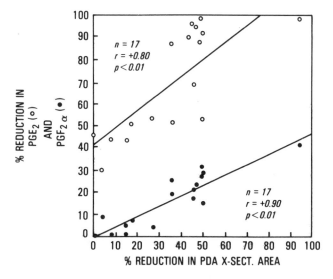

FIG. 4. A significant correlation existed between the reduction in ductus arteriosus cross sectional area, and the indomethacin induced reduction in circulating levels of PGE_2 and $PGF_{2\alpha}$.

pressures. However, constant infusions of imidazole at 2 and 4 mg/kg/min blunted the ductal constriction induced by high doses of indomethacin (Fig. 5). Figure 5 illustrates the dose relation of the imidazole blockade of indomethacin-induced ductal constriction. In the absence of imidazole, indomethacin caused an average reduction in the cross sectional area of the ductus of 54 ± 4%. The concurrent infusion of 2 mg/kg/min of imidazole lessened the indomethacin constrictor response to 27 ± 4% ($p < 0.001$), while with an imidazole infusion rate of 4 mg/kg/min the indomethacin constriction was reduced to 11 ± 6% ($p < 0.001$, when compared to the lower imidazole dose). The action of imidazole on the indomethacin-induced

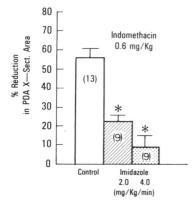

FIG. 5. The imidazole induced reversal is shown of the constrictor response of the ductus arteriosus to indomethacin. The numbers in brackets represent the number of animals studied. The height of each bar and the vertical line represent the mean ± SEM. The asterisks indicate the statistical significance of the imidazole action at each of the two doses given of the latter drug.

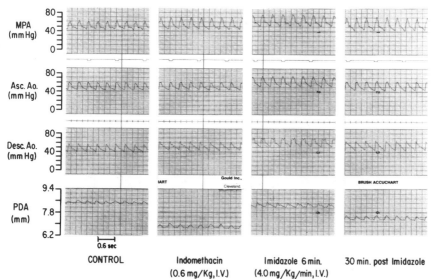

FIG. 6. A representative experiment in which indomethacin (0.6 mg/kg, i.v.) constricts the PDA **(lower panel)** and imidazole promptly reverses the indomethacin constriction in a fetal lamb, 120 days gestation, 8 days post-op. After discontinuing the imidazole infusion, the indomethacin induced constriction is once again evidenced. Pressures are recorded simultaneously from main pulmonary artery (MPA), ascending aorta (Asc Ao), and descending aorta (Desc Ao).

constriction was transient. The administration of imidazaole (4 mg/kg/min) following indomethacin (Fig. 6) promptly reversed ductal constriction within six min. However, within 30 min of discontinuing the imidazole, ductal constriction had returned to levels achieved after the administration of indomethacin alone.

Prostaglandins E_1, E_2, $F_{2\alpha}$, G_2, H_2 and I_2

This group of vasoactive agents was evaluated in a total of 55 experiments. When administered directly to the resting fetus at the doses employed (Table 1), none of these prostaglandins significantly influenced heart rate, blood pressure, or ductus arteriosus dimensions. However, when the ductus arteriosus was already constricted with any dose of indomethacin, PGE_1, PGE_2, PGI_2 and the ether analogue of PGH_2 promptly dilated the ductus arteriosus to control levels. In contrast, neither $PGF_{2\alpha}$, or PGG_2 were effective in reversing indomethacin constriction of the ductus arteriosus.

The responses to varying doses of PGI_2 were of particular interest. It was found that only relatively high doses of PGI_2 reversed the indomethacin-induced ductal constriction (Fig. 7, Table 1). Low doses of PGI_2 did not influence the caliber of the ductus arteriosus. This finding was independent of the path of injection, i.e., directly into the superior vena cava and, hence, into the lumen of the ductus arteriosus, or through a catheter implanted chronically into the left atrium which would be expected to deliver PGI_2 selectively to the vaso vasora of the ductus. Low doses of PGI_2, while not influencing the caliber of the indomethacin constricted ductus arteriosus, had profound effects on pulmonary and systemic arterial pressures, suggesting that PGI_2 caused significant pulmonary and systemic vasodilatation without influencing the ductus arteriosus.

Autonomic Nervous System Mediators and Blockers

Autonomic blocking agents were administered in doses that were shown to inhibit the effects of the agonists (Table 1). Although significant alterations in blood pressure and heart rate were observed in this series of experiments, with the possible exception of acetylcholine, no alterations occurred in the cross sectional area of the fetal ductus arteriosus. Acetycholine at high dose (1 µg/kg/min) caused substantial systemic and pulmonary hypotension which was associated with a $13 \pm 7\%$ decrease in the cross sectional area of the ductus arteriosus. This hemodynamic effect was reversed by atropine, but not PGE_1. Atropine per se was ineffective in reversing the indomethacin-induced constriction of the ductus arteriosus. Alpha and beta adrenergic agonists (methoxamine and norepinephrine, respectively) and (phentolamine and propranolol antagonists) had no influence on ductal caliber.

Angiotensin I and II, converting enzyme blocker (SQ 20881), serotonin, and methysergide did not influence the dimension of the ductus arteriosus directly, or interfere with the indomethacin-induced constriction of the ductus arteriosus. Aminophylline, adenosine, and dibutyryl cyclic AMP did not cause a signficant change in the dimensions of the ductus arteriosus, nor did they inhibit the ability of indomethacin to constrict the ductus arteriosus.

IMPLICATIONS OF THE *IN SITU* EXPERIMENTS

Attention was called 41 years ago to the unique oxygen sensitivity of the ductus arteriosus (39). Since then, many additional mechanisms have been proposed as the stimulants for muscular closure of the ductus arteriosus at birth. Prominent among these were autonomic and neural factors and the kinins (31).

Sympathetic and parasympathetic innervation of the ductus arteriosus have been demonstrated in several species (3,5), although studies of isolated patent ductus

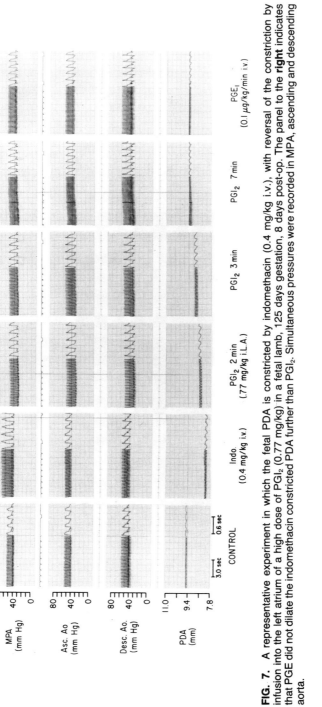

FIG. 7. A representative experiment in which the fetal PDA is constricted by indomethacin (0.4 mg/kg i.v.), with reversal of the constriction by infusion into the left atrium of a high dose of PGI₂ (0.77 mg/kg) in a fetal lamb, 125 days gestation, 8 days post-op. The panel to the **right** indicates that PGE did not dilate the indomethacin constricted PDA further than PGI₂. Simultaneous pressures were recorded in MPA, ascending and descending aorta.

arteriosus strips have demonstrated that the constrictor response is not affected by stimulation with, or blockade of, the adrenergic and cholinergic neurotransmitters (41,44). Other *in vitro* or *in vivo* investigations concerned with the influence of the autonomic nervous system in modulating the smooth muscle tone of the ductus arteriosus are inconclusive or contradictory. In the present study, despite hemodynamic perturbations, no changes were observed in the dimensions of the fetal ductus arteriosus upon administration directly of norepinephrine, propranolol, phentolamine or methoxamine. None of these drugs altered the responsiveness of the ductus arteriosus to prostaglandins or inhibitors of prostaglandin synthesis. Although the latter comment may be applied to atropine, acetylcholine administration resulted in a slight direct reduction in the cross sectional area of the fetal ductus, while concurrently lowering pulmonary and systemic blood pressures. The effect of acetylcholine was reversed by atropine and not PGE_1, and it must remain conjectural whether the cholinergic constriction of the ductus arteriosus was the result of a hydrostatic influence of hypotension, or a direct effect of the parasympathetic neurotransmitter.

Renovascular and tryptaminergic vasoactive agents did not appear to affect the ductus arteriosus or its responses when the prostaglandin milieu was altered. Some speculation exists that cyclic nucleotides might function as a link between hormonal stimulation and contractility of vascular smooth muscle (33,42). Evidence was sought, but not found, for a physiological role of cyclic nucleotides in the regulation of the contractility of the ductus arteriosus. The phosphodiesterase inhibitor, theophylline, and dibutyryl cyclic AMP did not influence the dimensions of the ductus arteriosus directly, nor did their administration alter the ability of indomethacin to constrict the ductus arteriosus. These same findings were observed with the cyclic nucleotide metabolite, adenosine. These experiments suggest, but do not prove, that cyclic nucleotides do not play a physiological role in modulating the smooth muscle tone of the ductus arteriosus. The major finding of these *in vivo* experiments was the exquisite sensitivity of the ductus arteriosus to changes in the prostaglandin environment. The ductus arteriosus appeared to be dilated maximally *in utero*, since direct infusion of prostaglandins could not cause further dilatation of the vascular channel. Intravenous doses of as little as 0.01 mg/kg of the prostaglandin synthetase inhibitor, indomethacin, caused significant constriction of the ductus arteriosus. PGE_1, PGE_2, PGH_2, and PGI_2 were all capable of reversing the constrictor response to indomethacin, in the absence of any alterations in fetal arterial pH, pO_2 or pCO_2.

The indomethacin constrictor response did not appear to be influenced by the age of the fetus, since animals at 95 days (0.65 gestation) showed reductions in ductus arteriosus cross sectional area to varying doses of the PG synthesis inhibitor comparable to that of animals observed close to term.

This last observation conflicts with those isolated ductus arteriosus studies suggesting that the prostaglandin mechanism responsible for ductus arteriosus patency is most active at about 0.6 to 0.7 gestation and abates thereafter (12,22). Several workers have suggested that opposite the response to oxygen, the isolated ductus arteriosus from fetal lambs about 100 days gestational age has a significantly increased response to indomethacin in comparison with near-term animals (10,12,21,22).

We have no ready explanation for the contrast between *in vivo* and *in vitro* findings. The *in situ* age independent equivalency of indomethacin constriction may suggest that a balance exists between the maturation of the vascular smooth muscle of the ductus arteriosus, the development of specific receptors for prostaglandins, and/or an alteration in the sensitivity of the vessel to, or in the synthesis and degradation of, both locally produced and circulating relaxing and contracting substances.

PGI_2 was found to be less potent than PGE_1 in reversing indomethacin-mediated ductual closure. Since PGI_2 is not metabolized as rapidly as PGE_1, it might be expected to have a longer half-life *in vivo* which could offset any differences at the receptor level. We would conclude that ductal prostaglandin receptors respond more readily to PGE_1 than PGI_2. Another explanation is that PGE_1, being slightly less polar than PGI_2, may gain access more readily to ductal receptors. Of course, it should be noted that PGE_1 would not be expected to occur in significant amounts in mammalian organisms. Thus, PGE_2 may have greater physiological significance. These findings are generally compatible with studies of isolated fetal lamb ductus arteriosus which suggest that PGE_2 is the most potent ductus arteriosus relaxing agent known (19,42). It has been suggested that PGI_2 per se only contributes to ductus patency by supplementing the PGE_2 action on muscle cells, and by preventing platelet adhesions on the luminal surface (22). Coceani has pointed out that 6 keto PGE_1 is a very potent ductus arteriosus relaxing agent, and it should be recognized that PGI_2 may indeed have a more central function in controlling ductus arteriosus contractility if future investigations demonstrate the presence, in ductus arteriosus tissue, of an enzyme system for the conversion of the PGI_2 metabolite, 6 keto PGF_1 to 6 keto PGE_1 (22).

Our results would argue that both locally generated and circulating prostaglandin components are involved in ductal patency and closure. The dilatory effects of PGE_2 and PGI_2, the former exhibiting the ability to act as a circulating hormone, appear to be important in ductal patency. Differences in endogenous prostaglandin synthesis might be expected to remove this dilatory influence, as might maturational alterations in prostaglandin receptors within the ductus. In addition, one may speculate that a lesser pulmonary degradation of PGI_2 than PGE_2 allows a sufficiently long half-life of PGI_2 in the circulation to consider it analogous to PGE_2 as a circulating hormone. Constriction of the ductus would appear to be the result of an active unknown process. It is of interest that imidazole is an inhibitor of thromboxane synthase and its effect in reversing indomethacin-mediated ductal closure may relate to this activity, although experiments in isolated ductal tissue exposed to a thromboxane generating system suggested that thromboxane A_2 has no direct effect on the ductus arteriosus (16). Further studies are needed to resolve this question.

BIOCHEMICAL STUDIES OF PROSTAGLANDIN BIOSYNTHESIS AND CATABOLISM IN FETAL AND NEONATAL VASCULAR AND LUNG TISSUES

Prostaglandin Biosynthesis in Fetal Blood Vessels

Despite the fact that a direct correlation existed between the fall in circulating levels of prostaglandins in the fetus and changes in the caliber of the ductus arteriosus

(Fig. 4), our *in situ* data did not answer the central question of whether ductal reactivity is more importantly associated with alterations in prostaglandin synthetase activity within the ductus itself, or with changes in circulating levels of the prostaglandins. Additional studies were performed, principally by R. A. Skidgel in our laboratories, that were designed to examine the hypothesis that the ductus arteriosus is unique in comparison to other fetal blood vessels in its ability to synthesize a vasodilator (to maintain patency), or at the time of birth a vasoconstrictor (for closure) prostaglandin (31,62).

Skidgel's experiments have shown that fetal blood vessels are capable of synthesizing prostacyclin from endoperoxide or arachadonic acid. Interestingly, the ductus arteriosus was less active in converting PGH_2 to prostacyclin than other arterial vessels (confirmed by both complete utilization and initial rate assays) (Table 2). While endoperoxide metabolic activity of the ductus was intermediate to that of the arteries and veins, the ductus arteriosus was at least as active as other fetal vessels in converting arachidonic acid to prostaglandin products. This indicated relatively high cyclo-oxygenase activity. There was no evidence for thromboxane A_2 formation in the ductus arteriosus, umbilical or other blood vessels. Quite importantly, the ductus arteriosus and other fetal arteries did not have the capacity to synthesize PGE_2, PGD_2, or $PGF_{2\alpha}$ enzymatically from PGH_2.

Most current theories on ductal patency focus on the role of endogenous production of prostaglandins by the ductus. Studies performed on ductal strips or rings *in vitro* have shown PGE_2 to be the most potent prostaglandin in causing relaxation, with PGI_2 being much less active (19,20,42). This had led Coceani et al (22) and Clyman and his associates (12) to hypothesize that ductal PGI_2 biosynthesis is responsible for maintaining its patency *in utero*. However, the results from this study, as well as others (51,53,66) appear to prove that the ductus does not contain the enzymatic capacity to synthesize PGE_2. Thus, if ductal patency is maintained by PGE_2 it might be coming from another source. One possibility is the fetal lung, and this will be explored.

While isolated ductus studies suggest that PGI_2 is not involved in maintaining ductal patency, there may be significant differences between the response of the ductus to exogenous prostaglandins and endogenously synthesized prostaglandins. Additionally, the trauma of removing the tissue, cutting it into rings or strips, and allowing it to equilibrate in a hypoxic or anoxic muscle bath for one to five hr could alter the tissues' responsiveness to prostaglandins. Thus, caution must be observed in extrapolating results that were obtained under nonphysiological conditions. The possiblity still exists that under normal conditions endogenously synthesized prostacyclin may play a role in the maintenance of ductus patency, since biochemical studies show that the ductus has significant cyclo-oxygenase activity and probably adequate prostacyclin synthase activity for this function.

The fetal lamb ductus arteriosus appears to be dilated maximally *in utero* and constricts at birth, or upon administration of prostaglandin synthetase inhibitors (27,31). Since indomethacin, aspirin and ibuprofen (agents used to constrict the ductus arteriosus in humans or animals) all interfere primarily with formation of

TABLE 2. Products of PGH_2 metabolism by fetal blood vessel homogenates

							p values[c]	
N[a]	Vessel	6-keto-PGF$_{1\alpha}$	PGF$_{2\alpha}$	PGE$_2$	PGD$_2$	HHT	Ductus arteriosus	Vena cava
6	Aorta	73.0 ± 2.1	7.7 ± 1.2	5.0 ± 0.5	3.6 ± 0.9	11.2 ± 1.1	$p < 0.01$	$p < 0.001$
6	Pulmonary artery	72.8 ± 3.6	7.5 ± 0.8	5.2 ± 2.0	3.3 ± 0.7	11.2 ± 1.6	$p < 0.02$	$p < 0.001$
5	Umbilical vessels	72.0 ± 4.2	7.7 ± 1.6	9.0 ± 2.5	2.4 ± 0.7	8.8 ± 1.8	$p < 0.05$	$p < 0.01$
5	Ductus arteriosus	56.6 ± 4.0	11.8 ± 2.5	7.8 ± 0.6	4.2 ± 0.3	19.6 ± 1.6		$p < 0.02$
3	Vena cava	30.5 ± 7.1	10.6 ± 0.9	25.3 ± 1.6	13.2 ± 5.2	20.4 ± 1.9	$p < 0.02$	—

Blood vessels were homogenized and all incubations contained equivalent amounts of protein (250 μg) and [1-^{14}C]-PGH$_2$ (25,000 dpm).
[a]Number of different fetal tissues examined.
[b]Expressed as percent ± SE.
[c]Statistical significance was tested by Student's t-test for non-paired means and refers to tests for significance between the ductus arteriosus or vena cava and the other tissues.

PGH_2, these agents would be expected to decrease the rate of formation of PGI_2. However, it appears unlikely that the mechanism of selective closure of the ductus by prostaglandin synthetase inhibitors solely involves the depression of PGI_2 synthesis.

At birth, the lower prostacyclin synthase activities seen in the ductus could lead to lower PGI_2 production in comparison to other vessels. It is unlikely, however, that this alone could allow the ductus to close, but it might enchance the sensitivity of the ductus to a vasoconstrictor in comparison to other vessels. Thus, it is possible that patency of the ductus arteriosus may be coupled directly to production of PGI_2, and that a *positive vasoconstrictor* process is necessary for ductal closure. While it has been hypothesized that the ductus closes at birth due to a direct constrictor effect of oxygen (24), it is also possible that a prostaglandin could be involved. Although the physiological changes which take place at birth could be a potent stimulus for prostaglandin biosynthesis, it is unlikely that the source of a constrictor prostaglandin would be the fetal vasculature, since no evidence for this was found in biochemical studies. A more likely source for such a protaglandin is the lung, since it is intimately involved with the circulatory changes which take place at birth and is known to actively synthesize prostaglandins.

Prostaglandin Endoperoxide Metabolism in Fetal and Neonatal Lungs

Pace-Asciak showed that the ability of fetal sheep lung to synthesize prostaglandins was present at very early gestational ages (52). He initially studied the synthesis of PGE_2 and $PGF_{2\alpha}$ from arachidonic acid, and he recently described preliminary findings showing that the fetal lung could make thromboxane and prostacyclin, although the development aspects of their synthesis were not studied (54). In our laboratory, studies were undertaken to determine whether there were developmental changes in the PGH_2 metabolizing ability of fetal and newborn sheep lungs (62). Homogenates of perfused lungs from fetal and newborn lambs of various ages (115 days gestation to 11 day-old newborn) were incubated with either 2 nM or 11 nM $[1-^{14}C]$-PGH_2 and the products analyzed by thin layer chromatography. The fetal lung was shown to have the capacity to enzymatically convert the intermediate endoperoxide, PGH_2, to three prostaglandin products—PGE_2, prostacyclin, and thromboxane. Pronounced changes were observed with thromboxane synthase which exhibited a developmental dependency, very low at 115 to 130 days gestation and significantly increased (5- to 6-fold) by term (Fig. 8). Prostacyclin synthase activity was relatively low and constant throughout gestation with the enzyme-exhibiting saturation at low concentrations of PGH_2.

Formation of PGE_2 did not show saturation with variation of substrate concentration at any age. This reflects, in part, the fact that PGE_2 is formed non-enzymatically by breakdown of PGH_2. Thromboxane synthase activity was very low in early fetuses at all substrate concentrations, but became a major product by 144 days gestation at higher substrate levels and did not level off at all at 6 hr after birth. Changes in the enzyme constants during development were defined by measuring

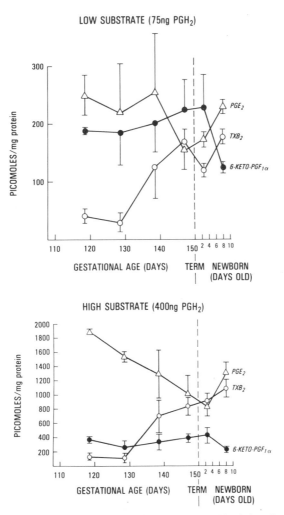

FIG. 8. Results of the incubation of two μM PGH$_2$ with fetal and lamb lung homogenates (250 μg protein) at various ages **(top)** and the incubation of 11 μM PGH$_2$ with fetal and lamb lung homogenates (250 μg protein) at various ages **(bottom)**. Each point is the mean ± SEM of the results obtained from 2 to 4 animals.

initial rates of PG formation from PGH$_2$ (Fig. 9). The apparent K_m values for prostacyclin synthase (29mM), thromboxane synthase (100 μM) and PGH$_2$-PGE$_2$ isomerase (275 μM) did not change with fetal age. Similarily, the V_{max} for the PGH$_2$-PGE$_2$ isomerase was very high (68,000-76,000 pmoles/min/mg/protein) and did not change significantly with fetal age. However, prostacyclin synthase activity (V_{max}) was much higher (5-fold) in the early gestation fetal lung than late gestation or newborn lung, while the V_{max} for thromboxane synthase was 2- to 3-fold higher in the late gestation and newborn lung than in the 115 day-gestation fetal lung.

Arachidonic Acid Metabolism in Fetal and Neonatal Lungs

The type of prostagladin produced by the lung *in vivo* will depend on substrate (PGH_2) levels, cofactor (reduced glutathione) levels and the relative activities of the PGH_2 metabolizing enzymes. The substrate (PGH_2) concentration *in vivo* will, in turn, be determined by the activity of the cyclo-oxygenase enzyme (prostaglandin endoperoxide synthetase) which will convert the arachidonic acid to PGH. It was thus important to determine the ability of fetal lungs to metabolize arachidonic acid via the cyclo-oxygenase enzyme. Other investigators have studied the ability of fetal lung homogenates from calf, sheep, and rabbits to convert arachidonic acid to prostaglandin products (3,52,58). However, true cyclo-oxygenase activity was not being measured in these studies because relatively long time points (5 to 10 min) were used. Since cyclo-oxygenase activity has been shown to be linear for only 30 sec (due to self-inactivation) (43,45), long incubations cannot yield meaningful kinetic data.

Conversion of arachidonic acid to prostaglandins was monitored (62) in lung microsomes from fetal, newborn and adult sheep. Since cyclo-oxygenase (prostaglandin endoperoxide synthetase) activity was measured by the conversion of [1-^{14}C]-arachidonic acid to prostaglandins, it was necessary to determine whether significant levels of endogenous arachidonic acid were present in the microsomal samples used. Free arachidonic acid concentrations in lung microsomes were measured by high pressure liquid chromatography and were found to be very low and variant with fetal and newborn age. Lung microsome cyclo-oxgenase activity was found to be constant at all gestational ages and increased after birth to two times the fetal level at 11 days of age, and four to five times the fetal level in the adult (Fig. 10). PGE_2 was the major product of arachidonic acid metabolism with other prostaglandins (i.e., 6 keto $PGF_{1\alpha}$, $PGF_{2\alpha}$, and TXB_2) being produced in smaller amounts at about the same proportion. The proportions of the various prostaglandins produced by the lung did not change significantly during fetal development or after birth (Table 3). It is generally presumed that, *in vivo*, the cyclo-oxygenase enzyme is always active, ready to convert any arachidonic acid released from membrane phospholipids into prostaglandins. If correct, since cyclo-oxygenase activity was found to be similar at all gestational ages, changes in total prostaglandin production would have to result from changes in phospholipase activity. Arachidonic acid release, in turn, is known to be stimulated by anything that causes membrane pertubation (48). Thus, total prostaglandin production *in vivo* will be determined by many factors other than cyclo-oxygenase activity, and could change dramatically in the absence of any apparent difference in cyclo-oxygenase activity (56).

Prostaglandin Catabolism in Fetal and Neonatal Lungs

Prostaglandin levels in a tissue can be regulated either by changes in biosynthetic activity or by changes in prostaglandin metabolism. In the absence of any change in activity of the biosynthetic enzymes, circulating prostaglandin levels could increase or decrease due to changes in catabolic activity. The initial step in the metabolism and inactivation of prostaglandins is oxidation of the ^{C}15 alcohol (1). This reaction is catalyzed by 15-hydroxyprostaglandin dehydrogenase, an enzyme found in many tissues and in high concentrations in the lung and kidney (2). The dehydrogenase enzyme has been shown to be short-lived with a half-life of only 47 to 75 min (4). This indicates that, because of its rapid synthesis and degradation, 15-hydroxyprostaglandin dehydrogenase activity could increase or decrease rapidly in response to the metabolic needs of the organ. Several studies have shown the activity of this enzyme to vary widely in organs of the fetus and mother during gestation (51,54). In addition, the activity seems to be organ-specific and possibly related to local metabolic and/or catabolic needs of the tissue at a specific point during organogenesis (54). Since the lung is a major source of 15-hydroxyprosta-glandin dehydrogenase, changes in activity during gestation could be important in relation to pulmonary maturation.

In addition, since the lung is a major site for catabolism of circulating prosta-glandins (55), catabolic activity could be important in regulating the levels of circulating prostaglandins, especially at birth (at which time there is a remarkable increase in pulmonary blood flow) and postnatally. Thus, abnormalities in fetal pulmonary PGDH activity may cause abnormalities in those cardiovascular changes (though to be controlled by prostaglandins) which take place at birth (e.g., closure of the ductus arteriosus). For these reasons, it was considered important to delineate the changes which take place in the activity of this enzyme during fetal and neonatal development in the lamb.

The activity of 15-OH prostaglandin dehydrogenase (PGDH) was measured by Skidgel in fetal and newborn lamb lungs at different stages of development (62). The assay followed the conversion of $[1-^{14}C]$-PGE$_2$ to its metabolite $[1-^{14}C]$-15 keto PGE$_2$ which was detected and quantified by thin layer radiochromatography. In the presence of 4 nM NAD$^+$ (a required co-factor) and 10 nM/ml PGE$_2$ the reaction was linear for 40 min at 24°C. Pulmonary prostaglandin dehydrogenase activity was found to vary greatly with fetal and newborn age (Fig. 11). At early gestational ages (115 to 130 days) PGDH activity was high, decreasing to one-third the activity at late gestation (143 to 146 days) and to one-twentieth the activity at term (6 hr newborn). After birth there was a dramatic rise in activity, reaching the same levels seen in the early gestational fetus by 2 days postpartum. Control experiments showed the low PGDH activity at term to be due to a lack of enzyme, and not due to endogenous inhibitors or utilization of NAD$^+$ by another pathway. The results of these studies indicate that PGDH, with its rapid turnover rate of 45 to 75 min, may be quickly synthetized or degraded in response to metabolic changes in an organ.

Pulmonary prostaglandins could certainly play a role in the cardiocirculatory changes which take place at birth. The low levels of PGDH at term are compatible with the hypothesis that these low levels are required to allow significant amounts of prostaglandins to be released into the circulation at birth which, in turn, cause changes to take place in the cardiovascular system. The pronounced increase in

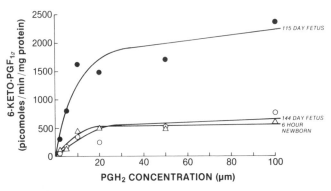

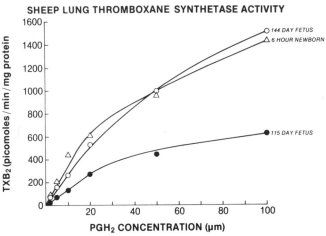

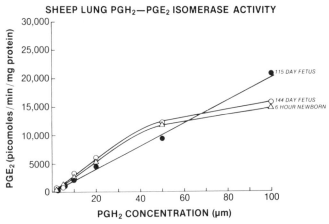

FIG. 9. Each panel shows the results of the effect of increasing PGH$_2$ concentrations on the initial rate of synthesis of PGI$_2$, TXB$_2$, and PGE$_2$ in fetal and newborn lamb lung homogenates.

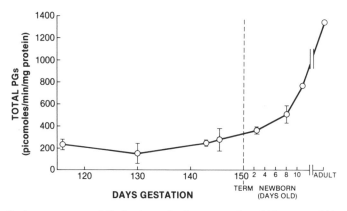

FIG. 10. Cyclooxygenase activity is shown by the conversion of 30 nM arachidonic acid to prostaglandins in fetal, newborn, and adult sheep lung microsomes.

TABLE 3. *Relative amounts of prostaglandins synthesized from arachidonic acid[a]*

Age group[b]	N	6-keto-PGF$_{1\alpha}$	PGF$_{2\alpha}$	PGs synthesized[c] TXB$_2$	PGE$_2$	Total
116 day fetus	2	46 ± 3	56 ± 11	39 ± 5	91 ± 31	232 ± 49
130 day fetus	2	33 ± 42	29 ± 8	37 ± 18	51 ± 25	151 ± 92
143 day fetus	5	38 ± 11	34 ± 3	43 ± 4	125 ± 12	246 ± 12
145 day fetus	3	57 ± 38	61 ± 20	72 ± 28	91 ± 21	280 ± 103
2 day-old newborn	4	59 ± 5	62 ± 12	56 ± 4	185 ± 18	362 ± 30
6 day-old newborn	2	73 ± 13	53 ± 15	86 ± 13	298 ± 39	510 ± 80
11 day-old newborn	1	104	95	100	470	769
Adult	1	382	158	251	556	1347

[a]Sheep lung microsomes (150 μg protein) were incubated in the presence of 1 mM GSH and 30 μM [1-^{14}C]-arachidonic acid under conditions described in Methods.
[b]Age groups: 116 Day = 115 day and 117 day, 130 day = 130 day (2), 143 day = 143 day (2) and 144 day (3), 145 day = 145 day (2) and 146 day, 2 day newborn = 6 hr newborn, 1 day newborn, 2 day newborn and 4 day newborn, 6 day-old newborn = 5 day and 7 day newborns, 11 day-old newborn = 11 day newborn, Adult = pregnant ewe.
[c]Results expressed as the mean ± SEM (pmoles/min/mg protein).

PGDH activity shortly after birth could be required to decrease prostaglandin levels and allow transition to the adult cardiovascular pattern, or could be an adaptation to the increase in pulmonary cyclo-oxygenase activity which is seen at that same time.

CONSIDERATIONS CONCERNING THE CONTROL OF THE DUCTUS ARTERIOSUS CIRCULATION

Ductus Arteriosus Patency

For many years it was assumed that patency of the fetal ductus arteriosus was passive and related to hemodynamic factors *in utero*. It is now quite clear that

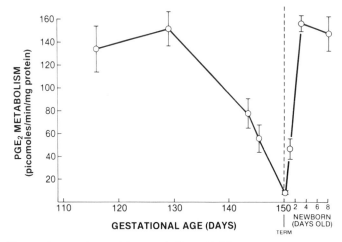

FIG. 11. The results are shown of the metabolism of PGE₂ (PGDH activity) by homogenates of fetal and newborn lamb lungs of various ages.

ductal patency is an active condition related to endogenous synthesis of a vasodilator prostaglandin, PGI_2. It is also likely that circulating PGE_2 acts in fetal life as a hormone since we (30) and others (7) have shown that high levels of PGE_2 exist in the fetus, in contrast to the newborn or adult. The high *in utero* PGE_2 levels may result from many factors, one of the more important of which is likely to be the minor role played by the lung of the fetus as a site of PGE_2 degradation, since *in utero* only a small fraction of the total cardiac output traverses the lung.

The data for the role of endogenous prostaglandins in maintaining ductal patency *in utero* are quite interesting. PGI_2 has been found by us, (28,31) and others (53,57) to be the major prostaglandin synthesized by the ductus arteriosus from fetal lambs and calves. This has led to the speculation that the production of intramural PGI_2 is responsible for ductal patency *in utero*. Coceani et al. (22) have disagreed with this speculation by virtue of their findings and the findings of Clyman et al. (11) that PGI_2 is three orders of magnitude less active than PGE_2 in causing relaxation of isolated ductal strips studied in a myograph. These workers hypothesize that endogenous synthesis of PGE_2 is responsible for maintaining ductal patency. However, other investigators have not shown the ductus to be capable of enzymatically synthesizing PGE_2. In our own laboratory experience, using ductal homogenates or microsomes, the evidence suggested that the ductus cannot enzymatically convert PGH_2 to PGE_2. If PGE_2 is to have any role in the maintenance of ductal patency, it must come from a source other than the ductus arteriosus.

It can be argued that *in vitro* studies showing the relative inactivity of PGI_2 in relaxing the ductus were not truly physiological, since ductal strips or rings were employed. However, in our own *in vivo* experiments, PGI_2 also was less potent in relaxing the ductus arteriosus when compared to PGE_2. Although the issue cannot be resolved at present, one important possibility that may help explain ductal patency is that the ductus may have an increased ability to synthesize hydroperoxy fatty acids in comparison to other blood vessels.

Preliminary data are consistent with the possibility that the ductus arteriosus contains functional lipoxygenase(s) (58), and Skidgel's studies (62) suggested that arachidonic acid could be converted by ductus tissue, via a lipoxygenase enzyme, to hydroperoxy and hydroxy fatty acids. The extreme sensitivity of prostacyclin synthase to inhibition by hydroperoxy fatty acids has been well documented (34,47). In addition, it is known that when both the cyclo-oxygenase and lipoxygenase enzymes are present, inhibition of cyclo-oxygenase leads to a substantial increase in the products of the lipoxygenase pathway (35).

Even if subsequent studies don't show the ductus to selectively produce greater quantities of hydroxy fatty acids than other blood vessels, the ductus would be expected to be more sensitive to hydroperoxy fatty acids, since we and others have shown that the ductus possesses significantly lower prostacyclin synthase activity than other arteries. Thus, exposure to similar concentrations of hydroperoxy fatty acids would be expected to more profoundly affect ductus prostacyclin synthase activity. Whether this is an important mechanism for ductus arteriosus closure at birth is conjectural, although the physiological changes which take place at birth (e.g., increased oxygen tension, increased membrane pertubation leading to arachidonic acid release, etc.) would be expected to increase the formation of hydroperoxy fatty acids in the ductus itself, and possibly from other sources such as platelets or the lung. Under these circumstances, ductal prostacyclin synthesis would decrease leading either to constriction directly, or to an enhancement of the sensitivity of the ductus to other constrictor agents such as oxygen or thromboxanes. Of course, this is a highly speculative hypothesis that can only be substantiated in the future by a comprehensive characterization of the lipoxygenase pathway(s) in the ductus and other tissues.

Ductus Arteriosus Constriction

Current theories of ductal closure relate to prostaglandins and the action of oxygen (12,22). One schema for ductal closure holds that oxygen promotes the conversion of arachidonic acid to $PGF_{2\alpha}$, which then causes contraction of ductus arteriosus smooth muscle (64). This theory has not been confirmed by *in vitro* (20) or the current *in vivo* studies of the ductus arteriosus, or by biochemical analyses.

An alternative hypothesis suggests that ductal closure may result from an oxygen-related decrease in the sensitivity of the ductus arteriosus to endogenously produced PGE_2 (15). Initial reports suggested that PGE_1 and PGE_2 caused relaxation of the lamb ductus arteriosus *in vitro* in low, but not elevated, oxygen tensions (15). However, more recent laboratory studies (12), and the observations of the clinical administration of PGE_1 to hypoxemia babies (37,49,50) suggest that prostaglandins *in vivo* relax the ductus arteriosus, even in the elevated oxygen tensions of postnatal life.

The data generated by our own laboratory experiences suggests that a *positive vasoconstrictor* process is necessary for ductal closure. We have proposed that the constriction may only be evidenced when PGI_2 formation within the ductus, and/or circulating PGE_2 levels (PGE_2 derived from the lung or placenta or other organs) are reduced or inhibited (27). Our results indicate that formation of significant amounts of TXA_2 within the ductus arteriosus (or any of the other vessels examined) is highly unlikely. A more likely source of TXA_2 *in vivo* is the lung. Although Coceani and his associates (18) could not demonstrate an effect of their TXA_2 generating system on *in vitro* ductal strips, it is quite possible that their experimental methods may have precluded seeing such an action.

There is provocative evidence that prostaglandins synthesized and released by the lung may play a role in the transitional circulatory alterations that occur at the time of birth. We and others (54) have shown that prostaglandin dehydrogenase activity in the sheep lung decreases to very low levels at term. Since the lung is a major site for metabolism of circulating prostaglandins, a decrease in their metabolism at birth could correlate with an increased role for circulating prostaglandins at birth, possibly of pulmonary origin. The rapid increase in lung PGDH activity seen shortly after birth (6) would suggest that this role for circulating prostaglandins may be restricted specifically to the time of birth.

The onset of pulmonary ventilation at birth is the physiological event most closely associated with functional closure of the ductus and the other birth related changes in the fetal circulation. The onset of respiration at birth could also be a potent stimulus for the release of prostaglandins from the lung. *In utero* the lung is exposed to relatively low levels of oxygen, low blood flow, and little mechanical trauma, i.e., no significant lung expansion or deflation. At birth, high levels of oxygen, a markedly increased magnitude of pulmonary blood flow, and expansion of lungs (known to be a potent stimulus for arachidonic acid release and PG synthesis and release (23)) could all contribute to a potential outpouring of prostaglandins from the lung. If this is important in causing the ductus arteriosus to close, then the biosynthetic capacity of the lung to make various types of prostaglandins may be important in determining this cardiocirculatory change. Indeed, our laboratory results show that there is a major developmental shift in the lung's ability to synthesize certain types of prostaglandins. At early fetal ages the lung was shown to possess an increased ability to synthesize PGI_2 and a decreased ability to synthesize thromboxane when compared to the mature fetus. This was due most likely to two factors: (1) a decrease in the V_{max} of thromboxane synthase at early fetal ages and an increase in the V_{max} of prostacyclin synthase and (2) increased levels of endogenous glutathione at early fetal ages. Thromboxane synthase activity increased 5- to 6-fold by term; the enhanced thromboxane synthetizing ability of the lung was even more pronounced in the 6 hr newborn lamb lung.

Since TXA_2 is considered a highly potent vasoconstrictor (59), it is tempting to speculate that pulmonary production of TXA_2 at birth is a contributing factor to closure of the ductus at that time. In this regard, it should be recognized that delivery of pulmonary prostaglandins to the ductus arteriosus at birth can be expected to occur via two pathways. With the onset of pulmonary ventilation and increased pulmonary blood flow, essentially all vasovasorum flow would be derived from the pulmonary perfusate. In addition, blood entering the lumen of the ductus would be derived for the first time from the pulmonary circulation, as the direction of ductal shunting reverses from the normal *in utero* right-to-left direction to a left-to-right pattern after the onset of pulmonary ventilation.

If our thromboxane hypothesis is to have any validity there are at least three arguments to which we must respond. First, it is known that TXA_2 is extremely unstable with a half-life of only 30 sec in buffer, putting in doubt its ability to act as a circulating hormone. However, in the presence of plasma proteins the stability of TXA_2 is greatly enhanced, extending its half-life to four min—long enough to have systemic effects (59,63). Also, if TXA_2 plays a role in closure of the ductus arteriosus, why don't other blood vessels constrict? It is clear that PGE_2 is the major prostaglandin produced by the lung at all gestational ages, with significant amounts of PGI_2 also being produced. Since these are both vasodilators their release from the lung at birth could be expected to antagonize the actions of TXA_2 on most vascular smooth muscle. The ductus would be expected to be more responsive than most blood vessels to TXA_2 because of its greater smooth muscle mass compared to other blood vessels, its sensitivity to direct constriction by oxygen, and because of its lower endogenous prostacyclin synthase activity. Third, if TXA_2 is released from the lungs in significant quantities why isn't there a massive aggregation of platelets? The answer probably resides in two factors: (1) along with release of TXA_2 there would probably be an almost equal release of PGI_2, which is well known to totally inhibit platelet aggregation (34), and (2) fetal and neonatal platelets appear to be much less responsive than adult platelets in their aggregatory response to many aggregating agents (59,63).

If TXA_2 is important for closure of the ductus arteriosus, it is also possible that patency of the ductus arteriosus in preterm neonates may be related to the relative inability of their immature lungs to synthesize thromboxanes. Hence, the onset of pulmonary ventilation in these preterm babies may not cause the normal magnitude of release of TXA_2, thus allowing the ductus to remain open. Ductus arteriosus patency in the preterm infant does appear to be coupled with developmental processes since those neonatal disorders most often associated with ductal patency are also disorders of maturation, i.e., prematurity, respiratory distress syndrome. Also, it is of interest to consider that corticosteroids, which promote *in utero* lung maturation, may also result in a lesser incidence of patent ductus arteriosus in the premature infant, and may promote a more mature ductal constrictor response (13,46).

ACKNOWLEDGMENTS

Supported by US Public Health Grant HL 25476 and HL06003 from the National Heart, Blood and Lung Institute. Drs. Benson and Zednikova supported by Los Angeles Heart Association Grants LA 650F2-1 and LA 669F2-1, respectively.

REFERENCES

1. Änggård, E., and Samuelsson, B. (1964): Prostaglandins and related factors 28. Metabolism of prostaglandin E_1 in Guinea pig lung: The structures of two metabolites. *J. Biol. Chem.*, 239:4097–4102.

2. Änggård, E., Larsson, C., and Samuelsson, B. (1971): The distribution of 15-hydroxy prostaglandin dehydrogenase and prostaglandin-13-reductase in tissues of the swine. *Acta Physiol. Scand.*, 81:396–404.
3. Aronson, S., Gennser, G., Owman, C., et al. (1970): Innervation and contractile response of the human ductus arteriosus. *Eur. J. Pharmacol.*, 11:178–186.
4. Blackwell, G. J., Flower, R. J., and Vane, J. R. (1975): Rapid reduction of PG 15-hydroxy-dehydroxygenase activity after treatment with protein synthesis inhibitors. *Br. J. Pharmacol.*, 55:233–238.
5. Boreus, L. O., Malmfors, T., McMurphy, D. M., et al. (1969): Demonstration of adrenergic receptor function and innervation in the ductus arteriosus of the fetal lamb. *Acta Physiol. Scand.*, 77:316–321.
6. Bustos, R., Ballego, G., Giussi, G., Rosas, R., and Isa, J. C. (1978): Inhibition of fetal lung maturation by indomethacin in pregnant rabbits. *J. Perinat. Med.*, 6:240–245.
7. Challis, J. R. G., Dilley, S. R., Robinson, J. S., et al. (1976): Prostaglandins in the circulation of the fetal lamb. *Prostaglandins*, 11:1041–1052.
8. Clyman, R. I., Heymann, M. A., and Rudolph, A. M. (1977): Ductus arteriosus responses to prostaglandin E_1 at high and low oxygen concentrations. *Prostaglandins*, 13:219–223.
9. Clyman, R. I., and Rudolph, A. M. (1978): Patent ductus arteriosus: A new light on an old problem. *Pediatr. Res.*, 12:92–94.
10. Clyman, R. I., Mauray, F., Heymann, M. A., et al. (1978): Ductus arteriosus: developmental response to oxygen and indomethacin. *Prostaglandins*, 15:923–998.
11. Clyman, R. I., Mauray, F., Roman, C., et al. (1978): PGE_2 is a more potent vasodilator of the lamb ductus arteriosus than is either PGI_2 or 6-keto-$PGF_{1\alpha}$. *Prostaglandins*, 16:259–264.
12. Clyman, R. I. (1980): Ontogeny of the ductus arteriosus response to prostaglandins and inhibitors of their synthesis. *Semin. Perinatol.*, 4:115–124.
13. Clyman, R. I., Ballard, P. L., Sniderman, S., Ballard, R., Roth, R., Heymann, M. A., and Granberg, J. P. (1980): Prenatal administration of betamethasone for prevention of patent ductus arteriosus. American Academy of Pediatrics. (Abstract) pg. 9.
14. Coceani, F., and Olley, P. M. (1973): The response of the ductus arteriosus to prostaglandins. *Can. J. Physiol. Pharmacol.*, 51:220–225.
15. Coceani, F., Olley, P. M., and Bodach, E. (1975): Lamb ductus arteriosus: Effect of prostaglandin synthesis inhibitors on the muscle tone and the response to prostaglandin E_2. *Prostaglandins*, 9:299–308.
16. Coceani, F., Bishai, I., White, E., et al. (1978): Actions of prostaglandins, endoperoxides and thromboxanes on the lamb ductus arterious. *Am. J. Physiol.*, 234:H117–122.
17. Coceani, F., Bodach, E., White, E., et al. (1978): Prostaglandin I_2 is less relaxant than prostaglandin E_2 on the lamb ductus arteriosus. *Prostaglandins*, 15:551–556.
18. Coceani, F., Bishai, I., Bodach, E., et al. (1978): On the evidence implicating PGE_2 rather than prostacyclin in the patency of the fetal ductus arteriosus, In: *Prostacyclin*, edited by J. R. Vane, and S. Bergstrom, pp. 247–252. New York, Raven Press.
19. Coceani, F., Bodach, E., White, E., et al. (1978): Prostaglandin I_2 is less relaxant than prostaglandin E_2 on the lamb ductus arteriosus. *Prostaglandins*, 15:551–556.
20. Coceani, F., Olley, P. M., Bishai, E., et al. (1978): Significance of the prostaglandin system to the control of muscle tone of the ductus arteriosus, In: *Advances in Prostaglandin and Thromboxane Research*, Vol. 4, edited by F. Coceani and P. M. Olley, pp. 325–333. New York, Raven Press.
21. Coceani, F. Bodach, E. Dumbrille, A. et al. (1979): Effect of PGE_2 and PGI_2 on the ductus arteriosus from immature fetal lambs. Fourth International Prostaglandin Conference, Washington, D.C. (Abstract) p. 21.
22. Coceani, F., and Olley, P. M. (1980): Role of prostaglandins, prostacyclin and thromboxanes in the control of prenatal patency and postnatal closure of the ductus arteriosus. *Semin. Perinatol.*, 4:109–113.
23. Edmonds, J. R., Berry, E., and Wyllie, J. H. (1969): Release of prostaglandins caused by distention of the lungs. *Br. J. Surg.*, 56:622–623.
24. Fay, F. (1971): Guinea pig ductus arteriosus. I. Cellular and metabolic basis for oxygen sensitivity. *Am. J. Physiol.*, 221:470–479.
25. Friedman, W. F. (1972): The intrinsic physiological properties of the developing heart. *Prog. Cardiovasc. Dis.*, 15:87.
26. Friedman, W. F., Hirschklau, M. J., Printz, M. P. et al. (1976): Pharmacologic closure of the patent ductus arteriosus in the preterm infant. *N. Engl. J. Med.*, 295:526–529.

27. Friedman, W. F., Molony, D. A. and Kirkpatrick, S. E. (1978): Prostaglandins: Physiological and clinical correlations, In: *Advances in Pediatrics*, Vol. 25, edited by L. Barnes, pp. 151–204. Chicago, Yearbook.
28. Friedman, W. F. (1978): Studies of the response of the ductus arteriosus. In: *The Ductus Arteriosus*, edited by M. A. Heymann, and A. M. Rudolph, pp. 35–43. Proceedings of the Seventy-fifth Ross Conference on Pediatric Research. Ross Laboratories, Columbus.
29. Friedman, W. F. (1978): Prostaglandins and the patent ductus arteriosus. Proceedings of the 7th International Congress of Pharmacology. In: *Advances in Pharmacology & Therapeutics*, Vol. 8, Drug-Action Modification—Comparative Pharmacology, edited by G. Olive. Pergamon Press, Oxford, England.
30. Friedman, W. F., Printz, M. P., and Kirkpatrick, S. E. (1978): Blockers of prostaglandin synthesis: a novel therapy in the management of the premature infant with patent ductus arteriosus, In: *Advances in Prostaglandin and Thromboxane Research*, Vol. 4, edited by F. Coceani, and P. M. Olley, pp. 373–381. New York, Raven Press.
31. Friedman, W. F., Fitzpatrick, K. M., Merritt, T. A., and Feldman, B. H. (1978): The patent ductus arteriosus. *Clin. Perinatol.*, 5:411–436.
32. Friedman, W. F., Kurlinski, J., Jacob, J., et al. (1980): The inhibition of prostaglandin and prostacyclin synthetase in the clinical management of patent ductus arteriosus. *Semin. Perinatol.*, 4:125–133.
33. Greenberg, S., Kadowitz, P. J., Long, J. P., and Wilson, W. R. (1976): Studies on the nature of a prostaglandin receptor in canine and rabbit vascular smooth muscle. *Circ. Res.*, 39:66.
34. Gryglewski, R. J., Bunting, S., Moncada, S., et al. (1976): Arterial walls are protected against deposition of platelet thrombi by a substance (prostaglandin X) which they make from prostaglandin endoperoxides. *Prostaglandins*, 12:685–713.
35. Hamberg, M., and Samuelsson, B. (1974): Prostaglandin endoperoxides. Novel transformation of arachidonic acid in human platelets. *Proc. Nat. Acad. Sci. USA*, 71:3400–3404.
36. Heymann, M. A., and Rudolph, A. M. (1976): Effect of acetylsalicylic acid on the ductus arteriosus and circulation in fetal lambs *in utero*. *Circ. Res.*, 38:418–422.
37. Heymann, M. A., and Rudolph, A. M. (1978): Effects of prostaglandins and blockers of prostaglandin synthesis on the ductus arteriosus: Animal and human studies, In: *Advances in Prostaglandin and Thromboxane Research*, Vol. 4, edited by F. Coceani, and P. M. Olley, pp. 363–372. New York, Raven Press.
38. Heymann, M. A., Berman, W., Jr., Rudolph, A. M., et al. (1979): Dilatation of the ductus arteriosus by prostaglandin E_1 in aortic arch abnormalities. *Circulation*, 59:169–173.
39. Kennedy, J. A., and Clark, S. L. (1941): Observations on the ductus arteriosus of the Guinea pig in relation to its method of closure. *Anat. Rec.*, 37:349–355.
40. Kirkpatrick, S. E., Pitlick, P. T., Friedman, W. F., et al. (1976): The importance of the Frank-Starling relationship as a determinant of fetal cardiac output. *Am. J. Physiol.*, 231:495–501.
41. Kovalcik, V. (1963): The response of the isolated ductus arteriosus to oxygen and anoxia. *J. Physiol. (Lond.)*, 169:185–197.
42. Kuehl, F. A. (1974): Prostaglandins, cyclic nucleotides and cell function. *Prostaglandins*, 5:325–330.
43. Marnett, L. J., Wlodawer, P., and Samuelsson, B. (1975): Co-oxygenation of organic substrates by the prostaglandin synthetase of sheep vesicular gland. *J. Biol. Chem.*, 250:8510–8517.
44. McMurphy, D. M. Heymann, M. A., Rudolph, A. M., et al. (1972): Developmental changes in constriction of the ductus arteriosus: Responses to oxygen and vasoactive agents in the isolated ductus arteriosus of the fetal lamb. *Pediatr. Res.*, 6:231–238.
45. Miyamoto, T., Ogino, M., Yamamoto, S., and Hayaishi, O. (1976): Purification of prostaglandin endoperoxide synthetase from bovine vesicular gland microsomes. *J. Biol. Chem.*, 251:2629–2636.
46. Momma, K., Nishihara, S., Ota, Y., and Takao, A. (1980): Constriction of the fetal ductus arteriosus by glucocorticoid hormones. World Congress of Pediatric Cardiology (Abstract), pg. 64.
47. Moncada, S., Gryglewski, R. J., Bunting, S., and Vane, J. R. (1976): A lipid peroxide inhibits the enzyme in blood vessel microsomes that generates from prostaglandin endoperoxides the substance which prevents platelet aggregation. *Prostaglandins*, 12:715–737.
48. Moncada, S., Bunting, S., Mullane, K., Thorogood, P. and, Vane, J. R. (1977): Imidazole: a selective inhibitor of thromboxane synthetase. *Prostaglandins*, 13:611–615.

49. Olley, P. M., Coceani, F., and Bodach, E. (1976): E type prostaglandins: a new emergency therapy for certain cyanotic heart malformations. *Circulation*, 53:728–731.

50. Olley, P. M., Coceani, F., and Rowe, R. D. (1978): The role of prostaglandin E_1 and E_2 in the management of neonatal heart disease, In: *Advances in Prostaglandin and Thromboxane Research*, Vol. 4, edited by F. Coceani, and P. M. Olley, pp. 325–333. New York, Raven Press.

51. Pace-Asciak, C., and Miller, D. (1973): Prostaglandins during development. *Prostaglandins*, 4:351–363.

52. Pace-Asciak, C. R. (1977): Prostaglandin biosynthesis and metabolism in the developing fetal sheep lung. *Prostaglandins*, 13:649–660.

53. Pace-Asciak, C. R., and Rangaraj, G. (1977): The 6 keto prostaglandin $F_{1\alpha}$ pathway in the lamb ductus arteriosus. *Biochem. Biophys. Acta*, 486:583–585.

54. Pace-Asciak, C. R. (1978): Prostaglandin biosynthesis and catabolism in several organs of developing fetal and neonatal animals. In: *Advances in Prostaglandin and Thromboxane Research*, Vol. 4, edited by F. Coceani and P. M. Olley, pp. 45–59. Raven Press, New York.

55. Piper, P. J., Vane, J. R., and Wyllie, J. H. (1970): Inactivation of prostaglandins by the lungs. *Nature*, 225:600–604.

56. Piper, P., and Vane, J. (1971): The release of prostaglandins from lung and other tissues. *Ann. N.Y. Acad. Sci.*, 180:363–385.

57. Powell, W. S., and Solomon, S. (1977): Formation of 6-oxoprostaglandin $F_{1\alpha}$ by arteries of the fetal calf. *Biochem. Biophys. Res. Commun.*, 75:815–822.

58. Powell, W. S., and Solomon, S. (1978): Biosynthesis of prostaglandins and thromboxanes in fetal tissues, In: *Advances in Prostaglandin and Thromboxane Research*, Vol. 4, edited by F. Coceani, and P. M. Olley, pp. 61–74. New York, Raven Press.

59. Samuelsson, B., Folco, G., Granstrom, E., Kindahl, H., and Malmsten, C. (1978): Prostaglandins and thromboxanes: Biochemical and physiological considerations, In: *Advances in Prostaglandin and Thromboxane Research*, Vol. 4, edited by F., Coceani, and P. M. Olley, pp. 1–25. Raven Press, New York.

60. Sharpe, G. L., Larsson, K. S., and Thalme, B. (1975): Studies on the closure of the ductus arteriosus. XII: *In utero* effects of indomethacin and sodium salicylate in rats and rabbits. *Prostaglandins*, 9:585–596.

61. Sharpe, G. L., and Larsson, K. S. (1975): Studies on the closure of the ductus arteriosus. X. *In vivo* effects of prostaglandins. *Prostaglandins*, 9:703–709.

62. Skidgel, R. A. (1979): Prostaglandin biosynthesis and catabolism in fetal and neonatal tissues. Doctoral dissertation, Univ. of Calif., San Diego, pp. 1–273.

63. Smith, J. B., Ingerman, C., and Sliver, M. J. (1976): Persistence of thromboxane A_2-like material and platelet release-inducing activity in plasma. *J. Clin. Invest.*, 58:1119–1122.

64. Starling, M. B., and Elliott, R. B. (1974): The effects of prostaglandins, prostaglandin inhibitors, and oxygen on the closure of the ductus arteriosus, pulmonary arteries, and umbilical vessels *in vitro*. *Prostaglandins*, 8:187–203.

65. Starling, M. B., Neutze, J. M., Elliott, R. L., et al. (1977): Studies on the effects of prostaglandins E_1, E_2, A_1, and A_2 on the ductus arteriosus of swine *in vivo*. *Prostaglandins*, 12:355–361.

66. Terragno, N. A., Mc Giff, J. C., and Smigel, M. (1978): Patterns of prostaglandin: Production in the bovine fetal and maternal vasculature. *Prostaglandins*, 16:846–854.

Prostaglandins and the Cardiovascular System,
edited by John A. Oates. Raven Press,
New York © 1982.

Participation of Prostaglandins in the Regulation of Peripheral Vascular Resistance

Åke Wennmalm

Department of Clinical Physiology, Huddinge University Hospital, Huddinge, Sweden

The concept of a role for cardiovascular prostaglandins (PG) in the regulation of blood pressure and peripheral vascular resistance has led to several investigations. Although most investigators appear somewhat doubtful as to whether PGs play a major role in these respects under normal conditions, data favoring a role for certain PG in pathophysiological states are accumulating, as will be evident from this chapter. The regulation of vascular resistance is a complex interplay between central, local, and humoral factors. Endogenously formed PG might theoretically act at a number of levels in this regulatory process. A short overview follows of currently accepted principles in the control of systemic vascular resistance.

The main determinants of systemic vascular resistance are the precapillary resistance vessels (small arteries and arterioles), the average B.P. drop in this vascular section being about 60 mmHg under resting conditions. The resistance (degree of contraction) in these vessels is a function of the basal myogenic tone in their walls together with superimposed local metabolic and extrinsic neurogenic and hormonal factors. The intrinsic myogenic tone is generated by the pacemaker activity in the noncontinuous smooth muscle layer in the precapillary sphincters and the metarterioles. In such vessels an irregular vasomotion is operating, due to the unsynchronized contraction pattern in the individual single-unit smooth muscle cells. These muscle cells are stretch sensitive, increasing their spontaneous activity in response to distension. However, a rise in arterial pressure does not evoke a vicious positive feedback vasoconstriction, probably due to the continuous production of vasodilator metabolites in the perfused tissue.

The locally generated vascular tone may, therefore, be seen as a balance between vasoconstricting and vasodilating forces. This balance probably meets the local demands for perfusion of the tissue and may be regarded as an autoregulation of capillary flow. An increase in arterial pressure augments the myogenic tone mechanically, due to the increased transmural pressure. The increased B.P. also facilitates the flow, thereby washing out locally formed metabolites and elevating tissue pO_2 more efficiently. The increased B.P. gives rise to two vasoconstrictor mechanisms, one mechanical and one chemical, which cooperate to limit the flow and restore the capillary pressure. A fall in B.P. activates the opposite mechanisms.

The B.P. stretch influence on the myogenic tone decreases and the lowered flow attenuates the washout of metabolites. Both factors tend to relax the vascular tone, thereby promoting a reestablishment of the blood flow. The ultimate decrease in blood pressure is elicited by the complete abolition of flow that follows arterial occlusion.

The absence of transmural pressure in this case is combined with a progressive accumulation of vasodilator metabolites and an impoverishment of tissue oxygen, all of which lead to a relaxation of vascular smooth muscle that approaches totality. If the B.P. is reestablished, i.e., the arterial occlusion is released, a marked but brief increase in blood flow develops. This increase, generally referred to as reactive hyperemia, disappears when the transmural pressure in the vessels normalizes and the accumulated metabolites are washed out.

The basal vascular tone, originating from the mechanisms described, varies considerably between tissues. Therefore, in organs like the brain and kidney, which steadily operate at a more or less constant metabolic level, the basal vascular tone is very low, and consequently the vasodilator capacity is limited. In contrast, tissues like skeletal muscle, myocardium, and salivary glands have a high basal vascular tone, implying a considerable capacity to increase the perfusion rate (Fig. 1).

The chemical principles that favor a relaxation of myogenic tone comprise not only vasodilator metabolites but also the concentrations of oxygen, carbon dioxide, and hydrogen ions in the blood. A fall in arterial pO_2, as well as a rise in pCO_2 and H^+ concentrations, will cause vasodilation. Of the other products of tissue metabolism which are known to have vasodilator properties, most interest has been paid to lactate and adenosine. Further factors which have been suggested are a high potassium ion concentration, hyperosmolarity, and elevated concentration of inorganic phosphate. It appears likely that these factors' relative importance is tissue-

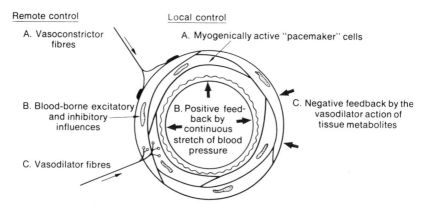

FIG. 1. Basic machinery of local vascular control: myogenic "pacemaker" activity, reinforced by the continuous stretch offered by the blood pressure, constitutes, via cell-to-cell excitation spread, the basal vascular tone, being steadily counteracted by the continuously produced tissue metabolites. Extrinsic excitatory and inhibitory factors, in the form of nervous and blood-borne influences modulate, and sometimes dominate, the local control system. (From B. Folkow and E. Neil, with permission.)

dependent. Thus, adenosine probably is very important in the regulation of coronary vascular resistance, and the local H^+ concentration plays a major role in the cerebral vessels. The possible contribution of locally formed PG to the regulation of peripheral resistance will be discussed later.

The most important neurogenic mechanism in the regulation of systemic vascular resistance is the sympathetic adrenergic vasoconstrictor system. Discharge in the adrenergic fibers to the resistance vessels leads to release of norepinephrine (NE) from the terminal fiber network that surrounds the outer layer of most types of vascular tissue. The NE activates α-adrenergic receptors in the smooth muscle cell membranes and the resultant smooth muscle contraction leads to vasoconstriction. Simplifying, the adrenergic vasoconstrictor effect can be seen physiologically as a function of five parameters: (a) the density of adrenergic fibers to the vessel; (b) the discharge rate in the fibers; (c) the amount of transmitter liberated per nerve impulse; (d) the active state of the adrenergic receptor; and (e) the amount of smooth muscle in the vessel wall.

The morphologically determined parameters, i.e., (a) and (e), may be characterized as follows. Skin vessels have a very dense vasoconstrictor fiber innervation, while other vascular regions like the coronary and cerebral vessels display a sparser network. Other regional circuits vary between these extremes. Besides these circuit differences, the consecutive vessels in a particular circuit differ in the number of fibers they receive, the essential resistance vessels (small arteries and metarterioles) usually having the richest supply. As one might expect, the thickness of the smooth muscle layer in the vessel wall corresponds closely to the density of the adrenergic innervation. The functional parameters, (b), (c), and (d), call for a few comments. The discharge rate in the sympathetic system is normally very low (1 to 4 Hz) and probably seldom exceeds 6 to 8 Hz. It is now generally accepted that the sympathetic discharge rate is not uniform but varies in a certain condition, between regions. The release of NE upon nerve discharge is probably a function of a basal amount-released-per-impulse rate, which agents like NE, adenosine, and PG modulate by coupling to specific receptors on the nerve terminals. On the other side of the synaptic cleft, the sensitivity of the α-adrenergic receptor is probably likewise modulated, to some extent by the same principles as presynaptically.

In addition to the sympatheic vasoconstrictor fibers, at least two families of vasodilator nerves have been described. Parasympathetic vasodilator nerves supply the salivary and some gastrointestinal glands and the external genitalia. It is unknown, however, whether the vasodilation which follows discharge in these fibers really is a consequence of the release of a transmitter substance that per se is smooth muscle relaxing and thereby serves as a vasodilator. At least in the salivary glands the vasodilation elicited by nerve discharge is a consequence of the gland's release of kallikrein, which converts plasma kininogen to smooth muscle relaxing kallidin. The other type of vasodilator fibers has been found in the skeletal muscle resistance vessels of some species, and is usually classified as sympathetic cholinergic. Such fibers have not yet been detected in primates and their physiological significance remains a question.

A number of humoral factors also have been attributed vasoregulatory function. The tendency is to minimize the importance of blood-borne principles in the normal regulation of peripheral resistance, and to look upon these compounds as emergency hormones, having significance only in pathophysiological states. Circulating adrenaline, liberated from the adrenal medulla, may, under conditions like heavy exercise, redistribute blood flow, besides having important metabolic functions. The resistance vessels in skeletal and cardiac muscle and liver have β-adrenergic receptors that respond to circulating adrenaline with relaxation. Thus adrenaline may redistribute blood flow from the kidneys and the gastrointestinal tract to the heart, working muscle, and liver. Another systemic vasoactive hormone that may also affect the overall vascular resistance is angiotensin, especially in certain states of kidney disease. The relation between adrenergic function, renin release, and conversion of angiotensinogen to angiotensin I is covered in a separate chapter in this volume and will not be treated further in this context. Other blood-borne compounds with vasoregulatory roles include the local hormones serotonin, histamin, and the kinins. There is increasing evidence that the latter compounds do not play any overall regulatory role in the cardiovascular system, but may reach significant concentrations due to local formation in pathological states, e.g., tissue damage or blood clotting.

From this simplified review of factors that may influence peripheral vascular resistance one can conclude that the distribution of cardiac output under resting conditions to a considerable extent is regulated locally. But the overall level of systemic B.P. that is required, at a given total peripheral resistance, to perfuse the tissues in accordance with their demands is regulated centrally. The aortic and carotid sinus baroreceptors play a key role here, but receptors in the heart, lungs, and venous circulation also converge towards the vasoregulatory center together with impulses from various cortical areas.

During physical activity, like exercise at various work loads, total systemic resistance is lowered markedly. The decrease comes mainly from a locally mediated relaxation of the resistance vessels in the working regions, neural and humoral factors playing a minor role under these circumstances. The decreased resistance results in an increased perfusion in the working circuit and more oxygen and substrate are delivered to the tissue. The facilitation of blood flow is further reinforced by a re-setting of the high-pressure circuit baroreceptors, allowing the mean systemic B.P. to be raised from a resting value of about 90 mmHg to a level between 100 and 120 mmHg, depending on the work load. The overall effect of these cardiovascular adjustments is a redistribution of flow that favors metabolically active regions by directing the increase in cardiac output towards them. In this connection, it should be remembered that although physical exercise is usually paralleled by increased activity in the sympathetic nervous system, the overall effect of exercise on the systemic resistance is not an increase (vasoconstriction) but rather a decrease (relaxation), due to locally regulated vasodilation.

PG AND MYOGENIC REGULATION

The early observation that PG of the E series have a hypotensive action stimulated a number of experiments to clarify the physiological role of these PG in the regulation of cardiovascular function. The distinction between pharmacological effect and the physiological function of PGs in tissues was not always maintained in these studies. With the discovery of prostacyclin, PGI_2, earlier called PGX (28,59), the role of endogenous PG in cardiovascular function was reevaluated. This important platelet anti-aggregatory prostanoid was early characterized as a vascular PG, based on its formation from arachidonate or PG endoperoxides in pig aortic microsomes.

That PGI_2 was not just one vascular PG, but rather *the* vascular PG, was established in various studies, both in intact tissues (16,40,60) and in isolated endothelial cells (56,96). It is now generally accepted that PGI_2 is quantitatively the most important PG produced in the systemic circulation, regardless of species and type of vessel. Generally the PGEs and prostacyclin bring about relaxation of vascular smooth muscle, leading to vasodilation in the intact vessel and lowered resistance in the organ. In contrast TxA_2, and also in many circuits $PGF_{2\alpha}$, induce contraction of vascular smooth muscle, leading to vasoconstriction and, in intact organs, an increased resistance. Many of the effects which PG and thromboxane (Tx) reportedly elicit in vascular tissue are of pharmacological interest only and the present account concentrates mainly on the effect of PGI_2.

Prostacyclin relaxes vascular strips from rabbit mesenteric and coeliac arteries, but has no effect on rabbit aorta (12). Human and bovine coronaries are relaxed by PGI_2 (65,77), as are coronary vessels from the cat (70), rat (50), rabbit (66), and guinea pig (84). In contrast, pig coronary arteries are contracted by PGI_2 (17) but appear to be the only exception. Also, in intact animals, lowered coronary resistance has been observed following administration of PGI_2 (5,18,21), even though the effect in such studies must have been counteracted by reflex compensatory mechanisms.

It is not clear whether these effects of exogenously applied PGI_2 in various vascular circuits reflect a vascular reaction that is physiologically significant. One way of evaluating the possible contribution of endogenous PGI_2 to the regulation of vascular tone is to study the effect of their withdrawal, to block the bioformation of PGs. Studies using this approach have yielded differing results, due at least in part to differences in technique. Kent et al. (46) reported an insignificant change in basal coronary flow in open-chest dogs following administration of indomethacin. Kaley's group failed to find any effect of indomethacin either on the resting arterioles' diameter in the isolated perfused rat cremaster muscle (57,58), or on vascular resistance in the constant rate blood-perfused gracilis muscle of anesthetized dogs (90). In some contrast, an increased vascular resistance at rest was observed in the denervated hind-leg of anesthetized dogs following indomethacin (41) and this was confirmed by other studies in a similar preparation (100). The observed differences are probably circumstantial. It is well known that PG bioformation in tissues is easily accelerated by mechanical, physical and chemical stimuli. In at least some of the studies the type of anesthesia, the extent of surgical trauma, and the degree of tissue hypoxia probably elevated the basal tissue production of PG and hence decreased the resting vascular tone.

The administration of indomethacin under such circumstances is obviously liable to elicit vascular reactions that do not reflect events in resting blood vessels. Other studies however, do not suffer from these technical pitfalls. In the human forearm the resting arterial blood flow was unaffected by therapeutical doses of indomethacin (47) or naproxen (20). It is of interest that in our laboratory human, resting calf blood flow fell slightly in response to indomethacin, during an unchanged forearm blood flow in the same subject (69). In view of the divergent results, it is too early to draw any definite conclusions concerning the contribution of endogenous PG to the regulation of basal vascular tone. But it does seem that such a contribution, if it occurs, is of limited magnitude. The final answer will have to await further studies under carefully controlled conditions.

From the possible role of endogenous PG in the maintenance of basal vascular tone we now turn to the physiologically more challenging significance of the prostanoids in the development of various types of hyperemia. Here the results are more consistent. The possible contribution of endogenous PG in functional (exercise-induced) or reactive (post-occlusive) hyperemia has been mainly investigated in cardiac and skeletal muscle. Kent et al. (46) observed in open-chest dogs that both indomethacin and meclofenamate reduced the vasodilator response to coronary arterial occlusion and hypoxia, and similar results were reported by Afonso et al. (2). However, it also was found that the hyperemic response to brief occlusions of the left coronary artery was unaffected in terms of the percentage repayment and peak increase as well as the duration of the hyperemia (25).

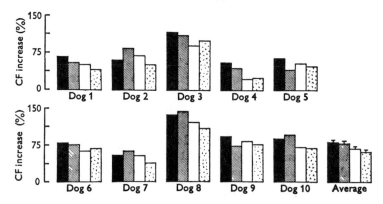

FIG. 2. Coronary vasodilator responses (expressed as percentage increases in coronary blood flow (CF) induced by hypoxia, before and 10, 30, and 60 min after indomethacin. Columns in the last block represent means ± SE of mean. At 10, 30, and 60 min after indomethacin coronary vasodilator responses to hypoxia were respectively −3.2% ($p < 0.5$), −16.5% ($p < 0.01$) and −23.1% ($p < 0.001$) less than the control one before indomethacin. Dogs no. 1, 2, and 7 received 8% oxygen in nitrogen and the remaining ones 5% oxygen in nitrogen. *Solid bar:* before indomethacin; *hatched bar:* 10 min after indomethacin; *white bar:* 30 min after indomethacin; *speckled bar:* 60 min. after indomethacin. From Afonso et al., ref. 2, with permission.

Similar data were reported by Hintze and Kaley (38), who found that while indomethacin or meclofenamate certainly decreased the peak dilation and volume of reactive hyperemia induced by brief coronary artery occlusions, they did not change the percentage flow debt repaid. These and other data appear to justify the conclusion that the role of coronary PG in the normal regulation of myocardial blood flow is negligible, while under conditions of more severe tissue hypoxia stimulation of cardiac PG biofor-mation may elicit a significantly improved myocardial perfusion.

Data favoring the concept of PG as local regulators of muscle blood flow also have been presented. In the denervated dog hindleg perfused with blood at a constant rate, indomethacin considerably attenuated the increase in vascular conductance that accompanies and follows muscular exercise (41). In a study on the regulation of human forearm blood flow performed in our laboratory, these data were supported in part. The forearm blood flow was recorded in the supine position in healthy subjects of both sexes, using venous occlusion plethysmography, during and after isometric forearm exercise (handgrip) and following dynamic forearm exercise (Fig. 3). The hyperemia which developed during and after isometric forearm work at a load of 15% of maximal strength was reduced after indomethacin to about 70% of control and the post-exercise hyperemia following dynamic work was diminished to about 60% (47). It should be stressed that isometric muscle work at more than 10% of maximal strength probably leads to a mechanical restriction of the local blood flow, so that this type of work from a circulatory point of view somewhat resembles arterial occlusion.

In a study on the constant-flow perfused gracilis muscle of anesthetized dogs, Weiner and coworkers (90) found that indomethacin significantly reduced the du-

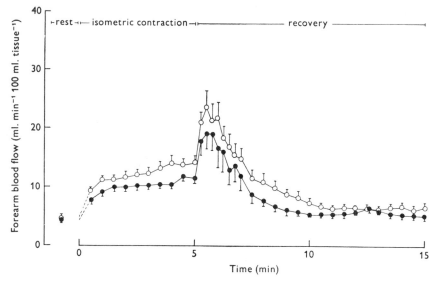

FIG. 3. Forearm blood flow at rest, during and after a sustained isometric contraction. Mean values and SE of mean for ten subjects before, *open circle*, and after indomethacin, *closed circle*. (From Kilbom and Wennmalm, ref. 47, with permission.)

ration of the vasodilation evoked by muscular contraction and in a similar series
the prolonged vasodilation after exercise was also diminished (63). However, other
data point to unaffected hyperemia in working muscle following PG synthesis
inhibition. Beaty and Donald (8) showed that steady-state exercise hyperemia of
canine hindlimb muscle was not reduced by meclofenamate or indomethacin and
others have reported no changes in canine muscle flow during electrically stimulated
exercise, both when constant flow (62) and free flow (100) was applied. In a recent
study in our laboratory, human leg blood flow, measured by a dye dilution technique,
was completely unchanged at three different intensities of leg exercise (69) (Fig.
4).

The most reasonable conclusion from all these studies, using different species,
muscle groups, and experimental conditions, is that no evidence at present favors
a role for local PG in exercise hyperemia. The picture is different for post-exercise
hyperemia and hyperemia in working muscle with limited blood flow (partial arterial
occlusion, constant flow technique, etc.). In these situations locally formed PG
may indeed be involved.

Least controversial is the issue of locally formed PG in reactive hyperemia. The
development of such hyperemia in the heart and its relation to PG synthesis inhibition
has been mentioned above. Reactive hyperemia probably does not constitute a
physiological reaction, but rather a mobilization of the tissue's maximal defense
against hypoxia. It is chiefly of interest because it uncovers vasoregulatory mechanisms which may be activated under pathophysiological conditions. A reduction
of reactive hyperemia following arterial occlusion has been found after PG synthesis
inhibition in rat, dog, and man. Messina and coworkers (57) reported that both
indomethacin and 5,8,11,14-eicosatetraynoic acid reduced the maximum increase
in diameter and duration of the vasodilator response following release of arterial
occlusion. The same group also found that indomethacin gave a diminished duration
of the vasodilation evoked by transient arterial occlusion in constant-flow perfused
gracilis muscle of anesthetized dogs. Studies in our laboratory yielded similar results
in man. The total forearm reactive hyperemia following 5 min of arterial occlusion
was reduced by 50 to 60% by indomethacin (47,69) and the corresponding figure

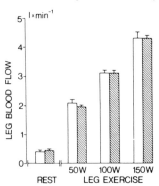

FIG. 4. Leg blood flow at rest and during dynamic
work. Mean values and SE of the mean for 6 subjects
before and after indomethacin. *White bar:* no drug;
hatched bar: indomethacin. (From Nowak and Wennmalm, ref. 69, with permission.)

in the calf (Fig. 5) was about 40% (69). The more unambiguous results for the contribution of locally formed PG in reactive compared to functional hyperemia suggest that the degree of substrate exhaustion in the tissue is pivotal. Kalsner (45) has shown that PG synthesis stimulation is clearly dependent on the local pO_2, and that an oxygen tension between 9 to 47 mmHg results in profound PG synthesis. It may be that tissue oxygen tension in working muscle under free-flow conditions never falls to a level at which PG formation accelerates significantly. Impoverishment of the tissue oxygen stores is obviously more complete under conditions of restricted or occluded blood flow and this fits well with the findings that reactive hyperemia is clearly dependent on an intact local PG formation.

PGs AND NEUROGENIC REGULATION

The neurogenic control of peripheral vascular resistance is maintained mainly via activity in the sympathetic adrenergic fibers on the systemic resistance vessels. Although vasodilator fibers do occur in some tissues and species, they are most probably of minor importance in the normal regulation of resistance. The central control of B.P. and hence peripheral resistance, is exercised by the so-called vasomotor center, a medullary complex of tonically active neurone pools, that exert a small excitatory drive on the resistance vessels via the vasoconstrictor fibers. In the vasomotor center, afferent activity from cardiovascular proprioceptors is integrated with cortico-hypothalamic influences and chemically mediated direct effects, yielding a final common vasoconstrictor discharge. The extent to which this afferent activity, central integration, and final efferent discharge are under the influence,

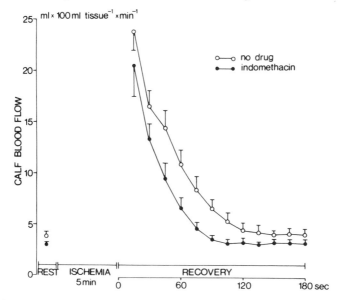

FIG. 5. Calf blood flow at rest and during the recovery period after 5 min arterial occlusion. Mean values and SE of the mean for 10 subjects before and after indomethacin. (From Nowak and Wennmalm, ref. 69, with permission.)

constant or transient, of locally or systemically formed PG is incompletely known. In a recent study in our laboratory we investigated whether inhibition of PG bio-formation in 12 healthy male and female volunteers could interfere with vasomotor regulation (95a).

The study included an orthostatic test, involving recording of heart rate and blood pressure at supine rest and during 8 min of unsupported standing, recording of the amplitude of respiratory sinus arrythmia during standardized breathing. It also recorded the amplitude of the heart rate lowering induced by external carotid stim-ulation (neck suction). All tests were performed before and after administration of indomethacin, 1 mg/kg B.W., rectally, 1 hr before the tests. As seen from Table 1, indomethacin in a therapeutical dose did not significantly affect the cardiovascular adjustment to standing up from supine position, as evidenced from the orthostatic test. The respiratory sinus arrythmia that probably is the result both of a direct intracardiac effect of atrial distension and of efferent vagal influence on the sinus node, was unaffected by the PG synthesis inhibitor. Finally, also evident from Table 1, neck suction, which distends the carotid sinus and mimics arterial hypertension, lowered the heart rate to the same extent before and after PG synthesis inhibition. These tests, which involve both afferent and efferent vasoregulatory pathways, both vagal and sympathetic fibers, and both extra- and intracardiac vasoregulatory mech-anisms, do not favor the concept of a significant role for PGs in the regulation of cardiovascular performance, apart from what will be presented in relation to their action in the sympathetic neuro-effector junction.

It is well known that PG of the E series inhibit the liberation of norepinephrine (NE) from discharging sympathetic neurons. This has been shown in various species and a number of preparations, and the reports have been reviewed repeatedly (32).

TABLE 1. *Effect of the PG synthesis inhibitor, indomethacin, on some clinically used tests of vasoregulatory function in healthy humans*

	Before indomethacin	After indomethacin
Orthostatic test		
Heart rate (beats/min)		
Basal	62	62
After standing 8 min	85	82
Syst./diast. blood pressure (mm Hg)		
Basal	110/75	105/65
After standing 8 min	110/70	120/75
Respiratory sinus arrythmia		
amplitude in beats/min	9.4	9.2
Carotid stimulation (heart rate lowering during neck suction)		
amplitude (beats/min)	11.4	9.2
Respiratory sinus arrythmia during carotid stimulation		
amplitude (beats/min)	1.5	0.5

Besides PG of the E series, it has been shown that prostacyclin interferes with transmitter liberation from sympathetic nerves. But these results are contradictory. In one study in our laboratory the interstitial effluent from isolated perfused hearts was found to contain a heat-labile platelet antiaggregatory product (probably PGI_2) that failed to inhibit adrenergic neurotransmission (93). In another series, PGI_2 was found to be about 700 times less efficient than PGE_2 in this respect (94). The lack of, or weak, effect of PGI_2 on NE release from sympathetic nerves observed in our laboratory was confirmed by Hedqvist (33) (Fig. 6), studying liberation of ^{3}H-NE in response to nerve stimulation from labelled perfused rabbit kidneys. There is also indirect evidence that PGI_2 does not inhibit NE release in vascular tissue from neonatal lambs (99). However, Herman et al. (37), studying the effect of prosta-cyclin in canine isolated veins, found that the compound reduced NE-reduced contractions without affecting the electrically induced responses and suggested a dual effect of PGI_2. This was depression of the responsiveness to NE of the smooth muscle and enhancement of the release of transmitter.

In contrast, Weitzell et al. (91) reported inhibition by PGI_2 of NE release in rabbit pulmonary arteries and Armstrong et al. (7) observed a similar effect in rabbit mesenterial veins, but not arteries.

Growing interest has been focused on various aspects of the pharmacology of PGD_2, mainly because this PG appears to be formed in substantial amounts in the brain (1). Indirect evidence for an effect of PGD_2 on sympathetic transmitter release has been reported by Hemker and Aiken (34). They observed that intracarotid arterial injection of PGD_2 in anaesthetized cats depressed sympathetic transmission to the nictitating membrane without depressing the effects of exogenous NE. In another study these authors had similar results with PGD_3 in this preparation (35).

Irrespective of which PG are in fact capable of inhibiting sympathetic transmitter release, this pharmacological effect of PG appears to have a physiological equiv-alent, i.e., synaptic inhibition of sympathetic transmitter release most probably occurs under normal conditions. The basis for this assumption is as follows. The

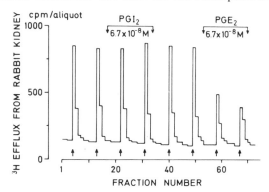

FIG. 6. Perfused rabbit kidney, loaded with ^{3}H-(-)-NA. Efflux of tracer from the kidney, resting and in response to nerve stimulation (5 Hz, 75 pulses, at arrows). Effects of PGI_2 and PGE_2 (6.7×10^{-8} M). Time in min = fraction numbers. (From Hedqvist, ref. 33, with permission.)

release of transmitter from sympathetically stimulated organs is increased following inhibition of PG formation (14,31,83). Indomethacin also increases the excretion of NE into the urine in rats, cold-stressed (85) or kept at room temperature (Fig. 7) (42), and facilitates the NE turnover rate in a variety of sympathetically innervated tissues in the rat (22). Also, some data indicate that a PG-mediated inhibition of NE release operates in humans. Stjärne and Gripe (86) studied isolated superfused field-stimulated specimens of peripheral arteries and veins obtained by biopsy from normotensive humans and obtained evidence suggesting that NE liberation in human vasoconstrictor nerves normally is restricted by two separate local feed-back mechanisms. One is dependent and the other independent of PGE. The most careful study presented so far on the possible occurrence of a PG-mediated transmitter control, also in humans and *in vivo*, yielded inconclusive results. Güllner and co-workers (30) found that treatment of normotensive subjects with indomethacin for 7 days resulted in a decrease in plasma NE, both under basal conditions and posturally as well as after 5 min of handgrip compression. The number of α-adrenergic receptors, as evidenced by platelet α-receptor density, was unaffected. The authors suggested that the withdrawal of vascular (vasodilating) PG via baroreceptor feedback caused lowering of the plasma NE concentration.

Their reasoning is correct provided the role of vascular PG is confined to regulation of myogenic tone in the resistance vessels. In that case, lack of vascular (vasodilator) PG would mean that less NE release is required to maintain a given B.P. level and plasma NE (if it does in fact reflect NE release in vasoconstrictor nerves) would fall. But, if vascular PG also have a role as inhibitors of NE release, inhibition of PG formation would hardly result in lowered plasma NE levels. Withdrawal of PG would then result in an unchanged plasma NE concentration, since the

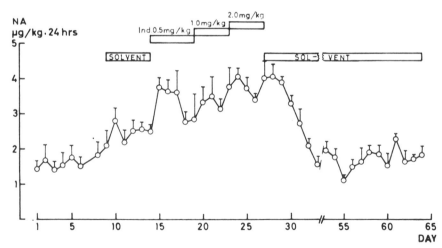

FIG. 7. Renal excretion of norepinephrine (NA). Each point represents mean ± SE of 5 urine samples; every sample consists of the 24-hr urine from 2 rats. Daily injections of indomethacin or drug solvent indicated by horizontal columns. (From Junstad and Wennmalm, ref. 42, with permission.)

increased NE release would elevate the systemic B.P. and lead via the baroreceptor reflex to decreased sympathetic activity and therefore no normalization of plasma NE.

Obviously the re-setting of the B.P. regulating feed-back circuit indicated by the lowered plasma NE levels reported by Güllner and co-workers (30) strongly indicates that locally formed PG *do not* interfere with sympathetic neuroeffector transmission, either pre- or postjunctionally, but rather with a vasoconstrictor mechanism independent of sympathetic activity, i.e., basal myogenic tone. Should it be the case that locally formed PG affect vasoconstrictor tone *both* via basal myogenic tone and through sympathetic activity, the question is more complex and further studies are required before final conclusions can be drawn.

With the discovery of prostacyclin as the quantitatively most important PG in vascular tissue (28), a tendency developed to regard this significant compound as the only vascular PG of interest. For example, Armstrong el al. (7) argued that "The finding that prostacyclin and not PGE_2 is the principal prostaglandin produced by certain blood vessels necessitates a re-interpretation of Hedqvist's hypothesis concerning the operation of a negative feedback mechanism..." and suggested that "... prostacyclin and not PGE_2 should be considered as the principal candidate for such a role..." Two objections can be raised to this reasoning. First, formation of PGI_2 in vascular tissue appears to be located mainly or entirely to the endothelium (36,54), the nerve-terminal carrying adventitia or muscle layer being devoid of PGI_2-synthetizing capacity. Second, the ability of PGI_2 to inhibit NE release from sympathetic nerves is doubtful and yet inhibition of PG bioformation results in increased NE liberation from discharging sympathetic neurons. Because of these data, both the *in vivo* existence of a local feed-back control of NE release by endogenous PGs and the chemical character of this PG must still be regarded as questions.

The postsynaptic effects of various PG, i.e., their interference with adrenergic alpha-receptor mediated responses, also have been studied extensively. Earlier reports in this field focused on the primary PGs but recently prostacyclin also has been studied. For the reasons mentioned, it is by no means obvious that PGE_2 is the only conceivable candidate for the role of modulator of adrenergic receptor mediated responses. At least, PGE_2 also should receive appropriate attention. The studies presented on the interference of PGA, PGB and PGE_1 with the vascular response to α-adrenergic agonists can, however, be regarded as of pharmacological interest only, since these PGs hardly occur in significant concentrations in vascular tissue under normal conditions.

In the dog hindlimb, perfused with blood at a constant rate, PGE_2 was found to inhibit the vasoconstrictor response to NE by 30 to 50% (43). In contrast, Greenberg and Long (27) reported increased contractile responses to NE in superfused strips of canine mesenteric and tibial arteries following adminstration of PGE_2. In the dog paw, representing mainly cutaneous vasculature, PGE_2 depressed the response to NE under conditions of constant flow maintained by a pump (101). In the same preparation, infusion of two structurally different PG synthesis inhibitors potentiated the pressor response to NE, indicating that endogenously synthesized PG antagonized the vasoconstrictor effect (101). However, when the dog paw was perfused without a pump, neither of these PG synthesis inhibitors changed the pressor response to NE, indicating that the experimental conditions per se may interfere with the results (80).

In the isolated perfused rat mesentery, PGE_2 was reported to inhibit the pressor responses to NE. In the same system indomethacin was devoid of effect (23). In conscious rats, both PGE_2 and PGI_2 attenuated pressor responses to NE, and indomethacin facilitated them in a dose-related manner, indicating that endogenous PG exerted a modulating action on the pressor responses (71).

In other studies, however, indomethacin or aspirin inhibited and PGE_2 restored the pressor-responses to NE in the perfused rat mesentery (15,39,55). Although these discrepancies are difficult to understand, it is obvious that when evaluating the effects of exogenous and endogenous PG on the vascular adrenergic responses, one has to take into account not only the experimental conditions and the species investigated, but also the vascular circuit being studied. The effect of PGI_2 on pressor responses to NE has also been investigated in other species. Hedqvist (33) reported that the vasoconstrictor response to NE or to sympathetic nerve stimulation in the rabbit kidney perfused with Tyrode solution was inhibited by PGI_2 (3 $\times$ $10^{-7}M$) to about 60% (Fig. 8), and Lippton et al. (52) found decreased pressor responses to NE in the feline mesenteric vascular bed following infusion of PGI_2. Both PGE_2 and PGI_2 decreased the vasoconstrictor responses to NE, sympathetic nerve stimulation, and angiotensin II, in the hindquarter of the rabbit, perfused with blood at a constant flow (26). In that study indomethacin was without consistent effect on the pressor responses, suggesting that locally formed PGs did not modulate the sensitivity of the vascular receptors.

It is quite clear that both PGE_2 and PGI_2 do possess the ability to modulate the vascular responses to α-adrenergic agonists in various tissues and species. Studies that conclusively extend this pharmacological potential to a physiological reality have not been presented. Perhaps a modulating action by locally formed PG is a

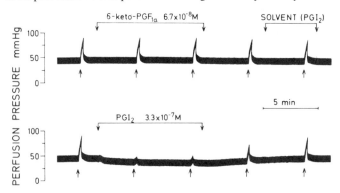

FIG. 8. Continuous recording of basal perfusion pressure and of vasoconstrictor responses to nerve stimulation (5 Hz, 75 pulses, at arrows) in a Tyrode's perfused rabbit kidney. Effects of 6-keto-$PGF_{1\alpha}$, PGI_2 solvent (0.05 M Tris buffer in 0.9% NaCl to give a buffer concentration of 3 μM in the perfusion stream), and PGI_2 (with the same buffer concentration as above). (From Hedqvist, ref. 33, with permission.)

transient phenomenon, appearing only when PG formation is accelerated, for example, by tissue hypoxia. If so, a decrease in the sensitivity of α-receptors caused by an increased local formation of PG would cooperate with the direct smooth muscle relaxing effect that these PG elicit on the resistance vessels. Vascular PG formation would then have the character of an emergency phenomenon. But if modulation of α-adrenergic responses is a normal task for locally formed PG, it may serve other purposes, e.g., differentiation, at a local level, of the vasoconstrictor response to a given sympathetic discharge rate.

PG AND BLOOD PRESSURE REGULATION

The concept of a role for PG in the regulation of blood pressure is presently under debate. The observation that arachidonate upon i.v. administration elicits a blood pressure drop, in rabbits (4) as well as in dogs (78), and that this effect is inhibited or abolished by PG synthesis inhibitors, strongly suggested that vascular tissue possesses the ability to produce significant amounts of vasodilator PGs. Furthermore, increased systemic B.P. has been reported following administration of indomethacin in rabbits (4), healthy men (92), and patients with mild essential hypertension (49), suggesting that circulation PG may elicit a modulatory tone in the peripheral vascular bed.

With the discovery of PGI_2 as the predominant vascular metabolite of arachidonate (59), the question of circulating PG as regulators of systemic B.P. attracted further interest. Prostaglandin I_2 is a vasodepressor, causing hypotension in dog (5), rat and rabbit (6), cat (51), and man (88). Gryglewski and co-workers (29), using the superfused rabbit Achilles tendon for continuous recording of the concentration of prostacyclin-like disaggregating activity in circulating cat blood, observed a consistently higher degree of disaggregating capacity in arterial blood than in mixed venous blood. They suggested that this was due to a continuous pulmonary release of prostacyclin into the systemic circulation. They did not suggest that the PGI_2 released from the lungs reached concentrations sufficient to modulate vascular resistance. Moncada et al. (61) obtained equivalent results in rabbits, using a technique very similar to that of Gryglewski et al., but they did not propose a vasoregulatory role for the PGI_2 released from the lungs either.

That PGI_2 released from the lungs could function as a circulating vasodilator and contribute to the regulation of blood vessel tone and B.P. has been suggested explicitly. Dusting et al. (19) proposed such a function for PGI_2 on the basis of its formation from arachidonate in the lungs of anesthetized dogs in combination with its passage through the lungs without inactivation. Lippton et al. (51) arrived at similar conclusions after studies in anesthetized cats. In contrast, Pace-Asciak et al. (72) recently presented evidence that does not support the concept of a vasodilator role for circulating PG. These authors infused anti-PGI_2-immunoglobulin i.v. into anesthetized rats and found that although much endogenous PGI_2 was in fact released into the circulation, the antibody administration had no effect on the systemic B.P.

The interplay between vascular PG and angiotensin should be mentioned. It is well known that angiotensin II, itself a vasoconstrictor agent, stimulates release of

PG from various tissues, including vascular endothelium. Infusion of angiotensin II in normal man elicits an increase in systemic B.P. that is significantly augmented following indomethacin (Fig. 9) (67), suggesting that endogenously formed PG modulate the vasoconstrictor effects of the drug. In the cat and dog i.v. injection of angiotensin II induced release of a PGI_2-like substance into the circulation, and this release was prevented by pretreatment with aspirin or saralasin (64,87). Also, injection of saralasin in cats lowered the circulating anti-aggregatory activity in their blood, implying that blocking the angiotensin receptor leads to a decreased prostacyclin release into the blood. According to this study, the renin-angiotensin system would be one of the factors responsible for the blood levels of PGI_2.

Data obtained in our laboratory (Wennmalm, *unpublished data*) demonstrate that infusion of angiotensin II decreases ADP-induced aggregability in the blood as tested shortly after sampling. This suggests that angiotensin elicits PGI_2 release into the circulation in humans also. In our study, the anti-aggregatory activity in the circulating blood deteriorated after 8 to 10 min of continued drug infusion, indicating rapid tachyphylaxis. Such rapid tachyphylaxis is certainly not compatible with the concept of the renin-angiotensin system as a normal determinant of plasma PGI_2 levels. Alternative mechanisms controlling the formation and release of circulating PGI_2 must be considered.

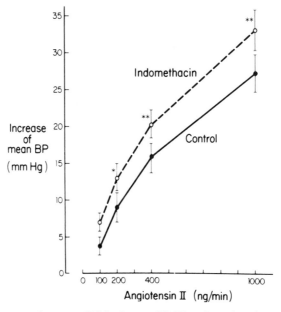

FIG. 9. The increase (mean $\pm$ SEM) of mean BP (diastolic + $\frac{1}{3}$ pulse pressure) is plotted against the infusion rate of angiotensin II. Each dose of angiotensin II was administered intravenously for 20 min. Control: *closed circles*; indomethacin: *open circles*. Indomethacin 150 mg was given in 3 divided doses over the prior 16 hr. Paired T test was used; $*p < 0.025$, $**p < 0.01$. Ten subjects were studied. (From Negus et al., ref. 67, with permission.)

Recently a stable metabolite of arachidonate, 6-keto-PGE$_1$, has been described that may prove important from a circulatory point of view. Formation of 6-keto-PGE$_1$ from PGE$_2$ or 6-keto-PGF$_{1\alpha}$ by a 9-hydroxy-PG-dehydrogenase has been demonstrated in the perfused rabbit liver (98). 6-keto-PGE$_1$, in analogy with PGI$_2$, inhibits platelet aggregation and decreases systemic vascular resistance (53,76) and it escapes pulmonary metabolism (76). In the feline mesenteric vascular bed 6-keto-PGE$_1$ inhibits vasoconstrictor responses to sympathetic nerve stimulation, NE, and angiotensin II (53). It is not known whether the metabolic pathway from PGI$_2$/6-keto-PGF$_{1\alpha}$ to 6-keto-PGE$_1$ operates *in vivo*.

Wong et al. (97) reported that 7% of the PGI$_2$ metabolized by the perfused rabbit liver appeared as 6-keto-PGE$_1$ and it was suggested that conversion of PGI$_2$ to 6-keto-PGE$_1$ might account for the unexpected duration of the effect of PGI$_2$ reported in some studies (76). Quantitative studies on plasma levels of 6-keto-PGE$_1$ and on PGI$_2$ metabolism *in vivo* are required before this hypothesis can be evaluated.

PG AND REGIONAL VASCULAR RESISTANCE

Coronary Circulation

The flow through the coronary arteries is autoregulated over a wide range of perfusion pressures. This autoregulation, which is present also in isolated hearts, plays the important role of adjusting the flow through the coronary vascular bed to the demands from the metabolic activity, and hence the mechanical performance, of the myocardium. It is generally assumed that this autoregulation is regulated in some way by products generated by metabolism in the cardiac muscle cells, but the nature of these products is still somewhat controversial. The vasodilator principle that has attracted most attention as a regulator of coronary tone is no doubt adenosine (79).

Adenosine is a breakdown product of adenine nucleotides and as such is continuously produced by the working heart. Although most cardiac physiologists do accept adenosine as a major determinator of coronary blood flow, considerable interest is still being shown in the possible role of PG in the regulation of coronary tone. This arises from the pharmacological action of the major cardiac PG, namely PGI$_2$, that powerfully relaxes isolated strips of coronary vessels and increases coronary flow in most species (50,65,70,77,84). In this context it should be noteed that the coronary flow in healthy humans was not increased by i.v infusion of PGI$_2$ in a dose sufficient to induce general hemodynamic effects (43c), while the coronary vascular resistance in patients with angina pectoris in fact was decreased by such infusion (8b).

The possible contribution of endogenously formed PG to the physiological or pathophysiological regulation of coronary flow *in situ* has been investigated assessing the effect of PG synthesis inhibitors on basal and stimulated coronary flow. Since the experimental conditions applied, and the parameters studied, differ between various investigations divergent results have been obtained that makes general conclusions difficult to draw. In open-chest mongrel dogs, the basal coronary flow decreased from 28 to 24 ml/min following administration of indomethacin at a dose of 5 mg/kg BW (38), and from 37 to 26 ml/min following a dose of 10 mg/kg BW (48). In contrast, the basal flow in a similar series was reported unaffected by indomethacin at a dose of about 7 mg/kg BW (42 vs 43 ml/min, ref. 2). Failure of indomethacin at a dose of 2 to 5 mg/kg BW to affect coronary flow also was reported in two other series using slightly different techniques, but in those investigations (3,25) the flow figures reported before drug administration were considerably higher, 122 and 79 ml/min, respectively, indicating that basal conditions were not prevailing.

The coronary flow response to hypoxia or ischemia appears even more complex when judged from the discussed studies. The reported differences are, in part, illusory. When comparing the results from various studies, the magnitude of the induced ischemia (the duration of the coronary arterial occlusion) or hypoxia (the oxygen percentage in the breathing air) must be taken into account, as well as the fact that the coronary response to hypoxia can be expressed as elevation either of peak or mean coronary flow (absolute or relative to the basal flow) while the response to ischemia can be expressed in either of the terms peak reactive hyperemia, duration of the hyperemia, total reactive hyperemia or percentage repayment of flow debt.

In open-chest mongrel dogs coronary arterial hypoxia resulting from breathing 5 to 8% O_2 in N_2 elevated the coronary flow from 42 to 76 ml/min before, and from 43 to 70 ml/min after indomethacin, at a dose of 7 mg/min (2). In another study a similar degree of hypoxia induced a peak increase in coronary flow that was 42 ml/min before and 35 ml/min after indomethacin at a dose of 5 mg/kg BW (38). In the latter study, however, the basal coronary flow also was reduced by indomethacin, implying that the total hyperemia (expressed as the area under the mean flow curve above the baseline) was not significantly affected by the PG synthesis inhibitor. The responses to coronary arterial occlusion during 5 sec to 10 min have also been studied in open-chest dogs before and after indomethacin (2 to 5 mg/kg BW). Reductions in the absolute magnitude of the peak post-occlusive flow following indomethacin (329 vs 267 ml/min, and 150 vs 103 ml/min, respectively) were reported (3,48). However, when the peak post-occlusive flow figures were expressed in percent of the basal flow in these studies the percentage increases before and after drug were 170 vs 152%, and 305 vs 296%, respectively. The latter figures on the effect of indomethacin are less impressive than the absolute increments and seem to accord with results from other studies (25,38) in which indomethacin failed to affect the percentage peak increase and the percent flow debt repaid following coronary arterial occlusion.

No studies have been presented up to now on the effect of indomethacin on coronary flow in healthy humans. A few studies in patients with ischemic heart disease have, however, been reported recently. It was found in these studies that indomethacin significantly impairs the coronary blood flow (19b, 22b). This observation might seem to support a role for endogenous PG in the coronary flow regulation. However, another PG synthesis inhibitor, naproxen, does not elicit a similar effect on the coronary flow (19b). The observed action by indomethacin may consequently be a direct vasoconstrictor effect, not operating via inhibition of cyclo-oxygenase. If so, locally formed PGs are not involved in coronary flow regulation, at least not in patients with coronary artery disease. This conclusion is indirectly supported by some studies which fail to show any efflux of 6-keto-PGF$_{1\alpha}$ from the coronary circulation in patients with ischemic heart disease, both in the basal state and during pacing induced angina pectoris (19b, 38b). Perhaps the cardiac ischemia induced during angina pectoris is too short-lasting to efficiently stimulate cardiac (coronary) PGI$_2$ formation. Evidence pointing in that direction has been obtained from studies of cardiac efflux of 6-keto-PGF$_{1\alpha}$ from human hearts during cardioplegia. Under those circumstances, involving 60–90 min of severe cardiac ischemia, a considerable increase in the cardiac production of PGI$_2$ develops (19c). This production of PGI$_2$, as judged from the coronary efflux of 6-keto-PGF$_{1\alpha}$, does not reach a maximum until about 60 min after the onset of the ischemia.

To sum up the available knowledge there is probably reason to conclude that cardiac PGs are not involved in the autoregulation of coronary flow in healthy subjects or in subjects with short-lasting myocardial ischemia (angina pectoris). Under conditions of long-lasting myocardial ischemia (as in acute myocardial infarction) increased formation of PGI$_2$ may take place in the coronary vessels. Whether such an increased production of PGI$_2$ is beneficial to the ischemic heart, e.g., by limiting infarct size, remains to be studied.

Skeletal Muscle Circulation

Data on the possible contribution of endogenous PG to the regulation of skeletal muscle vascular resistance have been mentioned earlier in this chapter. The following is a summary.

The resting blood flow in the perfused rat cremaster muscle has been reported to be unaffected by PG synthesis inhibition (57,58) and similar results have been obtained in the perfused gracilis muscle of the dog (90). In contrast, an increased vascular resistance at rest was observed in the denervated hind-limb of the dog following indomethacin (41,100). Most probably it was the techniques used rather than the species, which contributed to the different results. In human volunteers, forearm resting arterial blood flow is not changed by indomethacin (47) or naproxen (20), however, calf flow under similar circumstances has been reported slightly decreased (69). These data indicate that resting flow in skeletal muscle is regulated to only a minor degree, if at all, by locally formed PG.

The increase in muscle blood flow during and following muscular exercise may, under certain circumstances, be influenced to some degree by locally formed PG. Indomethacin considerably attenuated the increase in vascular conductance accompanying and following muscular exercise in the denervated dog hindleg (41), and also reduced the vasodilatation following exercise in the dog gracilis muscle (90) and anterior calf muscle (63). In contrast, steady-state exercise hyperemia of canine hindlimb muscle was not reduced following PG synthesis inhibition (8) and neither was the increase in canine hindlimb muscle blood flow during electrically stimulated exercise at constant flow (62) and free flow (100). Furthermore, human leg blood flow at three different leg muscle work loads was unaffected following indomethacin (69). These data do not support anything but, possibly, a small role for vascular PG in the developement of hyperemia in exercising muscle. In post-exercise hyperemia the picture differs, and in that situation locally formed PG may well be involved.

Splanchnic Circulation

Few data are available in the literature on the possible involvement of PG in the splanchnic circulation. Bunting et al. (12), in one of the first reports on prostacyclin, stated that this compound relaxed strips of coeliac and mesenteric arteries, being more potent than the parent endoperoxide, but less potent than PGE_2. Lippton and co-workers (52), studying the perfusion pressure in the constant-flow perfused feline mesenteric vascular bed in response to PGI_2 and 6-keto-$PGF_{1\alpha}$, observed a dose- and time-related pressure drop following infusion of PGI_2 (0.3 to 1 μg/min), amounting to about 40% after 30 min of infusion. Recent evidence indicate that the splanchnic vascular resistance bed in man is also very sensitive to the vasodilator effect of PGI_2 (43b).

In rat isolated perfused mesenteric blood vessels, addition of indomethacin to the perfusion fluid (10 to 60 μg/ml) did not alter the basal perfusion pressure (15). Spirally cut strips of rabbit mesenteric arteries did, however, increase their basal tension after addition of indomethacin (5×10^{-6}M) to the superfusion fluid. Both these experiments were performed under rather artificial conditions and extrapolation of the results to *in vivo* conditions is hardly justified (neither was it done by the authors). In anesthetized dogs indomethacin reduced the basal flow in the left gastric artery by almost 50%, suggesting that a basal production of vasodilator PGs contributes considerably to the gastric blood flow (24).

A slight hint of a possible regulation of basal splanchnic blood flow by locally formed PG in humans has been obtained in our laboratory (68). In awake volunteers investigated in the supine position, splanchnic blood flow was measured (using hepatic elimination of indocyanine green dye) before and after an i.v. infusion of indomethacin (Fig. 10). A significant increase in splanchnic vascular resistance, amounting to 16%, was obtained following administration of the drug. The mechanism behind this increase is unknown, and both myogenic and neurogenic factors may be involved. As in most vascular circuits, the exact role of locally formed PG in the mesenteric vascular bed is unclear. The data referred to, however, indicate that the splanchnic circulatory bed may be one of the regions in which local PG are involved even in the regulation of basal vascular tone.

Skin Blood Flow

The cutaneous vasculature, unlike e.g., the cerebral or muscle vascular circuits, is not primarily designed to meet the local metabolic demands of the perfused tissue. Instead it serves the important purpose of regulating heat elimination from the body.

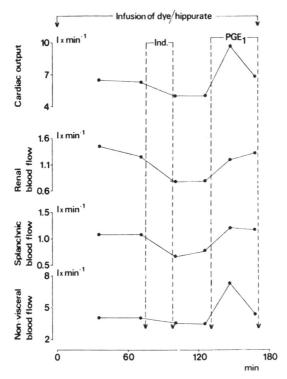

FIG. 10. Typical experiment demonstrating the effect of indomethacin (IND; 50 mg infused i.v. during 20 min) and of prostaglandin E_1 (PGE$_1$; 160 μg infused i.v. during 40 min) on cardiac output, and on renal, splanchnic, and non-visceral blood flow in a healthy male volunteer, aged 35. (From Nowak and Wennmalm, ref. 68, with permission.)

Homeothermic animals without fur, like humans, depend to a considerable extent on the proper adjustment of their skin blood flow for heat regulation. Furry animals must rely upon other mechanisms like panting. It is evident that data on skin circulation in most laboratory animals are of little or no interest in evaluating the cutaneous blood flow in humans. This section will therefore be limited to an overview of the data available from studies in man.

At the first infusion of PG in man it was observed that the subjects got a feeling of warmth and oppression in the head and chest and flushing in the face (9). There is no doubt that these symptoms were due at least in part to cutaneous vasodilation. Later Carlson and co-workers (13) observed that i.v. infusion of PGE$_2$ at a rate of 0.13 to 0.56 μg/min/kg B.W. produced a face flush in all subjects, again indicating cutaneous vasodilation.

Not surprisingly, PGI$_2$ is also a cutaneous vasodilator in humans. Szczeklik and co-workers (88) reported on skin flush in humans, both after i.v. administration and following inhalation (89) of PGI$_2$. It is not possible to conclude whether this observation carries physiological significance. To our knowledge no data have been reported on human skin blood flow and its dependence on locally formed PG. In

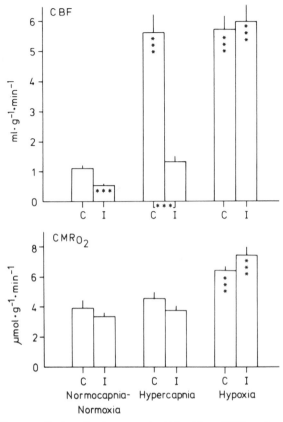

FIG. 11. The influence of indomethacin on cerebral blood flow (CBF) and cerebral metabolic rate for oxygen (CMR_{O_2}) under control conditions as well as in hypercapnia and in hypoxia. Values given are mean ± SE for indomethacin injected animals (I) as compared to the corresponding control situation (C). *** $p < 0.001$. Statistical symbols within bars indicate differences from normocapnic-normoxic controls, while those below bars indicate differences between indomethacin-injected and control groups. (From Sakabe and Siesjö, ref. 82, with permission.)

a study under completion in our laboratory, cutaneous blood flow (as reflected by basal finger tip flow measured plethsymographically in a temperature controlled environment) was not significantly affected by pre-treatment with indomethacin (Wennmalm, submitted for publication). This observation does not indicate involvement of PG formed in cutaneous vessels in the regulation of human skin blood flow. It need hardly be said that further investigations are required in this field, especially with regard to the interference of locally formed PG with sympathetic neurotransmission in the skin vessels.

Cerebral Circulation

The blood flow through the brain is maintained at a constant level in the approximate arterial pressure range 60 to 160 mmHg. This phenomenon, commonly

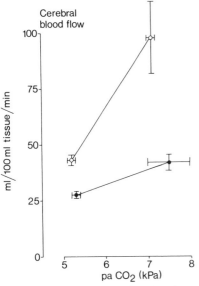

FIG. 12. Effect of indomethacin on basal and CO_2-stimulated cerebral blood flow in healthy human subjects. *Open circles:* values obtained before indomethacin; *closed circles:* figures obtained 60 to 70 min after indomethacin was given. All figures are expressed as mean ± SE. (From Wennmalm, et al., ref. 95, with permission.)

referred to as autoregulation, has been explained by either a myogenic or a metabolic influence exerted by systemic blood pressure variations on the smooth muscle in the cerebral resistance vessels. Cerebral autoregulation thus conforms to the common type of autoregulation described earlier in this chapter. The metabolite usually referred to in the regulation of vascular resistance by those favoring the concept of a metabolically controlled autoregulation is the hydrogen ion. Cerebral blood flow is considerably increased by hypoxia or hypercapnia and it is believed that the facilitated flow under these conditions is based on an increased hydrogen ion concentration, caused in turn by the impaired oxygen supply or increased pCO_2 in the medium surrounding the resistance vessels.

Pickard and co-workers (74) have demonstrated that PGE_2 and $PGF_{2\alpha}$ act as vasoconstrictors in anesthetized baboons. In contrast PGI_2 dilates all cerebral vessels, including the distal branches, in doses which produce no major cardiovascular changes (11). The significance of this observation is strengthened by the findings that human cerebral arteries can generate prostacyclin from an exogenous precursor (10) and that the formation of PGI_2 in the human brain seems to be oriented towards the prostacyclin pathway in the vascular bed but not in extravascular tissue (81).

There are no data available to indicate involvement of local PG in the regulation of cerebral blood flow. In anesthetized baboons, indomethacin reduced the cerebral blood flow by almost 40%, and considerably reduced the flow response to hypercapnia (73). Similar data have been obtained in rats (82). In contrast to the pronounced effect of indomethacin on basal cerebral blood flow and on the flow response to hypercapnia, this drug failed to affect the cerebrovascular response to changes in perfusion pressure induced by angiotensin or controlled hemorrhage, indicating that autoregulation of flow was not inhibited by indomethacin (75). Furthermore, the increase in cerebral flow in rats induced by hypoxia is also main-

326 *PROSTAGLANDINS AND VASCULAR RESISTANCE*

tained following indomethacin (Fig. 11) (82). The effect of the PG synthesis inhibitor in blocking the cerebral blood flow to hypercapnia consequently appears
specific, inasmuch as autoregulation and flow response to hypoxia were unaffected.
Recent studies to confirm these data in man have, however, yielded notable
results. Although the inhibitory effect of indomethacin on basal and CO_2-stimulated
cerebral flow was found to operate also in man (95), some other PG synthesis
inhibitors investigated did not produce a similar effect. Thus, both aspirin and
naproxen completely lacked effect on basal and CO_2-stimulated cerebral blood flow,
at doses known to inhibit vascular formation of PGI_2. Furthermore, no release of
PG precursor or of PGI_2 metabolites was detectable in the cerebral circulation in
these experiments, either in the basal state or during inhalation of CO_2 (95b). These
data consequently suggest, firstly, that the observed effect of indomethacin in animal
and human studies is a direct effect of the drug not due to inhibition of PG bioformation, and secondly, that locally formed PG do not participate in the regulation
of basal or CO_2-stimulated cerebral blood flow.

REFERENCES

1. Abdel-Halim, M. S., Hamberg, M., Sjöquist, B. and Änggård, E. (1977): Identification of prostaglandin D_2 as a major prostaglandin in homogenates of rat brain. *Prostaglandins*, 14:633–643.
2. Afonso, S., Bandow, G. T., and Rowe, G. G. (1974): Indomethacin and the prostaglandin hypothesis of coronary blood flow regulation. *J. Physiol.*, 241:299–308.
3. Alexander, R. W., Kent, K. M., Pisano, J. J., Keiser, H. R., and Cooper, T. (1975): Regulation
of postocclusive hyperemia by endogenously synthetized prostaglandins in the dog heart. *J. Clin.
Invest.*, 55:1174–1181.
4. Änggård, E., and Larsson, C. (1973): Prostaglandin mediated hypotensive effects of arachidonic
acid in the rabbit. *Acta Physiol. Scand. [Suppl.]*, 396:18.
5. Armstrong, J. M., Chapple, D., Dusting, G. J., Hughes, R., Moncada, S., and Vane, J. R. (1977):
Cardiovascular actions of prostacylcin (PGI_2) in chloralose anaesthetized dogs. *Br. J. Pharmacol.*,
61:136P.
6. Armstrong, J. M., Lattimer, N., Moncada, S., and Vane, J. R. (1978): Comparison of the vasodepressor effects of prostacyclin and 6-oxo-prostaglandin $F_{1\alpha}$ with those of prostaglandin E_2 in
rats and rabbits. *Br. J. Pharmacol.*, 62:125–130.
7. Armstrong, J. M., Thirsk, G., and Salmon, J. A. (1979): Effects of prostacyclin (PGI_2), 6-oxo-
$PGF_{1\alpha}$ and PGE_2 on sympathetic nerve function in mesenteric arteries and veins of the rabbit *in
vitro*. *Hypertension*, 1:309–315.
8. Beaty, O., and Donald, D. E. (1979): Contribution of prostaglandins to muscle blood flow in
anesthetized dogs at rest, during exercise, and following inflow occlusion. *Circ. Res.*, 44:67–74.
8b.Bergman, G., Atkinson, L., Richardson, P. J., Daly, K., Rothman, M., Jackson, G. and Jewitt,
D. E. (1981): Prostacyclin: Haemodynamic and metabolic effects in patients with coronary artery
disease. *Lancet* I:569–572.
9. Bergström, S., Dunér, H., v. Euler, U. S., Pernow, B., and Sjövall, J. (1959): Observations on
the effects of infusion of prostaglandin E in man. *Acta Physiol. Scand.*, 45:145–151.
10. Boullin, D. J., Bunting, S., Blaso, W. P., Hunt, T. M., and Moncada, S. (1979): Responses of
human and baboon arteries to prostaglandin endoperoxides and biologically generated and synthetic
prostacyclin: Their relevance to cerebral arterial spasm in man. *Br. J. Clin. Pharmacol.*, 7:139–
147.
11. Boullin, D. J. (1980): Vasospasm and prostacyclin—a new hypothesis and possibilities for therapy.
In: *Cerebral Vasospasm*, pp. 209–230. John Wiley & Sons Ltd., England.
12. Bunting, S., Gryglewski, R., Moncada, S., and Vane, J. R. (1976): Arterial walls generate from
prostaglandin endoperoxides a substance (prostaglandin X) which relaxes strips of mesenteric and
coeliac arteries and inhibits platelet aggregation. *Prostaglandins*, 12:897–914.
13. Carlson, L. A., Ekelund, L. G., and Orö, L. (1970): Clinical, metabolic and cardiovascular effects
of different prostaglandins in man. *Acta Med. Scand.*, 188:553–559.

14. Chanh, P. C., Junstad, M., and Wennmalm, Å. (1972): Augmented noradrenaline release following nerve stimulation after inhibition of prostaglandin synthesis with indomethacin. *Acta Physiol. Scand.*, 86:563–567.
15. Coupar, I. M., and McLennan, P. L. (1978): The influence of prostaglandins on noradrenaline-induced vasoconstriction in isolated perfused mesenteric blood vessels of the rat. *Br. J. Pharmacol.*, 62:51–59.
16. De Deckere, E. A. M., Nugteren, D. H., and Ten Hoor, F. (1977): Prostacyclin is the major prostaglandin released from the isolated perfused rabbit and rat heart. *Nature*, 268:160–163.
17. Dusting, G. J., Moncada, S., and Vane, J. R. (1977): Prostacyclin (PGI_2) is a weak contractor of coronary arteries of the pig. *Eur. J. Pharmacol.*, 45:301–304.
18. Dusting, G. J., Moncada, S., Mullane, K. M., and Vane, J. R. (1978): Implications of prostacyclin generation for modulation of vascular tone. *Clin. Sci. Mol. Med.* 55:195s–198s.
19. Dusting, G. J., Chapple, D. J., Hughes, R., Moncada, S., and Vane, J. R. (1978): Prostacyclin (PGI_2) induces coronary vasodilatation in anaesthetized dogs. *Cardiovasc. Res.*, 12:720–730.
19b. Edlund, A., Berglund, B., Kaijser, L., Patrono, C., Sollevi, A. and Wennmalm, Å. (1982): Release of adenosine and PGI_2 from ischemic human hearts. In: *Advances in Prostaglandin, Thromboxane and Leukotrine Research*, edited by B. Samuelsson and R. Paoletti, Raven Press, New York. *(in press)*.
19c. Edlund, A., Bomfim, W., Kaijser, L., Olin, C., Patrono, C., Pinca, E. and Wennmalm, Å. (1982): Cardiac formation of prostacyclin during cardioplegia in man. *Prostaglandins (in press)*.
20. Eklund, B., Kaijser, L., Nowak, J., and Wennmalm, Å. (1979): Prostaglandins contribute to the vasodilation induced by nicotinic acid. *Prostaglandins*, 17:821–830.
21. Fitzpatrick, T. M., Alter, I., Corey, E. J., Ramwell, P. W., Rose, J. C., and Kot, P. A. (1978): Cardiovascular responses to PGI_2 (prostacyclin) in the dog. *Circ. Res.*, 42:192–194.
22. Fredholm, B. B., and Hedqvist, P. (1975): Indomethacin-induced increase in noradrenaline turn-over in some rat organs. *Br. J. Pharmacol.*, 54:295–300.
22b. Friedman, P. L., Brown, E. J., Gunther, S., Alexander, R. W., Barry, W. H., Mudge, G. H., and Grossman, W. (1981): Coronary vasoconstrictor effect of indomethacin in patients with coronary-artery disease. *New Engl. J. Med.*, 305:1171-1175.
23. George, A. J. (1977): The effects of prostaglandin perfusion on the vascular responses to nerve stimulation and sympathomimetic amines. *Pharmac. Res. Commun.*, 9:397–414.
24. Gerkens, J. F., Flexner, Ch., Oates, J. A., and Shand, D. G. (1977): Prostaglandin and histamine involvement in the gastric vasodilator action of pentagastrin. *J. Pharmacol. Exp. Ther.*, 201:421–426.
25. Giles, R. W., and Wilcken, D. E. L. (1977): Reactive hyperaemia in the dog heart: inter-relations between adenosine, ATP, and aminophylline and the effect of indomethacin. *Cardiovasc. Res.*, 11:113–121.
26. Gottlieb, A. L., Lippton, H. L., Parey, S. E., Paustian, P. W., and Kadowitz, P. J. (1980): Block-ade of vasoconstrictor responses by prostacyclin (PGI_2), PGE_2 and PGE_1 in the rabbit hindquarters vascular bed. *Prostaglandins Med.*, 4:1–11.
27. Greenberg, S., and Long, J. P. (1973): Enhancement of vascular smooth muscle responses to vasoactive stimuli by prostaglandin E_1 and E_2. *Arch. Int. Pharmacodyn. Ther.*, 206:94–104.
28. Gryglewski, R. J., Bunting, S., Moncada, S., Flower, R. J., and Vane, J. R. (1976): Arterial walls are protected against deposition of platelet thrombi by a substance (prostaglandin X) which they make from prostaglandin endoperoxides. *Prostaglandins*, 12:685–714.
29. Gryglewski, R. J., Korbut, R., and Ocetkiewicz, A. (1978): Generation of prostacyclin by lungs in vivo and its release into the arterial circulation. *Nature*, 273:765–767.
30. Güllner, H-G., Lake, C. R., Bartter, F. C., and Kafka, M. S. (1979): Effect of inhibition of prostaglandin synthesis on sympathetic nervous system function in man. *J. Clin. Endocrinol. Metab.*, 49:552–556.
31. Hedqvist, P., Stjärne, L., and Wennmalm, Å. (1971): Facilitation of sympathetic neurotransmission in the cat spleen after inhibition of prostaglandin synthesis. *Acta Physiol. Scand.*, 83:430–432.
32. Hedqvist, P. (1977): Basic mechanisms of prostaglandin action on autonomic neurotransmission. *Am. Rev. Pharmacol. Toxicol.*, 17:259–279.
33. Hedqvist, P. (1979): Actions of prostacyclin (PGI_2) on adrenergic neuroeffector transmission in the rabbit kidney. *Prostaglandins*, 17:249–258.
34. Hemker, D. P., and Aiken, J. W. (1980a): Modulation of autonomic neurotransmission by PGD_2: comparison with effects of other prostaglandins in anesthetized cats. *Prostaglandins*, 20:321–332.

35. Hemker, D. P., and Aiken, J. W. (1980b): Effects of prostaglandin D_3 on nerve transmission in nictitating membrane of cats. *Eur. J. Pharmacol.*, 67:155–158.
36. Herman, A. G., Moncada, S., and Vane, J. R. (1977): Formation of prostacyclin (PGI_2) by different layers of the arterial wall. *Arch. Int. Pharmacodyn. Ther.*, 227:162–163.
37. Herman, A. G., Verbeuren, T. J., Moncada, S., and Vanhoutte, P. M. (1978): Effect of prostacyclin on myogenic activity and adrenergic neuroeffector interaction in canine isolated veins. *Prostaglandins*, 16:911–921.
38. Hintze, T. H., and Kaley, G. (1977): Prostaglandins and the control of blood flow in the canine myocardium. *Circ. Res.*, 40:313–320.
38b. Hirsh, P. D., Hillis, D., Campbell, W. B., Firth, B. G., and Willerson, J. T. (1981): Release of prostaglandins and thromboxane into the coronary circulation in patients with ischemic heart disease. *New Engl. J. Med.*, 304:685–691.
39. Horrobin, D. F., Manku, M. S., and Nassar, B. A. (1974): Aspirin and arteriolar responses to noradrenaline. *Lancet*, II:567–568.
40. Isakson, P. C., Raz, A., Denny, S. E., Pure, E., and Needleman, P. (1977): A novel prostaglandin is the major product of arachidonic acid metabolism in rabbit heart. *Proc. Natl. Acad. Sci. USA*, 74:101–105.
41. Janczewska, H., and Herbaczyńska-Cedro, K. (1974): Effect of indomethacin on vascular responses to vasoactive agents in working skeletal muscles in the dog. *Pol. J. Pharmacol. Pharm.*, 26:159–166.
42. Junstad, M., and Wennmalm, Å. (1972): Increased renal excretion of noradrenaline in rats after treatment with prostaglandin synthesis inhibitor indomethacin. *Acta Physiol. Scand.*, 85:573–576.
43. Kadowitz, P. J. (1972): Effect of prostaglandins E_1, E_2 and A_2 on vascular resistance and responses to noradrenaline, nerve stimulation and angiotensin in the dog hindlimb. *Br. J. Pharmacol.*, 46:395–400.
43b. Kaijser, L., Eklund, B., and Joreteg, P. (1982): Hemodynamic effects of PGE_1 and PGI_2 in man. In: *Prostaglandins in Cardiovascular and Thrombotic Disorders*, edited by K. K. Wu and E. C. Rossi, Pathotox, Chicago *(in press)*.
43c. Kaijser, L., Joreteg, P. and Eklund, B. (1982): Effect of prostacyclin on coronary flow in humans. *Prostaglandins (in press)*.
44. Kaijser, L., Nowak, J., Patrono, C. and Wennmalm, Å. (1982): Release of prostacyclin into the coronary venous blood in patients with arterial disease. In: *Advances in Myocardiology*. Univ. Park Press, Baltimore. *(Submitted)*.
45. Kalsner, S. (1977): The effect of hypoxia on prostaglandin output and on tone in isolated coronary arteries. *Can. J. Physiol. Pharmacol.*, 55:882–887.
46. Kent, K. M., Alexander, R. W., Pisano, J. J., Keiser, H. R., and Cooper, T. (1973): Prostaglandin-dependent coronary vasodilator responses. *The Physiologist*, 16:361.
47. Kilbom, Å., and Wennmalm, Å. (1976): Endogenous prostaglandins as local regulators of blood flow in man: Effect of indomethacin on reactive and functional hyperaemia. *J. Physiol.*, 257:109–121.
48. Kraemer, R. J., Phernetton, T. M., and Folts, J. D. (1976): Prostaglandin-like substances in coronary venous blood following myocardial ischemia. *J. Pharmacol. Exp. Ther.*, 199:611–619.
49. Lee, J. B. (1976): The renal prostaglandins and blood pressure regulation. In: *Advances in Prostaglandin and Thromboxane Research*, Vol. 2, edited by B. Samuelsson, and R. Paoletti, pp. 573–585. Raven Press, New York.
50. Link, H. B., Rösen, R., and Schrör, K. (1978): Prostacyclin: A potent coronary dilating agent in the rat isolated heart. *Proc. Physiol. Soc.*, 106–107P.
51. Lippton, H. L., Paustian, P. W., Mellion, B. T., Nelson, P. K., Feigen, L. P., Chapnick, B. M., Human, A. L., and Kadowitz, P. J. (1979): Cardiovascular actions of prostacyclin (PGI_2) in the cat. *Arch. Int. Pharmacodyn. Ther.*, 241:121–130.
52. Lippton, H. L., Chapnick, B. M., Hyman, A. L., and Kadowitz, P. J. (1979): Inhibition of vasoconstrictor responses by prostacyclin (PGI_2) in the feline mesenteric vascular bed. *Arch. Int. Pharmacodyn. Ther.*, 241:214–223.
53. Lippton, H. L., Chapnick, B. M., Hyman, A. L., and Kadowitz, P. J. (1980): Inhibition of vasoconstrictor responses by 6-keto-PGE_1 in the feline mesenteric vascular bed. *Prostaglandins*, 19:299–310.
54. MacIntyre, D. E., Pearson, J. D., and Gordon, J. L. (1978): Localisation and stimulation of prostacyclin production in vascular cells. *Nature*, 271:549–551.

55. Manku, M. S., and Horrobin, D. F. (1976): Indomethacin inhibits responses to all vasoconstrictors in the rat mesentric vascular bed: Restoration of responses by prostaglandin E_2. *Prostaglandins*, 12:369–376.
56. Marcus, A. J., Weksler, B. B., and Jaffe, E. A. (1978): Enzymatic conversion of prostaglandin endoperoxide H_2 and arachidonic acid to prostacyclin by cultured human endothelial cells. *J. Biol. Chem.*, 253:7138–7141.
57. Messina, E. J., Weiner, R., and Kaley, G. (1977): Arteriolar reactive hyperemia: modification by inhibitors of prostaglandin synthesis. *Am. J. Physiol.*, 232:H571–H575.
58. Messina, E. J., Rodenburg, J., Slomiany, B. L., Roberts, A. M., Hintze, T. H. and Kaley, G. (1980): Microcirculatory effects of arachidonic acid and a prostaglandin endoperoxide (PGH_2) *Microvasc. Res.*, 19:288–296.
59. Moncada, S., Gryglewski, R., Bunting, S., and Vane, J. R. (1976): An enzyme isolated from arteries transforms prostaglandin endoperoxides to an unstable substance that inhibits platelet aggregation. *Nature*, 263:663–665.
60. Moncada, S., Higgs, E. A., and Vane, J. R. (1977): Human arterial and venous tissues generate prostacyclin (Prostaglandin X), a potent inhibitor of platelet aggregation. *Lancet*, I:18–20.
61. Moncada, S., Korbut, R., Bunting, S., and Vane, J. R. (1978): Prostacyclin is a circulating hormone. *Nature*, 273:767–768.
62. Morganroth, M. L., Mohrman, D. E., and Sparks, H. V. (1975): Prolonged vasodilation following fatiguing exercise of dog skeletal muscle. *Am. J. Physiol.*, 229:38–43.
63. Morganroth, M. L., Young, E. W., and Sparks, H. V. (1977): Prostaglandin and histaminergic mediation of prolonged vasodilation after exercise. *Am. J. Physiol.*, 233:H27–H33.
64. Mullane, K. M., and Moncada, S. (1980): Prostacyclin release and the modulation of some vasoactive hormones. *Prostaglandins*, 20:25–49.
65. Needleman, P., Kulkarni, P. S., and Raz, A. (1977): Coronary tone modulation: Formation and actions of prostaglandins, endoperoxides, and thromboxanes. *Science*, 195:409–412.
66. Needleman, P., Bronson, S. D., Wyche, A., and Sivakoff, M. (1978): Cardiac and renal prostaglandin I_2. Biosynthesis and biological effects in isolated perfused rabbit tissues. *J. Clin. Invest.*, 61:839–849.
67. Negus, P., Tannen, R. L., and Dunn, M. J. (1976): Indomethacin potentiates the vasoconstrictor actions of angiotensin II in normal man. *Prostaglandins*, 12:175–180.
68. Nowak, J., and Wennmalm, Å. (1978): Influence of indomethacin and of prostaglandin E_1 on total and regional blood flow in man. *Acta Physiol. Scand.*, 102:484–491.
69. Nowak, J., and Wennmalm, Å. (1979): A study on the role of endogenous prostaglandins in the development of exercise-induced and post-occlusive hyperemia in human limbs. *Acta Physiol. Scand.*, 106:365–369.
70. Ogletree, M. L., Smith, B. J., and Lefer, A. M. (1978): Actions of prostaglandins on isolated perfused cat coronary arteries. *Am. J. Physiol.*, 235:H400–H406.
71. Okuno, T., Kondo, K., Suzuki, H., and Saruta, T. (1980): Effects of prostaglandins E_2, I_2 and $F_{2\alpha}$, arachidonic acid and indomethacin on pressor responses to norepinephrine in conscious rats. *Prostaglandins*, 19:855–864.
72. Pace-Asciak, C. R., Carrara, M. C., Levine, L., and Nicolaou, K. C. (1980): PGI_2-specific antibodies administered *in vivo* suggest against a role for endogenous PGI_2 as a circulating hormone in the normotensive and spontaneously hypertensive rat. *Prostaglandins*, 20:1053–1060.
73. Pickard, J. D., and Mackenzie, E. T. (1973): Inhibition of prostaglandin synthesis and the response of baboon cerebral circulation of carbon dioxide. *Nature*, 245:187–188.
74. Pickard, J. D., MacDonell, L. A., MacKenzie, E. T., and Harper, A. M. (1977): Response of the cerebral circulation in baboons to changing perfusion pressure after indomethacin. *Circ. Res.*, 40:198–203.
75. Pickard, J. D., MacDonell, L. A., MacKenzie, E. T., and Harper, A. M. (1977): Prostaglandin-induced effects in the primate cerebral circulation. *Eur. J. Pharmacol.*, 43:343–351.
76. Quilley, C. P., Wong, P. Y. K., and McGiff, J. C. (1979): Hypotensive and renovascular actions of 6-keto-prostaglandin E_1, a metabolite of prostacyclin. *Eur. J. Pharmacol.*, 57:273–276.
77. Raz, A., Isakson, P. C., Minkes, M. S., and Needleman, P. (1977): Characterization of a novel metabolic pathway of arachidonate in coronary arteries which generates a potent endogenous coronary vasodilator. *J. Biol. Chem.*, 252:1123–1126.
78. Rose, J. C., Johnson, M., Ramwell, P. W., and Kot, P. A. (1974): Effects of arachidonic acid on systemic arterial pressure, myocardial contractility and platelets in the dog. *Proc. Soc. Exp. Biol. Med.*, 147:652–655.

79. Rubio, R., and Berne, R. M. (1975): Regulation of coronary blood flow. *Prog. in Cardiovasc. Dis.*, 18:105–122.
80. Ryan, M. J., Kraft, E., Sugawara, K., and Zimmerman, B. G. (1977): Influence of prostaglandin precursors and synthesis inhibitors in vascular bed perfused without a pump. *J. Pharmac. Exp. Ther.*, 200:606–613.
81. Saeed Abdel-Halim, M., von Holst, H., Meyerson, B., Sachs, C., and Änggård, E. (1980): Prostaglandin profiles in tissue and blood vessels from human brain. *J. Neurochem.*, 34:1331–1333.
82. Sakabe, T., and Siesjö, B. K. (1979): The effect of indomethacin on the blood flow-metabolism couple in the brain under normal, hypercapnic and hypoxic conditions. *Acta Physiol. Scand.*, 107:283–284.
83. Samuelsson, B., and Wennmalm, Å. (1971): Increased nerve stimulation induced release of noradrenaline from the rabbit heart after inhibition of prostaglandin synthesis. *Acta Physiol. Scand.*, 83:163–168.
84. Schrör, K., Moncada, S., Ubatuba, F. B., and Vane, J. R. (1978): Transformation of arachidonic acid and prostaglandin endoperoxides by the guinea pig heart, formation of RCS and prostacyclin. *Eur. J. Pharmacol.*, 47:103–114.
85. Stjärne, L., (1972): Enhancement by indomethacin of cold-induced hypersecretion of noradrenaline in the rat *in vivo*—by suppression of PGE-mediated feed-back control. *Acta Physiol. Scand.*, 86:388–397.
86. Stjärne, L., and Gripe, K. (1973): Prostaglandin-dependent and -independent feedback control of noradrenaline secretion in vasoconstrictor nerves of normotensive human subjects. A preliminary report. *Naunyn Schmiedeberg's Arch. Pharmacol.*, 280:441–446.
87. Swies, J., Radomski, M., and Gryglewski, R. J. (1979): Angiotensin-induced release of prostacyclin (PGI$_2$) into circulation of anaesthetized cats. *Pharmacol. Res. Commun.*, 11:649–655.
88. Szczeklik, A., Gryglewski, R. J., Nizankowski, R., Musial, J., Pieton, R., and Mruk, J. (1978): Circulatory and anti-platelet effects of intravenous prostacyclin in healthy men. *Pharmacol. Res. Commun.*, 10:545–556.
89. Szczeklik, A., Gryglewski, R. J., Nizankowska, E., Nizankowski, R., and Musial, J. (1978): Pulmonary and anti-platelet effects of intravenous and inhaled prostacyclin in man. *Prostaglandins*, 16:651–660.
90. Weiner, R., Messina, E. J., Rodenburg, J., and Kaley, G. (1977): Indomethacin reduces skeletal muscle vasodilation induced by exercise and ischemia. *Artery*, 3:52–58.
91. Weitzell, R., Steppeler, A., and Starke, K. (1978): Effects of prostaglandin E$_2$, prostaglandin I$_2$ and 6-keto-prostaglandin F$_{1\alpha}$ on adrenergic neurotransmission in the pulmonary artery of the rabbit. *Eur. J. Pharmacol.* 52:137–141.
92. Wennmalm, Å. (1974): Hypertensive effect of the prostaglandin synthesis inhibitor indomethacin. *IRCS*, 2:1099.
93. Wennmalm, Å. (1978): Prostaglandin-mediated inhibition of noradrenaline release: III. Separation of prostaglandins released from stimulated hearts and analysis of their neurosecretion inhibitory capacity. *Prostaglandins*, 15:113–121.
94. Wennmalm, Å. (1978): Prostaglandin-mediated inhibition of noradrenaline release: V. A comparison of the neuroinhibitory effect of three prostaglandins: E$_2$, I$_2$, and 6-keto-PGF$_{1\alpha}$. *Prostaglandins Med.*, 1:49–54.
95. Wennmalm, Å., Eriksson, S., and Wahren, J. (1981): Effect of indomethacin on basal and carbon dioxide stimulated cerebral blood flow in man. *Clin. Physiol.*, 1:227–234.
95a. Wennmalm, Å. (1982): Effect of indomethacin on some cardiovascular reflexes in man. *Acta Physiol. Scand. (in press)*.
95b. Wennmalm, Å., Eriksson, S., Hagenfeldt, L., Law, D., Patrono, C., and Pinca, E. (1982): Effect of prostaglandin synthesis inhibitors on basal and carbon dioxide stimulated cerebral blood flow in man. In: *Advances in Prostaglandin, Thromboxane and Leukotriene Research*, edited by B. Samuelsson and R. Paoletti, Raven Press, New York *(in press)*.
96. Willems, Ch., and van Aken, W. G. (1979): Production of prostacyclin by vascular endothelial cells. *Haemostasis*, 8:266–273.
97. Wong, P. Y. K., McGiff, J. C., Sun, F. F., and Lee, W. H. (1979): 6-keto-prostaglandin E$_1$ inhibits the aggregation of human platelets. *Eur. J. Pharmacol.*, 60:245–248.
98. Wong, P. Y. K., Malik, K. U., Desiderio, D. M., McGiff, J. C. and Sun, F. F. (1980): Hepatic metabolism of prostacyclin (PGI$_2$) in the rabbit: formation of a potent novel inhibitor of platelet aggregation. *Biochem. Biophys. Res. Commun.*, 93:486–494.

99. Yabek, S. M., and Avner, B. P. (1980): Effects of prostacyclin (PGI$_2$) and indomethacin on neonatal lamb mesenteric and renal artery responses to electrical stimulation and norepinephrine. *Prostaglandins*, 19:23–30.

100. Young, H. E., and Sparks, H. V. (1980): Prostaglandin and exercise hyperemia of dog skeletal muscle. *Am. J. Physiol.*, 238:H191–H195.

101. Zimmerman, B. G., Ryan, M. J., Gomer, S., and Kraft, E. (1973): Effect of the prostaglandin synthesis inhibitors indomethacin and eicosa-5,8,11,14-tetraynoic acid on adrenergic responses in dog cutaneous vasculature. *J. Pharmacol. Exp. Ther.*, 187:315–323.

Prostaglandins and the Cardiovascular System,
edited by John A. Oates. Raven Press,
New York © 1982.

Action and Metabolism of Prostaglandins in the Pulmonary Circulation

P. J. Kadowitz, H. L. Lippton, D. B. McNamara,
E. W. Spannhake, and A. L. Hyman

*Departments of Pharmacology and Surgery, Tulane University School of Medicine,
New Orleans, Louisiana 70112*

Arachidonic acid is the precursor of the bisenoic prostaglandins and can be obtained from the diet or by desaturation and chain elongation of the dietary essential fatty acid linoleic acid (10,42,43,117,118,176). Arachidonic acid is transported in a protein bound state and incorporated into phospholipid in cell membranes of all body tissue (146). The presence of arachidonic acid and other long-chain unsaturated fatty acids in extracellular and intracellular membranes permits a more efficient interaction between the cell and its external environment (111,148,177). The C_{20}-polyenoic fatty acids appear necessary for metabolic activities that depend on respiration and oxidative phosphorylation suggesting that arachidonic acid is essential for organisms that utilize oxygen (35,111,148,177). Stimulation of phospholipase by a variety of stimuli promotes the release of arachidonic acid from cell membranes (36,118,179). This is apparently the rate-limiting step that determines in large measure the amount of substrate available for the synthesis of prostaglandins (98,100,142). The cyclooxygenase enzyme complex that converts arachidonic acid to prostaglandins is present in virtually every organ system of the body, but some such as the lung and seminal glands have the greatest capacity to form prostaglandins (22). The 15-hydroxy prostaglandin dehydrogenase (PGDH) enzyme system initiates the breakdown of prostaglandins by catalyzing the oxidation of the hydroxyl group at the C15 position (2,3,101,127–129). The relative metabolic activity of this enzyme complex in the lung determines the extent to which the activity of prostaglandins is limited to the organ alone, as opposed to systemic effects resulting from release of these agents. The pulmonary PGDH activity is high, thus the lung serves importantly as a metabolic organ. Since prostaglandins are readily formed in the lung and released into the systemic circulation, the lung can be viewed as an endocrine organ as well (9,178). The metabolism of prostaglandins is largely limited by the availability of the transport system enabling uptake of PGs from the pulmonary vascular bed into the cells which metabolize these substances (11,12). The pulmonary vascular and airway responses to the PGs appear to be of major physiologic and pathophysiologic importance, since the magnitude of the response to these substances exceeds that of other vasoactive substances in the lung (69). Difficulty in synthesis and characterization of the more active prostanoids and identification of agents that block specifically at critical points in the arachidonic acid cascade have hampered research in experimental animals. Since clinical studies regarding the action of hormones are, at best, incomplete, our present appreciation of their pulmonary effects is based on basic laboratory experiments. It is important to realize that this appreciation is not based on observations executed in man and that much more information is needed to clarify further the clinical role of the prostaglandins in a variety of pulmonary disease states. Moreover, formidable barriers to the clinical investigation of this role are presented by the need for sorting out the complex relationships between the effects of these agents on airway and vascular smooth muscle within the lung.

PATHWAYS OF PROSTAGLANDIN SYNTHESIS AND METABOLISM

The prostaglandins have a cyclopentane ring and 2 adjacent carbon side chains, one of which possesses the carboxyl group at the terminal position. The general pathway of PG synthesis is reasonably well established. The three fatty acid precursors for the PGs are: 8,11,14-eicosatrienoic acid (dihomo-γ-linolenic acid or 20:3), 5,8,11,14-eicosatetraenoic acid (arachidonic acid or 20:4) and 5,8,11,14,17-eicosapentaenoic acid (20:5) (37). These fatty acids can be derived from breakdown of cell membrane phospholipids and from nonesterified fatty acids, plasma triglycerides, and cholestrol esters through the normal enzymatic actions of phospholipase A and other lipolytic pathways (37). The prostaglandins (PGs) designated by the subscript "1" are derived from linolenic acid; those with the subscript "2", from arachidonic acid, and those with the subscript "3" from eicosapentaenoic acid. The bisenoic PGs constitute almost all the body PGs, and their biologic activities have been extensively investigated (69,155). Only a small amount of the monoenoic PGs is present, but some attention has been devoted to these substances (69–71,80). Little, if any, of the 3 series prostaglandin is normally found in the body (130). The amount of eicosapentaenoic acid in the body and the eicosapentaenoic/arachidonic acid ratio can be increased by a diet rich in marine oils (130). In regard to biologic activity the 3 series precursor has bronchoconstrictor activity (103).

The oxidative conversion of C-20 fatty acids to PGs is carried out by multienzyme, membrane-bound complex labeled PG synthetase. Several enzymes are probably involved; the cyclooxygenase is responsible for the formation of the endoperoxide intermediate PGG_2, which has the hydroperoxide group in the 15 position, then to the endoperoxide PGH_2 which has the hydroxyl group in the 15 position. These endoperoxides have marked biologic activity *in vitro*, but are quickly metabolized *in vivo*, so that the magnitude of their direct action on the pulmonary vascular bed does not seem to be great (72,81). Their major importance is their pivotal position as intermediates from which a variety of PGs and non-PGs of varying biologic potency can be derived. Abundant evidence is at hand to indicate that the activity and distribution of the various terminal enzymes, capable of transforming endoperoxides, vary in activity from organ to organ. This enzyme profile determines characteristic responses of an organ system to increased or decreased PG synthesis. In addition, the functional state of the enzyme system within an organ probably varies considerably with the metabolic state of the organ itself. On the other hand, the arachidonic acid released from membrane phospholipids of specifically activated platelets, mastocytoma cells, and leukocytes may be transformed by the lipoxygenase system into an array of non-PG metabolites, including the leukotrienes, that exhibit yet another spectrum of profound biologic activity (15,16,55,126,135,156,157,174,181,183).

Specific terminal enzymes rapidly transform the endoperoxide intermediates into diverse vasoactive products including prostacyclin (PGI_2), thromboxane A_2 (TXA_2), and the primary PGs $PGF_{2\alpha}$, PGE_2, and PGD_2 (PGA_2 and its isomer PGB_2 are dehydration products of PGE_2 and may not be present under physiologic conditions) in the lung (4). The lung also takes up and metabolizes PGs rapidly and selectively, but does not store them. The principal enzyme for pulmonary metabolism of PGs is 15-hydroxy prostaglandin dehydrogenase (PGDH), which catalyzes the oxidation of the hydroxyl group at C15, leading to the formation of a 15-keto-PG, an intermediate in the formation of 13,14-dihydro-15-keto-PG. In one transit through the lung, inactivation of exogenous PGEs is almost complete and inactivation of circulating $PGF_{2\alpha}$ is slightly less, however, PGA_2 is metabolized to a much lesser extent (115). Curiously, the major metabolite of the endoperoxides, PGI_2, is not removed to any substantial extent by the lung (6,73). Metabolism of the PGs in the lung is a function of a selective transport system in the capillary endothelial plasma membrane. Further, this system may function well to regulate systemic plasma levels of PGs under most physiologic states, but it is easily saturated in humans and experimental animals under stressful circumstances (66,96), and intravenously administered PGs readily reach the systemic circulation by exceeding the transport system's capacity.

Of the derivatives of arachidonic acid, PGI_2 is the major vasoactive product formed in vascular tissue (30,79,154). The large expanse of pulmonary vascular endothelium provides the lung with an enormous potential for its production. Although the enzyme is also found in connective tissue, it is not present in platelets, and these formed elements do not produce prostacyclin (119). PGI_2 is a potent pulmonary and systemic vasodilator, and is the only metabolic product of arachidonic acid that dilates the mature pulmonary vascular bed (73,82). This pulmonary vasodilating activity of PGI_2 is not readily apparent under physiologic circumstances because the pulmonary blood vessels have little tone when the animal breathes room air, and the vascular bed has extensive recruiting capacity. The vasodilating capacity in response to PGI_2 is readily demonstrated in pulmonary hypertensive states induced by adenosine diphosphate as seen in Fig. 1 or vasoconstrictor drugs as illustrated in Fig. 2. Furthermore, PGI_2 inhibits intrapulmonary platelet aggregation and disaggregates ADP-induced platelet clumps, both *in vitro* and *in vivo* (73). Recent studies in cats have also demonstrated that PGI_2 has modest bronchodilating activity

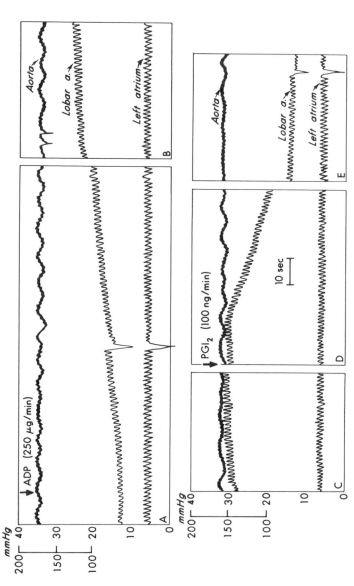

FIG. 1. Tracings from an experiment showing reversal of the pulmonary vascular hypertensive effects of ADP by PGI$_2$ in the intact-chest cat. In panels **A–C**, intralobar infusion of ADP, 250 µg/min, increases lobar arterial (*a*) pressure while having minimal effects on aortic and left atrial pressures. When a steady state pressure was attained in the lobar artery during continuous ADP infusion (panel **D**) PGI$_2$ was infused into the perfused lobar artery. Panel **E** shows that the PGI$_2$ infusion reversed the hypertensive response to ADP which was infused throughout (**A–E**).

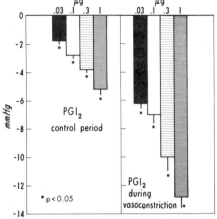

FIG. 2. Decrease in lobar arterial pressure with PGI$_2$. Bar graph illustrating dose-response relationships for PGI$_2$ in the feline pulmonary vascular bed under normal resting conditions (control period, *left panel*) and when vasoconstrictor tone was elevated by infusion of a stable prostaglandin endoperoxide analog (*right panel*). In these studies pulmonary lobar blood flow was maintained constant with a pump and pulmonary vasodilator responses to PGI$_2$ were enhanced when tone in the bed was elevated by the PGH$_2$ analog.

when tone in the airways has been increased (163). Although PGI$_2$ is not metabolized by the pulmonary vascular bed, it is unstable at physiologic pH (31,106). Its activity persists for 3 to 8 min *in vitro* before being hydrolyzed to the stable metabolite, 6-keto-F$_{1\alpha}$ (31). This metabolite has weak pulmonary vasoconstrictor activity and possesses little, if any, other biologic activity (79,82). The stability of this metabolite (6-keto-PGF$_{1\alpha}$), however, does permit it to serve as an indicator of *in vivo* or *in vitro* formation of its unstable parent compound, PGI$_2$ (118). Stable analogs of PGI$_2$ have been synthesized and their pulmonary vascular effects have been reported (72). Since present studies indicate that PGI$_2$ has the capacity to dilate the constricted pulmonary vascular bed, prevent intrapulmonary platelet aggregation induced by adenosine diphosphate, and dilate constricted airways, this agent would appear to have potential clinical application in the treatment of pulmonary hypertensive and thromboembolic diseases. Although sporadic case reports of its use under these circumstances have been reported (186), the clinical uses of this agent are not well documented and much more investigation is needed.

The other major metabolite of the endoperoxide intermediate PGH$_2$ found in the lung is TXA$_2$, the oxane intermediate between PGG$_2$ and thromboxane B$_2$ (TXB$_2$) (56,158). Although TXA$_2$ is a product of the cyclooxygenase pathway, its chemical structure differs somewhat from PGs and is best described as an eicosanoid (56). This substance is approximately ten times as potent as the endoperoxides in inducing platelet aggregation and the platelet release reaction (56). Furthermore, TXA$_2$ is known to be the most potent component of the incompletely defined rabbit aortic contracting substance (RCS) derived from the cyclooxygenase system in platelets and sensitized guinea pig lung (57). Indeed, recent experiments suggest that the potent effects of PG endoperoxides on platelets and isolated vascular smooth muscle may be due to conversion of the endoperoxide intermediate to TXA$_2$ (52). Thus, TXA$_2$ would be expected to elicit severe pulmonary hypertension by directly constricting the pulmonary vascular bed and by mechanically obstructing the microcirculation with platelet aggregates. Although the effects of TXA$_2$ on the pulmonary circulation are uncertain, several PGH$_2$ analogs which are believed to mimic TXA$_2$

have marked pressor activity in the pulmonary vascular bed (81,83,164). Since TXA$_2$ may promote bronchoconstriction by contracting airway smooth muscle, TXA$_2$ could further increase pulmonary vascular pressure by producing alveolar hypoxia. These impressions, however, are based on *in vitro* observations, since the 30 to 60 sec half-life of TXA$_2$ has not permitted a concise demonstration of its *in vivo* effects on the pulmonary circulation under carefully controlled conditions (57,186). Since TXA$_2$ is the major component of RCS released from isolated guinea pig lungs during anaphylactic challenge, mechanical stimulation, and a variety of chemical stimuli (9), it may be an important endogenous pulmonary vasoconstrictor generated under a host of pathologic conditions. Furthermore, the pulmonary vasoconstriction accompanying endotoxic shock, and the pulmonary embolism induced by protamine, thrombin, and collagen is associated with platelet clumping and is inhibited by cyclooxygenase inhibitors such as aspirin and indomethacin (118). Therefore, prostaglandin-like substances detected in arterial blood during endotoxic shock contain TXA$_2$, which could account for a part of the pulmonary hypertensive response (32).

A dynamic balance between the TXA$_2$ formed in the platelet and the PGI$_2$ formed in the inner walls of blood vessels has been suggested as the mechanism preventing adhesion of the platelets to vessel endothelium and eventual thrombosis within the vessel (54). In keeping with this concept, Moncada and co-workers have demonstrated a decreasing ability of concentric layers of blood vessel wall to inhibit platelet clumping on moving from the inner to outer layers (119). This inhibition reflects the distribution of PGI$_2$ biosynthetic capacity, since the greatest synthesis occurs in the endothelial and subendothelial regions (119). The demonstration of greater arterial capacity to produce PGI$_2$ may explain, in part, the increased resistance of arteries to thrombi as compared to veins (160). In addition, lipid peroxides in vascular lesions associated with arteriosclerotic disease can inhibit intramural PGI$_2$ synthesis, but not TXA$_2$ formation by platelets. This may promote platelet aggregation and adhesion to the arteriosclerotic lesion leading to eventual thrombosis (120,121). This interesting yin-yang hypothesis with respect to the TXA$_2$/PGI$_2$ systems leads to a rationale for blocking the TXA$_2$ pathway without affecting PGI$_2$ formation.

In addition to TXA$_2$ and PGI$_2$, primary prostaglandins PGE$_2$, PGF$_{2\alpha}$, and PGD$_2$ are formed from the endoperoxide intermediates in the lung (4). PGF$_{2\alpha}$ is a potent pulmonary vasoconstrictor in most species, but the magnitude of the response varies among species (71,74,84–86). For example, the intact feline pulmonary vascular bed is more responsive than the intact simian lung (72). The segments of the pulmonary vascular bed responding to PGF$_{2\alpha}$ in intact species also vary: in the dog, both the pulmonary veins and upstream vessels participate, but in the swine and lamb, apparently only arterial segments are constricted (71,84–86). PGF$_{2\alpha}$ acts on vascular smooth muscle in vessel walls and not on formed elements because vasoconstrictor effects are similar in intact lungs perfused with dextran or blood (74,84). PGF$_{2\alpha}$ does not aggregate platelets (75). The remarkable pulmonary vasoconstrictor effect of PGF$_{2\alpha}$ is in marked contrast to its almost insignificant effect on systemic arterial pressure or systemic vascular resistance (71,74,84). Comparative pressor responses to the primary PGs, TXB_2, and arachidonic acid in the feline pulmonary vascular bed are illustrated in Fig. 3. $PGF_{2\alpha}$ had marked pressor activity whereas arachidonic acid had the least activity. $PGF_{2\alpha}$ is also a potent bronchoconstrictor in humans and laboratory animals (113,114,165,184). Airway resistance is increased and compliance is decreased in intact paralyzed dogs ventilated at a constant volume and rate (165). The decreased compliance appears to be caused by small airway constriction rather than by pulmonary vascular congestion induced from venous hypertension (165). Additionally, the volume of blood in the pulmonary vascular bed is decreased by infusion of $PGF_{2\alpha}$ (71). $PGF_{2\alpha}$ is largely inactivated in one passage through the lung (87). The importance of intrapulmonary metabolism was well illustrated in experiments in isolated feline lungs (109). In those experiments, the pulmonary vascular pressor response to $PGF_{2\alpha}$ was considerably greater during forward flow than during retrograde flow, presumably because of intrapulmonary metabolism of $PGF_{2\alpha}$. Apparently in this species the pulmonary veins are not as responsive as the arterial segment. Furthermore, the 15-methyl analog of $PGF_2\alpha$, which is not a substrate for the dehydrogenase system, produces about twice the pulmonary vasopressor response as does $PGF_2\alpha$ in experimental animals (88). This analog also causes transient breathlessness in pregnant women (187) and is a potent bronchoconstrictor agent in the dog (166).

The effects of PGE_2 have been extensively investigated in several species and the airway responses have been reported in man (19,85,86,153). PGE_2 causes a

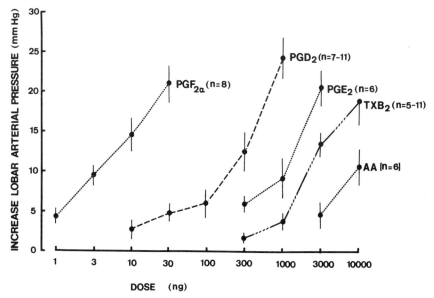

FIG. 3. Dose-response relationships comparing increases in lobar arterial pressure in response to bolus injections of graded doses of $PGF_{2\alpha}$, PGD_2, PGE_2, thromboxane (TX) B_2 and arachidonic acid in the intact-chest cat. The number of animals studied is indicated *(n)* and blood flow to the left lower lobe was held constant with a pump.

mild pulmonary vasoconstrictor response in the dog, and this response is about one-thirtieth of that seen with $PGF_{2\alpha}$ (89). This response to PGE_2 resulted from the direct effect of this agent on vascular smooth muscle and not formed elements in those experiments; other studies have suggested that PGE_2 enhances phase 2 of platelet aggregation induced by adenosine diphosphate, *in vitro* (159). In contrast, a pulmonary vasodilator response to PGE_2 has been shown in isolated perfused calf and fetal goat lungs (20,102,172). The reasons for these divergent responses in adult and fetal experimental animals is not apparent, but may be related to the very high initial tone as well as other factors in fetal lung vessels. This difference seems to have important clinical implications. Since nonsteroidal antiinflammatory drugs (NSAID) cross the placenta freely, they inhibit fetal cyclooxygenase from producing PGE_2 and PGI_2 (21). These PGs promote patency of the fetal ductus arteriosus and decrease pulmonary vascular resistance in the neonate (24,152). Indeed, the syndrome of primary pulmonary hypertension of the newborn is thought to be related to maternal ingestion of NSAID (26,110,150), and a caveat has been issued against the use of NSAID during pregnancy (145). On the other hand, the ability of NSAID to promote closure of the patent ductus arteriosus has been used with varying success rates during the first two weeks of life (44,67).

PGD_2, the other naturally occurring prostaglandin, has vasoconstrictor effects that approach that of $PGF_{2\alpha}$ in some species (90,167,185). In intact dogs, PGD_2 is more active than $PGF_{2\alpha}$ in decreasing dynamic lung compliance, tidal volume, and expiratory air flow and in increasing airway resistance (167,185). Although PGD_2 is an isomer of PGE_2, its pulmonary vascular and bronchial actions are much greater than E_2 and its systemic vasodilator activity is much less (167,185). Moreover, PGD_2 has potent antiaggregating ability *in vitro*, but the effects of this agent on intrapulmonary platelet aggregation are unknown (134). The pulmonary hypertensive effect is presumed to be produced by its direct vasoconstrictor activity, although this has not been studied in intact animals.

In addition to their actions on smooth muscle, prostaglandins have been shown to alter both the release of and response to norepinephrine from sympathetic nerve terminals in the peripheral vascular bed (63,64,107,108). Through such a mechanism, prostaglandins may be involved in the regulation of vasomotor tone in the systemic circulation (107,108). Evidence has accumulated that the pulmonary vascular bed is innervated by the sympathetic nervous system; however, the physiologic function of this extensive innervation in regulating the pulmonary circulation is uncertain (41,91,92,97). It is conceivable that prostaglandins released peripherally and/or by the lung, may affect the release of and response to norepinephrine from adrenergic nerve terminals in pulmonary vessels (93). In turn, prostaglandins may influence vasomotor tone in the pulmonary vascular bed through the modulation of adrenergic neurotransmission.

In contrast to prostaglandin formation by the cyclooxygenase system, arachidonic acid may be metabolized by the lipoxygenase system present in human lung platelets and leukocytes including alveolar macrophages and neutrophils (15,16,55,135,174,181,183). Mammalian lipoxygenases can be classified into several groups according to the product specificity observed when arachidonic acid is used as a substrate. The platelet lipoxygenase metabolizes arachidonic acid to yield 12-hydroperoxy-5,8,10,14-eicosatetraenoic acid (12-HPETE) whereas leukocytes possess the lipoxygenase enzymes which produces 5-HPETE and 15-HPETE (15,135,174,183). The latter metabolites are precursors of a recently characterized group of biologically active substances termed leukotrienes that appear to be potent mediators of immediate and subacute hypersensitivity reactions (157). For example, leukotrienes (LT) C_4 and D_4 are peptide-HETE's containing glutathione and cysteine-glycine, respectively, and have been identified as major constituents of "slow reacting substance" of anaphylaxis (SRS-A) (7,8,104,157). Further identification of LTs has been shown in basophilic leukemia cells (123,139), macrophages (174), eosinophils (46), mastocytoma cells (62), and lungs (124), and it is uncertain if these substances have a general distribution similar to prostaglandins or are limited to organ systems more directly involved in allergic reactions (17). Since SRS-A (LTs) are released from a variety of tissues including skin (53), nasal polyps (95), vascular smooth muscle (105), heart (105), and cat paw (5), speculation has arisen suggesting that LTs may have a broad distribution in mammals (17). These agents are potent contractors of smooth muscle, especially in pulmonary airways, and alter the permeability and tone of the microvasculature in skin and other tissues (27,65). The effects of LTC_4 and LTD_4 on cutaneous vascular smooth muscle and on vascular endothelial cells differ quantitatively: LTD_4 has greater activity in its ability to induce plasma exudation in the skin and LTC_4 is a more potent vasoconstrictor in the cutaneous circulation (140). LTC_4 and LTD_4 on a molar basis are approximately 200-fold to 2,000-fold more potent than histamine in inducing contraction of parenchymal strips of guinea pig lung and are 30-fold to 100-fold more potent than histamine in constriction of segments of guinea pig trachea (28,65). Furthermore, LTC_4 and LTD_4 are at least 1,000-fold more potent than histamine in causing contraction of isolated human bronchi and these effects are not influenced by muscarinic and histamine-1 receptor antagonists, including atropine and mepyramine (27,65). However, the biologic activity of LTs appears to vary among species since isolated guinea pig bronchi and ilea produce significant contraction in the presence of LTC_4 and LTD_4, whereas rabbit bronchial and duodenal strips do not contract to these arachidonic acid metabolites (29,65). Thus, leukotrienes must seriously be considered as possible pathophysiological mediators causing both the bronchospasm and mucosal edema of bronchial asthma in man. In contrast to LTC_4 and LTD_4, LTB_4, particularly the isomer containing a *cis* double bond, is by far the most potent chemotactic factor for human polymorphonuclear leukocytes, whereas LTA_4 and the two dihydroxy HETE epimers are less active in this respect and LTC_4 is essentially inactive (39,47). LTB_4, 5-HETE and 12-HETE enhance migration of neutrophils and eosinophils and increase the intracellular concentrations of cyclic GMP (guanosine 3',5'-cyclic monophosphate) in neutrophils (7,8,27,28,41,47–50,65,93,104). The chemical synthesis of an LT containing cysteine (LTE_4) has been demonstrated and this component of SRS-A has recently been reported to induce an increase in vascular permeability in rat skin, constrict isolated guinea pig

ilea, and produce bronchoconstriction in guinea pigs when administered intravenously (149,189). Neutrophils have been shown to aggregate in response to a number
of substances including arachidonic acid, lanthanum complement (C5a), f-met-
leuphenylalanine, and A23187, a calcium ionophore; however, unlike platelets,
this aggregatory response appears to be due to the formation of lipoxygenase products (14,25,33,40,60,116,136,137). Since neutrophil aggregation may depend on
the lipoxygenase activity present in leukocytes, pulmonary leukostasis may result
from embolization of neutrophils primarily aggregated in the venous circulation by
lipoxygenase products (25). Such a mechanism may be involved in the pulmonary
vasoconstriction that accompanies endotoxic shock. The formation of neutrophil
aggregates during complement activation may be responsible for emboli formation
that may play a role in this hypertensive response. Thus, leukocytes, similar to
thrombocytes, possess enzymes that convert arachidonic acid to products that may
promote the formation of emboli by white blood cells. Present knowledge may
indicate that the relative rate of conversion of arachidonic acid to cyclooxygenase
and lipoxygenase products in the lung may be crucial in determining the pulmonary
response to any given stimulus. The lipoxygenase system has been the subject of
recent reviews (17,51,156,157). Present evidence suggests that several lipoxygenase
derivatives may produce feedback inhibition of enzyme systems and, thus, serve a
potential regulatory role in the metabolism of arachidonic acid. 12-HETE produced
by platelets inhibits prostacyclin synthetase in vascular endothelium and can decrease the formation of PGI_2 in the cyclooxygenase pathway, whereas 15-HETE
produced by neutrophils inhibits 5-lipoxygenase in leukocytes and may influence
the intracellular formation of SRS-A (121,175). SRS-A has been shown to release
thromboxane from perfused guinea pig lung, a property which is also shown by
rabbit aorta contracting substance-releasing factors (RCS-RF1), a peptide released
from guinea pig lungs during anaphylaxis (58,133,143,190). Recently, a novel
substance found in peritoneal anaphylactic fluid has been reported to release arachidonic acid and thromboxane from guinea pig lung (190). Further study into the
interrelationship between prostaglandins, thromboxanes, and leukotrienes in immediate hypersensitivity may indicate that an arachidonic acid metabolite or its
derivative might be of potential therapeutic value in the treatment of inflammatory
processes and allergic responses such as anaphylaxia and asthma. Since lipoxygenase derivatives are mediators of both cellular and humoral components of human
allergic reactions and possess potent contractile and vasoactive components, they
may have great importance in hypersensitivity states. At present, no data relating
to the effect of these derivatives of the lipoxygenase pathway on the pulmonary
circulation in the intact animal are available. Furthermore, specific inhibitors of the
platelet lipoxygenase system have only recently been reported; however, the actions
of these substances *in vivo* are uncertain (170,182,192). NSAID (aspirin, indomethacin), which block cyclooxygenase, have been shown not to block the lipoxygenase pathway and may actually enhance this process (15,59,161). In addition
to NSAID, corticosteroids have been shown to inhibit both thrombocyte and granulocyte aggregations suggesting that these substances may prove to be efficacious

in the treatment of pulmonary disorders such as adult respiratory distress syndrome (ARDS) and thromboembolism (61,132,141). The physiologic states under which these agents act in the intact pulmonary circulation are not clear since, in NSAID-treated animals, arachidonic acid, injected in even large doses, causes no demonstrable effect on the pulmonary circulation or pulmonary airways. The effects of arachidonic acid before and after administration of indomethacin are illustrated in Fig. 4. In the dog, intravenous injections of arachidonic acid increase transpulmonary and pulmonary arterial pressure and decrease aortic pressure. It is evident in Fig. 4 that pulmonary responses to large doses of arachidonic acid are completely blocked by indomethacin. This experiment may indicate that the lipoxygenase pathway is not active under resting conditions in the lung since indomethacin should shunt more arachidonic acid into this pathway (156).

Relatively speaking, little, if any, monoenoic PGs are present in the body, and their metabolic derivatives play a minor role in maintaining the physiologic state (23,75). However, the monoenoic derivatives have important differences from the biosenoic PGs. The pulmonary vasoconstrictor response to dihomo-γ-linolenic acid is only about one-tenth the response to arachidonic acid (70,191). The difference may, in part, be related to differences in specificity of the cyclooxygenase, but it probably reflects the lesser pressor potency of $PGF_1\alpha$ and TXA_1 as compared to $PGF_{2\alpha}$ and TXA_2, and the marked dilator effect of PGE_1 as compared to the modest constrictor effect of PGE_2. Furthermore, TXA_1, if formed, probably has little vasopressor activity (131), whereas, TXA_2 has a powerful vasoconstrictor effect, as

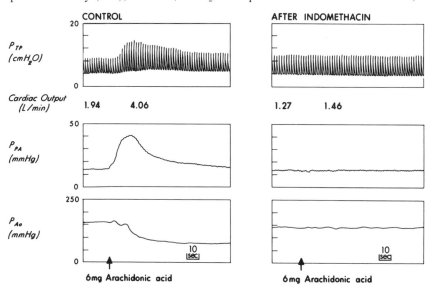

FIG. 4. Records from an experiment illustrating the effects of arachidonic acid (6 mg) on transpulmonary pressure P_{TP}, mean pulmonary arterial pressure P_{PA}, and mean aortic pressure P_{Ao} before and after indomethacin, 2.5 mg/kg in the intact-chest dog. Arachidonic acid was injected rapidly into the superior vena cava. Cardiac output was measured at the peak of the increase in P_{PA} by the thermodilution technique.

well as platelet-aggregating activity. Of clinical significance is one metabolic product of dihomo-γ-linolenic acid, PGE_1. This derivative is a potent vasodilator in the systemic and pulmonary beds and inhibits platelet aggregation (34,71,84). It is about one-third as potent as PGI_2 (106). About 95% of PGE_1 is metabolized in one passage through the lung, so that in smaller doses the pulmonary vasodilator effect of intravenous injections is more apparent than the systemic effect (69). This may be a possible advantage over PGI_2, which is not metabolized in the lung. In large doses, however, the 15-PGDH enzyme is saturated and the systemic hypotensive effects of PGE_1 are readily observed (69). PGE_1, like PGI_2, will disaggregate ADP-induced platelet clumping and reverse the pulmonary hypertensive response to ADP (34,76). PGE_1 has been used successfully to manage persistent pulmonary hypertension following corrective surgery for congenital heart disease (138). Prostaglandin 6-keto-E_1 is a chemically stable substance which has many of the biologic properties of PGE_1 and PGI_2 and may be useful in the treatment of pulmonary hypertensive and thromboembolic disorders (77,144). This substance can be formed in the liver by the 9-hydroxy-prostaglandin dehydrogenase pathway and has bronchodilator activity (168,193).

PROSTAGLANDINS IN HEALTH AND DISEASE

The continuous process of formation, metabolism, and release of PGs in the lung is delicately balanced in the normal physiologic state. This balance appears to be easily disturbed by an enormous variety of physiologic and pathologic stimuli to which the lung is subjected. The factors involved in these metabolic alterations and their relation to pathophysiologic processes in the lung are currently under investigation to learn the extent of the role of PGs in pulmonary disease and to devise new therapeutic approaches. Investigation of the relation of PGs to pathogenic mechanisms is complex, and data are often difficult to interpret. Identification of PGs in the venous effluent or in the tissues of an organ involved in a disease process does not establish causality. For example, Prinzmetal's variant angina has been thought to be due to increased TXA_2 production causing coronary arterial spasm and intraarterial platelet aggregation. Indeed, the levels of TXB_2 in coronary sinus blood are elevated markedly in variant angina (68,147). However, after suppression of TXA_2 formation with low-dose aspirin, or indomethacin and dipyrimadole, the frequency, severity, and duration of angina was unchanged, even though coronary sinus blood TXB_2 levels remained very low (112,147). The multiplicity of causes of coronary arterial spasm was suggested by the observation that relief of symptoms was afforded to only one in six patients with variant angina by infusions of PGI_2 (112). In bronchial asthma and other allergic states, PG metabolism may not be a cardinal factor since the clinical status of these patients is not appreciably improved by administration of indomethacin (162). If, in clinical practice, NSAID shift the metabolism of arachidonic acid away from the cyclooxygenase-PG cascade to the lipoxygenase-leukotriene pathway, one may suspect that these agents would aggravate such allergic states. The interesting but unusual groups of patients in whom asthma is provoked by aspirin may be an example of the lipoxygenase (leukotriene) effect, or of the response to removal of bronchodilator PGE_2, or both. A relationship, however, has not been documented. The hypoxic pulmonary vasoconstrictor effect is not PG-dependent, since NSAID do not inhibit the response (171,173,188). On the contrary, the response has occasionally been enhanced (171,173,188), suggesting that a vasodilator PG is normally generated in the lung to partly offset the vasoconstriction.

The role of PGs in the function of pulmonary circulation remains unclear. At present, their major role seems to be that of a mediator or modulator of physiologic or pharmacologic responses, although evidence has accumulated that the lung is maintained in a dilated state by continuous formation of a dilator PG (94). In most species, the major product of arachidonic metabolism in the pulmonary circulation is the vasodilator and platelet inhibitor, PGI_2. This metabolic product contributes to maintenance of the normal vasodilated state of the lung vessels. These vessels constrict when PGI_2 formation is blocked by NSAID. Moreover, PGI_2 may modulate pulmonary vasoconstrictor responses to other agents (1,171,173,180). Other studies have indicated that the vasodilator response to bradykinin (125) and to hydralazine (151) is mediated by vasodilator prostaglandins. However, this dilating and modulating effect may not be universal since vascular tone in the cat lung, at least, is not affected by NSAID. On the other hand, arachidonic acid, when released from cell membranes in very large quantities may, through its TXA_2 derivative, act as a vasoconstrictor. This is suggested by recent experiments which showed that as the arachidonic acid substrate is increased, it exceeds the level of saturation of PGI_2 synthetase but not that of TXA_2 synthetase (158). Thus, at low doses arachidonic acid causes vasodilation, but at higher doses, the net effect is vasoconstriction (78,169). A biochemical mechanism for the divergent responses to arachidonic acid is suggested by recent studies in our laboratory. A typical radiochromatographic scan obtained following thin-layer chromatography of the products of incubation of $(1\text{-}^{14}C)$ PGH_2 with cat lung microsomes is shown in Fig. 5. The endoperoxide metabolites were identified by co-migration with authentic PG standards. A characteristic pattern of three major peaks can be seen (Fig. 5). The two more polar peaks co-chromatographed with standard TXB_2 and 6-keto-$PGF_{1\alpha}$ the stable breakdown products of TXA_2 and PGI_2, respectively. The fastest running peak, which moved slightly behind the compound DL-12-hydroxystearic acid, was 12L-hydroxyl-5,8,10-hepadecatrienoic acid (HHT), formed by the action of thromboxane synthetase. TXB_2 and 6-keto-$PGF_1z\alpha$ were not found in the incubation mixture of PGH_2 with heat-inactivated microsomes (Fig. 5). Instead PGH_2 appeared to undergo decomposition to PGD_2, PGE_2, and $PGF_{2\alpha}$. The TXB_2 peak was abolished and HHT formation was lowered in the presence of 20 mM imidazole (Fig. 5), an inhibitor of thromboxane synthetase. Addition of 10 mM tranylcypromine, an inhibitor of prostacyclin synthetase, to an incubation mixture resulted in the disappearance of 6-keto-$PGF_{1\alpha}$, as well as a decrease in the production of both TXB_2 and HHT (Fig. 5). The effects of varying PGH_2 concentration on the formation of TXB_2 and 6-keto-$PGF_{1\alpha}$ are illustrated in Fig. 6. A hyperbolic curve was observed

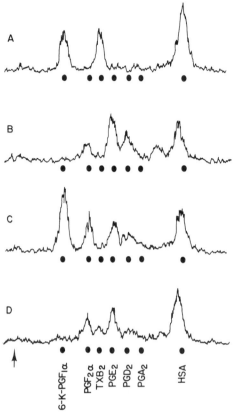

FIG. 5. Radiochromatogram of the products isolated from incubation of 5 μM PGH$_2$ with 300 μg microsomal protein from cat lung in 100 μl 0.1 M potassium phosphate buffer, pH 7.4, for 2 min at 37°C. **A:** Cat lung microsomes; TXB$_2$ and 6-keto-PGF$_{1\alpha}$ conversion 23.4% and 17.2%, respectively. **B:** Microsomes boiled for 10 min. **C:** Microsomes + 20 mM imidazole. **D:** Microsomes + 10 mM tranylcypromine. Migration of authentic PG standards are indicated. HSA denotes DL-12-hydroxy-stearic acid. The *arrow* indicates the origin.

for the production of 6-keto-PGF$_{1\alpha}$ and prostacyclin synthetase became saturated with PGH$_2$ at the substrate concentration of about 60 μM. TXB$_2$ production increased linearly with increasing PGH$_2$ concentration reaching saturation only after the substrate concentration of 100 μM. More TXB$_2$ was formed than 6-keto-PGF$_{1\alpha}$ except at concentrations of PGH$_2$ below 10 μM. The maximum formation of TXB$_2$ was about seven times more than that of 6-keto-PGF$_{1\alpha}$ after saturation of both enzymes with substrate. These biochemical studies show that metabolism of PGH$_2$ varies depending on substrate availability. Prostacyclin synthetase became saturated at a lower substrate concentration than thromboxane synthetase, and thromboxane biosynthesis dominated the metabolism of the endoperoxide except at low PGH$_2$ concentration (10 μM) where prostacyclin formation occurred to a similar extent. Our studies show that arachidonic acid, when delivered at high concentration, causes increased pulmonary arterial pressure and pulmonary vascular resistance in the

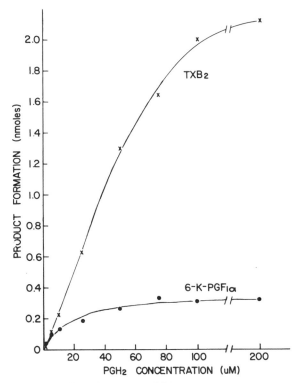

FIG. 6. Graph showing the effect of increasing PGH$_2$ concentration on product formation by cat lung microsomes. Incubation conditions as in Fig. 5. Amount of product was calculated from area under peak on the radiochromatogram.

intact-chest cat, whereas vasodilation can occur at lower doses and with low infusion rates of the precursor acid. Our results offer a possible explanation for these divergent responses. Administration of high concentrations of arachidonic acid may result in production of large amounts of PGH$_2$, leading to the predominant formation of TXA$_2$ relative to PGI$_2$, with subsequent pulmonary vasoconstriction. However, at low concentrations of PGH$_2$, which could occur at lower doses or infusion rates of arachidonic acid, PGI$_2$ production may be equivalent to or slightly less than TXA$_2$. Consequently, due to the longer half-life of PGI$_2$ (5 min versus 30 sec for TXA$_2$), pulmonary vasodilation could result (158). TXA$_2$ and the primary PGs may both contribute to this constriction.

Prostaglandins play a relatively small role in the therapy of lung diseases. PGE$_1$ and PGI$_2$ can retard closure of the patent ductus arteriosus, and PGE$_1$ has been used in congenital cardiac lesions causing pulmonary hypoperfusion (152). PGE$_1$ has also been used effectively in infants with pulmonary hypertension which persists postoperatively after correction of congenital cardiac defects. Many physicians have successfully used pharmacologic dilators such as the readily available nitroprusside and alpha-adrenergic antagonists with equal success. A major thrust of research in prostaglandins is in the development of clinically applicable blocking agents, selective enough to inhibit specific enzymes along the metabolic cascade of arachidonic acid. Although the NSAID are available, they block the conversion of arachidonic acid to both the constrictor TXA_2 and primary PGs by the cyclooxygenase pathway and the dilator, PGI_2 (118). Furthermore, they tend to shift arachidonic acid metabolism to the leukotriene pathway (55). Corticosteroids also inhibit PG synthesis nonselectively, primarily by inhibiting the release of arachidonic acid (38). Local anesthetics, tetracaine and procaine, inhibit phospholipase from releasing arachidonic acid as well (99). *In vitro* selective inhibition of PGI_2 formation is readily produced by 15-hydroperoxy arachidonic acid, which does not affect other metabolites of the endoperoxides (18). The selective ability of this agent to alter arachidonic acid metabolism in the intact pulmonary circulation has not been reported. Moreover, the imidazoles selectively inhibit TXA_2 formation from the endoperoxides *in vitro* (122,158). The effect of this group of agents *in vivo* is unclear. On the other hand, PG metabolism can be retarded by blocking uptake transport mechanisms in vascular endothelium. Probenecid and bromcresol green are active in the lung (13). The diuretic, furosemide, has been reported to increase the release of arachidonic acid and thereby increase production of the naturetic PG, PGE_2 (45), and perhaps PGI_2.

In summary, this review indicates that the products of arachidonic acid metabolism via the cyclooxygenase and lipoxygenase pathways have a remarkable spectrum of biologic activity. An appreciation of this diversity is fundamental to the deductions that can be made from studies employing general inhibitors of the cyclooxygenase and lipoxygenase pathways, and to considerations of any role of these highly active products in the pathogenesis and treatment of pulmonary disease.

ACKNOWLEDGEMENTS

This work was supported in part by NIH grants HL11802, HL15580, HL18070, and HL22945.

REFERENCES

1. Anderson, W. H., Krzanowski, J. J., Polson, J. B. and Szentivanyi, A. (1980): Prostaglandins as mediators of tachyphylaxis to histamine in canine tracheal smooth muscle. *Adv. Prostaglandin Thromboxane Res.*, 7:995.
2. Anggard, E. and Samuelsson, B. (1966): Purification and properties of a 15-hydroxy prostaglandin dehyrogenase from swine lung. *Arkh. Kemi*, 25:293.
3. Anggard, E. (1971): Studies on the analysis and metabolism of the prostaglandins. *Ann. N.Y. Acad. Sci.*, 180:200.
4. Anggard, E. and Samuelsson, B. (1965): Biosynthesis of prostaglandin from arachidonic acid in guinea pig lung. *J. Biol. Chem.*, 240:2518.
5. Anggard, E., Bergqvist, U., Hogberg, B., Johansson, K., Thon, I.-L. and Uvnas, B. (1963): Biologically active principles occurring on histamine release from cat paw, guinea pig lung and isolated rat mast cells. *Acta Physiol. Scand.*, 59:97.
6. Armstrong, J. M., Lattimer, N., Moncada, S. and Vane, J. R. (1978): Comparison of the vasodepressor effects of prostacyclin and 6-oxo-prostaglandin F_1 alpha with those of prostaglandin E_2 in rats and rabbits. *Br. J. Pharmacol.*, 62:125.

7. Bach, M. K., Brashler, J. R., Hammarstrom, S. and Samuelsson, B. (1980): Identfication of leukotriene C as a major component of slow reacting substance from rat mononuclear cells. *J. Immunol.*, 125:115.
8. Bach, M. K., Brashler, J. R., Hammarstrom, S., and Samuelsson, B. (1980): Identification of a component of rat mononuclear cell SRS as leukotriene D. *Biochem. Biophys. Res. Commun.*, 93:1121.
9. Bahlke, Y. S. and Vane, J. R. (1974): Pharmacokinetic function of the pulmonary circulation. *Physiol. Rev.*, 54:1007.
10. Bergstrom, S., Danielson, H. and Samuelsson, B. (1964): The enzymatic formation of prostaglandin E_2 from arachidonic acid. Prostaglandins and related factors. *Biochim. Biophys. Acta*, 90:207.
11. Bito, L. Z., Barvody, R. A. and Reitz, M. E. (1977): Dependence of pulmonary prostaglandin metabolism on carrier-mediated processes. *Am. J. Physiol.*, 232:E382.
12. Bito, LZ. (1972): Accumulation and apparent active transport of PGs by some rabbit tissue *in vitro. J. Physiol. (London)* 221:371.
13. Bito, L. Z. and Baroody, R. A. (1975): Inhibition of pulmonary prostaglandin metabolism by inhibitors of prostaglandin biotransport (probenemil and bromcresal green). *Prostaglandins*, 10:633.
14. Bokoch, G. M. and Reed, P. W. (1980): Stimulation of arachidonic acid metabolism in the polymorphonuclear leukocyte by an N-formylated peptide. *J. Biol. Chem.*, 255:10223.
15. Borgeat, P., Hamberg, M. and Samuelsson, B. (1976): Transformation of arachidonic acid and homo-γ-linolenic acid by rabbit polymorphonuclear leukocytes. Monohydroxy acids from novel lipoxygenases. *J. Biol. Chem.*, 251:7816.
16. Borgeat, P. and Samuelsson, B. (1979): Arachidonic acid metabolism in polymorphonuclear leukocytes: effects of ionophore A23187. *Proc. Natl. Acad. Sci. USA*, 76:2148.
17. Borgeat, P. and Sirois, P. (1981): Leukotrienes: A major step in the understanding of immediate hypersensitivity reactions *J. Med. Chem.*, 24:121.
18. Bunting, S., Gryglewski, R., Moncada, S. and Vane, J. R. (1976): Arterial walls generate from prostaglandin endoperoxides a substance (PGX) which relaxes strips of mesenteric and coeliac arteries and inhibits platelet aggregation. *Prostaglandins*, 12:897.
19. Carlson, L. A., Ekelund, L. G. and Oro, L. (1970): Clinical metabolic and cardiovascular effects of different prostaglandins in man. *Acta Med. Scand.*, 188:553.
20. Cassin, S., Tyler, T. and Wallis, R. (1975): The effects of prostaglandin E on fetal pulmonary vascular resistance. *Proc. Soc. Exp. Biol. Med.*, 148:584.
21. Cassin, S. (1980): Role of prostaglandins and thromboxanes in the control of pulmonary circulation in the fetus and newborn. *Semin. Perinatol.* 4:101.
22. Christ, E. J., and VanDorp, D. A. (1972): Comparative aspects of prostaglandins. *Adv. Biosc.*, 9:35.
23. Christ, E. J. and Van Dorp, D. A. (1973): Comparative aspects of prostaglandin biosynthesis in animal tissue. *Adv. Biosci., Suppl.*, 9:35.
24. Coceani, F. and Olley, P. M. (1973): The response of the ductus arteriosus to prostaglandins. *Can. J. Physiol. Pharmacol.*, 51:200.
25. Craddock, P. R. Hammerschmidt, D., White, J. G., Dalmasso, A. P. and Jacob, H. S. (1977): Complement (C5a)-induced granulocyte aggregation *in vitro. J. Clin. Invest.*, 60:260.
26. Csaba, I. F., Sulyok, E. and Ertl, T. (1978): Relationship of maternal treatment with indomethacin to persistance of fetal circulation syndrome. *J. Pediatr.*, 92:484.
27. Dahlen, S.-E., Hedqvist, P., Hammerstrom, S. and Samuelsson, B. (1980): Leukotrienes are potent constrictors of human bronchi. *Nature*, 288:484.
28. Drazen, J. M., Austen, K. F. and Lewis, R. A. (1980): Comparative airway and vascular activities of leukotrienes C-1 and D *in vivo* and *in vitro. Proc. Natl. Acad. Sci. USA*, 77:4354.
29. Drazen, J. M., Lewis, R. A., Wasserman, S. I., Orange, R. P. and Austen, K. F. (1979): Differential effects of a partially purified preparation of slow-reacting substance of anaphylaxis on guinea pig trachea spirals and parenchymal strips. *J. Clin. Invest.*, 63:1.
30. Dusting, G. J., Moncada, S., Mullane, K. M. and Vane, J. R. (1978): Biotransformation of arachidonic acid in the circulation of the dog. *Br. J. Pharmacol.*, 63:359.
31. Dusting, G. J., Moncada, S. and Vane, J. R. (1977): Prostacyclin (PGX) is the endogenous metabolite responsible for relaxation of coronary arteries induced by arachidonic acid. *Prostaglandins*, 13:3.
32. Dusting, G. J., Moncada, S. and Vane, J. R. (1979): Prostaglandins, their intermediates and precursors: cardiovascular actions and regulatory roles in normal and abnormal circulatory systems. *Prog. Cardiovas. Dis.*, 21:405.

33. Dutilh, C. E., Haddeman, E., Jouvenaz, G. H., TenHoor, F. and Nugteren, D. H. (1979): Study of the two pathways for arachidonate oxygenation in blood platelets. *Lipids*, 14:241.
34. Emmons, P. R., Hampton, J. R., Harrison, M. J. C., Honour, A. J. and Mitchell, J. R. A. (1967): Effect of prostaglandin E₁ on platelet behavior *in vitro* and *in vivo*. *Br. Med. J.*, 2:468.
35. Erwin, J. and Bloch, K. (1963): Polyunsaturated fatty acids in some photosynthetic microorganisms. *Biochem. Z.*, 338:496.
36. Flower, R. J. and Blackwell, G. J. (1976): The importance of phospholipase-A₂ in prostaglandin biosynthesis. *Biochem. Pharmacol.*, 25:285.
37. Flower, R. J. and Vane, J. R. (1974): Inhibition of prostaglandin biosynthesis. *Biochem. Pharmacol.*, 23:1439.
38. Flower, R. J. (1974): Drugs which inhibit prostaglandin biosynthesis. *Pharmacol. Rev.*, 26:33.
39. Ford-Hutchinson, A. W., Bray, M. A., Cunningham, F. M., Davidson, E. M. and Smith, M. J. H. (1981): Isomers of leukotriene B₄ possess different biological potencies. *Prostaglandins*, 21:143.
40. Ford-Hutchinson, A. W., Bray, M. A. and Smith, M. J. H. (1979): The aggregation of rat neutrophils by arachidonic acid: a possible bioassay for lipoxygenase activity. *J. Pharm. Pharmacol.*, 31:868.
41. Fox, B., Bull, T. B. and Guz, A. (1980): Innervation of alveolar walls in the human lung: An electron microscopic study. *J. Anat.*, 131:683.
42. Friedman, Z., Marks, K. H., Maisels, M. J., Thorson, R. and Naeye, R. (1978): Effect of parenteral fat emulsion on the pulmonary and reticuloendothelial systems in the newborn infant. *Pediatr.*, 61:694.
43. Friedman, Z., Danon, A., Stahlman, M. T. and Oates, J. A. (1976): Rapid onset of essential fatty acid deficiency in the newborn. *Pediatr.*, 58:640.
44. Friedman, W. F., Hirshklau, M. J., Printz, M. P., Pitlick, P. T., and Kirkpatrick, S. E. (1976): Pharmacological closure of the patent ductus arteriosus in premature infant. *N. Engl. J. Med.*, 295:526.
45. Gerber, J. G. and Nies, A. S. (1980): Furosemide-induced renal vasodilation: The role of the release of arachidonic acid. In: *Advances in Prostaglandin and Thromboxane Research*. Vol. 7, edited by B. Samuelsson, P. W. Ramwell, and R. Paoletti. Raven Press, New York.
46. Goetzl, E. J., Weller, P. F. and Sun, F. F. (1980): The regulation of human eosinophil function by endogenous mono-hydroxy-eicosatetraenoic acids. *J. Immunol.*, 124:926.
47. Goetzl, E. J. and Pickett, W. C. (1982): The human PMN leukocyte chemotactic activity of complex hydroxy-eicosatetraenoic acids (HETEs). *J. Immunol. (in press).*
48. Goetzl, E. J., Woods, J. M. and Gorman, R. R. (1977): Stimulation of human eosinophil and neutrophil polymorphonuclear leukocyte chemotaxis and random migration by 12-L-hydroxy-5,8,10,14-eiosatetraenoic acid. *J. Clin. Invest.*, 59:179.
49. Goetzl, E. J. (1982): In: *The Eosinophil: Chemical, Biochemical and Functional Aspects*. Edited by A. Mahmoud and K. F. Austen, Grune and Stratton, New York, *in press*.
50. Goetzl, E. J., Brash, A. R., Oates, J. A. and Hubbard, W. C. (1979): Functional determinants of the monohydroxy eicosatetraenoic acids (HETEs) which stimulate human neutrophil (N) and eosinophil (E) chemotaxis. *Fed. Proc.*, 38:4539A.
51. Goetzl, E. J. (1980): Mediators of immediate hypersensitivity derived from arachidonic acid. *N. Engl. J. Med.*, 303:822.
52. Gorman, R. R., Fitzpatrick, F. A. and Miller, O. V. (1978): Reciprocal regulation of human platelet cAMP levels by thromboxane A₂ and prostacyclin (PGI₂). In: *Advances in Cyclic Nucleotide Research*. Vol. 9, edited by W. J. George, L. J. Ignarro, P. Greengard, and G. A. Robison, Raven Press, New York.
53. Greaves, M. W., Yamamoto, S. and Fairley, V. M. (1972): IgE-mediated hypersensitivity in human skin studied using a new *in vitro* method. *Immunol.*, 23:239.
54. Gryglewski, R. J., Bunting, S., Moncada, S., Flower, R. J. and Vane, J. R. (1976): Arterial walls are protected against deposition of platelet thrombi by a substance (PGX) which they make from PG endoperoxides. *Prostaglandins*, 12:685.
55. Hamberg, M. and Samuelsson, B. (1974): Prostaglandin endoperoxides. Novel transformations of arachidonic acid in human platelets. *Proc. Natl. Acad. Sci. USA*, 71:3400.
56. Hamberg, M., Svensson, Y. and Samuelsson, B. (1975): Thromboxanes: A new group of biologically active compounds derived from prostaglandin endoperoxides. *Natl. Acad. Sci. USA*, 72:2994.
57. Hamberg, M., Svensson, Y. and Samuelsson, B. (1976): Novel transformation of prostaglandin endoperoxides: Formation of thromboxanes. In: *Advances in Prostaglandin and Thromboxane Research*. Vol. 1, edited by B. Samuelsson and R. Paoletti, p. 19. Raven Press, New York.

58. Hamberg, M., Svensson, J. and Samuelsson, B. (1975): Thromboxanes: A new group of biologically active compounds derived from prostaglandin endoperoxides. *Proc. Natl. Acad. Sci. USA*, 72:2994.
59. Hamberg, M., Svensson, J. and Samuelsson, B. (1974): Prostaglandin endoperoxides. A new concept concerning the mode of action and release of prostaglandins. *Proc. Natl. Acad. Sci. USA*, 71:3824.
60. Hammerschmidt, D. E., Harris, P. D., Wayland, J. H., Craddock, P. R., and Jacob, H. S. (1981) Complement-induced granulocyte aggregation *in vivo*. *Am. J. Pathol.* 102:146.
61. Hammerschmidt, D. E., White, J. G., Craddock, P. R. and Jacob, H. S. (1979): Corticosteroids inhibit complement-induced granulocyte aggregation. *J. Clin. Invest.*, 63:798.
62. Hammarstrom, S., Murphy, R. C., Samuelsson, B., Clark, D. A., Mioskowski, C., and Corey, E. J. (1979): Structure of leukotriene C. Identification of the amino acid part. *Biochem. Biophys. Res. Commun.*, 91:1266.
63. Hedqvist, P. and Brundin, J. (1969): Inhibition by prostaglandin E_1 of noradrenaline release and of effector response to nerve stimulation in the cat spleen. *Life Sci.*, 8:389.
64. Hedqvist, P. (1977): Basic methods of prostaglandin action on autonomic neurotransmission. *Ann. Rev. Pharmacol. Toxicol.*, 17:259.
65. Hedqvist, P. Dahlen, S.-E., Gustafsson, L., Hammerstrom, S. and Samuelsson, B. (1980): Biological profile of leukotriene C_4 and D_4. *Acta Physiol. Scand.*, 110:331.
66. Hertelendy, F., Woods, R. and Jaffe, B. M. (1973): PGE levels in blood during labor. *Prostaglandins*, 3:223.
67. Heymann, M. A., Rudolph, A. M. and Silverman, N. H. (1976): Closure of the ductus arteriosus in premature infants by inhibition of PG synthesis. *N. Engl. J. Med.*, 295:530.
68. Hirsch, P. D., Hillis, L. D., Campbell, W. B., Firth, B. G. and Willerson, J. T. (1980): Transcardiac thromboxane concentrations in patients with and without ischemic heart disease. *Circulation*, 22(III):310.
69. Hyman, A. L., Spannhake, E. W. and Kadowitz, P. J. (1978): Prostaglandins and the lung. *Am. Rev. Resp. Dis.*, 117:111.
70. Hyman, A. L., Spannhake, E. W., Chapnick, B. M., McNamara, D. B., Mathe, A. A. and Kadowitz, P. J. (1978): Effect of dihomo-γ-linolenic acid on the canine pulmonary vascular bed. *Am. J. Physiol.*, 234(2):H133.
71. Hyman, A. L. (1969): The active responses of the pulmonary veins in intact dogs to prostaglandins $F_{2\alpha}$ and E_1. *J. Pharmacol. Exp. Ther.*, 165:267.
72. Hyman A. L., Kadowitz, P. J., Lands, W. E. M., Crawford, C. G., Fried, J. and Barton, J. (1978): Unusual pulmonary vasodilator activity of a novel prostacyclin analog: comparison with endoperoxides and prostanoids. *Proc. Natl. Acad. Sci. USA*, 12:5711.
73. Hyman, A. L. and Kadowitz, P. J. (1979): Pulmonary vasodilator activity of prostacyclin (PGI_2) in the cat. *Circ. Res.*, 42:404.
74. Hyman, A. L., Chapnick, B. M., Kadowitz, P. J., Lands, W. E. M., Crawford, C. G., Fried, J. and Barton, J. (1977): Unusual pulmonary vasodilator activity of 13,14-dehydroprostacyclin methyl ester. Comparison with endoperoxides and other prostanoids. *Proc. Natl. Acad. Sci. USA*, 12:5711.
75. Hyman, A. L., Spannhake, E. W., Chapnick, B. M., McNamara, D. B., Mathe, A. A. and Kadowitz, P. J. (1978): Effect of dihomo-γ-linolenic acid on the canine pulmonary vascular bed. *Am. J. Physiol.*, 234:H133.
76. Hyman, A. L., Woolverton, W. C., Pennington, D. G. and Jaques, W. E. (1971): Pulmonary vascular responses to adenosine phosphate. *J. Pharmacol. Exp. Ther.*, 178:549.
77. Hyman, A. L. and Kadowitz, P. J. (1980): Vasodilator actions of prostaglandin 6-keto-PGE_1 in the pulmonary vascular bed. *J. Pharmacol. Exp. Ther.*, 213:468.
78. Hyman, A. L., Spannhake, E. W. and Kadowitz, P. J. (1980): Divergent actions of arachidonic acid in the feline pulmonary bed. *Am. J. Physiol.*, 239:1140.
79. Johnson, R. A., Morton, D. R., Kinner, J. H., Gorman, R. R., McGuire, J. C., Sun, F. F., Whittaker, N., Bunting, S., Salmon, J., Moncada, S. and Vane, J. R. (1976): The chemical structure of prostaglandin X (prostacyclin). *Prostaglandins*, 12:915.
80. Kadowitz, P. J., Joiner, P. D. and Hyman, A. L. (1975): Physiological and pharmacological roles of prostaglandins. *Ann. Rev. Pharmacol.*, 15:285.
81. Kadowitz, P. J., Gruetter, C. A., McNamara, D. B., Gorman, R. R., Spannhake, E. W. and Hyman, A. L. (1977): Comparative effects of the endoperoxide PGH_2 and an analog on the pulmonary vascular bed. *J. Appl. Physiol.*, 42:953.

82. Kadowitz, P. J., Chapnick, B. M., Feigen, L. P., Hyman, A. L., Nelson, P. K. and Spannhake, E. W. (1978): Pulmonary and systemic effects of a newly discovered prostaglandin, PGI₂. *J. Appl. Physiol.*, 45:408.

83. Kadowitz, P. J. and Hyman, A. L. (1977): Influence of prostaglandin endoperoxide analog on the canine pulmonary vascular bed. *Circ. Res.*, 40:282.

84. Kadowitz, P. J., Joiner, P. D., Hyman, A. L. and George, W. J. (1975): Influence of prostaglandin E₁ and F₂ₐ on pulmonary vascular resistance, isolated lobar vessels, and cyclic nucleotide levels. *J. Pharmacol. Exp. Ther.*, 192:677.

85. Kadowitz, P. J., Joiner, P. D. and Hyman, A. L. (1973): Effects of prostaglandins E₁ and F₂ₐ on the swine pulmonary circulation. *Proc. Soc. Exp. Biol. Med.*, 145:53.

86. Kadowitz, P. J., Joiner, P. D. and Hyman, A. L. (1974): Influence of prostaglandins E₁ and F₂ₐ on the pulmonary vascular resistance in the sheep. *Proc. Soc. Exp. Biol. Med.*, 145:1258.

87. Kadowitz, P. J., Spannhake, E. W., Greenberg, S., Feigen, L. P. and Hyman, A. L. (1977): Comparative effects of arachidonic acid, bisenoic prostaglandins, and an endoperoxide analog on the pulmonary vascular bed. *Can. J. Physiol. Pharmacol.*, 55:1369.

88. Kadowitz, P. J., Joiner, P. D., Matthews, C. S. and Hyman, A. L. (1975): Effects of the 15-methyl analogs of prostaglandin E₂ and F₂ₐ on the pulmonary circulation in intact dogs. *J. Clin. Invest.*, 55:937.

89. Kadowitz, P. J., Joiner, P. D. and Hyman, A. L. (1975): Effects of prostaglandin E₂ on pulmonary vascular resistance in the intact dog, swine, and lamb. *Eur. J. Pharmacol.*, 31:72.

90. Kadowitz, P. J. and Hyman, A. L. (1980): Comparative effects of thromboxane B₂ on the canine and feline pulmonary vascular bed. *J. Pharmacol. Exp. Ther.*, 213:300.

91. Kadowitz, P. J., Joiner, P. D. and Hyman, A. L. (1975): Influence of sympathetic stimulation and vasoactive substances on the canine pulmonary veins. *J. Clin. Invest.*, 56:354.

92. Kadowitz, P. J., Knight, D. S., Hebbs, R. G., Ellison, J. P., Joiner, P. D., Brody, M. J. and Hyman A. L. (1976): Influence of 5- and 6-hydroxydopamine on adrenergic transmission and nerve terminal morphology in the canine pulmonary vascular bed. *Circ. Res.*, 39:191.

93. Kadowitz, P. J., George, W. J., Joiner, P. D. and Hyman, A. L. (1980): Effect of prostaglandins E₁ and F₂ₐ on adrenergic responses in the pulmonary circulation. In: *Advances in the Biosciences.* edited by S. Bergstrom, International Conference on Prostaglandins, Vienna, Pergamon Press, New York.

94. Kadowitz, P. J., Chapnick, B. M., Joiner, P. D. and Hyman, A. L. (1975): Influence of inhibitors of prostaglandin synthesis on the canine pulmonary vascular bed. *Am. J. Physiol.*, 229:941.

95. Kaliner, M., Wasserman, S. I., and Austen, F. (1973): Immunologic release of chemical mediators from human nasal polyps. *New Eng. J. Med.*, 289:277.

96. Karim, S. M. M. (1968): Appearance of PGF₂ₐ in human blood during labor. *Br. Med. J.*, 4:618.

97. Knight, D. S., Ellison, J. P., Hebbs, R. G., Hyman, A. L. and Kadowitz, P. J. (1981): A light and electron microscopic study of the innervation of pulmonary arteries in the cat. *Anat. Rec.*, 201:513–521.

98. Kunze, H. and Vogt, H. (1971): Significance of phospholipase A for prostaglandin formation. *Ann. N.Y. Acad. Sci.*, 180:123.

99. Kunze, H., Bohn, E. and Vogt, W. (1974): Effects of local anaesthetics on prostaglandin bio-synthesis *in vitro. Biochim. Biophys. Acta.*, 360:260.

100. Lands, W. E. M. and Samuelsson, B. (1968): Phospholipid precursor of prostaglandins. *Biochim. Biophys. Acta.*, 164:426.

101. Larsson, C. and Anggard, E. (1970): Distribution of prostaglandin metabolizing enzymes in tissues of the swine. *Acta Pharmacol. Toxicol. (Kbh)*, 1:61.

102. Leffler, C., Tyler, T. and Cassin, S. (1977): Pulmonary vascular responses of newborn goats to aerosolized prostaglandin E₂. *Proc. Soc. Exp. Med. Biol.*, 155:9.

103. Levin, J. R., Spannhake, E. W., Hyman, A. L. and Kadowitz, P. J. (1982): Analysis of airway responses to dihomo-γ-linolenic acid in the cat. *J. Pharmacol. (in press).*

104. Lewis, R. A., Austen, K. F., Drazen, J. M., Clark, D. A., Marfat, A. and Corey, E. J. (1980): Slow reacting substances of anaphylaxis: Identification of leukotrienes C-1 and D from human and rat sources. *Proc. Natl. Acad. Sci. USA*, 77:3710.

105. Liebeg, R., Bernauer, W. and Peskar, B. A. (1975): Prostaglandin slow-reacting substance, and histamine release from anaphylactic guinea-pig hearts, and its pharmacological modification. *Naunyn-Schmiedeberg's Arch. Pharmacol.*, 289:65.

106. Lippton, H. L., Paustian, P. W., Mellion, B. T., Nelson, P. K., Feigen, L. P., Chapnick, B. M., Hyman, A. L. and Kadowitz, P. J. (1979): Cardiovascular actions of prostacyclin (PGI₂) in the cat. *Arch. Int. Pharmacodyn. Ther.*, 241:121.

107. Lippton, H. L., Chapnick, B. M., Hyman, A. L. and Kadowitz, P. J. (1979): Inhibition of vasoconstrictor responses by prostacyclin (PGI₂) in the feline mesenteric vascular bed. *Arch. Int. Pharmacodyn. Ther.*, 241:214.
108. Lippton, H. L., Chapnick, B. M. and Kadowitz, P. J. (1981): Influence of prostaglandins on vasoconstrictor responses in the hindquarters vascular bed of the cat. *Prostaglandins Med.*, 6:183–202.
109. Lonigro, A. J. and Dawson, C. A. (1975): Vascular responses to PGF₂ₐ in isolated cat lungs. *Circ. Res.*, 36:706.
110. Manchester, D., Margolis, H. S. and Sheldon, R. E. (1975): Possible association between maternal indomethacin therapy and primary pulmonary hypertension of the newborn. *Am. J. Obstet. Gynecol.*, 126:467.
111. Marcus, A. J. (1978): The role of lipids in platelet function: with particular reference to the arachidonic acid pathway. *J. Lipid Res.*, 19:793.
112. Maseri, A. (1980): In: *Proceedings of Workshop on Platelet-Active Drugs in the Secondary Prevention of Cardiovascular Events.* Circulation: 62 (Part II, Suppl. V,) p. V44.
113. Mathe, A. A., Hedqvist, P., Holmgren, A. and Svanborg, N. (1973): Bronchial hyperactivity to PGF₂ₐ and histamine in patients with asthma. *Br. Med. J.*, 1:193.
114. Mathe, A. A. and Hedqvist, P. (1975): Effects of prostaglandins F₂ₐ and E₂ on airway conductance in healthy subjects and asthmatic patients. *Am. Rev. Respir. Dis.*, 111:313.
115. McGiff, J. C., Terragno, N. A., Strand, J. C., Lee, J. B., Lonigro, A. J. and Ng, K. K. F. (1969): Selective passage of prostaglandins by the lung. *Nature*, 223:742.
116. McGillen, J. J. and Phair, J. P. (1979): Adherence, augmented adherence, and aggregation of polymorphonuclear leukocytes. *J. Infect. Dis.*, 139:69.
117. Mohrhauer, H. and Holman, R. T. (1963): The effect of dose level of essential fatty acids upon fatty acid composition of the rat liver. *J. Lipid Res.*, 4:151.
118. Moncada, S. and Vane, J. R. (1979): Pharmacology and endogenous roles of prostaglandin endoperoxides, thromboxane A₂, and prostacyclin. *Pharmacol. Rev.*, 30:293.
119. Moncada, S., Herman, A. H., Higgs, E. A. and Vane, J. R. (1977): Differential formation of prostacyclin (PGX or PGI₂) by layers of the arterial wall. An explanation for the anti-thrombotic properties of vascular endothelium. *Thromb. Res.*, 11:323.
120. Moncada, S., Gryglewski, R. J., Bunting, S. and Vane, J. R. (1976): A lipid peroxide inhibits the enzyme in blood vessel microsomes that generates from prostaglandin endoperoxides the substance (PGX) which prevents platelet aggregation. *Prostaglandins*, 12:715.
121. Moncada, S. and Vane, J. R. (1978): Unstable metabolites of arachidonic acid and their role in hemostasis and thrombosis. *Br. Med. Bull.*, 34:129.
122. Moncada, S., Bunting, S., Mullane, K., Thorogood, P. and Vane, J. R. (1977): Imidazole: a selective inhibitor of thromboxane synthetase. *Prostaglandins*, 13:611.
123. Morris, H. R., Taylor, G. W., Piper, P. J., Samhoun, M. N. and Tippins, J. R. (1980): Slow reacting substances (SRSs): the structure identification of SRSs from rat basophil leukaemia (RBL-1) cells. *Prostaglandins*, 19:185.
124. Morris, H. R., Taylor, G. W., Piper, P. J. and Tippins, J. R. (1980): Structure of slow-reacting substance of anaphylaxis from guinea-pig lung. *Nature*, 285:104.
125. Mullane, K. M. and Moncada, S. (1980): Prostacyclin release and the modulation of some vasoactive hormones. *Prostaglandins*, 20:25.
126. Murphy, R. C., Hammerstrom, S. and Samuelsson, B. (1979): Leukotriene C: A slow-reacting substance from murine mastocytoma cells. *Proc. Natl. Acad. Sci. USA*, 76:4275.
127. Nakano, J., Anggard, E. and Samuelsson, B. (1969): 15-Hydroxy-prostanoate dehydrogenase. Prostaglandins as substrates and inhibitors. *Eur. J. Biochem.*, 11:386.
128. Nakano, J., Montague, B. and Darrow, B. (1971): Metabolism of prostaglandin E₁ in human plasma, uterus and placenta in swine ovary and rat testicle. *Biochem. Pharmacol.*, 20:2512.
129. Nakano, J. and Morsy, N. H. (1971): Beta-oxidations of prostaglandins E₁ and E₂ in rat lung and kidney homogenates. *Clin. Res.*, 19:142.
130. Needleman, P., Whitaker, M. O., Wyche, A., Watters, K., Sprecher, H. and Raz, A. (1980): Manipulation of platelet aggregation by prostaglandins and their fatty acid precursors: Pharmacological basis for a therapeutic approach. *Prostaglandins*, 19:165.
131. Needleman, P., Minkes, M. and Raz, A. (1976): Thromboxanes: selective biosynthesis and distinct biological properties. *Science*, 193:163.
132. Nelson, W. R. and Taylor, G. A. (1975): *In vitro* inhibition of endotoxin-induced platelet aggregation with hydrocortisone sodium succinate (Solu-Cortef). *Scand. J. Haematol.*, 15:33.

133. Niikamp, F. P., Flower, R. J., Moncada, S. and Vane, J. R. (1976): Partial purification of rabbit aorta contracting substance-releasing factor and inhbition of its activity by anti-inflammatory steroids. *Nature*, 263:479.
134. Nishizawa, E. E., Miller, W. L., Gorman, R. R., Bundy, G. L., Svensson, J. and Hamberg, M. (1975): Prostaglandin D_2 as a potent antithrombotic agent. *Prostaglandins*, 9:109.
135. Nugteren, D. H. (1975): Arachidonate lipoxygenase in blood platelets. *Biochem. Biophys. Acta*, 380:299.
136. O'Flaherty, J. T., Showell, H. J., Becker, E. L. and Ward, P. A. (1979): Neutrophil aggregation and degranulation. *Am. J. Pathology*, 95:433.
137. O'Flaherty, J. T., Showell, H. J., Becker, E. L. and Ward, P. A. (1978): Substances which aggregate neutrophils. *Am. J. Pathology*, 92:155.
138. Ollwy, P. M., Coceani, F. and Bodach, E. (1976): E-type prostaglandins: A new emergency therapy for certain cyanotic congenital heart malformations. *Circulation*, 53:728.
139. Orning, L., Hammarstrom, S. and Samuelsson, B. (1980): Leukotriene D: a slow reacting substance from rat basophilic leukemia cells. *Proc. Natl. Acad. Sci. USA*, 77:2014.
140. Peck, M. J., Piper, P. J. and Williams, T. J. (1981): The effect of leukotrienes C_4 and D_4 on the microvasculature of guinea-pig skin. *Prostaglandins*, 21:315.
141. Pierce, C. H., Oshiro, G. and Nickerson, M. (1974): Effects of methylprednisolone sodium succinate (MP) on platelet aggregation (abstract). *Circulation*, 49 (Suppl. I):289.
142. Piper, P. J. and Vane, J. R. (1971): The release of prostaglandins from lung and other tissues. *Ann. N.Y. Acad. Sci.*, 180:363.
143. Piper, P. J. and Vane, J. R. (1969): Release of additional factors in anaphylaxis and its antagonism by antiinflammatory drugs. *Nature*, 223:29.
144. Pontecorvo, E. G., Myers, C. B., Lippton, H. L. and Kadowitz, P. J. (1981): Inhibition of platelet aggregation by 6-keto-PGE_1; lack of an effect on cGMP levels. *Prostaglandins Med.*, 6:473.
145. PG-Synthetase Inhibitors in Obstetrics and After. Leading Editorial, *Lancet*, 2:185.
146. Ramwell, P. W., Leovey, E. M. K. and Sintetos, A. L. (1977): Regulation of the arachidonic acid cascade. *Biol. Reprod.*, 16:70.
147. Robertson, R. M., Bernard, Y., Maas, R. L., Roberts, L. J., II, Friesinger, G. C. and Oates, J. A. (1980): Variant angina: The role of TXA_2. *Circulation*, 62 (Suppl. III):310.
148. Rosenberg, A. (1967): *Euglena gracilis:* a novel lipid energy reserve and arachidonic acid enrichment during fasting. *Science*, 157:1189.
149. Rosenberger, M. and Neukom, C. (1980): Total synthesis of (5S,6R,7E,11Z,14Z)-5-hydroxy-6-((2R-amino-2-carboxyethyl)thiol)-7,9,11,14-eicosatetraenoic acid, a potent SRS-A. *J. Am. Chem. Soc.*, 102:5426.
150. Rubaltelli, F. F., Chiozza, M. L., Zanardo, V. and Cantanitti, F. (1979): Effect on neonate of maternal treatment with indomethacin. *J. Pediatr.*, 94:161.
151. Rubin, L. J. and Lazar, J. D. (1981): Influence of prostaglandin synthesis inhibitors on the pulmonary vasodilatory effects of hydralazine in dogs with hypoxic pulmonary vasoconstriction. *J. Clin. Invest.*, 67:193.
152. Rudolph, A. M. (1978): Effects of PG and PG synthetase inhibition on fetal circulation. In: *Pre-Term Labor*. edited by A. Anderson, R. Beard, M. Brudenell and P. Dunn, p. 231, London Royal College of Obstetrics & Gynaecology.
153. Said, S. I. (1967): Some respiratory effects of prostaglandins E_2 and F_2. In: *Prostaglandin Symposium, Worchester Foundation for Experimental Biology*. edited by P. W. Ramwell and J. E. Shaw, p. 267, Interscience, New York.
154. Salmon, J. A., Smith, D. R., Flower, R. J., Moncada, S. and Vane J. R. (1978): Further studies on the enzymatic conversion of prostaglandin endoperoxide into prostacyclin by porcine aorta microsomes. *Biochim. Biophys. Acta*, 523:250.
155. Samuelsson, B., Granstrom, E., Green, K., Hamberg, M. and Hammarstrom, S. (1975): *Prostaglandins Ann. Rev. Biochem.*, 44:669.
156. Samuelsson, B., Borgeat, P., Hammarstrom, S. and Murphy, C. (1980): Leukotrienes: A new group of biologically active compounds. In: *Advances in Prostaglandin and Thromboxane Research*, edited by B. Samuelsson, P. Ramwell and R. Paoletti, p. 1, Raven Press, New York.
157. Samuelsson, B., Hammerstrom, S., Murphy, R. C. and Borgeat, P. (1980): Leukotrienes and slow reacting substance of anaphylaxis (SRS-A). *Allergy*, 35:375.
158. She, H. S., McNamara, D. B., Spannhake, E. W., Hyman, A. L. and Kadowitz, P. J. (1981): Metabolism of prostaglandin endoperoxide by microsomes from cat lung. *Prostaglandins*, 21:531.

159. Shio, H. and Ramwell, P. (1972): Effects of prostaglandins E$_2$ and aspirin on the secondary aggregation of human platelets. *Nature (New Biol.)*, 236:45.
160. Skidgel, R. A. and Printz, M. P. (1978): PGI$_2$ production in rat blood vessels: diminished PGI$_2$ formation in veins compared to arteries. *Prostaglandins*, 16:1.
161. Smith, R. L. and Weidemann, M. J. (1980): Reactive oxygen reduction associated with arachidonic acid metabolism by peritoneal macrophages. *Biochem. Biophys. Res. Commun.*, 97:973.
162. Smith, A. P. and Cuthbert, M. F. (1976): The response of normal and asthmatic subjects to PGE$_2$ and PGF$_{2\alpha}$ by different routes and their significance in asthma. In: *Advances in Prostaglandin and Thromboxane Research*. Vol. 1, edited by B. Samuelsson and R. Paoletti, p. 449, Raven Press, New York.
163. Spannhake, E. W., Levin, J. L., Mellion, B. T., Hyman, A. L., and Kadowitz, P. J. (1980): Reversal of 5-HT induced bronchoconstriction by PGI$_2$: Distribution of central over peripheral actions. *J. Appl. Physiol.*, 49:521.
164. Spannhake, E. W., Lemen, R. J., Wegmann, M. J., Hyman, A. L. and Kadowitz, P. J. (1978): Analysis of the airway effects of a PGH$_2$ analog in the anesthetized dog. *J. Appl. Physiol.*, 44:406.
165. Spannhake, E. W., Hyman A. L. and Kadowitz, P. J. (1980): Dissimilar *in vivo* effects of arachidoic acid on canine pulmonary vascular beds and airways. In: *Advances in Prostaglandin and Thromboxane Research*. Vol. 7, edited B. Samuelsson, P. Ramwell and R. Paoletti, p. 937, Raven Press, New York.
166. Spannhake, E. W., Mercier, R. R., Hyman, A. L. and Kadowitz, P. J. (1978): 15-(S)-15 methyl PGF$_{2\alpha}$ elicits marked peripheral airway constriction in the intact dog. *J. Pharmacol. Exp. Ther.*, 207:83.
167. Spannhake, E. W., Lemen, R. J., Wegmann, M. J., Hyman, A. L. and Kadowitz, P. J. (1978): Effects of arachidonic acid and prostaglandins on lung function in intact dogs. *J. Appl. Physiol.*, 44:397.
168. Spannhake, E. W., Levin, J. L., Hyman, A. L. and Kadowitz, P. J. (1981): 6-keto-PGE$_1$ exhibits more potent bronchodilator activity in the cat than its precursor, PGI$_2$. *Prostaglandins*, 21:267.
169. Spannhake, E. W., Hyman, A. L. and Kadowitz, P. J. (1980): Dependence of the airway and pulmonary vascular effects of arachidonic acid upon route and rate of administration. *J. Pharmacol. Exp. Ther.*, 212:584.
170. Sun, F. F., McGuire, J. C., Morton, D. R., Pike, J. E., Sprecher, H. and Kunau, W. H. (1981): Inhibition of platelet arachidonic acid 12-lipoxygenase by acetylenic acid compounds. *Prostaglandins*, 21:333.
171. Tucker, A. and Reeves, J. T. (1975): Nonsustained pulmonary vasoconstriction during acute hypoxia in anesthetized dogs. *Am. J. Physiol.*, 228:756.
172. Tyler, T., Leffler, C., Wallis, R. and Cassin, S. (1975): Effects of prostaglaninds of the E series on pulmonary and systemic circulations of newborn goats during normoxia and hypoxia. *Prostaglandins*, 10:963.
173. Vaage, J., Bjertnaes, J. and Hauge, A. (1975): The pulmonary vasoconstrictor response to hypoxia: Effects of inhibitors of prostaglandin biosynthesis. *Acta Physiol. Scand.*, 95:95.
174. Valone, F. H., Franklin, M., Sun, F. F. and Goetzl, E. (1980): Alveoloar macrophage lipoxygenase products of arachidonic acid: Isolation and recognition as the predominant constituents of the neutrophil chemotactic activity elaborated by alveolar macrophages. *Cell. Immunol.*, 54:390.
175. Vanderhoek, J. Y., Bryant, R. W. and Bailey, J. M. (1980): Ihibition of leukotriene biosynthesis by the leukocyte product 15-hydroxy-5,8,11,13-eicosatetraenoic acid. *J. Biol. Chem.*, 255:10064.
176. VanDorp, D. A., Beerthuis, R. K., Nugteren, D. H. and Vonheman, H. (1964): The biosynthesis of prostaglandins. *Biochim. Biophys. Acta*, 90:204.
177. VanDorp, D. A. (1976): Essential fatty acids and prostaglandins. *Acta Biol. Med. Ger.*, 35:1041.
178. Vane, J. R. (1972): The role of the lungs in metabolism of vasoactive substances. In: *Pharmacology and Pharmacokinetics*. Edited by T. Teorell, R. L. Dedrick, and P. G. Condliffe, p. 195, Plenum Press, New York.
179. Vigo, C., Lewis, G. P. and Piper, P. J. (1980): Mechanisms of inhibition of phospholipase A$_2$. *Biochem. Pharmacol.*, 29:623.
180. Voelkle, N. F., Gerber, J. G., McMurty, I. G., Reeves, J. T., and Nies, A. S. (1980): Release of dilator prostaglandins from rat lung during angiotensin II-induced vasoconstriction. *Adv. Prostaglandin and Thromb. Res.*, 7:957.
181. Walker, J. L. (1980): Interrelationships of SRSA production and arachidonic acid metabolism in human lung tissue. In: *Advances in Prostaglandin and Thromboxane Research*. Vol. 6, edited by B. Samuelsson, P. W. Ramwell and R. Paoletti, Raven Press, New York.

182. Wallach, D. P. and Brown, V. R. (1981): A novel preparation of human platelet lipoxygenase: characteristics and inhibition by a variety of phenyl hydrazones and comparisons with other lipoxygenases. *Biochem. Biophys. Acta*, 663:361.

183. Walsh, C. E., Dechatelet, L. R., Thomas, M. J., O'Flaherty, J. T. and Waite, M. (1981): Effect of phagocytosis and ionophores on release and metabolism of arachidonic acid from human neutrophils. *Lipids*, 16:120.

184. Wasserman, M. A. (1975): Bronchopulmonary effects of $PGF_{2\alpha}$ and three of its metabolites in the dog. *Prostaglandins*, 9:959.

185. Wasserman, M. A., Ducharme, D. W., Griffin, R. L., DeGraef, G. L. and Robertson, F. G. (1977): Bronchopulmonary and cardiovascular effects of PGD_2 in the dog. *Prostaglandins*, 13:255.

186. Watkins, W. D., Peterson, M. B., Crone, R. K., Shannon, D. C. and Levine, L. (1980): Prostacyclin and prostaglandin E_1 for severe idiopathic pulmonary artery hypertension. *Lancet*, I:1083.

187. Weir, E. K., Geer, B. E., Smith, S. C., Silvers, G. W., Droegemweller, W., Reeves, J. T., and Grover, R. F. (1979): 15-Methylation augments the cardiovascular effects of prostaglandin $PGF_{2\alpha}$. *Prostaglandins*, 9:369.

188. Weir, E. K., McMurty, I. F., Tucker, A., Reeves, J. T. and Grover, R. F. (1976): Prostaglandin synthesis inhibitors do not decrease hypoxic pulmonary vasoconstriction. *J. Appl. Physiol.*, 41:714.

189. Welton, A. F., Crowley, H. J., Miller, D. A. and Yaremko, B. (1981): Biological activities of a chemically synthesized form of leukotriene E_4. *Prostaglandins*, 21:287.

190. Whelan, C. J. (1980): The partial purification of slow reacting substance of anaphylaxis from rat peritoneal anaphylactic fluid and its separation from an arachidonic acid releasing substance. *Biochem. Pharmacol.*, 29:319.

191. Wicks, T. C., Ramwell, P. W., Rose, J. C., and Kot, P. A. (1977): Vascular responses to the monoenoic prostaglandin precursor dihomo-γ-linolenic acid in the perfused canine lung. *J. Pharmacol. Exp. Ther.* 201:417.

192. Wilhelm, T. E., Sankarappa, S. K., VanRollins, M. and Sprecher, H. (1981): Selective inhibitors of platelet lipoxygenase: 4,7,10,13-icosatetraynoic acid and 5,8,11,14-henicosatetraynoic acid. *Prostaglandins*, 21:323.

193. Wong, PY.-K., Malik, K. U., Desiderio, D. M., McGiff, J. C., and Sun, F. F. (1980): Hepatic metabolism of prostacyclin (PGI_2) in the rabbit: formation of a novel inhibitor of platelet aggregation. *Biochem. Biophys. Res. Commun.*, 93:486.

Prostaglandins and the Cardiovascular System,
edited by John A. Oates. Raven Press,
New York © 1982.

Metabolites of Arachidonic Acid in the Pathophysiology of the Pulmonary Circulation

Kenneth L. Brigham, John H. Newman, James R. Snapper,
and Martin L. Ogletree

*Pulmonary Circulation Center and Pulmonary Division, Department of Medicine,
Vanderbilt University School of Medicine, Nashville, Tennessee 37232*

Although there is no conclusive proof that metabolites of arachidonic acid mediate important changes in the function of the human lungs, there is an increasing body of experimental data to suggest it. There are several general reasons to suspect these substances as important mediators of changes in lung function: the lung contains the enzyme systems necessary for metabolism of arachidonate to biologically active metabolites; increased amounts of such metabolites emerge from the lung in response to insults that alter its function; exogenous administration of several arachidonate metabolites alters lung function. The circumstantial evidence is strong. In addition, studies using inhibitors of specific pathways of arachidonate metabolism lend credence to the idea that endogenous generation of arachidonate metabolites is necessary for some responses of both the pulmonary circulation and the airways to pathological stimuli.

Although this chapter deals primarily with the pathophysiology of the lung circulation, there is good reason to believe that arachidonate products are also important mediators of airway dysfunction. The relatively recent demonstration that the bronchoconstrictor, slow reacting substance of anaphylaxis (SRS-A), is a mixture of leukotrienes has called attention to that fact. Also, cyclooxygenase products of arachidonate may mediate severe bronchoconstriction in at least some experimental circumstances (24). In fact, in many circumstances discussed below, bronchoconstriction occurs coincident with vasoconstriction, and the two responses may share common mediators.

Arachidonate metabolites may be important mediators of airway abnormalities, but this chapter will concentrate on lung circulation. Specifically, we will discuss three areas where there is increasing evidence implicating arachidonate metabolites as mediators: pulmonary vasoconstriction; altered pulmonary vasoreactivity (especially the depression of vasoconstriction in response to alveolar hypoxia); and increased lung microvascular permeability.

PULMONARY VASOCONSTRICTION

Several of the cyclooxygenase products of arachidonic acid cause pulmonary vasoconstriction when infused into experimental animals. Vasoconstriction is the dominant pulmonary vascular effect of arachidonate infused into animals; the effect is inhibited by cyclooxygenase inhibitors (18). It is not entirely clear which of the cyclooxygenase products is the major pulmonary vasoconstrictor. The endoperoxide intermediate, PGH_2 is an extremely potent vasoconstrictor, as are structural analogs of that compound (3). Circumstantial evidence seems to implicate TxA_2 as an important pulmonary vasoconstrictor, as PGH_2 is metabolized partly to that potent, short-lived vasoconstrictor, and PGH_2 analogs appear to mimic TxA_2 in biological activity in smooth muscle preparations *in vitro* (8).

Vasoconstriction is a common response of the lung to injury (1,7,10). We have used a chronically instrumented sheep preparation to investigate the pathogenetic role of arachidonate metabolites in pulmonary vasoconstriction resulting from several insults. The advantages of the preparation are that it permits measurements of lung vascular function and collection of lymph, predominately from the lungs, in unanesthetized animals (25). Lung lymph may be a particularly good fluid in which to measure arachidonate metabolites produced in the lung, since we have demonstrated that concentrations of these substances are much higher in lymph than in either pulmonary arterial or left atrial blood plasma following several insults (12).

When gram-negative bacterial endotoxin is infused into sheep, marked pulmonary vasoconstriction results (4). The time course of this response is shown in Fig. 1. There is a marked increase in pulmonary vascular resistance within the first hour after endotoxin, then resistance declines toward baseline, but often remains elevated for several hours. Coincident with the increase in pulmonary vascular resistance is an increase in the concentrations of both TxB_2 (the principal metabolite of TxA_2), and 6-keto $PGF_{1\alpha}$ (the principal prostacyclin metabolite) in lung lymph (12); this is also illustrated in Fig. 1. Although not shown, blood concentrations of prostaglandin and thromboxane metabolites increased less than concentrations in lung lymph. These data suggest that there is production of thromboxane and prostacyclin specifically in the lung. As Fig. 1 illustrates, there is temporal coincidence of the increase in pulmonary vascular resistance and the increase in lung lymph TxB_2 concentration.

The initial, marked pulmonary vasoconstriction following endotoxemia in sheep is inhibited by drugs that inhibit the cyclooxygenase pathway of arachidonate metabolism (1,19,24). This is illustrated in Fig. 2 which shows pulmonary vascular pressures after endotoxin infusion in the same sheep in the presence and absence of cyclooxygenase inhibition. Cyclooxygenase inhibition largely affected the early rise in pulmonary artery pressure following endotoxin. These data strongly suggest that the early, marked pulmonary vasoconstriction following gram-negative endotoxin infusion in unanesthetized sheep is mediated by some cyclooxygenase product of arachidonic acid, possibly TxA_2.

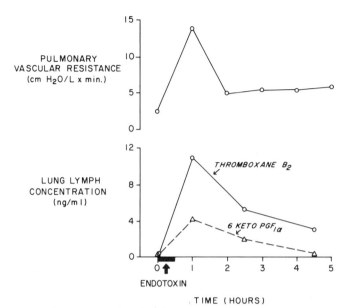

FIG. 1. Effects of intravenous *E. coli* endotoxin on pulmonary vascular resistance and lung lymph concentrations of TxB$_2$ and 6-keto-PGF$_{1\alpha}$ in unanesthetized sheep (Snapper, Ogletree, and coworkers, *unpublished*).

The relationship between vasoconstriction in the lung and arachidonate metabolites is not limited to endotoxin. For example, phorbol myristate acetate, a substance which activates granulocytes (9), also causes pulmonary hypertension with a time course similar to the endotoxin response (15). As shown in Fig. 3, pulmonary hypertension caused by phorbol myristate acetate is accompanied by increased concentrations of TxB$_2$ in lung lymph. As with endotoxin, the early rise in pulmonary artery pressure is attenuated by cyclooxygenase inhibition (16).

It is tempting to postulate that lipoxygenase products of arachidonate are also important mediators of pulmonary hypertension. Some of these substances are smooth muscle constrictors (21), and some preliminary work suggests that they may be pulmonary vasoconstrictors. As discussed later, we have shown increased lung lymph concentrations of lipoxygenase metabolites after endotoxin, particularly in the late phase of the reaction. However, demonstration of their pathophysiologic importance as pulmonary vasoconstrictors must await further study.

In summary, several different insults to the lung, delivered via the circulation, cause marked pulmonary vasoconstriction. The vasoconstriction is accompanied by increased production and release of cyclooxygenase products of arachidonic acid in the lung. The pulmonary hypertension is inhibited by drugs that inhibit cyclooxygenase. These data strongly implicate cyclooxygenase metabolites of arachidonate as mediators of the pulmonary hypertension. Although it is tempting to speculate that lipoxygenase products of arachidonate may also be important mediators of

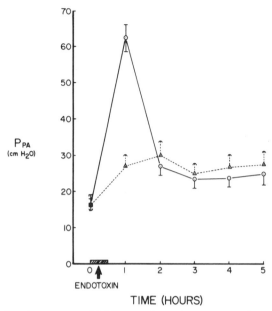

FIG. 2. Effects of cyclooxygenase inhibition on the pulmonary vascular response to *E. coli* endotoxemia in unanesthetized sheep (Snapper and coworkers, *unpublished*).

pulmonary vasoconstriction, there is not yet sufficient information to document their pathophysiologic significance.

PULMONARY VASOREACTIVITY

Although the lung vasculature constricts in response to a number of mediators including prostaglandins, presumably the most important physiologic vasoconstrictor response is that which occurs with alveolar hypoxia. This response, hypoxic vasoconstriction, can be localized to injured lung, reducing perfusion to poorly ventilated regions thereby improving ventilation–perfusion matching and preserving blood oxygenation. Endogenous production of constrictor prostaglandins was suspected earlier as the mechanism of this response, but the bulk of available evidence opposes that hypothesis. The mechanism of hypoxic vasoconstriction is unknown and may result from a direct effect on small pulmonary arteries rather than involving a humoral mediator (26).

However, prostaglandins may be important modulators of hypoxic vasoconstriction. Under some circumstances, the hypoxic constrictor response in the lung is lost; sometimes the response can be restored by arachidonate cyclooxygenase inhibitors.

Weir et al. (27) showed that several hours after infusion of sublethal doses of endotoxin into dogs, ventilation with hypoxic gas failed to elicit pulmonary vasoconstriction. When the animals then were treated with the cyclooxygenase inhibitor meclofenamate, the response was restored to baseline levels.

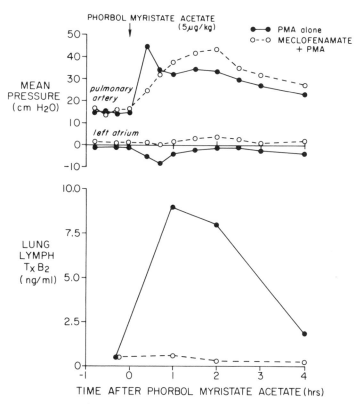

FIG. 3. Effects of intravenous phorbol myristate acetate on pulmonary vascular pressures and lung lymph TxB$_2$ concentrations in unanesthetized sheep, with and without cyclooxygenase inhibition (Loyd, Newman, Ogletree, and coworkers, *unpublished*).

Newman et al. (17) found that lungs isolated from rats who had breathed high concentrations of oxygen for several days did not vasoconstrict when ventilated with hypoxic gas. They also found that the hypoxic response was restored by adding meclofenamate to the perfusate.

Studies like these have led to the hypothesis that endogenous production of the potent pulmonary vasodilator, prostacyclin, may be responsible for the loss of hypoxic vasoconstriction. Support for this hypothesis has been provided by the recent observation that when arachidonic acid was infused into the lung circulation during hypoxic vasoconstriction, it produced dilation, contrary to the effects of arachidonate under baseline conditions where it is a potent vasoconstrictor (13,18). In those same studies, increased concentrations of 6-keto PGF$_{1\alpha}$ (the principal prostacyclin metabolite) were demonstrated in the effluent from the hypoxic lung during arachidonate infusion, suggesting preferential synthesis of prostacyclin under those conditions (13).

A number of insults to the lung that cause acute vasoconstriction also cause increased production of prostacyclin by the lung. For example, Fig. 1 shows pulmonary vascular resistance and lung lymph concentrations of 6-keto $PGF_{1\alpha}$ following endotoxemia in sheep. Coincident with the marked pulmonary vasoconstriction after endotoxin was a marked increase in lymph concentrations of the prostacyclin metabolite. Other stimuli that cause pulmonary vasoconstriction also increase lung prostacyclin production, raising the question whether this dilator prostaglandin serves a physiologic function. Since lung lymph concentrations of other arachidonate metabolites also increase, the increase in prostacyclin could be nonspecific. Also, lung production of prostacyclin has not been evaluated carefully in a sufficient number of conditions to permit a general hypothesis about the physiologic significance of this response.

PULMONARY MICROVASCULAR PERMEABILITY

In the past few years, there has been increasing interest in the pathogenesis of increased permeability of lung microvessels. This interest stems from the recognition of noncardiogenic pulmonary edema (the adult respiratory distress syndrome, ARDS) as a major cause of morbidity and mortality in humans. Since patients with this syndrome have pulmonary edema and respiratory failure with normal or low pulmonary artery wedge pressures, and, in contrast to patients with heart failure, their edema fluid is rich in proteins (23), it is inferred that increased permeability of lung exchange vessels to fluid and protein is the cause of the edema. How does the increase in capillary permeability come about?

The search for the factor(s) responsible for increased microvascular permeability has addressed a number of potential mediators including those derived from oxygenation of arachidonic acid. Interest in metabolites of arachidonic acid stems from their known formation by the lung and by granulocytes that appear to participate in ARDS and from their demonstrated capability to increase capillary permeability experimentally (28).

Most evidence suggests that cyclooxygenase products of arachidonic acid do not increase permeability in the lung circulation when infused intravenously (6). As shown in Fig. 4, infusion of arachidonic acid into unanesthetized sheep causes pulmonary hypertension and increases lung lymph flow, but lymph protein concentration falls. This is like the response to increased hydrostatic pressure in the lung circulation (22), and unlike responses to interventions that increase vascular permeability (5). Figure 5 shows relationships between lung lymph/plasma protein concentrations and lung lymph flow; responses to mechanically increased pressure and to arachidonate infusion are shown. When pressure is increased simulating heart failure, lymph flow increases and lymph protein concentration falls; arachidonate infusion causes a similar response. Thus, the effects of arachidonic acid on lung fluid balance are entirely explained as an increase in capillary pressure with no change in vascular permeability. Figure 5 also shows that the response to arachidonate is entirely inhibited by cyclooxygenase inhibition, suggesting that the vasoconstriction results from generation of prostaglandins or thromboxane *in vivo*.

The demonstrated effects of arachidonate are consistent with a large number of studies of specific metabolites. The endoperoxide intermediate, PGH_2 and its cyclic

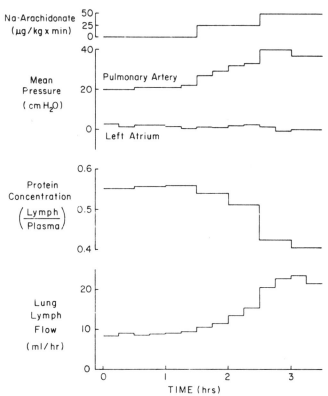

FIG. 4.   Effects of intravenous arachidonate on pulmonary vascular pressures and lung lymph in a sheep (from ref. 18).

ether analog are potent pulmonary vasoconstrictors, but do not increase permeability (6). The same is true for PGE_2, $PGF_{2\alpha}$, and PGD_2 (6). Similarly, prostacyclin is a potent pulmonary vasodilator, but its effects on lung fluid balance appear to result from effects on vascular pressures and changes in perfused lung vascular surface area.

Data relevant to possible effects of lipoxygenase products of arachidonate on lung vascular permeability are less clear. SRS-A, a mixture of leukotrienes, increases capillary permeability in a systemic vascular bed (28). As illustrated in Figure 6, we have shown increased lung lymph concentrations of a lipoxygenase metabolite coincident with the onset of increased lung vascular permeability following endotoxin infusion in sheep (20). The time course of the response seems to associate lipoxygenase products with the period of increased vascular permeability. Also, several interventions that increase lung vascular permeability in animals depend on the interaction of granulocytes with the lung microcirculation (11,14). Granulocytes could be a source of lipoxygenation metabolites (2). The chemotactic activity of several lipoxygenation products could be important in activating granulocytes, causing or perpetuating pulmonary leukostasis. All of these observations

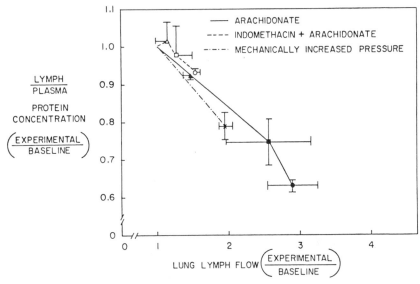

FIG. 5. Relationship between lung lymph/plasma protein concentration and lymph flow in unanesthetized sheep. Responses to increased hydrostatic pressure and to arachidonate infusion alone and with cyclooxygenase inhibition are shown. All studies were done in unanesthetized sheep (from ref. 2).

are suggestive, but there is as yet no conclusive evidence implicating lipoxygenase metabolites of arachidonate as mediators of increased lung vascular permeability.

SUMMARY

There is clear evidence that cyclooxygenase products of arachidonate (probably thromboxane) are potent pulmonary vasoconstrictors and mediate the acute pulmonary vasoconstriction that occurs in the lung in response to a variety of inflammatory stimuli. Such substances may not be entirely responsible for the more prolonged and less severe vasoconstriction which inflammatory stimuli cause. Although hypoxic pulmonary vasoconstriction, probably an important homeostatic mechanism, is not mediated by arachidonate metabolites (certainly not cyclooxygenase metabolites), endogenous production of prostacyclin may be the cause of the loss of hypoxic pulmonary vasoconstriction in some pathologic circumstances. This could prove to be an important phenomenon in human disease, since loss of hypoxic vasoconstriction may play a major role in respiratory failure. Cyclooxygenase products of arachidonic acid do not appear to affect lung vascular permeability directly and probably do not mediate such changes. It remains possible that lipoxygenation products of arachidonate may be important mediators of pulmonary hypertension and increased lung vascular permeability.

ACKNOWLEDGMENTS

This work was supported by National Heart, Lung and Blood Institute Grants HL 19153 (SCOR in Pulmonary Vascular Diseases), HL 00702, HL 27274, HL 26198.

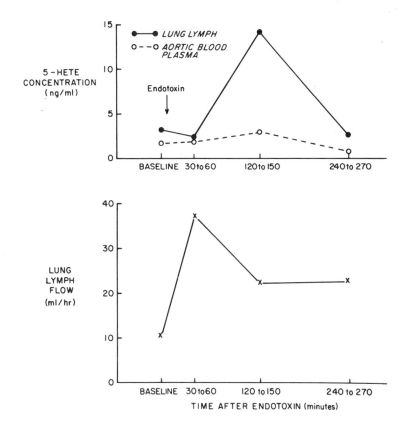

FIG. 6. Effects of intravenous *E. coli* endotoxin on lung lymph flow and lymph 5-HETE concentrations in unanesthetized sheep (Ogletree and coworkers, *unpublished*).

REFERENCES

1. Anderson, F., Theofilos, T., Jubiz, W., and Duida, H. (1975): Prostaglandin E and F levels during endotoxin induced pulmonary hypertension in calves. *Am. J. Physiol.*, 184:333.
2. Borgeat, P., and Samuelsson, B. (1979): Transformation of arachidonic acid by polymorphonuclear leukocytes. *J. Biol. Chem.*, 254:2643.
3. Bowers, R., Ellis, E., Brigham, K., and Oates, J. (1979): Effects of prostaglandin cyclic endoperoxides on the lung circulation of sheep. *J. Clin. Invest.*, 66:131.
4. Brigham, K., Bowers, R., and Haynes, J. (1979): Increased sheep lung vascular permeability caused by E. coli endotoxin. *Circ. Res.*, 45:292.
5. Brigham, K., Harris, T., Bowers, R., and Roselli, R. (1979): Lung vascular permeability: Inferences from measurements of plasma to lung lymph protein transport. *Lymphology*, 12:177.
6. Brigham, K., and Ogletree, M. (1982): Effects of prostaglandins and related compounds on lung vascular permeability. *Bull. Eur. Physiopathol. Resp*, 17:703–722.
7. Brigham, K., Woolverton, W., Blake, L., and Staub, N. (1974): Increased sheep lung vascular permeability caused by Pseudomonas bacteremia. *J. Clin. Invest.*, 54:792.
8. Coleman, R., Humphrey, P., Kennedy, I., Levy, G., and Lumley, P. (1981): Comparison of the actions of U-46619, a prostaglandin H₂-analog, with those of prostaglandin H₂ and thromboxane A₂ on some isolated smooth muscle preparations. *Br. J. Pharmacol.*, 73:773.
9. De Chatelet, L., Shirley, P., and Johnston, R. (1980): Effect of phorbol myristate acetate on the oxidative metabolism of human polymorphonuclear leukocytes. *Blood*, 47:545.
10. Demling, R., Gee, M., and Flynn, J. (1980): Changes in lung vascular permeability and lung lymph prostaglandins after endotoxin in sheep. *Am. Rev. Resp. Dis.*, 121:429.

11. Flick, M., Perel, A., and Staub, N. (1981): Leukocytes are required for increased lung micro-vascular permeability after microembolization in sheep. *Circ. Res.*, 48:344.
12. Frolich, J., Ogletree, M., and Brigham, K. (1980): Pulmonary hypertension correlated to pulmonary thromboxane synthesis. *Adv. Prost. Thrombox. Res.*, 7:745.
13. Gerber, J., Voelkel, N., Nies, A., McMurtry, I., and Reeves, J. (1980): Moderations of hypoxic vasoconstriction by infused arachidonate acid: Role of PGI$_2$. *J. Appl. Physiol.*, 49:107.
14. Heflin, C., and Brigham, K. (1981): Granulocyte depletion attenuates increased lung vascular permeability after endotoxemia in sheep. *J. Clin. Invest.*, 68:1253–1260.
15. Loyd, J., Newman, J., English, D., Ogletree, M., and Brigham, K. (1982): Pulmonary hypertension and increased lung vascular permeability caused by phorbol myristate acetate in unanesthetized sheep. *J. Appl. Physiol. (in press)*.
16. Newman, J., Loyd, J., Ogletree, M., and Brigham, K. (1982): Effects of meclofenamate on the pulmonary vascular response to phorbol myristate acetate in awake sheep. *Am. Rev. Resp. Dis. (abstr.)*, 125(4):282.
17. Newman, J., McMurtry, I, and Reeves, J. (1981): Vascular responses of lungs from rats exposed to high oxygen tensions. *Prostaglandins*, 22:11.
18. Ogletree, M., and Brigham, K. (1980): Arachidonate increased pulmonary vascular resistance without changing lung vascular permeability in unanesthetized sheep. *J. Appl. Physiol.*, 48:581–586.
19. Ogletree, M., and Brigham, K. (1979): Indomethacin augments endotoxin induced increased lung vascular permeability in sheep. *Am. Rev. Resp. Dis.*, 119:383.
20. Ogletree, M., Oates, J., Brigham, K., and Hubbard, W. (1982): Evidence for pulmonary release of 5-hydroxyeicosatetraenoic acid (5-HETE) during endotoxemia in unanesthetized sheep. *Prostaglandins*, 23:459–468.
21. Orange, R., and Austen, K. (1969): Slow reacting substance of anaphylaxis. *Adv. Immunol.*, 10:106.
22. Parker, R., Roselli, R., Harris, T., and Brigham, K. (1981): Effects of graded increase in pulmonary vascular pressures on lung fluid balance in unanesthetized sheep. *Circ. Res.*, 49(5):1164–1172.
23. Snapper, J. (1981): Septic pulmonary edema. *Sem. Resp. Med.*, 3:92.
24. Snapper, J., Ogletree, M., Hutchison, A., and Brigham, K. (1981): Meclofenamate prevents increased resistance of the lung (R$_L$) following endotoxemia in unanesthetized sheep. *Am. Rev. Resp. Dis.*, 123:200.
25. Staub, N., Bland, R., Brigham, K., Demling, R., Erdmann, J., and Woolverton, W. (1975): Preparation of chronic lung lymph fistulas in sheep. *J. Surg. Res.*, 19:315.
26. Tucker, A., McMurtry, I., Grover, R., and Reeves, J. (1976): Attenuation of hypoxic pulmonary vasoconstriction by calcium antagonists in isolated rat lungs. *Circ. Res.*, 38:99.
27. Weir, K., Mlczoch, J., Reeves, J., and Grover, R. (1976): Endotoxemia and the prevention of hypoxic pulmonary vasoconstriction. *J. Lab. Clin. Med.*, 88:975.
28. Williams, T., and Piper, P. (1980): The action of chemically pure SRS-A on the microcirculation *in vivo*. *Prostaglandins*, 19:779.

Prostaglandins and the Cardiovascular System,
edited by John A. Oates. Raven Press,
New York © 1982.

Prostaglandins and the Cerebral Circulation

*Bo K. Siesjö and **Bengt Nilsson

*Laboratory of Experimental Brain Research, and **Department of Neurology,
University Hospital, S-221 85 Lund, Sweden*

It has been known for more than 15 years that cerebral tissues synthetize prostaglandins (PGs) and related substances in response to the appropriate stimuli (53,59,60). The substances identified include PGE_2, $PGF_{2\alpha}$ and PGD_2, as well as thromboxane B_2, and 6-keto-$PGF_{1\alpha}$, the stable metabolites of thromboxane A_2 and prostacyclin, respectively. Like in other tissues, the major part of the prostaglandins formed seems to emanate from parenchymal cells, although most of the prostacyclin is produced by vascular tissue (2). It is generally believed that the fatty acid precursors of prostaglandins are released by the action of phospholipase A_2 on phospholipids, chiefly inosine and serine phosphoglyceride (36).

Less has been known about the physiological and pathophysiological roles of prostaglandins in the brain. Administration of prostaglandins, chiefly via the intraventricular route, has given relatively marked behavioral effects (27,28,47,59), and there is indication that prostaglandins modulate the intensity and duration of seizures (18,27). Actions of prostaglandins have also been assessed at the level of single cells; for example, prostaglandins of the E type have been found to antagonize the effect of noradrenaline on Purkinje cells (25).

Prostaglandins are known to influence cerebrovascular tone. Initial interest was centered on the possibility that such substances could contribute to cerebral vasospasm in pathological conditions such as ischemia (15,58,61). However, results reported strongly indicate that prostaglandins and related substances are important modulators of normal cerebrovascular tone, and that they could constitute some of the otherwise unknown factors coupling cerebral metabolism and blood flow. It is the purpose of the present chapter to briefly review this information, and to attempt an assessment of the role of prostaglandins in the regulation of cerebral blood flow (CBF) under normal and pathological conditions. In order to facilitate such an assessment, we will begin by briefly considering current views on the coupling of cerebral function, metabolism, and blood flow.

COUPLING OF BRAIN FUNCTION, METABOLISM AND BLOOD FLOW UNDER NORMAL AND PATHOLOGICAL CONDITIONS

Under normal conditions, the cells of the brain use glucose as the main fuel. At least 90% of the glucose extracted from the blood is oxidized to CO_2 and water

367

and the aerobic spillover of lactate is small. In starvation, or in other conditions leading to accumulation of ketone bodies in the blood, a significant part of the oxidative metabolism of the brain may be covered by acetoacetate and β-hydroxybutyrate but the end products of these oxidations are similar, CO_2 and water. In pathological states involving a reduced oxygen supply (hypoxia and ischemia), or a paroxysmal neuronal activity (seizures), glycolysis is stimulated and lactic acid accumulates. Whether we are dealing with a normal or a pathologically altered metabolism the functional activity releases H^+ ions.

A major fraction of the energy consumed by brain cells is spent in recharging the ionic batteries of the cells following the transmembrane fluxes of K^+, Na^+, Cl^- and Ca^{2+} that are associated with neuronal activity. Although the changes vary with the type of activity, activation of neuronal circuits usually leads to increases in the extracellular concentration of K^+, and to decreases in those of Na^+ and Ca^{2+}. On the inside of excitable membranes, activation of the membrane-bound Na^+-K^+-ATPase must lead to hydrolysis of ATP with accumulation of ADP and P_i. Any increase in ADP should cause a shift in the adenylate kinase equilibrium, favoring accumulation of AMP (ADP + ADP $\rightleftharpoons$ ATP + AMP). This, in turn, can be expected to cause some dephosphorylation of AMP to the vasoactive nucleoside adenosine which can then be translocated to the extracellular fluids.

Normally, alterations in the overall functional activity of the brain leads to changes in cerebral oxygen consumption (CMR_{O_2}) and these, in turn, are associated with corresponding alterations in CBF. The coupling of metabolism and blood flow can be exemplified by results obtained in one species, the rat, with a [133]Xenon modification of the original Kety and Schmidt (31) technique (Fig. 1). A corresponding coupling between metabolic rate (glucose consumption) and blood flow is observed within the brain when these variables are determined for a variety of cerebral structures by autoradiographic techniques (52,56).

Possible Coupling Factors Involved in the Regulation of CBF

The tight relationship betwen metabolic rate and blood flow has inspired an intense search for coupling mechanisms. In this search, particular attention has been attached to the fact that two conditions, hypercapnia and hypoxia, lead to marked increases in CBF with little or no change in CMR_{O_2}. The fact that both these conditions (and epileptic seizures) lead to acidification of the tissue has inspired some authors to propose that extracellular pH is the main determinant of vascular resistance (32,33). Others have emphasized the role of adenosine, which was reported to accumulate during hypoxia and epileptic seizures (50). Still others have taken the view that cerebrovascular tone is set by an interaction of several factors, with changes in extracellular [K^+] and [Ca^{2+}] playing a significant role (8).

A recent series of results from our own laboratory has challenged the hypothesis that CBF is regulated by the error signals discussed. These results can be summarized as follows (41,54): (1) in hypoxia and epileptic seizures, marked vascular dilatation may occur *before* the extracellular fluid is acidified, and in the absence of detectable

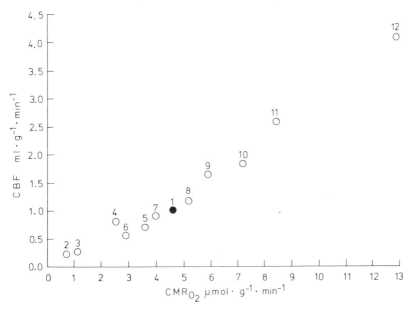

FIG. 1. Relationship between cerebral oxygen consumption (CMR_{O_2}) and cerebral blood flow (CBF) during different functional states. Decreases in CMR_{O_2} from control (1) were induced in ventilated rats by barbiturate anesthesia, by hypothermia, or combinations thereof, and increases in CMR_{O_2} by hyperthermia, immobilization stress, and drug-induced seizures. (From Nilsson et al., ref. 41 with permission.)

accumulation of adenosine, although seizure activity is accompanied by an increase of extracellular K^+ activity; (2) There are several conditions such as hypoglycemia, and the hypermetabolic states induced by large i.v. doses of amphetamine and adrenaline, in which CBF increases in the absence of changes in extracellular pH or K^+ activity; (3) There are no results to suggest that K^+, Ca^{2+}, or adenosine can explain the increase in CBF during hypercapnia but it has been more difficult to exclude an effect of pH. However, a recent series of results suggest that measures that modulate neurotransmission in the brain markedly alter the cerebral circulatory response to hypercapnia (54). In these experiments, ventilated rats were either infused with isoprenaline (8 $mg \cdot kg^{-1} \cdot min^{-1}$) or treated with propranolol (2.5 $mg \cdot kg^{-1}$) or with diazepam (2.25 $mg \cdot kg^{-1}$). Although none of these measures altered CMR_{O_2} under normocapnic conditions the increase of CBF induced by hypercapnia was markedly affected (Fig. 2). It should be emphasized that these differences were unrelated to changes in blood pressure.

The Participation of Prostaglandins

The results quoted emphasize the need to assess the possible role played by neurotransmitters and neurohormones. At present, there is little indication that biogenic amines are direct coupling factors. Although adrenaline and noradrenaline, as well as dopamine agonists, when administered in such a way that the blood-

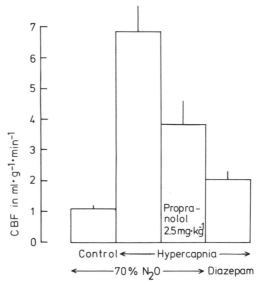

FIG. 2. Influence of hypercapnia (PaCO$_2$ about 80 mm Hg) on CBF and CMR$_{O_2}$ in control animals (70% N$_2$0) as well as in rats given propranolol (2.5 mg kg^{-1}) or diazepam (2.25 mg kg^{-1}) prior to induction of hypercapnia. (From Siesjö et al., ref. 54 with permission.)

brain barrier is circumvented, increase CBF, and serotonin has the opposite effect, the changes in CBF are associated with corresponding alterations in CMR$_{O_2}$ (7,12,24,34,35,38). Furthermore, the changes in CBF exemplified in Fig. 2 were associated with alterations in CMR$_{O_2}$. It seems possible that the measures described primarily alter CMR$_{O_2}$ and that CBF is adjusted to the metabolic needs by other coupling factors.

Results have been published that implicate prostaglandin-like substances in the control of CBF. Admittedly, these results represent a restricted approach since they mainly concern the circulatory effects of cyclooxygenase inhibitors. Nevertheless, they provide challenging hints of the control of CBF since they seem to uncouple metabolic rate and blood flow. The results will be described below.

Effect of Cyclo-Oxygenase Inhibitors Under Normo- and Hypercapnic Conditions

In a pioneer study, Pickard and MacKenzie (43), working on baboons under phencyclidine-N$_2$O anesthesia, administered indomethacin by intravenous (10 mg·kg^{-1}) or intracarotid (0.04 to 0.2 mg·kg^{-1}·min^{-1}) routes and measured CBF by a [133]Xenon clearance technique. They found that the drug reduced control CBF by an average of 38% with no significant change in CMR$_{O_2}$, and markedly attenuated the circulatory response to induced hypercapnia. These results were confirmed by Sakabe and Siesjö (51), and Dahlgren el al. (13), who worked on paralyzed and artificially ventilated rats and measured CBF with the modified Kety and Schmidt technique. In this species, indomethacin (10 mg·kg^{-1}) reduced resting CBF to 50% of control without affecting CMR_{O_2}. Similar results were obtained in animals with local anesthesia, excluding an interaction between the general anesthetic (N_2O) and indomethacin. The similarity in response in baboons and rats is illustrated in Fig. 3. If allowance is made for the difference in control CBF between the two species the circulatory responses in normocapnia and hypercapnia are strikingly similar.

Recent results provide further information on the effect of indomethacin. In the rat, the [133]Xenon CBF data have been validated by autoradiographic measurements of local CBF (13). As Fig. 4 shows, indomethacin (10 mg·kg[-1]) reduced local CBF to 40 to 80% of control, most cortical structures having flow rates of 40 to 50% of control. The *relative* reduction in CBF was similar in normo- and hypercapnia. In that study, dose response curves showed that significant reductions in CBF were obtained with 1 mg·kg[-1] and that maximal responses required 3 to 5 mg·kg[-1]. There was a striking similarity between this dose response and that previously reported by Abdel-Halim et al. (1) who determined prostaglandin formation in brain tissue *in vitro* following *in vivo* administration of indomethacin (Fig. 5). It could also be shown that, following i.v. injection of indomethacin, CBF started decreasing within 10 sec, the maximal response being obtained within about 2 min. The results suggest that indomethacin inhibited cyclo-oxygenase in a compartment in fast diffusion equilibrium with the blood. It is tempting to conclude that this compartment are the endothelial cells of the vasculature, and that the effects on CBF were due to inhibition of prostacyclin synthesis. Evidence that this is so will be reviewed.

At first sight, the results of Fig. 4 may be interpreted to show that indomethacin does not influence the CO_2 response to hypercapnia. However, *relative* changes in CBF do not give adequate information on CO_2 responsiveness which is best expressed by the ratio $\Delta CBF/\Delta P_{CO_2}$. From results illustrated in Fig. 3 one can calculate

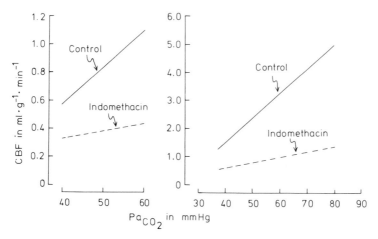

FIG. 3. Infulence on indomethacin (10 mg/kg[-1]) on control CBF in baboons *(left)* and rats *(right)*, as well as on the CBF response to induced hypercapnia. (From Pickard and MacKenzie, ref. 43, and Sakabe and Siesjö, ref. 51 with permission.)

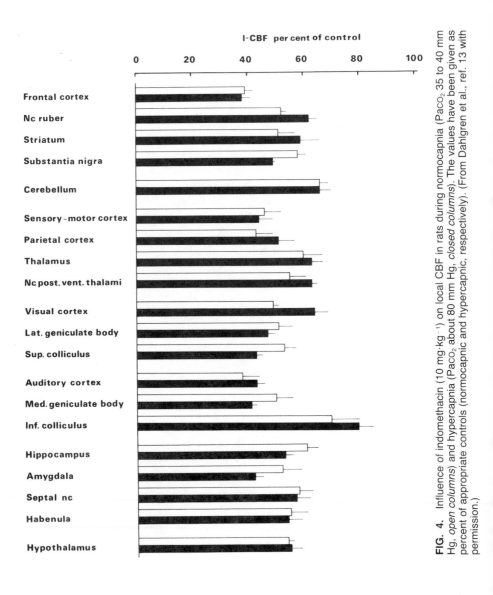

FIG. 4. Influence of indomethacin (10 mg·kg⁻¹) on local CBF in rats during normocapnia ($PaCO_2$ 35 to 40 mm Hg, *open columns*) and hypercapnia ($PaCO_2$ about 80 mm Hg, *closed columns*). The values have been given as percent of appropriate controls (normocapnic and hypercapnic, respectively). (From Dahlgren et al., ref. 13 with permission.)

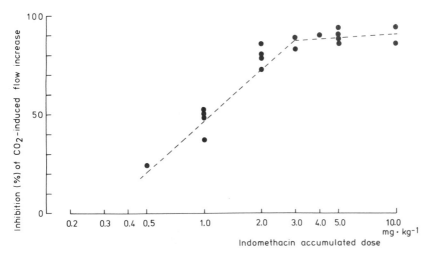

FIG. 5. Dose-related attenuation by i.v. indomethacin of CO_2-induced CBF increase, *closed circles* (From Dahlgren et al., ref. 13). *Broken line:* the dose-related inhibition of prostaglandin synthesis in rat brain (From Abdel-Halim et al. ref. 1.)

that indomethacin reduces this ratio from 0.09 to 0.02 $ml \cdot g^{-1} \cdot min^{-1} \cdot mmHg^{-1}$. Corresponding figures for local CBF in frontal, parietal and sensorimotor cortex were, for control, 0.06 to 0.08 and, for indomethacin-injected animals, 0.02 to 0.03 $ml \cdot g^{-1} \cdot min^{-1} \cdot mmHg^{-1}$. Thus, indomethacin reduces CO_2 responsiveness at least three-fold (43).

Although it seems difficult to question the validity of the data obtained in baboons and rats, nonconfirmative results have nevertheless been published. In these studies, qualitative estimates of CBF were obtained in rabbits with a thermocouple technique (11) and in cats by measurements of pial arteriolar diameter (57). In none of the studies did indomethacin affect resting CBF, or the circulatory response to hypercapnia. The results are open to criticism, though. First, none of the techniques used give quantitative estimates of CBF and both are invasive and thereby potentially traumatic. Second, the animals were anesthetized with barbiturates, drugs that by themselves lower resting CBF as well as the response to hypercapnia (19,21). These facts may have masked any effect of indomethacin present. However, we cannot exclude the possibility that appreciable species differences exist (baboons-rats versus rabbits-cats). Unfortunately, there is little information on circulatory effects of other cyclooxygenase inhibitors.

Pickard et al. (46) recently infused sodium salicylate into their baboon preparation (50 or 200 $mg \cdot kg^{-1}$) and determined CBF-CMR_{O_2}. The drug failed to alter resting CBF but the authors concluded that sodium salicylate in the lower dose (50 $mg \cdot kg^{-1}$) attenuated the CO_2 response. Two facts hamper the interpretation. First, absolute CBF values were not greatly different in control and salicylate-infused animals during the moderate hypercapnia induced. Second, at both doses the drug increased CMR_{O_2}, with 200 $mg \cdot kg^{-1}$ as much as 60% above control. Previous experiments, in which even a higher dose of the drug was infused in goats (salicylate intoxication) showed that both CMR_{O_2} and CBF increased, an effect that was attributed to the ability of the drug to act as an uncoupler of oxidative phosphorylation (5). Obviously, sodium salicylate has different effects than those elicited by indomethacin, effects that may be partly unrelated to inhibition of the cyclooxygenase.

We conclude that indomethacin increases resting cerebrovascular tone, and markedly attenuates the circulatory response to hypercapnia. One question immediately arises: are cyclo-oxygenase products also responsible for the modulation of cerebrovascular tone in other situations? Results reported a few years ago suggest that this is not so. Pickard et al. (44) found that, in the baboon, indomethacin failed to affect the normal autoregulatory response, i.e. the relative constancy of CBF with changes in perfusion pressure. Obviously, mechanisms responsible for autoregulation differ from those maintaining cerebrovascular tone in normo- and hypercapnia. We will proceed examining the effect of indomethacin in other situations.

Effects of Indomethacin on the Hyperemia Associated with Hypoxia, Hypoglycemia, and Status Epilepticus

Since indomethacin reduces absolute CBF values under hypercapnic conditions, it must be asked whether or not it curtails the increase in CBF in other high flow conditions. Sakabe and Siesjö (51) found that although indomethacin reduced absolute CBF during hypercapnia it failed to alter CBF during hypoxia (arterial P_{O_2} about 25 mmHg). As a result, indomethacin-injected animals exposed to hypoxia increased their CBF close to 10-fold. The data show that indomethacin does not generally affect the reactivity of the cerebral vessels, and they suggest that mechanisms causing vasodilation in hypercapnia and hypoxia are at least partly dissimilar.

Similar negative results have been obtained in insulin-induced hypoglycemia (42) and during bicuculline-induced status epilepticus (30). In general, local CBF increased to similar levels in control and indomethacin-injected animals. An example of that is shown in Fig. 6. The results emphasize the complexity of the regulation of CBF in normal and pathological conditions.

What Prostaglandin-Like Substances are Involved?

Since indomethacin exerts its effects in doses of close to 1 mg·kg^{-1} we may hypothesize that the drug primarily acts by blocking production of prostaglandin-like substances (16). If so, the question remains what substances are involved. Pickard et al. (45) approached this problem by studying circulatory and metabolic effects in the baboon brain of prostaglandins infused via the intracarotid route, without or with previous osmotic opening of the blood-brain barrier. The results show that both $PGF_{2\alpha}$ and PGE_2 reduced both CMR_{O_2} and CBF, PGE_2 having the most pronounced effects (Fig. 7). It could also be shown that osmotic opening of the barrier by prior infusion of hyperosmolar urea enhanced the effect of PGE_2 infusion so that the effect of a dose of 10^{-7}g·kg^{-1}·min^{-1} became similar to that recorded with 10^{-6} g·kg^{-1}·min^{-1} without prior disruption of the barrier. Attempts

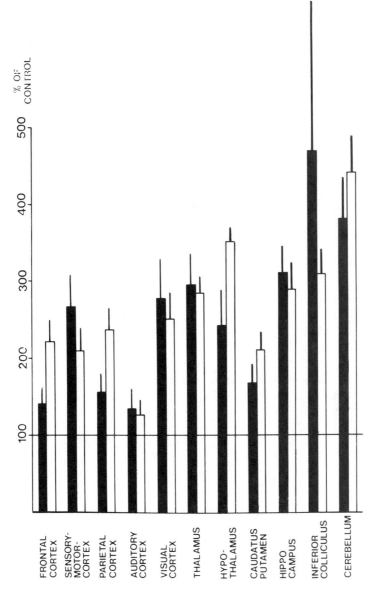

FIG. 6. Increase of CBF in different structures during severe hypoglycemia related to the values obtained in normoglycemic animals. *Closed columns:* animals pretreated with indomethacin 10 mg/kg i.v.; *open columns:* untreated animals. (From Nilsson et al., ref. 42.)

to separate the effects on CBF and CMR_{O_2} (by induced hypo- and hypercapnia) failed and the authors tentatively concluded that the effects on CBF were secondary to metabolic depression.

The circulatory and metabolic effects of PGE_2 and $PGF_{2\alpha}$ suggest that none of these prostaglandins are involved in the circulatory effects observed following

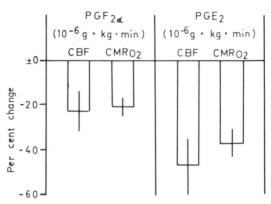

FIG. 7. Influence of intracarotid infusion of prostaglandins on CBF and CMR_{O_2} in anesthetized baboons. The values, which are means ± SEM are given as percent changes from control. (From Pickard et al. ref. 44.)

indomethacin administration. In view of the observed effects of prostacyclin on other vascular beds, for example, that of the heart (14,39,55), it is tempting to conclude that the cerebrovascular effects of indomethacin are secondary to inhibition of prostacyclin synthesis in the endothelial cells of the vasculature of the brain. This conclusion receives some support from recent experiments with intracarotid infusion of prostacyclin (46). In these, it could be shown that prostacyclin increased resting CBF, and reversed the indomethacin-induced vasoconstriction.

The Possible Role of Prostaglandin-Like Substances in Pathological States

There is a growing suspicion that massive accumulation of free fatty acids precipitates an arachidonic acid cascade that can lead to untoward effects such as cell edema, thrombosis, and vasoconstriction (17,37). Theoretically, such effects can be secondary not only to enhanced oxidation of arachidonic acid via the fatty acid cyclooxygenase pathway but also via the lipoxygenase pathway, the latter leading to formation of leukotrienes (9,40). In the following, though, we will confine the discussion to the cyclooxygenase pathway.

Arachidonic acid accumulates in the brain during ischemia (6), hypoglycemia (4), and epileptic seizures (6,10,36), three conditions that, when sufficiently severe and prolonged, lead to neuronal cell damage. In the latter two conditions oxygen is present during the insult, favoring oxidation of arachidonic acid. In ischemia, such reactions should occur first in the recirculation period when oxygen supply is reinstituted and arachidonic acid concentration only gradually decreases (48). This conclusion is amply corroborated by the results reported by Gaudet and Levine (20) who recorded a spurt of prostaglandin synthesis when recirculation was reinstated in gerbils with induced cerebral ischemia. It is of interest that both ischemia (29) and hypoglycemia (3) are accompanied by a delayed hypoperfusion, that is by a reduction of CBF to low levels that gradually develops during the recovery periods. It should also be mentioned that during bicuculline-induced status epilepticus, an initial hyperemia is followed by a secondary reduction in CBF that may be quite pronounced in some regions (M. Ingvar and B. K. Siesjö, in preparation).

It has been proposed that prostaglandin-like substances are involved in the delayed hypoperfusion that follows prolonged ischemia. Hallenbeck and Furlow (22,23) induced cerebrospinal fluid compression ischemia for 35 min in dogs, and assessed postischemic perfusion by a ^{14}C-antipyrine autoradiographic method. After 30 min of reperfusion, untreated dogs showed reduced CBF with focal areas of greatly impaired flow. Animals receiving indomethacin (1.5 to 5 mg/kg) prior to induction of ischemia, or a combination of indomethacin and prostacyclin (30 to 130 $\mu \cdot kg^{-1} \cdot min^{-1}$) 5 min after the start of reperfusion showed significantly enhanced post-ischemic perfusion rates. The authors concluded that an imbalance in prostaglandin pathways at the blood-endothelial interface was at least partly responsible for the impaired reperfusion, and emphasized the potential therapeutic implications of the results.

The general validity of these interesting and provocative results is not known at present. Pretreatment of rats with indomethacin has failed to ameliorate the post-hypoglycemic decrease in CBF (42). It cannot be excluded that any oxidative damage triggered by accumulation of arachidonic acid is secondary to oxidation of the acid via the lipoxygenase pathway. However, the results reported by Hallenbeck and Furlow (22) will no doubt inspire an intense exploration of vascular effects of an aberrant arachidonic acid metabolism.

CONCLUDING REMARKS AND PERSPECTIVES

There is little doubt that indomethacin, presumably by inhibiting endothelial prostacyclin synthesis, increases normal cerebrovascular tone and reduces the CBF response to hypercapnia without any significant effects on cerebral metabolic rate. This indicates that, under normal conditions, cyclooxygenase products participate in the regulation of CBF. However, results obtained with indomethacin demonstrate that the mechanisms controlling cerebrovascular tone in normo- and hypercapnia are different from those responsible for autoregulation, or for the increase in cerebral blood flow occurring in hypoxia, hypoglycemia, and epileptic seizures. It seems futile to attempt formulating a unitary theory of cerebrovascular regulation in the brain.

In view of the fact that indomethacin increases normal cerebrovascular tone at constant CMR_{O_2} one may speculate that cyclooxygenase products constitute factors coupling cerebral metabolism and flow. If so, the possibility exists that activity in single cells releases transmitters that not only affect recognition sites at postsynaptic neuronal membranes but also sites at the vascular wall, leading to release of ar-achidonic acid and activation of the cyclooxygenase pathway. Possibly, such in-formation transmission in parallel could either involve the release of a single transmitter or of two neurotransmitters/neurohormones, one of which acts on a postsynaptic neuronal site and the other on vascular receptors (26). However, it is equally possible that prostaglandin-like substances constitute cybernenes, substances that more diffusively adjust the external milieu of neuronal circuits in which cell-to-cell information transfer is conveyed by conventional transmitters (49).

Results suggesting a role for cyclooxygenase products in adverse circulatory and cellular reactions during pathological states constitute a challenge to those exploring mechanisms of cell damage in the brain. These reactions, which may depend on the fact that such states are accompanied by accumulation of free fatty acids, including arachidonic acid, could prove important not only in adversely effecting nutrient blood flow but also cell metabolism. However, in view of the fact that lipoxygenase products are potentially toxic, further research also should be directed towards other aspects of an arachidonic acid cascade than those confined to cyclooxygenase products.

ACKNOWLEDGMENTS

This study was supported by grants from the Swedish Medical Research Council project No. 14X-263 and from US PHS grant No. 5 ROl NSO7838.

REFERENCES

1. Abdel-Halim, M. S., Sjöquist, B., and Änggård, E. (1978): Inhibition of prostaglandin synthesis in rat brain. *Acta Pharmacol. Toxicol.*, 43:266–272.
2. Abdel-Halim, M. S., Lundén, I., Cseh, G., and Änggård, E. (1980): Prostaglandin profiles in nervous tissue and blood vessels of the brain in various animals. *Prostaglandins*, 19:249–258.
3. Abdul-Rahman, A., Agardh, C.-D., and Siesjö, B. K. (1980): Local cerebral blood flow in the rat during severe hypoglycemia, and in the recovery period following glucose injection. *Acta Physiol. Scand.*, 109:307–314.
4. Agardh, C. D., Westerberg, E., and Siesjö, B. K. (1980): Severe hypoglycemia leads to accumulation of arachidonic acid in brain tissue. *Acta Physiol. Scand.*, 109:115–116.
5. Alexander, S. C., and Smith, A. L. (1969): Cerebral blood flow and metabolism during acute salicylate intoxication in the goat. *J. Appl. Physiol.*, 26:745–751.
6. Bazán, N. G. (1976): Free arachidonic acid and other lipids in the nervous system during early ischemia and after electroshock. In: *Function and Metabolism of Phospholipids in the Central and Peripheral Nervous System*, edited by G. Porcellati, L. Amaducci, and C. Galli *Adv. Exp. Med. Biol.*, 72:317–335. Plenum Press, N.Y., London.
7. Berntman, L., Dahlgren, N.,and Siesjö, B. K. (1978): Influence of intravenously administered catecholamines on cerebral oxygen consumption and blood flow in the rat. *Acta Physiol. Scand.*, 104:101–108.
8. Betz, E. (1972): Cerebral blood flow: Its measurement and regulation. *Physiol. Rev.*, 52:595–630.
9. Borgeat, P., and Samuelsson, B. (1979): Transformation of arachidonic acid by rabbit polymorphonuclear leukocytes. Formation of a novel dihydroxyeicosatetraenoic acid. *J. Biol. Chem.*, 254:2643–2646.
10. Chapman, A., Ingvar, M., and Siesjö, B. K. (1980): Free fatty acids in the brain in bicuculline-induced status epilepticus. *Acta Physiol. Scand.*, 110:335–336.
11. Cuypers, J., Cuevas, A., and Duisburg, R. (1978): Effect of indomethacin on CO_2-induced hyperaemia (CO_2-response) in the rabbit brain. *Neurochirurgia*, 21:62–66.
12. Dahlgren, N., Rosén, I., Sakabe, T., and Siesjö, B. K. (1980a): Cerebral functional metabolic and circulatory effects of intravenous infusion of adrenaline in the rat. *Brain Res.*, 184:143–152.
13. Dahlgren, N., Nilsson, B., Sakabe, T., and Siesjö, B. K. (1980b): The effect of indomethacin on cerebral blood flow and oxygen consumption in the rat at normal and increased carbon dioxide tensions. *Acta Physiol. Scand.*, 111:475–485.
14. Dusting, G. J., Moncada, S., and Vane, J. R. (1977): Prostacyclin (PGX) is the endogenous metabolite responsible for relaxation of coronary arteries induced by arachidonic acid. *Prostaglandins*, 13:3–15.

15. Ellis, E. F., Enoch, P. W., and Kontos, H. A. (1979): Vasodilation of cat cerebral arterioles by prostaglandins D_2, E_2, G_2, and I_2. *Am. J. Physiol.*, 237:H381–H385.
16. Flower, R. J. (1974): Drugs which inhibit prostaglandin synthesis. *Pharmacol. Rev.*, 26:33–67.
17. Flower, R. J. (1979): Biosynthesis of prostaglandins. In: *Oxygen Free Radicals and Tissue Damage*. Ciba Foundation Symp. 65 (new series). pp. 120–142. Excerpta Medica, Amsterdam, Oxford, New York.
18. Folco, G. C., Longiave, D., and Bosisio, E. (1977): Relations between prostaglandin E_2, $F_{2\alpha}$, and cyclic nucleotide levels in rat brain and induction of convulsions. *Prostaglandins*, 13:893–900.
19. Fujishima, M., Scheinberg, P., Busto, R., and Reinmuth, O. M. (1971): The relation between cerebral oxygen consumption and cerebral vascular reactivity to carbon dioxide. *Stroke*, 2:251–257.
20. Gaudet, R. J., and Levine, L. (1979): Transient cerebral ischemia and brain prostaglandins. *Biochem. Biophys. Res. Commun.*, 86:893–901.
21. Grubb, R. L., Jr., Raichle, M. E., Eichling, J. O., and Ter-Pogossian, M. M. (1974): The effects of changes in Pa_{CO_2} on cerebral blood volume, blood flow and vascular mean transit time. *Stroke*, 5:630–639.
22. Hallenbeck, J. M., and Furlow, T. W., Jr. (1979a): Prostaglandin I_2 and indomethacin prevent impairment of post-ischemic brain reperfusion in the dog. *Stroke*, 10:629–637.
23. Hallenbeck, J. M., and Furlow, T. W., Jr. (1979b): Prostaglandins influence nutrient perfusion in brain during the postischemic period. In: *Prostacyclin* edited by J. R. Vane and S. Bergström, pp. 299–310. Raven Press, New York.
24. Harper, A. M., and MacKenzie, E. T. (1977): Cerebral circulatory and metabolic effects of 5-hydroxytryptamine in anaesthetized baboons. *J. Physiol. (Lond.)*, 271:721–733.
25. Hoffer, B. J., Siggins, G. R., and Bloom, F. E. (1969): Prostaglandins E_1 and E_2 antagonize norepinephrine effects on cerebellar Purkinje cells. Microelectrophoretic study. *Science*, 166:1418–1420.
26. Hökfelt, T., Johansson, O., Ljungdahl, Å., Lundberg, J. M., and Schultzberg, M. (1980): Peptidergic neurones. *Nature*, 284:515–521.
27. Horton, E. W. (1972): In: *Prostaglandins*, pp. 120–122. Springer-Verlag, Berlin, Heidelberg, New York.
28. Horton, E. W., and Main, I. H. M. (1965): Differences in the effects of prostaglandin $F_{2\alpha}$ constituent of cerebral tissue and prostaglandin E_1. 4:65–69.
29. Hossman, K.-A., Sakaki, S., and Kimoto, K. (1976): Cerebral uptake of glucose and oxygen in the cat brain after prolonged ischemia. *Stroke*, 7:301–305.
30. Ingvar, M., Nilsson, B., and Siesjö, B. K. (1980): Local cerebral blood flow in the brain during bicuculline-induced seizures and the modulating influence of inhibition of prostaglandin synthesis. *Acta Physiol. Scand.*, 111:205–212.
31. Kety, S. S., and Schmidt, C. F. (1948): The nitrous oxide method for the quantitative determination of cerebral blood flow in man: theory, procedure and normal values. *J. Clin. Invest.*, 27:476–483.
32. Kogure, K., Scheinberg, P., Reinmuth, O. M., Fujishima, M., and Busto, R. (1970): Mechanisms of cerebral vasodilatation in hypoxia. *J. Appl. Physiol.*, 29:223–229.
33. Lassen, N. A. (1968): Brain extracellular pH: the main factor controlling cerebral blood flow. *Scand. J. Clin. Lab. Invest.*, 22:247–251.
34. MacKenzie, E. T., McCullough, J., and Harper, A. M. (1976a): Influence of endogenous norepinephrine on cerebral blood flow and metabolism. *Am. J. Physiol.*, 231:489–494.
35. MacKenzie, E. T., McCulloch, J., O'Kean, M., Pickard, J. D., and Harper, A. M. (1976b): Cerebral circulation and norepinephrine: relevance of the blood-brain barrier. *Amer. J. Physiol.*, 231:483–488.
36. Marion, J., and Wolfe, L. S. (1978): Increase *in vivo* of unesterified fatty acids, prostaglandin $F_{2\alpha}$ but not thromboxane B_2 in rat brain during drug induced convulsions. *Prostaglandins*, 16:99–110.
37. Markelonis, J., and Garbus, J. (1975): Alterations of intracellular oxidative metabolism as stimuli evoking prostaglandin biosynthesis. A review of prostaglandins in cell injury and an hypothesis. *Prostaglandins*, 10:1087–1106.
38. McCulloch, J., and Harper, A. M. (1977): Cerebral circulation: effect of stimulation and blockade of dopamine receptors. *Am. J. Physiol.*, 233:H222–H227.
39. Moncada, S., and Vane, J. R. (1978): Unstable metabolites of arachidonic acid and their role in haemostasis and thrombosis. *Br. Med. Bull.*, 34:129–135.

40. Murphy, R., Hammerström, S., and Samuelsson, B. (1979): Leukotriene C: A slow-reacting substance from murine mastocytoma cells. *Proc. Natl. Acad. Sci. USA*, 76:4275–4279.
41. Nilsson, B., Rehncrona, S., and Siesjö, B. K. (1978): Coupling of cerebral metabolism and blood flow in epileptic seizures, hypoxia and hypoglycemia. In: *Cerebral Vascular Smooth Muscle and its Control*, edited by M. Purves, pp. 199–218. Excerpta Medica, Amsterdam, Oxford, New York.
42. Nilsson, B., Agardh, C. D., Ingvar, M., and Siesjö, B. K. (1980): Cerebrovascular response during and following severe insulin-induced hypoglycemia: CO_2-sensitivity, autoregulation, and influence of prostaglandin synthesis inhibition. *Acta Physiol. Scand.*, 111:455–463.
43. Pickard, J. D., and MacKenzie, E. T. (1973): Inhibition of prostaglandin synthesis and the response of baboon cerebral circulation to carbon dioxide. *Nature*, 245:187–188.
44. Pickard, J. D., MacDonnell, L. A., MacKenzie, E. T., and Harper, A. M. (1977a): Prostaglandin-induced effects in the primate cerebral circulation. *Eur. J. Pharmacol.*, 43:343–351.
45. Pickard, J. D., Durity, F., Welsh, F. A., Langfitt, T. W., Harper, A. M., and MacKenzie, E. T. (1977b): Osmotic opening of the blood brain barrier: value in pharmacological studies on the cerebral circulation. *Brain Res.*, 122:170–176.
46. Pickard, J., Tamura, A., Stewart, M., McGeorge, A., and Fitch, W. (1980): Prostacyclin, indomethacin and the cerebral circulation. *Brain Res.*, 197:425–431.
47. Potts, W. J., East, P. F., and Mueller, R. A. (1974): Behavioral effects. In: *The Prostaglandins*, Vol. 2, edited by P. W. Ramwell, pp. 157–173. Plenum Press, New York.
48. Rehncrona, S., Westerberg, E., Åkesson, B., and Siesjö, B. K. (1982): Brain cortical fatty acids and phospholipids during and following complete and severe incomplete ischemia. *J. Neurochem.*, 38:84–93.
49. Roberts, E. (1980): Prospectus. Epilepsy and antiepileptic drugs: A speculative synthesis. In: *Antiepileptic Drugs: Mechanisms of Action*, edtied by G. H. Glaser, J. K. Penry, and D. M. Woodburg, pp. 667–713. Raven Press, New York.
50. Rubio, R., Berne, R. M., Bockman, E. L., and Curnish, R. R. (1975): Relationship between adenosine concentration and oxygen supply in rat brain. *Amer. J. Physiol.*, 228:1896–1902.
51. Sakabe, T., and Siesjö, B. K. (1979): The effect of indomethacin on the blood flow — metabolism couple in the brain under normal, hypercapnia and hypoxic conditions. *Acta Physiol. Scand.*, 107:282–284.
52. Sakurada, O., Kennedy, C., Jehle, J., Brown, J. D., Carbin, C. L., and Sokoloff, L. (1978): Measurement of local cerebral blood flow with ¹⁴C-iodoantipyrine. *Am. J. Physiol.*, 234:H59–H66.
53. Samuelsson, B. (1964): Identification of a smooth muscle stimulating factor in bovine brain. *Biochem. Biophys. Acta*, 84:218.
54. Siesjö, B. K., Berntman, L., and Nilsson, B. (1980): Regulation of microcirculation in the brain *Microvasc. Res.*, 19:158–170.
55. Sivakoff, M., Pure, E., Hsueh, W., and Needleman, P. (1979): Prostaglandins and the heart. *Fed. Proc.*, 38:78–82.
56. Sokoloff, L. (1977): Relation between physiological function and energy metabolism in the central nervous system. *J. Neurochem.*, 29:13–26.
57. Wei, E. P., Ellis, E. F., and Kontos, H. A. (1980): Role of prostaglandins in pial arteriolar response to CO_2 and hypoxia. *Am. J. Physiol.*, 238:H226–H230.
58. White, R. P., Hagen, A. A., Morgan, H., Dawson, W. N., and Robertson, J. T. (1975): Experimental study of the genesis of cerebral vasospasm. *Stroke*, 6:52–57.
59. Wolfe, L. S., and Coceani, F. (1979): The role of prostaglandins in the central nervous system. *Ann. Rev. Physiol.*, 41:669–684.
60. Wolfe, L. S., Rostworowski, K., and Pappius, H. M. (1976): The endogenous synthesis of prostaglandins by brain tissue *in vitro. Can. J. Biochem.*, 54:629–640.
61. Yamamoto, Y. L., Feindel, W., Wolfe, L. S., Katoh, H., and Hodge, C. P. (1972): Experimental vasoconstriction of cerebral arteries by prostaglandins. *J. Neurosurg.*, 37:385–397.

Note added in proof

Results reported during the International Conference on Prostaglandins in Florence (1982, see abstract and lecture volumes) demonstrate that the CBF effects of indomethacin are species-dependent, and that the effects shown in rat and man are unrelated to cyclo-oxygenase inhibition. Thus, indomethacin fails to alter CBF in cats and rabbits (Busija and Heistad), and the CBF effects of indomethacin in man (Wennmalm et al.) and in the rat (Siesjö and Wieloch) are not observed with other cyclo-oxygenase inhibitors such as aspirin, diclofenac, naprosyn, and piroxicam.

Subject Index